READINGS IN BIOMEDICAL ETHICS:

A Canadian Focus

Edited by
EIKE-HENNER W. KLUGE
University of Victoria

Prentice Hall Canada Inc., Scarborough, Ontario

Canadian Cataloguing in Publication Data

Main entry under title:

Readings in biomedical ethics: a Canadian focus
1st ed.

ISBN 0-13-015181-5

1. Medical ethics - Canada. 2. Bioethics - Canada.
I. Kluge, Eike-Henner W.
R724.R4 1993 174.2 C93-093286-2

Prentice-Hall, Inc., Englewood Cliffs, New Jersey
Prentice-Hall International (UK) Limited, London
Prentice-Hall of Australia, Pty. Limited, Sydney
Prentice-Hall Hispanoamericana, S.A., Mexico City
Prentice-Hall of India Private Limited, New Delhi
Prentice-Hall of Japan, Inc., Tokyo
Simon & Schuster Asia Private Limited, Singapore
Editora Prentice-Hall do Brasil, Ltda., Rio de Janeiro

ISBN 0-13-015181-5

Acquisitions Editor: Marjorie Munroe
Developmental Editor: Maurice Esses
Production Editor: William Booth
Production Coordinator: Anna Orodi
Cover Design: Alex Li

1 2 3 4 5 RRD 97 96 95 94 93

Printed and bound in the United States of America

Table of Contents

Preface

The idea for this volume grew out of the experience of teaching bioethics to Canadian undergraduate and graduate students from a variety of backgrounds and with a variety of specializations, and from giving seminars to Canadian health care professionals about bioethical issues as they arise in the Canadian setting. Time and again, one of the most frustrating experiences that the students encountered — and in which I as instructor shared — was that almost without exception, the only reading materials that were readily available were anthologies from the US.

Of course, many of the issues that arise in the delivery of health care, in medical research and in the politics that surround health care delivery arise no matter what the country and no matter what the social perspective on health care. Furthermore, the ethical principles that guide — or more correctly perhaps, that should guide — the development and delivery of health care are not unique to a particular national perspective, whether that be Canadian or anything else. They are rooted in the fundamental ethical relations that apply to all people, as people.

However, the Canadian setting is in many respects different from that of other countries. Above all, it is quite different from the US, where most anthologies come from. Even when the issues are the same, the social reality and the political orientation in which they are embedded are often profoundly different. The issue of access to health care is a good example. Canada starts from the assumption that everyone has the right of equal access to appropriate health care, and the various levels of health care service are structured towards achieving this end.

This is not so in the US. In the US, health care is not perceived as a right but as a commodity that must be purchased. There is only token acceptance of the thesis that society should provide some minimum level of health care. As a result, over 35 million people in the US either have only inadequate access to health care or have no access at all. Given this difference, the ethics of health care resource allocation assumes an entirely different perspective.

Another example is informed consent. The socio-legal framework in the US is different from that in Canada. Specifically, the standard of disclosure in the US is attuned to what the reasonable person would want to know before making a choice. In Canada, the standard is more exacting. It requires the health care professional to take into account the special position of the patient, and to adjust the disclosure to what a reasonable person *in the patient's particular position* would want to know.[1] Furthermore, the Canadian approach demands that health care professionals use language that is appropriate to the level of understanding of the individual patient. Nothing like this is required in the US. Therefore, to rely on articles that are geared to the US context is to confuse the discussion — and to give a mistaken perception of the realities that are at stake. It is not that the ethics is or should be different in the two countries. The socio-legal realities are different. That is why the ethical orientation of the problems that arise is frequently fundamentally distinct. This difference is often very important. Still other examples where there is a profound difference, with equally profound implications, include: withdrawal of treatment, abortion, proxy decision-making, living wills. The list is long.

Still, many bioethical issues are independent of the socio-legal context in which they arise. Issues like that of competence, the physician-patient relationship, etc. immediately come to mind. Ethics is not national in nature, and the fact that something is accepted — or, for that matter, rejected — in a particular jurisdiction does not automatically make it ethical (or unethical).

The present anthology tries to reflect this. It contains a number of relevant (and classic) readings from the US, as well as from other countries, that deal with the ethics, pure and simple. In that sense, the volume allows the reader insight into the general field of bioethics independently of purely national Canadian considerations. It tries to strike a balance — with an admittedly strong slant in the direction of a Canadian perspective. Nevertheless, the book contains a larger proportion of Canadian authors. The legal cases it contains are almost exclusively Canadian, and the regulations, codes and other official guidelines that it contains are either Canadian or from the Commonwealth of Nations.

The volume may be used in several ways: as a companion to *Bioethics in a Canadian Context*, as a book of readings around which an instructor can develop a course of lectures, or as a resource book for students who want to read up on a variety of perspectives. Finally, it should also be useful to health care professionals who want to acquaint themselves with the current bioethical literature as it is being developed for the Canadian setting.

Notes

1. See *Reibl v. Hughes,* Chapter 5.

PART 1 HEALTH CARE AND BIOETHICAL PRINCIPLES

CHAPTER 1 HEALTH AS AN ETHICAL ISSUE

INTRODUCTION

What is truth? The question has occupied philosophers, lawyers and theologians since ancient times. *What is health?* must surely rank a close second in terms of difficulty. Time and again, physicians and philosophers have tried to define the notion, only to find that as their knowledge advanced, the definitions they had just settled on again seemed inadequate. And yet it is clear that, if health care is to be assigned its proper place in the sphere of social endeavours and the health care professions are to have a clearly defined role and mandate, the notion has to have an appropriate and acceptable definition.

The issue has become particularly pressing in the twentieth century, as society came to accept the position that it has an obligation to provide at least some level of health care services for its members. If the nature of health could not be satisfactorily defined, then the limits of this social obligation could not be drawn properly either. That, so it was felt, would have important implications in terms of social policy.

Furthermore, when people say that society has an obligation to provide at least some level of health care for its members, they are not only talking about health care services on an individual basis. They are also thinking of the sorts of services that usually fall under the rubric of public health measures. These are services that are designed to maintain, raise and promote the health of all of society, collectively. Here, too, the notion of health plays a central role. Therefore, without some common understanding of what exactly health is, these services could be identified only in a very haphazard way.

But there were also other reasons for seeking a definition. In most countries — Canada included — people may not legally consent to have grievous harm inflicted on them. Inflicting such harm constitutes grounds for bringing a charge of assault and battery. However, much of health care involves procedures that, *prima facie*, fall under this rubric. Surgical interventions, psychiatric therapy, dental work and even the most basic of nursing functions would all be implicated if they were not placed into a special category that would exempt them from this charge. Of course there is such a category: namely, the category of health care. However, in order for this category to be properly defined and delimited, what is needed is a proper definition of "health."

In other words, there has to be some way in which the notion of what harm a patient can legitimately agree to can be identified, and some way in which consent to such procedures can be legitimated. The concept of health assumes a fundamental role in all this.

For these and similar reasons, there began some time ago what can only be described as a hunt for an appropriate definition of "health." The lead was taken by the World Health Organization, with its 1958 definition of "health." It is included below. The reaction to this definition, however, was less than enthusiastic in some quarters. As a whole series of authors pointed out, the definition is extremely vague. For instance, what does "well-being" mean, or "infirmity?" It is also circular: it defines "health" in terms of its correlative, "disease." The notion of disease, however, could itself only be defined in terms of health; so this gets us nowhere. Furthermore, the definition is far too inclusive. It would have us classify social and moral problems as health problems. The selection from Callahan captures the thrust of most of this criticism very well.

Other definitions attempted to overcome these problems. For instance, health has been defined as "a state of physiological normalcy" or a "proper working order of the human body,"[1] as "the general condition of the body with respect to efficient or inefficient discharge of functions;" as "spiritual, moral or mental soundness or well-being,"[2] the ability to function "in a given physical and social environment,"[3] the "well-working of the organism as a whole," "an activity of the living body in accordance with its specific excellence,"[4] or simply as "a state of physical well-being."[5]

However, these definitions also ran into criticism. In fact, the very attempt to define health at all came to be criticized. On a general level, the criticism maintained that a proper definition is impossible because concepts like those of health and disease are inherently value-laden. They include not only descriptive components but also normative ones. Some people[6] have argued that this is inadequate. To say that something is a disease commits us to saying something about human nature and the nature of human well-being, and this involves choices among human goods. This, in turn, involves considerations of what counts as the proper human state, which of course involve value judgements in an integral fashion. Therefore, to call someone ill is to make a social judgement.

The selection by Whitbeck presents a version of this critique. Whitbeck maintains that the notion of health is necessarily value-laden, because it is used to categorize what we find good or appropriate in people's capacity to act or respond to a wide variety of situations. However, she sees nothing wrong with this. In fact, she sees this valuational approach to be a proper role played by the notion of health itself. Furthermore, by introducing the notion of capacity, she expands the discussion to include the notion of functional potential. She expands the discussion still further by proposing that the concept of wholeness should be involved as well, and by saying that the more encompassing a person's capacity to respond appropriately to a wide variety of situations is, and the greater a person's capacity to achieve her/his goals under the circumstances is, the healthier the individual. In that sense, for Whitbeck, there is no upper limit to health.

Nordenfeldt agrees that the notion of health is value-laden. Like Whitbeck, he sees nothing wrong with this. In fact, he maintains even more emphatically than Whitbeck that the notion of health is intimately tied to the values and goals that motivate people. He therefore takes the notion of health into the experiential realm, and maintains that any acceptable definition of health must take this parameter into account. However, he does not take the obvious step and make health an entirely subjective affair. The values he is talking about are not the values of individual people. Instead, the notion of health should be seen as a schema that allows a particular society to insert its own values. This would then make what counts as health relative from society to society. Nordenfeldt also attempts to show how this could be extended to animals.

Of course, there are other positions on health. The bio-statistical model proposed by Boorse is one of the best-known. It attempts to define the notion of health in terms of what is statistically normal for the species. Nordenfeldt's critique of this is well worth reading. He points to what he considers the ineluctably valuational aspect of the concept of health. Ultimately, however, we do have to come to grips with this position: Is it true that the notion of health is necessarily value-laden? The issue is important because it has been argued that if we cannot give a value-free definition of health, then we will always have to ask ourselves whether the health services that are provided by our society are so coloured by our values that they, in fact, amount to a cultural agenda. This would have to be of particular concern to Canadians because Canada, by choice and by Charter, is a multicultural society.

NOTES

1. Joel Feinberg, "Disease and Values," in Joel Feinberg, *Doing and Deserving: Essays in the Theory of Responsibility*. (Princeton: Princeton University Press, 1974), 253–55.
2. *Oxford English Dictionary*.
3. Réné Dubos, "Health as Ability to Function," in T.L. Beauchamp and L. Walters, eds., *Contemporary Issues in Bioethics*. (Belmont: Dickenson Publ. Co., 1978), 99.
4. Leon Kass, "Regarding the End of Medicine and the Pursuit of Health," in Beauchamp and Walters, ref. note 3, 108.
5. Callahan, "Thc WHO Definition of Health," included below. A somewhat more theoretical and developed analysis is offered by Ellen Idler, "Definition of Mental Health and Illness and Medical Sociology," *Society, Science and Medicine* 3A, 723–31. She claims that these and other definitions are based on a Parsonian model of illness and disease: one that defines it as "an abstract, biomedical conception of pathological abnormality in people's bodies, where this is indicated by certain abnormal signs and symptoms which can be measured, recorded, classified and analyzed." To be quite correct, so she argues, the concept should be modified so that "subjective reality plays a role in determining whether an individual becomes ill in the first place." For other attempts to define "health," see President's Commission for the Study of Ethical Problems in Medicine and Biomedical and Behavioral Research, *Securing Access to Health Care: A Report on the Ethical Implications of Differences in the Availability of Health Services*. (U.S. Government Printing Office: Washington D.C., 1983) 3 vols., vols. two and three.
6. Tristram Englehardt, Jr., "Human Well-Being and Medicine: Some Basic Value-Judgments in the Biomedical Science," from H.T. Engelhardt and D. Callahan, eds., *Science, Ethics and Medicine* (Institute of Society, Ethics and the life Sciences: 1976)

Preamble: Constitution of the World Health Organization

World Health Organization

The States Parties to this Constitution declare, in conformity with the Charter of the United Nations, that the following principles are basic to the happiness, harmonious relations and security of all peoples:

Health is a state of complete physical, mental and social well-being and not merely the absence of disease or infirmity.

The enjoyment of the highest attainable standard of health is one of the fundamental rights of every human being without distinction of race, religion, political belief, economic or social condition.

The health of all peoples is fundamental to the attainment of peace and security and is dependent upon the fullest co-operation of individuals and States.

The achievement of any State in the promotion and protection of health is of value to all.

Unequal development in different countries in the promotion of health and control of disease, especially communicable disease, is a common danger.

Healthy development of the child is of basic importance; the ability to live harmoniously in a changing total environment is essential to such development.

The extension to all peoples of the benefits of medical, psychological and related knowledge is essential to the fullest attainment of health.

Informed opinion and active co-operation on the part of the public are of the utmost importance in the improvement of the health of the people.

Governments have a responsibility for the health of their peoples which can be fulfilled only by the provision of adequate health and social measures.

Accepting these principles, and for the purpose of co-operation among themselves and with others to promote and protect the health of all peoples, the Contracting Parties agree to the present Constitution and hereby establish the World Health Organization as a specialized agency within the terms of Article 57 of the Charter of the United Nations.

Reproduced by permission of WHO from: *Basic Documents. Thirty-Ninth Edition.* Geneva: World Health Organization, 1992, pp. 1-2.

The WHO Definition of Health

Daniel Callahan

There is not much that can be called fun and games in medicine, perhaps because unlike other sports it is the only one in which everyone, participant and spectator, eventually gets killed playing. In the meantime, one of the grandest games is that version of king-of-the-hill where the aim of all players is to upset the World Health

Daniel Callahan, "The WHO Definition of Health," *The Hastings Center Studies,* 1:3 (1973).

Organization (WHO) definition of "health." That definition, in case anyone could possibly forget it, is, "Health is a state of complete physical, mental, and social well-being and not merely the absence of disease or infirmity." Fair game, indeed. Yet somehow, defying all comers, the WHO definition endures, though literally every other aspirant to the crown has managed to knock it off the hill at least once. One possible reason for its presence is that it provides such an irresistible straw man; few there are who can resist attacking it in the opening paragraphs of papers designed to move on to more profound reflections.

But there is another possible reason which deserves some exploration, however unsettling the implications. It may just be that the WHO definition has more than a grain of truth in it, of a kind which is as profoundly frustrating as it is enticingly attractive. At the very least it is a definition which implies that there is some intrinsic relationship between the good of the body and the good of the self. The attractiveness of this relationship is obvious: it thwarts any movement toward a dualism of self and body, a dualism which in any event immediately breaks down when one drops a brick on one's toe; and it impels the analyst to work toward a conception of health which in the end is resistant to clear and distinct categories, closer to the felt experience. All that, naturally, is very frustrating. It seems simply impossible to devise a concept of health which is rich enough to be nutritious and yet not so rich as to be indigestible.

One common objection to the WHO definition is, in effect, an assault upon any and all attempts to specify the meaning of very general concepts. Who can possibly define words as vague as "health," a venture as foolish as trying to define "peace," "justice," "happiness," and other systematically ambiguous notions? To this objection the "pragmatic" clinicians (as they often call themselves) add that, anyway, it is utterly unnecessary to know what "health" means in order to treat a patient running a high temperature. Not only that, it is also a harmful distraction to clutter medical judgment with philosophical puzzles.

Unfortunately for this line of argument, it is impossible to talk or think at all without employing general concepts; without them, cognition and language are impossible. More damagingly, it is rarely difficult to discover, with a bit of probing, that even the most "pragmatic" judgment (whatever *that* is) presupposes some general values and orientations, all of which can be translated into definitions of terms as general as "health" and "happiness." A failure to discern the operative underlying values, the conceptions of reality upon which they are based, and the definitions they entail, sets the stage for unexamined conduct and, beyond that, positive harm both to patients and to medicine in general.

But if these objections to any and all attempts to specify the meaning of "health" are common enough, the most specific complaint about the WHO definition is that its very generality, and particularly its association of health and general well-being as a positive ideal, has given rise to a variety of evils. Among them are the cultural tendency to define all social problems, from war to crime in the streets, as "health" problems; the blurring of lines of responsibility between and among the professions, and between the medical profession and the political order; the implicit denial of human freedom which results when failures to achieve social well-being are defined as forms of "sickness," somehow to be treated by medical means; and the general debasement of language which ensues upon the casual habit of labeling everyone from Adolf Hitler to student radicals to the brat next door as "sick." In short, the problem with the WHO definition is not that it represents an attempt to propose a general definition, but it is simply a bad one.

That is a valid line of objection, provided one can spell out in some detail just how the definition can or does entail some harmful consequences. Two lines of attack are possible against putatively hazardous social definitions of significant general concepts. One is by pointing out that the definition does not encompass all that a concept has commonly been taken to mean, either historically or at present, that it is a partial definition only. The task then is to come up with a fuller definition, one less subject to misuse. But there is still another way of objecting to socially significant definitions, and that is by pointing out some baneful effects of definitions generally accepted as adequate. Many of the objections to the WHO definition fall in the latter category, building upon the important insight that definitions of crucially important terms with a wide public use have ethical, social, and political implications; defining general terms is not an abstract exercise but a way of shaping the world metaphysically and structuring the world politically.

Wittgenstein's aphorism, "Don't look for the meaning, look for the use," is pertinent here. The ethical problem in defining the concept of "health" is to determine what the implications are of the various uses to which a concept of "health" can be put. We might well agree that there are some uses of "health" which will produce socially harmful results. To carry Wittgenstein a step further, "Don't look for the uses, look for the abuses." We might, then, examine some of the real or possible abuses to which the WHO definition leads, recognizing all the while that what we may term an "abuse" will itself rest upon some perceived *positive* good or value.

HISTORICAL ORIGIN AND CONTEXT

Before that task is undertaken, however, it is helpful to understand the historical origin and social context of the WHO definition. If abuses of that definition have developed, their seeds may be looked for in its earliest manifestations.

The World Health Organization came into existence between 1946 and 1948 as one of the first major activities of the United Nations. As an outcome of earlier work, an Interim Commission to establish the WHO sponsored an International Health Conference in New York in June and July of 1946. At that Conference, representatives of 61 nations signed the Constitution of the WHO, the very first clause of which presented the now famous definition of "health." The animating spirit behind the formation of the WHO was the belief that the improvement of world health would make an important contribution to world peace; health and peace were seen as inseparable. Just why this belief gained ground is not clear from the historical record of the WHO. While there have been many historical explanations of the origin of World War II, a lack of world health has not been prominent among them; nor, for that matter, did the early supporters of the WHO claim that the Second World War or any other war might have been averted had there been better health. More to the point, perhaps, was the conviction that health was intimately related to economic and cultural welfare; in turn, that welfare, so it was assumed, had a direct bearing on future peace. No less important was a fervent faith in the possibilities of medical science to achieve world health, enhanced by the development of powerful antibiotics and pesticides during the war.

A number of memorandums submitted to a spring 1946 Technical Preparatory Committee meeting of the WHO capture the flavor of the period. The Yugoslavian memorandum noted that "health is a prerequisite to freedom from want, to social security and happiness." France stated that "there cannot be any material security, social security, or well-being for individuals or nations without health ... the full responsibility of a free man can only be assumed by healthy individuals ... the spread of proper notions of hygiene among populations tends to improve the level of health and hence to increase their working power and raise their standard of living...." The United States contended that "international cooperation and joint action in the furtherance of all matters pertaining to health will raise the standards of living, will promote the freedom, the dignity, and the happiness of all peoples of the world."

In addition to those themes, perhaps the most significant initiative taken by the organizers of the WHO was to include mental health as part of its working definition. In its memorandum, Great Britain stated that "it should be clear that health includes mental health," but it was Dr. Brock Chisholm, soon to become the first director of the WHO, who personified what Dr. Chisholm himself called the "visionary" view of health. During the meeting of the Technical Preparatory Committee he argued that: "The world is sick and the ills are due to the perversion of man; his inability to live with himself. The microbe is not the enemy; science is sufficiently advanced to cope with it were it not for the barriers of superstition, ignorance, religious intolerance, misery and poverty....These psychological evils must be understood in order that a remedy might be prescribed, and the scope of the task before the Committee therefore knows no bounds."

In Dr. Chisholm's statement, put very succinctly, are all of those elements of the WHO definition which led eventually to its criticism: defining all the problems of the world as "sickness," affirming that science would be sufficient to cope with the causes of physical disease, asserting that only anachronistic attitudes stood in the way of a cure of both physical and psychological ills, and declaring that the cause of health can tolerate no limitations. To say that Dr. Chisholm's "vision" was grandiose is to understate the matter. Even allowing for hyperbole, it is clear that the stage was being set for a conception of "health" which would encompass literally every element and item of human happiness. One can hardly be surprised, given such a vision, that our ways of talking about "health" have become all but meaningless. Even though I believe the definition is not without its important insights, it is well to observe why, in part, we are so muddled at present about "health."

HEALTH AND HAPPINESS

Let us examine some of the principal objections to the WHO definition in more detail. One of them is that, by including the notion of "social well-being" under its rubric, it turns the enduring problem of human happiness into one more medical problem, to be dealt with by scientific means. That is surely an objectionable feature, if only because there exists no evidence whatever that medicine has anything more than a partial grasp of the sources of human misery. Despite Dr. Chisholm's optimism, medicine has not even found ways of dealing with more than a fraction of the whole range of physical diseases; campaigns, after all, are still being mounted against cancer and heart disease. Nor is there any special reason to think that future forays against those and other common diseases will bear rapid fruits. People will continue to die of disease for a long time to come, probably forever.

But perhaps, then, in the psychological and psychiatric sciences some progress has been made against what Dr. Chisholm called the "psychological ills," which lead to wars, hostility, and aggression? To be sure, there are many interesting psychological theories to be found about these "ills," and a few techniques which can, with some individuals, reduce or eliminate antisocial behavior. But so far as I can see, despite the mental health movement and the rise of the psychological sciences, war and human hostility are as much with us as ever. Quite apart from philosophical objections to the WHO definition, there was no empirical basis for the unbounded optimism which lay behind it at the time of its inception, and little has happened since to lend its limitless aspiration any firm support.

Common sense alone makes evident the fact that the absence of "disease or infirmity" by no means guarantees "social well-being." In one sense, those who drafted the WHO definition seem well aware of that. Isn't the whole point of their definition to show the inadequacy of negative definitions? But in another sense, it may be doubted that they really did grasp that point. For the third principle enunciated in the WHO Constitution says that "the health of all peoples is fundamental to the attainment of peace and security...." Why is it fundamental, at least to peace? The worst wars of the 20th century have been waged by countries with very high standards of health, by nations with superior life-expectancies for individuals and with comparatively low infant mortality rates. The greatest present threats to world peace come in great part (though not entirely) from developed countries, those which have combated disease and illness most effectively. There seems to be no historical correlation whatever between health and peace, and that is true even if one includes "mental health."

How are human beings to achieve happiness? That is the final and fundamental question. Obviously illness, whether mental or physical, makes happiness less possible in most cases. But that is only because they are only one symptom of a more basic restriction, that of human finitude, which sees infinite human desires constantly thwarted by the limitations of reality. "Complete" well-being might, conceivably, be attainable, but under one condition only: that people ceased expecting much from life. That does not seem about to happen. On the contrary, medical and psychological progress have been more than outstripped by rising demands and expectations. What is so odd about that, if it is indeed true that human desires are infinite? Whatever the answer to the question of human happiness, there is no particular reason to believe that medicine can do anything more than make a modest, finite contribution.

Another objection to the WHO definition is that, by implication, it makes the medical profession the gatekeeper for happiness and social well-being. Or if not exactly the gatekeeper (since political and economic support will be needed from sources other than medical), then the final magic-healer of human misery. Pushed far enough, the whole idea is absurd, and it is not necessary to believe that the organizers of the WHO would, if pressed, have been willing to go quite that far. But even if one pushes the pretension a little way, considerable fantasy results. The mental health movement is the best example, casting the psychological professional in the role of high priest.

At its humble best, that movement can do considerable good; people do suffer from psychological disabilities and there are some effective ways of helping them. But it would be sheer folly to believe that all, or even the most important, social evils stem from bad mental health: political injustice, economic scarcity, food shortages, unfavorable physical environments, have a far greater historical claim as sources of a failure to achieve "social well-being." To retort that all or most of these troubles can, nonetheless, be seen finally as symptoms of bad mental health is, at best, self-serving and, at worst, just plain foolish.

A significant part of the objection that the WHO definition places, at least by implication, too much power and authority in the hands of the medical profession need not be based on a fear of that power as such. There is no reason to think that the world would be any worse off if health professionals made all decisions than if any other group did; and no reason to think it would be any better off. That is not a very important point. More significant is that cultural development which, in its skepticism about "traditional" ways of solving social problems, would seek a technological and specifically a medical solution for human ills of all kinds. There is at least a hint in early WHO discussions that, since politicians and diplomats have failed in maintaining world peace, a more expert group should take over, armed with the scientific skills necessary to set things right; it is science which is best able to vanquish that old Enlightenment bogeyman, "superstition." More concretely, such an ideology has the practical effect of blurring the lines of appropriate authority and responsibility. If all problems — political, economic and social — reduce to matters of "health," then there ceases to be any ways to determine who should be responsible for what.

THE TYRANNY OF HEALTH

The problem of responsibility has at least two faces. One is that of a tendency to turn all problems of "social well-being" over to the medical professional, most pronounced in the instance of the incarceration of a large group of criminals in mental institutions rather than prisons. The abuses, both medical and legal, of that practice are, fortunately, now beginning to receive the attention they deserve, even if little corrective action has yet been taken. (Counterbalancing that development, however, are others, where some are seeking more "effective" ways of bringing science to bear on criminal behavior.)

The other face of the problem of responsibility is that of the way in which those who are sick, or purportedly sick, are to be evaluated in terms of their freedom and responsibility. Siegler and Osmond (*Hastings Center Studies,* Vol. 1, No. 3, 1973, pp. 41-58) discuss the "sick role," a leading feature of which is the ascription of blamelessness, of non-responsibility, to those who contract illness. There is no reason to object to this kind of ascription in many instances — one can hardly blame someone for contracting kidney disease — but, obviously enough, matters get out of hand when all physical, mental, and communal disorders are put under the heading of "sickness," and all sufferers (all of us, in the end) placed in the blameless "sick role." Not only are the concepts of "sickness" and "illness" drained of all content, it also becomes impossible to ascribe any freedom or responsibility to those caught up in the throes of sickness. The whole world is sick, and no one is responsible any longer for anything. That is determinism gone mad, a rather odd outcome of a development which began with attempts to bring unbenighted "reason" and free self-determination to bear for the release of the helpless captives of superstition and ignorance.

The final and most telling objection to the WHO definition has less to do with the definition itself than with one of its natural historical consequences. Thomas Szasz has been the most eloquent (and most single-minded) critic of that sleight-of-hand which has seen the concept of health moved from the medical to the moral arena. What can no longer be done in the name of "morality" can now be done in the name of "health": human beings labeled, incarcerated, and dismissed for their failure to toe the line of "normalcy" and "sanity."

At first glance, this analysis of the present situation might seem to be totally at odds with the tendency to put everyone in the blame-free "sick role." Actually, there is a fine, probably indistinguishable, line separating these two positions. For as soon as one treats all human disorders — war, crime, social unrest — as forms of illness, then one turns health into a normative concept, that which human beings must and ought to have if they are to live in peace with themselves and others. Health is no longer an optional matter, but the golden key to the relief of human misery. We *must* be well or we will all perish. "Health" can and must be imposed; there can be no room for the luxury of freedom when so much is at stake. Of course the matter is rarely put so bluntly, but it is to Szasz's great credit that he has discerned what actually happens when "health" is allowed to gain the cultural clout which morality once had. (That he carries the whole business too far in his embracing of the most extreme moral individualism is another story, which cannot be dealt with here.) Something is seriously amiss when the "right" to have healthy children is turned into a further right for children not to be born defective, and from there into an obligation not to bring unhealthy children into the world as a way of respecting the right of those children to health! Nor is everything altogether lucid when abortion decisions are made a matter of "medical judgment" (see *Roe vs. Wade*); when decisions to provide psychoactive drugs for the relief of the ordinary stress of living are defined as no less "medical judgment"; when patients are not allowed to die with dignity because of medical indications that they can, come what may, be kept alive; when prisoners, without their consent, are subjected to aversive conditioning to improve their mental health.

ABUSES OF LANGUAGE

In running through the litany of criticisms which have been directed at the WHO definition of "health," and what seem to have been some of its long-term implications and consequences, I might well be accused of beating a dead horse. My only defense is to assert, first, that the spirit of the WHO definition is by no means dead either in medicine or society. In fact, because of the usual cultural lag which requires many years for new ideas to gain wide social currency, it is only now coming into its own on a broad scale. (Everyone now talks about everybody and everything, from Watergate to Billy Graham to trash in the streets, as "sick.") Second, I believe that we are now in the midst of a nascent (if not actual) crisis about how "health" ought properly to be understood, with much dependent upon what conception of health emerges in the near future.

If the ideology which underlies the WHO definition has proved to contain many muddled and hazardous ingredients, it is not at all evident what should take its place. The virtue of the WHO definition is that it tried to place health in the broadest human context. Yet the assumption behind the main criticisms of the WHO definition seem perfectly valid. Those assumptions can be characterized as follows: (1) health is only a part of life, and the achievement of health only a part of the achievement of happiness; (2) medicine's role, however important, is limited; it can neither solve nor even cope with the great majority of social, political, and cultural problems; (3) human freedom and responsibility must be recognized, and any tendency to place all deviant, devilish, or displeasing human beings into the blameless sick-role must be resisted; (4) while it is good for human beings to be healthy, medicine is not morality; except in very limited contexts (plagues and epidemics) "medical judgment" should not be allowed to become moral judgment; to be healthy is not to be righteous; (5) it is important to keep clear and distinct the different roles of different professions, with a clearly circumscribed role for medicine, limited to those domains of life where the contribution of medicine is appropriate. Medicine can save some lives; it cannot save the life of society.

These assumptions, and the criticisms of the WHO definition which spring from them, have some important implications for the use of the words "health," "illness," "sick," and the like. It will be counted an abuse of language if the word "sick" is applied to all individual and communal problems, if all unacceptable conduct is spoken of in the language of medical pathologies, if moral issues and moral judgments are translated into the language of "health," if the lines of authority, responsibility, and expertise are so blurred that the health profession is allowed to pre-empt the rights and responsibilities of others by re-defining them in its own professional language.

Abuses of that kind have no possibility of being curbed in the absence of a definition of health which does not contain some intrinsic elements of limitation — that is, unless there is a definition which, when abused, is self-evidently *seen* as abused by those who know what health means. Unfortunately, it is in the nature of general definitions that they do not circumscribe their own meaning (or even explain it) and contain no built-in safeguards against misuse, e.g., our "peace with honor" in Southeast Asia — "peace," "honor"? Moreover, for a certain class of concepts — peace, honor, happiness, for example — it is difficult to keep them free in ordinary usage from a normative content. In our own usage, it would make no sense to talk of them in a way which implied they are not desirable or are merely neutral: by well-ingrained social custom (resting no doubt on some basic features of human nature) health, peace, and happiness are both desired and desirable — good. For those and other reasons, it is perfectly plausible to say the cultural task of defining terms, and settling on appropriate and inappropriate usages, is far more than a matter of getting our dictionary entries right. It is nothing less than a way of deciding what should be valued, how life should be understood, and what principles should guide individual and social conduct.

Health is not just a term to be defined. Intuitively, if we have lived at all, it is something we seek and value. We may not set the highest value on health — other goods may be valued as well — but it would strike me as incomprehensible should someone say that health was a matter of utter indifference to him; we would well doubt either his sanity or his maturity. The cultural problem, then, may be put this way. The acceptable range of uses of the term "health" should, at the minimum, capture the normative element in the concept as traditionally understood while, at the maximum, incorporate the insight (stemming from criticisms of the WHO definition) that the term "health" is abused if it becomes synonymous with virtue, social tranquillity, and ultimate happiness. Since there are no instruction manuals available on how one would go about reaching a goal of that sort, I will offer no advice on the subject. I have the horrible suspicion, as a matter of fact, that people either have a decent intuitive sense on such matters (reflected in the way they use language) or they do not; and if they do not, little can be done to instruct them. One is left with the pious hope that, somehow, over a long period of time, things will change.

IN DEFENSE OF WHO

Now that simply might be the end of the story, assuming some agreement can be reached that the WHO definition of "health" is plainly bad, full of snares, delusions, and false norms. But I am left uncomfortable with such a flat, simple conclusion. The nagging point about the definition is that, in badly put ways, it was probably on to something. It certainly recognized, however inchoately, that it is difficult to talk meaningfully of health solely in terms of "the absence of disease or infirmity." As a purely logical point, one must ask about what positive state of affairs disease and infirmity are an absence of — absent from what? One is left with the tautological proposition that health is the absence of non-health, a less than illuminating revelation. Could it not be said, though, that at least intuitively everyone knows what health is by means of the experiential contrast posed by states of illness and disease; that is, even if I cannot define health in any positive sense, I can surely know when I am sick (pain, high fever, etc.) and compare that condition with my previous states which contained no such conditions? Thus one could, in some recognizable sense, speak of illness as a deviation from a norm, even if it is not possible to specify that norm with any clarity.

But there are some problems with this approach, for all of its commonsense appeal. Sociologically, it is well known that what may be accounted sickness in one culture may not be so interpreted in another; one culture's (person's) deviation from the norm may not necessarily be another culture's (person's) deviation. In this as in other matters, commonsense intuition may be nothing but a reflection of different cultural and personal evaluations. In addition, there can be and usually are serious disputes about how great a deviation from the (unspecified) norm is necessary before the terms "sickness" and "illness" become appropriate. Am I to be put in the sick role because of my nagging case of itching athlete's foot, or must my toes start dropping off before I can so qualify? All general concepts have their borderline cases, and normally they need pose no real problems for the applicability of the concepts for the run of instances. But where "health" and "illness" are concerned, the number of borderline cases can be enormous, affected by age, attitudinal and cultural factors. Worse still, the fact that people can be afflicted by disease (even fatally afflicted) well before the manifestation of any overt symptoms is enough to discredit the adequacy of intuitions based on how one happens to feel at any given moment.

A number of these problems might be resolved by distinguishing between health as a norm and as an ideal. As a norm, it could be possible to speak in terms of deviation from some statistical standards, particularly if these standards were couched not only in terms of organic function but also in terms of behavioral functioning. Thus someone would be called "healthy" if his heart, lungs, kidneys (etc.) functioned at a certain level of efficiency and efficacy, if he was not suffering physical pain, and if his body was free of those pathological conditions which even if undetected or undetectable could impair organic function and eventually cause pain. There could still be dispute about what should count as a "pathological" condition, but at least it would be possible to draw up a large checklist of items subject to "scientific measurement"; then, having gone through that checklist in a physical exam, and passing all the tests, one could be pronounced "healthy." Neat, clean, simple.

All of this might be possible in a static culture, which ours is not. The problem is that any notion of a statistical norm will be superintended by some kind of ideal. Why, in the first place, should anyone care at all how his organs are functioning, much less how well they do so? There must be some reason for that, a reason which goes beyond theoretical interest in statistical distributions. Could it possibly be because certain departures from the norm carry with them unpleasant states, which few are likely to call "good": pain, discrimination, unhappiness? I would guess so. In the second place, why should society have any interest whatever in the way the organs of its citizens function? There must also be some reason for that, very possibly the insight that the organ functioning of individuals has some aggregate social implications. In our culture at least (and in every other culture I have ever heard of) it is simply impossible, finally, to draw any sharp distinction between conceptions of the human good and what are accounted significant and negatively evaluated deviations from statistical norms.

That is the whole point of saying, in defense of the WHO definition of health, that it discerned the intimate connection between the good of the body and the good of the self, not only the individual self but the social community of selves. No individual and no society would (save for speculative, scientific reasons only) have any interest whatever in the condition of human organs and bodies were it not for the obvious fact that those conditions can have an enormous impact on the whole of human life. People do, it has been noticed, die; and they die because something has gone wrong with their bodies. This can be annoying, especially if one would, at the moment of death, prefer to be busy doing other things. Consider two commonplace occurrences. The first I have alluded to already: dropping a heavy brick on one's foot. So far as I know, there is no culture where the pain which that event occasions is considered a good in itself. Why is that? Because (I presume) the pain which results can not only make it difficult or impossible to walk for a time but also because the pain, if intense enough, makes it impossible to think about anything else (or think at all) or to relate to anything or anyone other than the pain. For a time, I am "not myself" and that simply because my body is making such excessive demands on my attention that nothing is possible to me except to howl. I cannot, in sum, dissociate my "body" from my "self" in that situation; my self is my body and my body is my pain.

The other occurrence is no less commonplace. It is the assertion the old often make to the young, however great the psychological, economic, or other miseries of the latter: "at least you've got your health." They are saying in so many words that, if one is healthy, then there is some room for hope, some possibility of human recovery; and even more they are saying that, without good health, nothing is possible, however favorable the other conditions of life may be. Again, it is impossible to dissociate good of body and good of self. Put more formally, if health is not a sufficient condition for happiness, it is a necessary condition. At that very fundamental level, then, any sharp distinction between the good of bodies and the good of persons dissolves.

Are we not forced, therefore, to say that, if the complete absence of health (i.e., death) means the complete absence of self, then any diminishment of health must represent, correspondingly, a diminishment of self? That does not follow, for unless a disease or infirmity is severe, it may represent only a minor annoyance, diminishing our selfhood not a whit. And while it will not do to be overly sentimental about such things, it is probably the case that disease or infirmity can, in some cases, increase one's sense of selfhood (which is no reason to urge disease upon people for its possibly psychological benefits). The frequent reports of those who have recovered from a serious illness that it made them appreciate life in a far more intense way than they previously had are not to be dismissed (though one wishes an easier way could be found).

MODEST CONCLUSIONS

Two conclusions may be drawn. The first is that some minimal level of health is necessary if there is to be any possibility of human happiness. Only in exceptional circumstances can the good of self be long maintained in the absence of the good of the body. The second conclusion, however, is that one can be healthy without being in a state of "complete physical, mental, and social well-being." That conclusion can be justified in two ways: (a) because some degree of disease and infirmity is perfectly compatible with mental and social well-being; and (b) because it is doubtful that there ever was, or ever could be, more than a transient state of "complete physical, mental and social well-being," for individuals or societies; that's just not the way life is or could be. Its attractiveness as an ideal is vitiated by its practical impossibility of realization. Worse than that, it positively misleads, for health becomes a goal of such all-consuming importance that it simply begs to be thwarted in its realization. The demands which the word "complete" entail set the stage for the worst false consciousness of all: the demand that life deliver perfection. Practically speaking, this demand has led, in the field of health, to a constant escalation of expectation and requirement, never ending, never satisfied.

What, then, would be a good definition of "health"? I was afraid someone was going to ask me that question. I suggest we settle on the following: "Health is a state of physical well-being." That state need not be "complete," but it must be at least adequate, i.e., without significant impairment of function. It also need not encompass "mental" well-being; one can be healthy yet anxious, well yet depressed. And it surely ought not to encompass "social well-being," except insofar as that well-being will be impaired by the presence of large-scale, serious physical infirmities. Of course my definition is vague, but it would take some very fancy semantic footwork for it to be socially misused; that brat next door could not be called "sick" except when he is running a fever. This definition would not, though, preclude all social use of the language of "pathology" for other than physical disease. The image of a physically well body is a powerful one and, used carefully, it can be suggestive of the kind of wholeness and adequacy of function one might hope to see in other areas of life.

A Theory of Health

Caroline Whitbeck

I. THE INITIAL DEFINITION OF HEALTH

People generally recognize the value of having the psychophysiological capacity to act or respond appropriately in a wide variety of situations. By "appropriately," I mean in a way that is supportive of, or at least minimally destructive to, the agent's goals, projects, aspirations, and

C. Whitbeck, "A Theory of Health," in A.L. Caplan, H.T. Engelhardt, Jr. and J.J. McCartney, eds., *Concepts of Health and Disease: Interdisciplinary Perspectives* (Reading, Mass.: Addison-Wesley Publishing Co., 1981) pp. 611-626.

so forth.[1] This good, I claim, is the good of health. The absence of any restrictions on a person's goals, projects, and aspirations in this definition is intentional. Even if we consider such unusual goals as the wish to die, we would find that it, too, is more easily and surely attained by a person with a wide range of capabilities.

To understand *fully* the concept of health, we need more than a definition of the term, we need to understand how the concept of health relates to a host of others, including those of disease, injury, fitness, prevention, "health hazard," motivational disturbance, health promotion, and medical care.[2] In what follows, I develop such a philosophical theory of health, and argue that health is a concept of a different order from the concept of disease (and, *mutatis mutandis*, those of injury and impairment). Although medicine, in the broad sense, is the body of knowledge and practice concerned with the prevention of disease and the treatment of disease and injury (and, to some extent impairment), and diseases and injuries frequently *do* compromise the health of those who bear them, nonetheless, health promotion goes *beyond* the scope of medical care.

II. THE CONCEPT OF HEALTH AND PROPOSALS TO REFORM MEDICINE

If we bear in mind the human interest in health as here defined, we will have a perspective on the institution of medicine, in terms of which its scope and limits may be properly assessed. One implication of the theory outlined here is that *expertise* in medicine, even in the broad sense of medicine as we have defined, will not be relevant to many health decisions. The term "medicine" is used in a number of narrower senses, for example, to mean a discipline distinct from nursing, clinical nutrition, or public health. I refer to this as the "narrow sense." This is the sense in which we speak of "a license to practice medicine." Of course, the term is used still more narrowly to mean the nonsurgical specialties, or just one among these, internal medicine. When I speak of "medicine" without giving further qualification, I mean medicine in the broad sense, that is, all of those disciplines concerned with the treatment and prevention of disease and injury.

A number of recent proposals to change the emphasis or practice of medicine in both the broad and narrow sense of "medicine," have been couched in terms of "health." Although many of these proposed changes have merit, overuse of the term "health" has created new confusions about what health is. Among these proposed changes has been one to integrate a concern for prevention back into medicine in the narrow sense. Thus physicians are encouraged to help people recognize behavior that increases their risk of future disease and injury, by using some instrument like the Health Hazard Appraisal List. Unfortunately the new emphasis on recognizing the way in which certain ways of living predispose a person to injury or disease is often phrased as though it concerned health per se, whereas, in fact, it often involves *only* the prevention of disease and injury. (There are additional problems posed by the way in which this valuable re-emphasis on prevention is discussed. For example, the relevant variables are often termed "lifestyle variables" which makes it seem that *most* people have a wide range of choices in these matters, whereas, in fact, only the privileged have such a range of choices.)

Another proposal is one designed to combat the fragmentation of patient care, which has been one of the untoward side effects of the growth of specialty medicine. First nursing and, more recently, other provider groups have explicitly addressed the issue of developing a more comprehensive approach to patient care, because they have recognized that at present medical care often harms in one way while helping in another. Unfortunately, this proposal to make patient care more comprehensive has been phrased in terms of providing "health care." At the same time, greater appreciation of the fact that in developed nations most major illnesses are chronic illnesses, and thus not susceptible to cure, has led to greater attention to finding ways to care for people whose conditions can only be managed (as opposed to cured). Although such continuing care generally does enhance people's health, it does so only by coping with particular problems.

Until recently, the term "health" was hardly mentioned in medical circles — the term does not even appear in the index of many standard medical texts, such as Beeson and McDermott, *Textbook of Medicine*. Then, the only danger of conceptual confusion regarding health arose from the attempt to define health entirely in terms of medical concepts, such as those of disease and injury. This attempt generated the so-called "negative notion" of health, health as the absence of disease, injury, and impairment. The term "health," however, was only rarely used in this way. Even in such expressions as "restoring the patient to health," "health" often does not mean "the absence of disease." Instead, "restoring the patient to health" merely means restoring the patient to a *premorbid* level of functioning where "premorbid" refers only to *a particular episode* of illness, so that the "health" of the "restored" patient still includes all his or her chronic diseases as well as poor physical condition, neurotic malaise, and so forth.

If there are any clear assets for human beings, health (considered as the psychophysiological capacity to respond appropriately to a wide variety of situations) is one. This evaluation of health accords with the historical one. Those philosophers from Aristotle to Rawls who have believed that there are some "natural goods" for human beings have placed health among those goods. In contrast, it is easy to find conditions that are generally agreed to be cases of disease, injury, or impairment, which could hardly be counted as the loss of a natural good by those who use this category, but, indeed, which under plausible circumstances would *benefit* their bearers. Sterility and cowpox are examples that come quickly to mind. Indeed, as will be argued presently, the concepts of disease and health are value-laden in different respects.

My general thesis is that not only is health something over and above the absence of disease, injury, and impairment, but also that a high degree of health is compatible with some degree of disease, injury, and impairment. Moreover, the relationship between concepts of health and disease is an intimate one: people's interest in health, together with their aversion to pain, is the *origin* of their interest in having the means to prevent and effectively treat disease, injury, and impairment.

In taking the position that the concepts of health and disease are *not* complementary concepts, I differ with Engelhardt, Margolis, Boorse, and most recent writers on this subject, but concur with the ancient writers, for whom medicine and hygiene (the science of health promotion) were different disciplines.[3] To understand the intimate and complex relation between the concepts of health and disease, it is necessary to clarify what is meant by the terms "disease," and "impairment" and to elaborate the respects in which they are value-laden.

III. WAYS IN WHICH CONCEPTS MAY BE VALUE-LADEN

It is sometimes argued that the distinctions drawn in the language of a human community are, largely, the distinctions needed to carry out the projects recognized by that community, and as such, reflect the value commitments of that community. I think that there is something to the view that the distinctions made in a language reflect what the community using that language take to be important, and to the extent that it is correct, there is a sense in which all general terms are value-laden.[4] The assertion that the concept of health and the concept of disease are value-laden only in this particular sense, could not be an interesting claim about *these* two concepts.

Some terms, such as "discovery," (an act of) kindness," "hideous," "vicious," "sacred," "blunder," and "worthwhile," are value-laden in a very strong sense: to use these terms is to say that that to which they are applied is good or bad, valuable or worthless, in some way — aesthetically, ethically, religiously, prudentially, epistemically, or hedonistically. Health considered as the psychophysiological ability to act or respond appropriately, is a concept that is value-laden in this very strong sense.

I claim that the concept of disease[5] is value-laden in a third sense, which is distinct both from the very strong sense and from the weak sense in which all general terms may be said to be value-laden. I shall call this intermediary sense "the capability sense" and define it as follows: a concept or term will be said to be value-laden in the capability sense if, and only if, the concept or the definition of the term warrants the conclusion that people have an interest in *being able* to influence things of that type. The failure to recognize this third sense has obscured the understanding of the ways in which terms may be value-laden; the implicit assumption of most examinations of the extent to which concepts are value-laden has been that *either* a term is no more value-laden than the other general terms of a language, *or* it is value-laden in the very strong sense that application of the term implies the judgment that the particular to which it was applied is valuable (or worthless) in some respect.

In particular, people's interest in *being able* to prevent and treat diseases may be inferred from the concept of disease. Indeed, the interest in prevention and treatment is the basis of the distinction between disease processes and other atypical psychophysiological processes.

All human societies have devoted some of their resources to the development of medicinal or healing arts. This allocation represented the society's attempt to acquire these desired capabilities. Yet notice that, according to what I have argued, to say that a *particular* psychophysiological process is a case of disease is to say only that it is an instance of a kind of psychophysiological process that one wishes *to be able* to prevent or to treat effectively, not that the particular *case* of a disease itself is necessarily a misfortune for the bearer and hence necessarily something that is in the bearer's interest to have treated. The impairment, sterility, is one which people frequently go to some trouble and expense to acquire through medical intervention. The same was true of cases of cowpox before the development of smallpox vaccine. These examples of disease and impairment, which are commonly of net benefit to their bearer, together with the desirability of *being able* to prevent or treat diseases, shows that the concept is value-laden in what I have called, "the capability sense," rather than being value-laden in the very strong sense. The concepts of food, shelter, flood, and infestation are all capability-valued. One generally wishes *to be able* to produce or maintain a supply of food or shelter and *to be able* to prevent or eliminate infestations and floods, but on a given occasion it may not be in anyone's interest to produce or possess more food or shelter or to prevent or eliminate every infestation or flood.

Consider two identical physiological processes, one of which is counted as the early stages of a disease, and the other of which is regarded as a normal reaction to a vaccination. This disparity casts doubt on any attempt to define "disease" purely in terms of physiological functioning, and hence, on the claim that disease is value-laden only to the same extent as biological concepts.

The definition of *disease* that I have offered is that diseases are, first of all, psychophysiological processes; second, they compromise the ability to do what people commonly want and expect to be able to do; third, they are not necessary in order to do what people commonly want to be able to do; fourth, they are either statistically abnormal in those at risk or there is some other basis for a reasonable hope of finding means to effectively treat or prevent them.[6]

According to these criteria, what qualifies as a disease is relative to a societal context insofar as what people are understood as wanting to do is relative to societal context. Statistical abnormality in those at risk (worldwide), however, is *independent* of societal context. Therefore, a psychophysiological process may qualify as a disease even if a society fails to *recognize* its presence because of its near ubiquity in those at risk in that society. The last three characteristics provide the basis for the interest in *being able to do something about* processes of this sort. It is the desirability of *being able to do something about things* of this sort which is the valuational component of terms like "disease," "food," or "flood."

The value of having a capability with respect to things of some type does not presume *anything* about the worth of particular things of that type. It is therefore as misleading to say that calling something a case of disease is to assert a prima facie case for preventing or eliminating it, as it is to say that calling an item "food" is to make a prima facie case that we want to produce or provide it.

IV. THE AGENT AND THE PATIENT

Health is frequently pursued through a variety of intermediary goals. One is the prevention and termination of particular processes and states that compromise health. Sometimes the way diseases compromise health is taken to be so important that the person whose health is at stake is thought of as an actual or potential "patient," that is, one who bears, or is *afflicted* with, or *suffers* from the process or condition in question. The passivity that is central to the concept of a "patient" is the person's passivity vis-à-vis the disease. (Passivity of the patient in the treatment process or as the client of the health professionals may or may not also exist as part of the social role of being a patient.) Notice that in talking about people's health, and not just the actual or potential diseases that may compromise that health, it is misleading to start by viewing these persons as actual or potential patients or bearers of disease.

The notion of health as the capacity to act or respond appropriately explicates the positive conception of health, which has been particularly evident in the practice of the self-help and mutual aid movements of this century and the last. It is closely connected with the idea of wholeness, rather than with a high level of functioning in some isolated areas or in some limited respects. Deriving from "hale," which means whole, health, in the positive sense, connotes wholeness of a person. Wholeness of a person is more than the wholeness of an organism, although the wholeness of the organism contributes to the health or wholeness of the person. This sense of wholeness of a person implies the ability to engage in distinctively human activities. I will use the term "capabilities" hereafter to mean the ability to engage in activities that are characteristically intentional actions. In contrast, the term "capacity" is used for biological functioning, whether of organisms (as respiratory capacity) or of parts of organisms such as organs or cells (as the heart's capacity to pump blood).

To assess people's health, one must take into account their capabilities and not merely their biological capacities. Therefore, the notion of health or wholeness is closely associated with the notions of autonomy, with the ability to act to achieve one's purposes, and with the ability to live as a member of a human community. Accordingly, health, rather than being something that happens or fails to happen to a person in the way that diseases and injuries do, is the ability to act or participate autonomously and effectively in a wide range of activities. The term "wholeness" should not, however, suggest that there exists an upper limit, a state of optimum health. Such a suggestion would be foreign to the account given here since, presumably, people can always increase their ability to act appropriately in *some* situations. The absence of an upper limit on health does not make that concept any more obscure than concepts such as wealth, which also have no upper limit.

I will not address here the question of just what are the components of human life, because the theory of health that I am advancing does not require specification of these components. The best method is to begin by accepting an account of human life that is as broad as possible, since if some human activity is a mistaken, or stupid, or sloppy, or naive way of undertaking some other, quite different, human activity, this will eventually become clear as the two enterprises are examined further. However, if one starts from an assumption that some activity is just a mistaken way of doing something else and it turns out not to be, there will never be an opportunity to discover the error.[7]

It may be objected that some goals are themselves irrational and thus that it is odd to include such goals among those that the actions of a healthy person would contribute to attaining. To the extent that we believe that some goal is itself peculiar, however, or even irrational, we are inclined to say that it is something else that the person "really wants." The peculiar goal is only a means to some other end, and that if the further end were attained, the person would be satisfied and abandon the peculiar one. Thus if someone asserted that he or she wished to become miserable, one would assume either that this was only a means to some end, such as being so tranquil or resigned as to be beyond repulsion or attraction, or that this was an attempt to expiate some guilt, and if the guilt were lifted in some other way, the person would be satisfied. Nothing in this argument turns on a specification of the goals that are thought to be irrational or peculiar. The point is only that if we are willing to apply the term "irrational" to a goal, we are also inclined to say that the goal is only a means to some further end which we may regard as rational.

Therefore, it should not seem paradoxical to define health in terms of a person's ability to act or respond in a way that is supportive of the person's goals, projects, and aspirations.

The notion of health expounded here, while much broader than the notion of a mere absence of disease, is not as broad as the much criticized definition of the World Health Organization: "the state of complete physical, mental and social well-being and not merely the absence of disease or infirmity." By this definition, all elements of social well-being, including wealth, legal capacity, political power, and social prestige, are a *part* of health. Although there are important *causal* connections between the components of social well-being and health (for example, people with social advantages do tend to have less disease), people do not become healthier just by becoming wealthier or by gaining the right to vote. Thus, wealth, legal capacity, political power, and social prestige should *not* be considered a part of health, even if possession of them increases the likelihood that people will be healthier or less subject to disease.

Health as the ability to act or respond appropriately in a variety of situations requires more than many individual human capabilities and functional capacities. This conception requires the integration of such capabilities and capacities so that each is exercised in ways that serve the interests of the person in question. In particular, the psychophysiological changes that constitute a stress response will serve a person's interests in some situations but, in others, will simply be painful and taxing. (Contrast the situation in which a stress response permits someone to lift a heavy object that has fallen on someone else, with another situation in which the person undergoes these changes but no physical action is required and the person experiences the changes as anxiety and disturbed sleep.) Much more could be said about the compatibility or incompatibility of a person's projects and goals, and thus about the ease or difficulty with which appropriateness can be assessed in a particular case. But we have at least some idea of what it is to function or act in an appropriate way. We may then understand the claim that health is the capacity for a high level of integrated psychophysiological functioning, which enables the agent to act or respond to situations in a way that promotes the agent's projects and goals (and that promotes the availability of a wide range of responses in the future).

The failure of some writers on the concept of health to recognize the integration of functioning that characterizes health has led them to assume that an increase in health, in any positive sense of health, would be identical with an increase in isolated abilities, specifically *athletic* abilities. Such an approach to positive health predictably runs afoul of the fact that the development of a physique to perform some particular athletic feat with unusual excellence generally interferes with developing the physique to perform some *other* feat. The lesson to be learned from this fact is not that health cannot be conceived positively, but rather that an increase in health should not be confused with an increase in isolated capabilities and capacities. Although an increase in health cannot be identified with an increase in *isolated* capabilities, it is nonetheless possible to specify some significant components of health.

V. SIGNIFICANT COMPONENTS OF HEALTH

Consider the notion of physical fitness. In addition to being a significant component of capability/capacity

health (so that, other things equal, a more physically fit person is healthier, that is, is more able to respond appropriately in a wide range of situations), physical fitness is a concept that resembles the concept of health. That is, it is best characterized in general terms, which make no mention of the excellence with which a person performs specific feats. This may come as a surprise to those who measure fitness in terms of, say, the ability to run laps, and who confuse the concept of fitness with the procedure for measuring it. A high level of physical fitness is usually characterized as a state in which there is good muscle tone and improved circulation, bones are less brittle, and the person has greater cardiac reserve. It may be evident that one result of these changes, in addition to an increase in a variety of athletic abilities, is that an increase in the capacity to withstand a wide range of insults with a minimum of injury or to retard or forestall the development of a wide range of diseases. The consequence that being healthy (or having a high level of fitness) makes a person less liable to disease and injury is not an accidental feature of the concept of health that I have proposed. Since acting or responding in a way that minimizes disease and injury (that prevents its occurrence *or* lessens its severity) is a way of responding that generally promotes people's goals and projects, *any psychophysiological state* that makes one better able to ward off a wide variety of diseases and injury would for that reason be considered a significant component of health.

It is important to highlight two points implicit in what has just been said. First, it is *not* suggested that a significant component of health, such as fitness, is itself health. Quite to the contrary, the conception of health as a wholeness of the agent entails the *integration* of capabilities and capacities. Knowing that one person is more fit than another person does not by itself tell us which is healthier. Second, a decreased susceptibility to a specific disease, or injury, or to a narrow subclass of either, is not a significant component of health. Specific immunity is just that. Although immunity to a disease (say, measles) is useful in diminishing one's chance of becoming a patient, the capacity to respond in a desirable way only when exposed to measles virus is too specific to be a significant component of health in my theory. People who have lower risk of some specific type of injury may well have a greater life expectancy, but it is misleading to call them healthier. Such persons are only more likely to be healthy in the future than persons with greater risks. One may have increased risks for many reasons other than that of not being very healthy. For example, one may have a dangerous job. It is, therefore, misleading to use the Health Hazard Appraisal List in a way that puts not wearing seat belts on a par with smoking as an indication of being "less healthy," since smoking compromises health by compromising lung capacity *in addition* to increasing the risk of other diseases. Primary prevention, which increases safety, should be distinguished from primary prevention through promotion of health, since only the latter entails a change in psychophysiological state.

The distinction between a significant component of health, like fitness, and health itself, is important in other respects. If other things are equal, an increase in one significant component of health may make one healthier. But other things are rarely equal, and one can readily imagine a case in which a physically fit person would be less healthy than one who was out of condition. Suppose that the first was so ridden by phobias and neuroses that, in many situations, the most appropriate responses would be blocked by an anxiety reaction.

Compared to such a person, a less neurotic but out-of-condition individual would be better able to respond in most situations, regardless of whether we view neuroses as disease. Suppose, on the other hand, that a person with a high level of one or more significant components of health (that is, being physically fit, or being aware of her or his emotions, or having a realistic view of both and of him/herself and others, or being able to handle stressful situations well), has a sprained finger or acne. It seems clear that such a person would be healthier than another person who was out of condition, out of touch with feelings, had an unrealistic view of people, or stayed in a state of high anxiety long after a stressful situation, but had no detectable disease or injury.

These possibilities illustrate again the crucial point that not only is health something over and above the absence of disease, but a high level of health may be compatible with some degree of disease, injury, and impairment. One reason for choosing *not* to seek treatment or not following recommended treatment for some disease, injury, or impairment would be that undergoing the treatment excessively undermined the person's exercise of his or her capacities and capabilities, that is, the treatment would be detrimental to the person's health. This might occur not only in cases in which the treatment carried risk of further disease and injury, but in cases in which the treatment caused disruption of health maintenance routines, or resulted in loss of social supports (for example, because of travel required) or in other ways undermined the person's ability to deal with stress. Notice that refusal of treatment for health reasons contrasts with the refusal of treatment for economic or social reasons, although refusal of recommended treatment (often unfortunately called "noncompliance") for reasons such as these may also be a sensible decision.

VI. THE RELATION BETWEEN THE CONCEPTS OF HEALTH AND HAPPINESS

To recapitulate, health is a person's psychophysiological capacity to act or respond appropriately (in a way that is supportive of the person's goals, projects, and aspirations) in a wide variety of situations. Health encompasses certain significant components: among them, maintaining physical fitness, having a generally realistic view of situations, and having the ability to discharge negative feelings. The *net* effect of having a disease is frequently, although not invariably, to undermine a person's health. The institution of medicine is society's collective attempt to develop the means of preventing and treating conditions that are likely to undermine health.

The foregoing survey of the scope of the concept of health invites further statement about its limits. (The demarcation of health from such aspects of social well-being as wealth, social status, and legal capacity has already been discussed.) The distinction between health and happiness is particularly apropos. I argue that, to be happy, a person needs to be able to act in ways that serve *many goals, aspirations, and projects simultaneously.* The opportunity to do this is a function of at least four things: the range and relative importance of a person's goals, aspirations, and projects; the person's health (as previously characterized); the person's creativity; and the person's access to resources of all types (social, economic, and so forth). To consider creativity (as opposed to originality) as a significant component of health is consistent, at least, with the account of health we have given, although it is not entailed by it. The range and relative importance of a person's goals, aspirations, and projects, as well as a person's access to resources, however, are excluded from health in the presented theory. This demarcation accords with the intuition that having a diversity of interests, say, promoting social justice, pursuing truth, building close friendships, and living close to nature, can make it difficult to pursue all one's goals simultaneously, and can create unhappiness, yet does not compromise health. This demarcation is also consistent with the distinction between health and other social goods.

VII. CONDITIONS OF SELF-ALIENATION OR ALIENATED-SELF CONDITIONS

Other sorts of conditions, in *addition* to those of disease, injury, and impairment, *compromise a person's* ability to act or respond appropriately, but yet are not diseases, injuries, or impairments. These I call conditions of self-alienation, which may be classified into three or four general types. The first of them is what Thalberg has called "motivational disturbance," namely, a condition in which a person has thoughts, feelings, or attitudes, or expresses types of behavior that are experienced as being at odds with his or her beliefs, basic attitudes, and habits. The second is akrasia or "weakness of will," a situation in which the person fails to act as he or she has resolved to act. (Akrasia may or may not have motivational disturbance admixed in a given case.) The third is a self-deception, which has been most aptly characterized by Fingerette as the condition in which people systematically avoid avowing some aspect of their engagements in the world. (The cardinal sign of avowing is the act of spontaneously spelling out that aspect of the engagement to oneself or others.) Fourth is what I will call remorse/self-hatred, which encompasses everything from rejection and deidentification with an aspect of the self (remorse) to rejection of the self in its entirety or at least in its central aspects (self-hatred).

Although it is undoubtedly evident that many of the conditions that I have characterized here as conditions of self-alienation would be classified as neuroses from the point of view of psychoanalytically oriented psychotherapy, I wish to leave open the question of whether, and to what extent, psychoanalytic nosology is correct and, in particular, whether some of what are now termed neuroses may turn out to be diseases (like toxic psychoses[8]) or impairments (like mental retardation), whereas others will be self-alienation problems as defined here. Psychiatric nosology is fluid and is likely to remain so for the foreseeable future.

These conditions are not discussed in detail here, but several points about them should be noted. First, they are value-laden in the capability sense, that is, in the way that medical conditions (diseases, injuries, and impairments) are. Furthermore, alienated-self problems frequently, but not invariably, compromise health. In particular, self-deception might enable a person to behave appropriately under circumstances that were too painful to acknowledge immediately, and hence *contribute* to health in this instance. Remorse might be necessary for rapid change and growth, and hence could contribute to integrated development.

Second, in the many societies the institutions that address these problems most directly have been religious, even where medicine and religion have been separated. This latter point may be important to make since we may be so struck by the popularity in our own culture of psychoanalysis or other secular approaches, such as EST, which have dealt with these problems, that we may lose sight of other conceptions that historically have dealt with the same phenomena. Commonly, the adherents of one practice claim that alternative practices actually increase self-alienation problems in general, and self-deception in particular, but I will not examine those controversies here.

The third point about these conditions is that, although they may predispose a person to medical problems or may frequently be aggravated by medical problems, this is no reason to regard them as medical problems. In the absence of evidence that they ought to be considered diseases, injuries, or impairments, we have no reason to think that expertise in medicine will be relevant to preventing or treating these conditions. This is not to say that *the presence* of such conditions may be ignored by medical personnel in the course of treating medical problems. In view of their causal connections to medical problems, they need to be *taken into account* in devising any plan for *comprehensive* medical care, even if they cannot be eliminated by medical intervention. In this respect, having an alienated-self condition is like having low income, or undergoing a grief reaction.

The subject of alienated-self conditions raises the question of agent competence in deciding what actions will promote health. Although diseases, injuries, and impairment *can* make people incompetent (such as when a person is delirious due to fever, or acutely psychotic due to a brain tumor or due to the ingestion of toxic substances, or unconscious due to a concussion of the brain), these situations are relatively easy to recognize. Furthermore, the effects of disease are more often less severe, and make the person more vulnerable and more in need of support, rather than incompetent. Self-alienation, however, creates a different sort of problem in that, when severe, it does not make the person incapable of acting in any coherent way at all, but may distort a person's decisions so that they fail to reflect the person's (integrated) self-interest. The burden of proof must be on the side of those who say that a particular person is so self-alienated as to be unable to make decisions that promote her or his own health.

Suppose, however, that a person is so self-alienated as to choose against his or her own interests. Suppose, for example, that a person's self-hatred is so great that he or she elects to have a succession of mutilating surgical procedures that are not warranted by evidence of grave health risks. In such a case, both medical practitioners as well as those who care about the person, might have a moral duty to try to dissuade the person from the operations. Such cases, though, are relatively rare. Since numerous studies show that the various (lay and professional) forms of psychotherapy have about the same recovery rate, there is no reason to think that self-alienation is not at least as amenable to self-care and mutual aid approaches as it is to medically and non-medically oriented professional psychotherapies (although this will depend on the exact nature of the self-alienation). Certainly, the practice of self-care and mutual aid is especially conducive to enhanced self-esteem and reduced self-hatred.

VIII. THE ROLE OF MEDICINE IN HEALTH PROMOTION

Expertise in medicine — skill in the prevention of disease and the treatment of disease and injury — is not sufficient to make many decisions concerning health. What then is the role of medicine in health promotion? Because diseases and injuries frequently do compromise health, the ability to prevent disease and injury is an important component in an individual's or a society's attempts to promote people's health. However, I submit that the paradigm instance in which one person appropriately makes decisions about the promotion of another's health is not the situation in which a medical practitioner (nurse, physician, physical therapist) makes decisions about care of patients, but rather is the situation in which a parent reaches a decision on the care of a young child. Typically the parent considers such possible consequences of a course of action, as how it will affect the child's self-esteem, body awareness, trust of adults, relation to peers, and general comfort, as well as whether it will prevent disease or facilitate recovery from it. Now I am not suggesting that it would be appropriate for a practitioner, or any one else, to make decisions for another in the way in which the parent does for a child. Indeed, as I have argued, the person whose health is in question is in the best position to be aware of all of the factors involved. When that person is unconscious or otherwise incompetent to do so, those closest to the person and who care about him or her are in the best position to be aware of all of the factors that bear on their overall health. Of course, the person may not have anyone who cares about him or her deeply, in which case, there will be no good proxy to make the decision.

In some respects, consulting a medical practitioner is like consulting an architect: both have information about what can be done to achieve the ends of the client, what future options will be foreclosed by taking a given course of action, and the likely time and expense required for each option. The analogy breaks down, however, when the patient is significantly affected by fear, pain, or confusion due to the threat of disease or death or due to disease itself or to diagnostic and treatment procedures. Furthermore, those who care about the sick person may also be distraught. People generally are not fully articulate about all of the important factors in their lives, and those who are sick and stressed are still less so. Thus patients who are distraught cannot be expected to transfer all of the necessary information to a practitioner. Practitioners, therefore, need the skills to provide clients with support and an opportunity to discharge their pain and distress, so that they can make the momentous and often painful decisions with which they are faced. It is only when practitioners are themselves able to do this, or see that it is adequately done by others, that medical knowledge will be correctly applied, that is, applied in a way that promotes and enhances people's health.

IX. SUMMARY OF THE ARGUMENT

I might have called this chapter "a theory of health as the context for an adequate understanding of medicine," were that title not so long and awkward, since it gives a more precise specification of the subject. I began by observing that people generally recognize the value of having the psychophysiological capacity to act or respond appropriately in a wide variety of situations and claimed that this good is the good of health. I examined the ways in which the term "health," has been used in recent years, in order to unravel some of the confusions concerning it. I argued that whereas the term "health" is properly understood to be value-laden in the very strong sense, that is, to say something is healthy or that it promotes health, is to give a reason for saying that it is good. In contrast, the term "disease" is value-laden in a distinct and hitherto unrecognized sense, that is, when we apply it to a psychophysiological process, we judge that the process is one that would be good (for people) to *be able* to prevent or treat effectively. The concepts of health and disease are not complementary concepts, therefore, but turn out to be concepts of different orders. This point is brought out further by the contrast between disease as something that befalls its bearer and health as the integrated ability to engage effectively in a wide range of activities.

Although it is important to understand the integrated character of a high state of health, significant components of health can be identified. Among these are physical fitness, having a realistic view of oneself and others, and having the ability to handle stressful situations. Although the concept of health is much more than the absence of disease, and indeed a high level of health is compatible with having some disease, health contrasts both with other aspects of social well-being and with happiness. In addition to medical conditions, there is another class of conditions that often compromise health, which I call "self-alienation conditions." Because of the importance of the consideration of these and other factors that bear on a person's health and lie outside of the scope of medical expertise, decisions about the appropriateness of some medical intervention, that is, decisions about whether that intervention is likely to produce a net increase or enhancement in a person's health, cannot be decided on the basis of medical expertise alone. I argue that usually these are best made by the person whose health is at stake.

NOTES

I am most grateful to the Committee on the Status of Women of the American Philosophical Association for the invitation to present an earlier version of this paper at the Eastern Division Meetings in December 1977, to the late Jane English and other attenders and participants at that session for their comments and criticisms, and to the many people who have given me suggestions since that time, especially James Speer, Marilyn Thompson, Maradee Davis, Arthur Caplan, Edmund Erde, Joseph Margolis, and Christopher Boorse.

1. If one is able to respond appropriately, of course, one is also *able* to respond inappropriately.
2. In my discussion of medicine and medical concepts, such as the concept of disease, I assume to some extent the perspective of Western allopathic medical science. Specifically, I assume that medical science is generally correct in believing that certain sorts of things exist in nature: disease entities, microbes, cells, malignant cells, DNA, and so on. I do not assume, however, that every customary application of those concepts is correct. Thus, if it were true that pregnancy is frequently construed as a disease in medical theory and practice, I would not take that empirical fact about the explicit and implicit ascription of disease status as sufficient warrant to decide that pregnancy is a disease. Furthermore, although I do not assume anything about the existence or nonexistence of natural entities answering to the description of the theoretical terms in nonallopathic medicine, theoretical notions such as "chi," I accept on its own merits

any evidence for the efficacy of practices, like acupuncture, which are explained in terms of notions like "chi" in those nonallopathic traditions.

3. Today one scarcely hears "hygiene" used to mean the promotion of health except in such contexts as the "Natural Hygiene Movement." The term "hygienic" (and its cognate, "sanitary") have lost their connection with health and have come to mean merely clean (although modern usage dictionaries do not seem to have caught on to this fact). Sometimes, the cleanliness involved has at least a prophylactic function, as is the case with dental hygiene, but often "hygiene," and "sanitary" mean only clean, that is, free from matter that is regarded as ugly or taboo, but in no way is the meaning related to health or the prevention or treatment of disease. This is aptly illustrated by the application of the term "sanitary napkin" to a product which, like a table napkin, merely serves to keep clothes clean.
4. It is surprising how often people will speak as though value commitments are "subjective" in the pejorative sense of being preferences which may be based as easily on individual or collective whim as on considered judgment. Since one hears this from nonphilosophers as often as from philosophers, it is more than the legacy of the philosophical thesis of emotivism. However, since many, if not most, of the projects recognized in a human community are requisite for the survival of the community in its present form, the community's interest in these projects can hardly be viewed as capricious.
5. From here on when I speak of disease my remarks apply, *mutatis mutandis,* to injury and impairment as well. I take the latter concepts to be value-laden in the same way as those of disease. What is required to fulfill the *mutatis mutandis* clause is spelled out in my "Four Basic Concepts of Medical Science," *PSA 1978,* vol. 1, pp. 210-222. There I also delineate the confusions that may arise if the differences between disease, injuries, impairments, and symptoms are not recognized. The distinctions between these concepts, however, are not important for the present discussion.
6. I have explained and argued for this definition in "Four Basic Concepts of Medical Science" in *PSA 1978*, vol. 1, pp. 210-222.
7. This way of putting the matter assumes that any activity to which people have devoted a good deal of time and effort is, at worst, a mistaken way of doing something else, and not *just* a mistake.
8. I have argued elsewhere that it is unlikely that the separation of organic or somatic factors from psychosocial factors in the determination of the etiology of diseases, or the etiology of self-alienation, can be done so clearly and unequivocally that there will be any generally useful distinction to be marked by calling some diseases "mental" and others "physical," or "somatic."

REFERENCE

Whitbeck, Caroline, "Four Basic Concepts of Medical Science." *PSA 1978,* 1(1978):210-222.

Towards a New Philosophy of Health: A Welfare Notion of Health

Lennard Nordenfeldt

The General Idea

Let us recollect our main conclusions from the analyses of the two proposals on the vital goals of man.

The vital goals as determined by our basic needs: Prima facie merits

(i) This concept is a candidate for being a universal concept of health. It is not necessarily restricted to human beings. If there is some sense in talking about basic needs of humans there ought to be sense in ascribing basic needs to animals and plants as well.

(ii) It seems to admit a uniform application to all human beings. If the basic needs are general, it seems not to be necessary to make an investigation into any particular needs of an individual in order to determine his health.

Disadvantages

(iii) The notion of a basic need is, if at all defined, tied to the concepts of survival and health. But the latter concept cannot be used in a characterization of health itself.

(iv) If need is conceptually connected merely to survival it seems to cover too little. Man has vital goals far beyond survival.

We have observed that standard circumstances normally require one's participating in some professional activity in order to survive. Therefore, as a standard result of this conception, a person is healthy if, and only if, he can fulfil his professional duties. Then the result is not completely unreasonable. It gives us a technical notion of health roughly equivalent to the notion used by health insurance authorities.

Still, this notion covers too little. There are many uses of the term "health" which go far beyond this technical use.

This observation led us to scrutinize *the subject-goal conception of health.*

Prima facie merits

(i) This concept is extremely sensitive to the multiplicity of human goals and the variations in goal-setting among different persons. It therefore answers well to the basic complaints concerning the need-concept of health. It can thus explain that old people can be healthy and that some people who indeed manage to fulfil their professional duties may still be ill. The determination of health is completely dependent on the individual person's setting of goals.

Disadvantages

(ii) The SG-concept of health has a restricted application. It does not go

Lennard Nordenfeldt, "A Welfare Theory of Health," from Lennard Nordenfeldt, *On the Nature of Health: An Action-Theoretic Approach*. (Dordrecht: D. Reidel Publishing Co., 1987) pp. 76-80.

further than the realm of human beings; it cannot explain the health and illness of animals and plants.

(iii) The sensitivity of the SG-concept to individual goal-setting seems to be too great. We obtain counter-intuitive results both in the case where the subject sets too low and limited goals for himself, and in the case where he sets counter-productive or damaging goals.

We shall now suggest a conception of health which is different from that suggested by the need-theory and the SG-theory, but which retains important elements from both of them. The key notion in this conception is *welfare*; in the case of humans welfare will be equated with *happiness*. Happiness should then be understood as a technical concept covering more ground than does the ordinary concept of happiness.

The general idea is the following: The vital goals of man are those whose fulfilment is necessary and jointly sufficient for a minimal degree of welfare, i.e. happiness. To be healthy, then, is to have the ability to fulfil those goals which are necessary and jointly sufficient for a minimal degree of happiness. Observe, however, that this implies neither that health is sufficient for minimal happiness, nor that it is necessary. Health is not sufficient, since the ability to fulfil one's vital goals does not imply that one actually fulfils them. And health is not necessary, since the vital goals can be fulfilled by other means, for instance by the actions of someone else.

To relate health to happiness is to give credit both to the need-theory and the SG-theory. In a way it could be seen as a new way of specifying the goals of needs. Instead of relating needs to survival and health we now propose to relate them to happiness. Our suggestion also includes essential elements from the SG-theory. As we shall see in the subsequent analysis, happiness is conceptually related to the fulfilment of the agent's goals. It is important to note, however, that not all intended goals fulfil the requirements of being goals in the welfare sense. Moreover, there are some goals in the welfare sense which are not goals aimed at by the agent himself.

Is, then, the question of what the vital goals of man are a theoretically decidable question? Can any empirical investigation completely determine this? Superficially, it may seem so. If the fulfilment of the vital goals is necessary and jointly sufficient for minimal happiness, then our task must be to inquire what happiness requires. What does Jones need to be happy, and what does Smith need? The investigation may involve very difficult methodological problems, but it seems, in principle, to be a theoretically decidable question.

Our reply to this will be the following: the question of what the vital goals are is only partially theoretically decidable. Roughly, it is decidable to the extent that a modified SG-theory is correct. We can determine the vital goals by theoretical means to the extent that they are identical with the goals set by the agent himself.

The welfare-theory of health to be proposed here means, however, precisely that this cannot be the whole story. The question of what constitutes "real" happiness, as well as a minimal degree of such, can only be answered by a primary evaluation; it is not a question of science. Consider the following problem: a person with very low intelligence and a low degree of vitality sets very few and primitive goals. Assume that he is able to fulfil these goals and that the situation actually permits their fulfilment. From the point of view of mere goal-satisfaction this person is then a happy person.

It may, however, be contended that this is not enough. "Real" happiness presupposes a minimum of complexity and subtlety. A person who fulfils a very small and primitive set of goals does not fulfil the requirements of minimal *human* welfare, minimal human happiness. Thus, if his abilities do not supersede the ability to fulfil his primitive goals, then he cannot be healthy.

The problem here cannot, we believe, be solved by scientific means. It can only be solved by a decision founded on an evaluation of what should constitute minimal human happiness. Let us call this an evaluation of welfare. It is, as far as we can see, an evaluation *sui generis*. It should, for instance, be kept distinct from moral evaluation. An evaluation of welfare does not require that the vital goals have any particular moral status. The vital goals are primarily egocentric. They are goals the fulfilment of which gives the agent himself satisfaction. This is certainly compatible with the goals, being moral goals; but it is also compatible with their not being so.

The theory which we propose has profound consequences for the philosophy of health. A conceptual analysis cannot once and for all settle what the vital goals of health are. It can bring us precisely to the point we have reached in our discussion. It can tell us that the ultimate specification of the vital goals must be left to an evaluation of welfare.

The basic conception of health offered by the welfare-theory is the following:

> *A* is healthy if, and only if, *A* is able, given standard circumstances in his environment, to fulfil those goals which are necessary and jointly sufficient for his minimal happiness.

Depending on one's platform of values these vital goals can be specified in a number of ways. In this sense we can get a family of concepts of health consistent with our basic theory. The theory itself cannot decide which concept is to be preferred.

The important question, then, is: can anybody make this primary evaluation of welfare? Can we live with a great number of characterizations of happiness and thus a great number of characterizations of health? Such an idea might seem disastrous to the science of medicine and the general enterprise of health care. We shall say more about this later but let us now just offer the following words of caution.

Evaluation is not a fortuitous affair. It should be made with the same care and rigour as the making of a scientific investigation. Moreover, once the basic evaluations of what constitutes a minimally happy life have been made, then this has strictly logical implications for the particular applications of the terms "health" and "illness" in individual cases. Once a speaker has made an evaluation, he cannot rationally change criteria from one application of "health" to another.

Secondly, evaluations do not simply appear from nowhere; they are formed in social settings. People within the same culture will tend to make the same basic evaluations concerning the good life from a welfare point of view. This will in most cases result in a great deal of intersubjectivity in judgment. There will automatically be some common ground for "consensus"-discussions about minimal and desirable degrees of welfare.

Thirdly, and as a continuation of the last statement, welfare evaluations can be made explicit, and as in political affairs, be decided upon. In fact, this is partly being done — although normally implicitly — in the social policies of different countries. By legislating on social and medical matters a government declares what it considers to be desirable and what minimal levels of welfare it would tolerate without intervention. This amounts to, among other things, specifying what it considers to be the border between health and illness. (From now on the term "illness" will be used consistently as the term contradictory of "health". This means that we follow the proposals of Pörn's in this respect....).

Fourthly, there is a secondary use of the terms "health" and "illness" which is *not* evaluative. This is when we ascribe health to somebody *against the background of a standard previously decided upon.* Perhaps this is what most of us do most of the time. We may presuppose some technical concept of health or we may base our statement on what we take to be society's judgment about the minimal limits of happiness. If we do the latter we are not the evaluators; we make theoretical applications of standards given by others who are the primary evaluators.

Considerations such as these will enable us to see that the enterprise of health care is not really in danger. In order to see that medicine can remain a science we shall have to make some further reflections based on an analysis of the concepts of disease and impairment and similar concepts, as will be undertaken below.

FURTHER READINGS

Boorse, C.
"Health as a Theoretical Concept," *Philosophy of Science* 44 (1977) 542–573.

Burns, Chester R.
"The Nonnaturals: A Paradox in the Western Concept of Health," *The Journal of Medicine and Philosophy* 1: 3 (1976) 202–211.

Desai, P.N.
Health and Medicine in the Hindu Tradition. (New York: Crossroad, 1989)

Goldwyn, R.M.
"Deformity and the Human Ideal of Medicine," *Journal of Clinical Ethics* 1:3 (1990) 235-236.

Goosens, W.
"Values in Health and Medicine," *Philosophy of Science* 47 (1980) 100–115.

Idler, Ellen
"Definition of Mental Health and Illness and Medical Sociology," *Society, Science and Medicine* 3A, 723–31.

Klerman, Gerald L.
"Mental Illness, the Medical Model, and Psychiatry," *The Journal of Medicine and Philosophy* 2: 3 (1977) 222–243.

Sedgewick, Peter
"What is Illness?" *The Hastings Center Studies* 1: 3 (1973)

CHAPTER 2 MACRO-ALLOCATION AND THE RIGHT TO HEALTH CARE

INTRODUCTION

When it comes to health care, the belief of most Canadians can be summed up in three words: *universality*, *equality* and *portability*. That is to say, most Canadians believe that *everyone* has a right to health care. Access to appropriate health care should not depend on the condition of the individual or on her or his ability to pay, but should be open to everyone on an equitable basis. This is sometimes also expressed by saying that most Canadians believe that health care should be a socially insured service.

Furthermore, most Canadians also believe that everyone has the right to the *same level* of service, no matter what province they are in.

Finally, most Canadians believe that even though the insurance for these services is a provincial matter, it should be *portable*, so that no matter in what province the individual happens to find her- or himself, the services will be paid for.

Canadians have not always felt this way. Until the 1930s, they agreed with the citizens of most other countries that health care is a commodity like all others, and that those who could not afford to pay for it did not have a right to it. However, the experiences of the depression of the 1930s fostered a gradual change in this perspective, and by the 1940s, the outlook had changed fundamentally. First in Saskatchewan and then in other provinces, the now-prevailing attitude became politically dominant. It led to the establishment of universal health and hospital insurance in Saskatchewan in 1945[1] and successively in other provinces. It was reflected in the Hall Report of 1964, the Lalonde Report of 1974, (excerpts from which are included in the readings that follow) and ultimately led to the Canada Health Act of 1984, which was proclaimed in 1985. Today, all Canadian provinces and territories have a universal health care system, where physicians and hospitals provide services according to province-wide schedules, and where only certain services have to be paid for by patients themselves.[2]

Furthermore, not all countries share the current Canadian perspective; and even those who accept the general principles do not all share the conviction to the same degree. For instance, although the UK accepts the general principle of social responsibility for health care, it also believes that society does not have an obligation to provide all medically possible, or even all medically indicated, services to all of its citizens. It therefore allows the growth of private clinics and private hospitals for those who are able to pay.

Closer to home, the US has traditionally maintained that health care is a service like all other services, and that it should therefore be available only to those who can pay for it. While in recent years the U.S. government has moved towards a more socially responsible perspective by establishing Medicare and Medicaid programs, the fact remains that there are over 35 million uninsured people in the U.S. who have either inadequate access to health care, or none at all.[3]

The excerpt from the Canada Health Act that opens this Chapter outlines the government's perspective on the right to health care. It might be interesting to compare the philosophy expressed in it with that of the US.

However, while Canadians believe that there is a socially guaranteed right to health care, this belief may be difficult to translate into practice. The health care resources that are available to Canadians are limited. This is not the fault of politicians, nor is the fact of limitation peculiar to Canada. The fact of limitation lies in the nature of human society. Any society, no matter what its nature, has only a finite number of people and disposes of only a finite amount of resources.

Therefore, no matter how technologically advanced the society may be, the amount of goods, services and other things it can produce is finite. This finite amount has to be divided among the various services the society has to provide to its members as a matter of social obligation. Health care is only one of these obligations. Education, transportation and defence are others. All of them have to be funded from the same limited resource pool. This means that, although it may be possible to assign different proportions of the overall resources to each social service, the total amount will still be finite.

The fact of limitation may not pose much of a problem when health services are relatively cheap and the demand for them is slight. However, as the services become more expensive, as the number of people who demand them increases, and as the number of requests for the services themselves go up, so does the relative drain on the health care resource pool. Sooner or later, no matter how they are drawn, the limits of that resource pool are reached, and society has to make a decision. Who shall have when not all can have? What shall be available when not everything can be made available? What is the extent of the right to health care, particularly when resources are scarce? And who should decide?

There are various factors that can exacerbate the problem. For instance, demographic factors such as an increase in the mean age of the population: elderly people tend to consume more health care resources than younger ones. Then there is the cost-factor associated with the increasing technological sophistication of medicine and of health care itself. Transplantation saves many lives, but at a tremendous cost in terms of capital and operating costs for transplant centres, treatment and follow-up costs for transplant patients, and so on. Medical diagnostic tools and procedures like computer assisted tomography (CAT-scans), magnetic resonance imaging (MRI), positron emission tomography (PET scans), amniocentesis, PKU testing, etc. have improved the abilities of physicians to detect diseases and conditions. However, in many cases the cost in terms of capital expenditure costs has been tremendous, and the hidden down-stream costs for the health care system have been even greater: People who previously died because their illnesses were detected too late are now being diagnosed early enough that they can undergo treatment.

All of this has to be paid for, and it demands a commitment of resources where previously none was required. While it may not cost much to perform a test on a specific occasion, when such tests become routine they add up to a considerable total. Or we could look at the development and increased use of surgical procedures, such as bypass operations. They also have developmental costs attached to them, and their availability has to be funded. This funding has to include not only the material costs and salaries for physicians, nurses, technicians and so on, but also the additional costs generated by the fact that people who are very ill have been given a renewed lease on life. Death is very cheap; diagnosis and treatment are expensive.

Health care policy-makers and administrators and health care providers have to be aware that no matter how beneficial a particular health care service may be, it has to be paid for. Many health care consumers do not appreciate this fact, because they tend to look at health care delivery only from the perspective of the specific individuals who benefit from the service. However, administrators must not lose sight of the overall cost implications, because their job is to optimize the use of the resources that are available. By definition, therefore, they have to take a global perspective. In other words, their job is to find an acceptable way of solving the problem of macro-allocation.

Macro-allocation, then, deals with the distribution of health care resources at the level of groups of people and types of health care services. Important questions here include the following: Is there some ethical mechanism for distinguishing between types of health care services that should be funded as a matter of general health care for everyone — for example, appendectomies, public health measures such as immunizations, etc.? Is there a limit on the extent of allocation for a given area? What criteria are appropriate here? Who should make these decisions?

Various answers have been proposed. Some have suggested that cost/benefit analysis[4] provides the answer, others have focused on cost/effectiveness coefficients,[5] on quality-of-life years gained (QALYs)[6] and so on. So far, no clear favourite has emerged. However, there is a tendency on the part of provincial governments, hospital districts and the like to assume that efficiency and effectiveness are the primary determinants of just and fair allocation. As several commentators have pointed out,[7] this is not necessarily true. What should take their place?

In their article, Freedman and Baylis point out that there are certain assumptions that underlie most of the discussions of resource allocation in the Canadian setting. Most notable of these is the assumption that payment in government-funded health insurance programs should be limited only to those procedures that are medically required or indicated. Freedman and Baylis argue that such an approach results in serious inequities and dislocated service delivery.

Kluge addresses some of the practical problems raised by the necessity of allocation at the policy level. In an excerpt taken from a general discussion about the differences between the Canadian and the US approaches to health care, he makes some suggestions as to how the general ethical principles of equity and justice could be translated into quantifiable terms that could be used in the actual allocation process at the political level. Of course, there are other positions. The bibliography of suggested readings lists some of the more influential writings.

NOTES

1. It was enacted in the Saskatchewan Hospitalization Act, 1946, which followed the Health Services Act of 1945. The program outlined in this legislation did not become fully operative until an agreement was reached with the College of Physicians and Surgeons of Saskatchewan, with the so-called Saskatoon Agreement of 1962. See also Mr. Justice Emmett Hall, *Report of the Royal Commission on Health Services* (Ottawa: Queen's Printer, 1964) for a discussion of the evolution of health services in Canada.
2. The idea of equitable access, which underlies the Canada Health Act, is currently under threat because of the Government Expenditures Restraint Act (1990, effecitve 1991). It effectively removes federal transfer payments, and especially established programme financing (EPF), of which health care is one of the most important. The effect of this Act is that it will become impossible for the poorer Canadian provinces to provide the same degree of health care services to their residents as the richer provinces.
3. President's Commission for the Study of Ethical Problems in Medicine and Biomedical and Behavioral Research, *Securing Access to Health Care: A Report on the Ethical Implications of Differences in the Availability of Health Services.* (US Govt. Printing Office: Washington DC, 1983) 3 vols.

4. Cost/benefit analysis assigns numerical coefficients to the costs for a given treatment modality and to the financial benefits to society of the outcomes, and then compares the different modalities relative to each other. For a good discussion, see Michael Drummond, "Guidelines for Health Technology Assessment: Economic Evaluation," in David Feeny, Gordon Guyatt and Peter Tugwell, eds., *Health Care Technology: Effectiveness, Efficiency and Public Policy.* (Montréal: Institute for Research on Public Policy, 1986)
5. Cost/effectiveness analysis compares numerical coefficients assigned to costs as opposed to the amounts of resources (money) saved for comparable forms of treatment. For several good discussions, see M.F. Drummond, *Principles of Economic Appraisal in Health Care*, (Oxford: Oxford Medical Publications, 1980); R. Sugden and A. Williams, *The Principles of Practical Cost-Benefit Analysis.* (Oxford: Oxford University Press, 1978); H.E. Klarman, J.O. Francis, G.D.
6. QUALYs or Quality Adjusted Life Years calculations assign numerical coefficients to quality-of-life evaluations and compare them to the cost involved in bringing about the extended life-span. See Feeny, ref. note 15, for several good discussions from an economic perspective.
7. Drummond, ref. note 5.

Canada Health Act

PROGRAM CRITERIA

Program criteria

7. In order that a province may qualify for a full cash contribution referred to in section 5 for a fiscal year, the health care insurance plan of the province must, throughout the fiscal year, satisfy the criteria described in sections 8 to 12 respecting the following matters:

(*a*) public administration;

(*b*) comprehensiveness;

(*c*) universality;

(*d*) portability; and

(*e*) accessibility. 1984, c. 6, s. 7.

Public administration

8. (1) In order to satisfy the criterion respecting public administration,

(*a*) the health care insurance plan of a province must be administered and operated on a non-profit basis by a public authority appointed or designated by the government of the province;

(*b*) the public authority must be responsible to the provincial government for that administration and operation; and

(*c*) the public authority must be subject to audit

of its accounts and financial transactions by such authority as is charged by law with the audit of the accounts of the province.

Designation of agency permitted

(2) The criterion respecting public administration is not contravened by reason only that the public authority referred to in subsection (1) has the power to designate any agency

(*a*) to receive on its behalf any amounts payable under the provincial health care insurance plan; or

(*b*) to carry out on its behalf any responsibility in connection with the receipt or payment of accounts rendered for insured health services, if it is a condition of the designation that all those accounts are subject to assessment and approval by the public authority and that the public authority shall determine the amounts to be paid in respect thereof. 1984, c. 6, s. 8.

Comprehensiveness

9. In order to satisfy the criterion respecting comprehensiveness, the health care insurance plan of a province must insure all insured health services provided by hospitals, medical practitioners or dentists, and where the law of the province so permits, similar or additional services rendered by other health care practitioners. 1984, c. 6, s. 9.

Universality

10. In order to satisfy the criterion respecting universality, the health care insurance plan of a province must entitle one hundred per cent of the insured persons of the province to the insured health services provided for by the plan on uniform terms and conditions. 1984, c. 6, s. 10.

Portability

11. (1) In order to satisfy the criterion respecting portability, the health care insurance plan of a province

(*a*) must not impose any minimum period of residence in the province, or waiting period, in excess of three months before residents of the province are eligible for or entitled to insured health services;

(*b*) must provide for and be administered and operated so as to provide for the payment of amounts for the cost of insured health services provided to insured persons while temporarily absent from the province on the basis that

(i) where the insured health services are provided in Canada, payment for health services is at the rate that is approved by the health care insurance plan of the province in which the services are provided, unless the provinces concerned agree to apportion the cost between them in a different manner, or

(ii) where the insured

health services are provided out of Canada, payment is made on the basis of the amount that would have been paid by the province for similar services rendered in the province, with due regard, in the case of hospital services, to the size of the hospital, standards of service and other relevant factors; and

(*c*) must provide for and be administered and operated so as to provide for the payment, during any minimum period of residence, or any waiting period, imposed by the health care insurance plan of another province, of the cost of insured health services provided to persons who have ceased to be insured persons by reason of having become residents of that other province, on the same basis as though they had not ceased to be residents of the province.

Requirement for consent for elective insured health services permitted

(2) The criterion respecting portability is not contravened by a requirement of a provincial health care insurance plan that the prior consent of the public authority that administers and operates the plan must be obtained for elective insured health services provided to a resident of the province while temporarily absent from the province if the services in question were available on a substantially similar basis in the province.

Definition of "elective insured health services"

(3) For the purpose of subsection (2), "elective insured health services" means insured health services other than services that are provided in an emergency or in any other circumstance in which medical care is required without delay. 1984, c. 6, s. 11.

Accessibility

12. (1) In order to satisfy the criterion respecting accessibility, the health care insurance plan of a province

(*a*) must provide for insured health services on uniform terms and conditions and on a basis that does not impede or preclude, either directly or indirectly whether by charges made to insured persons or otherwise, reasonable access to those services by insured persons;

(*b*) must provide for payment for insured health services in accordance with a tariff or system of payment authorized by the law of the province;

(*c*) must provide for reasonable compensation for all insured health services rendered by medical practitioners or dentists; and

(*d*) must provide for the payment of amounts to hospitals, including hospitals owned or operated by Canada, in respect of the cost of insured health services.

Reasonable compensation

(2) In respect of any province in which extra-billing is not permitted, paragraph (1)(*c*) shall be deemed

to be complied with if the province has chosen to enter into, and has entered into, an agreement with the medical practitioners and dentists of the province that provides

(a) for negotiations relating to compensation for insured health services between the province and provincial organizations that represent practising medical practitioners or dentists in the province;

(b) for the settlement of disputes relating to compensation through, at the option of the appropriate provincial organizations referred to in paragraph *(a),* conciliation or binding arbitration by a panel that is equally representative of the provincial organizations and the province and that has an independent chairman; and

(c) that a decision of a panel referred to in paragraph *(b)* may not be altered except by an Act of the legislature of the province. 1984, c. 6, s. 12.

CONDITIONS FOR CASH CONTRIBUTIONS OR PAYMENTS

Conditions

13. In order that a province may qualify for a full cash contribution referred to in section 5 or payment of the full amount referred to in section 6 for a fiscal year, the government of the province

(a) shall, at the times and in the manner prescribed by the regulations, provide the Minister with such information, of a type prescribed by the regulations, as the Minister may reasonably require for the purposes of this Act; and

(b) shall give recognition to the contributions and payments by Canada under this Act in any public documents, or in any advertising or promotional material, relating to insured health services and extended health care services in the province. 1984, c. 6, s. 13.

DEFAULTS

Referral to Governor in Council

Consultation process

14. (1) Subject to subsection (3), where the Minister, after consultation in accordance with subsection (2) with the minister responsible for health care in a province, is of the opinion that

(a) the health care insurance plan of the province does not or has ceased to satisfy any one of the criteria described in sections 8 to 12, or

(b) the province has failed to comply with any condition set out in section 13,

and the province has not given an undertaking satisfactory to the Minister to remedy the default within a period that the Minister considers reasonable, the Minister shall refer the matter to the Governor in Council.

(2) Before referring a matter

to the Governor in Council under subsection (1) in respect of a province, the Minister shall

(*a*) send by registered mail to the minister responsible for health care in the province a notice of concern with respect to any problem foreseen;

(*b*) seek any additional information available from the province with respect to the problem through bilateral discussions, and make a report to the province within ninety days after sending the notice of concern; and

(*c*) if requested by the province, meet within a reasonable period of time to discuss the report.

Where no consultation can be achieved

(3) The Minister may act without consultation under subsection (1) if the Minister is of the opinion that a sufficient time has expired after reasonable efforts to achieve consultation and that consultation will not be achieved. 1984, c. 6, s. 14.

Order reducing or withholding contribution

15. (1) Where, on the referral of a matter under section 14, the Governor in Council is of the opinion that the health care insurance plan of a province does not or has ceased to satisfy any one of the criteria described in sections 8 to 12 or that a province has failed to comply with any condition set out in section 13, the Governor in Council may, by order,

(*a*) direct that any cash contribution or amount payable to that province for a fiscal year be reduced, in respect of each default, by an amount that the Governor in Council considers to be appropriate, having regard to the gravity of the default; or

(*b*) where the Governor in Council considers it appropriate, direct that the whole of any cash contribution or amount payable to that province for a fiscal year be withheld.

Amending orders

(2) The Governor in Council may, by order, repeal or amend any order made under subsection (1) where the Governor in Council is of the opinion that the repeal or amendment is warranted in the circumstances.

Notice of order

(3) A copy of each order made under this section together with a statement of any findings on which the order was based shall be sent forthwith by registered mail to the government of the province concerned and the Minister shall cause the order and statement to be laid before each House of Parliament on any of the first fifteen days on which that House is sitting after the order is made.

Commencement of order

(4) An order made under subsection (1) shall not come into force earlier than thirty days after a copy of the order has been sent to the government of the province concerned under subsection (3). 1984, c. 6, s. 15.

Reimposition of reductions or withholdings

16. In the case of a continuing failure to satisfy any of the criteria described in sections 8 to 12 or to comply with any condition set out in section 13, any reduction or withholding under section 15 of a cash contribution or an amount payable to a province for a fiscal year shall be reimposed for each succeeding fiscal year as long as the Minister is satisfied, after consultation with the minister responsible for health care in the province, that the default is continuing. 1984, c. 6, s. 16.

When reduction or withholding imposed

17. Any reduction or withholding under section 15 or 16 of a cash contribution or payment may be imposed in the fiscal year in which the default that gave rise to the reduction or withholding occurred or in the following fiscal year. 1984, c. 6, s. 17.

EXTRA-BILLING AND USER CHARGES

Extra-billing

18. In order that a province may qualify for a full cash contribution referred to in section 5 for a fiscal year, no payments may be permitted by the province for that fiscal year under the health care insurance plan of the province in respect of insured health services that have been subject to extra-billing by medical practitioners or dentists. 1984, c. 6, s. 18.

User charges

19.(1) In order that a province may qualify for a full cash contribution referred to in section 5 for a fiscal year, user charges must not be permitted by the province for that fiscal year under the health care insurance plan of the province.

Limitation

(2) Subsection (1) does not apply in respect of user charges for accommodation or meals provided to an in-patient who, in the opinion of the attending physician, requires chronic care and is more or less permanently resident in a hospital or other institution. 1984, c. 6, s. 19.

Deduction for extra-billing

20.(1) Where a province fails to comply with the condition set out in section 18, there shall be deducted from the cash contribution to the province for a fiscal year an amount that the Minister, on the basis of information provided in accordance with the regulations, determines to have been charged through extra-billing by medical practitioners or dentists in the province in that fiscal year or, where information is not provided in accordance with the regulations, an amount that the Minister estimates to have been so charged.

Deduction for user charges

(2) Where a province fails to comply with the condition set out in section 19, there shall be deducted from the cash contribution to the province for a fiscal year an

amount that the Minister, on the basis of information provided in accordance with the regulations, determines to have been charged in the province in respect of user charges to which section 19 applies in that fiscal year or, where information is not provided in accordance with the regulations, an amount that the Minister estimates to have been so charged.

Consultation with province

(3) The Minister shall not estimate an amount under subsection (1) or (2) without first undertaking to consult the minister responsible for health care in the province concerned.

Separate accounting in Public Accounts

(4) Any amount deducted under subsection (1) or (2) from a cash contribution in any of the three consecutive fiscal years the first of which commences on April 1, 1984 shall be accounted for separately in respect of each province in the Public Accounts for each of those fiscal years in and after which the amount is deducted.

Refund to province

(5) Where, in any of the three fiscal years referred to in subsection 4), extra-billing or user charges have, in the opinion of the Minister, been eliminated in a province, the total amount deducted in respect of extra-billing or user charges, as the case may be, shall be paid to the province.

Saving

(6) Nothing in this section restricts the power of the Governor in Council to make any order under section 15. 1984, c. 6, s. 20.

Purpose and Function in Government Funded Health Coverage

Benjamin Freedman and Françoise Baylis

ABSTRACT

Government-funded health insurance programs that claim to provide comprehensive funding of their clients' demands have commonly adopted a purposive (deductive) approach to the problem of health care funding. This involves determining the extent of covered benefits by seeking an "adequate" definition of health or health care. Payment is then limited to only those procedures medically required or indicated. In this paper we argue that the purposive approach is inadequate, and that attempted adherence to it results in a curious dislocation of service, serious inequities, and an

Benjamin Freedman and Françoise Baylis, "Purpose and Function In Government-funded Health Coverage." *Journal of Health Policy, Politics and Law* 1987 (Spring) 12:1; 97-112 *unhealthy contemplation of the definition of health. These problems are the result of structural deficiencies in the approach, and so will not be rectified by tinkering with the definitions adopted. As an alternative, we present an outline of a functional (inductive) approach, which seeks to identify which of the expectations of its clients the government health insurance system may realistically satisfy.*

Government-funded health insurance schemes are under increasing pressure to reconcile finite medical resources with seemingly infinite demands for medical services. Consequently, problems regarding the macroallocation of available resources must constantly be readdressed. The substantive macroallocational questions are familiar: What proportions of health care funding should be directed toward acute, chronic, or preventive care, or toward research in these respective areas? What, if any, provision should be made for the funding of novel therapies? When more than one approach to a disorder is available (e.g., medical or surgical treatment of angina pectoris), should the insurance program reward the use of the cheapest option (one assumption underlying the DRG system; see Wasserman 1983), the option which the physician believes is clinically preferable, or that which the patient prefers, perhaps on grounds of compatibility with lifestyle?

Questions such as these underline the need for a demarcation principle which government-funded health insurance programs could use to determine what should and should not be funded. The usefulness of such a principle is obvious, particularly from the government's perspective, when one considers how quickly new approaches to health care are adopted by health care providers (creating a demand for insurance reimbursement on their behalf). Current examples would include transportation, advanced diagnostic and imaging equipment, and expensive techniques for the treatment of infertility (most notoriously, *in vitro* fertilization). A demarcation principle would serve to limit the constantly expanding claims for health insurance coverage which feed upon (and, when successful, fuel) the unrealistic expectation that the government-funded health care system can guarantee everyone a long, happy, and productive life.

At present, the approach to funding adopted by government health care programs is eclectic. Aside from strictly medical concerns, attention is given to factors deriving from economics, politics, and public policy. Even within the mélange of compromise that constitutes health insurance, however, we may discern a basic theme of demarcation: absent special considerations, a purposive (deductive) approach is commonly used in deciding whether a specific service should be a covered benefit. The results of this theme may be reconstructed in almost syllogistic terms: the insurance scheme should fund that which yields, or leads to, health (major premise); the proposed service does (or does not) yield or lead to health (minor premise); therefore the proposed service should (should not) be reimbursed. Presented in this way, the deductive approach is, of course, an artificial reconstruction of a more complicated reality. In the cases that we will be presenting, however, it plausibly captures an important theme in insurance decision making as that is publicly presented.

The Preamble to the Ontario Health Insurance Plan's *Schedule of Benefits* (1983), for example, states at the outset that "Insured medical services are limited to the services which are medically necessary ..." (p. 1). This we understand to mean that only those services designed to restore health ("medically necessary") are to be funded. The purposive concept of medical necessity is therefore ostensibly an *exclusive* criterion of demarcation — that is, a necessary but not sufficient condition for coverage. However, medical necessity also serves as an *inclusive* criterion of demarcation. The fitting of contact lenses, for example, is not a covered benefit unless it is being done to correct aphakia, myopia greater than nine diopters, irregular astigmatism, or keratoconus (p. 20). Similarly, other services commonly sought for reasons of vanity or convenience are not covered benefits unless they are called for by some substantial degree of medical necessity. A case in point is cosmetic surgery, which is not an insured benefit "except where medically required" (p. 19).

The deductive model, idealized as it is, is a plausible — sometimes, the *only* plausible — reconstruction of a number of specific decisions on insurance coverage. Although it is initially appealing, we shall argue that this form of reasoning results in some obvious inequities and distortions in government coverage practice. An alternative approach, which may be termed functional or inductive, will be suggested. The functional approach would have us resolve the problem of demarcation by asking whether the specific service in question represents a demand which the health care system may efficiently satisfy. The question of whether the funded service supplies "health" or "health care" is thereby intentionally finessed.

The examples we shall be using are drawn largely from Canadian (and predominantly Ontarian) experiences. They are intended to serve for purposes of illustration alone. If successful, they point to problems and approaches generally prevalent among any government-funded insurance scheme which claims to comprehensively fund the health demands of the serviced population.

THE PURPOSIVE APPROACH

In ordinary language, "purpose" broadly refers to the end one has in view in acting in a certain way (i.e., "purposively"). The use of the term implies the conscious choice of both a goal and an action designed to achieve the stated goal. By extension, we may think of objects as purposively designed. For example, a television receiver is built with the end of it serving as a decoder of electronic impulses. In designing it, a certain size and shape are chosen on the grounds of fitness toward that end (Turkel 1984); any components which prove unreliable in achieving that end are either discarded or redesigned. Social institutions, such as traffic regulation, can also be construed as purposive. A panoply of elements (road markings, rules, etc.) are chosen subordinate to the primary goal of the swift and accident-free motion of traffic.

Similarly, some view medical practice as a purposive enterprise. It is usual to distinguish medical from nonmedical interventions — to demarcate medical practice — by referring to current beliefs concerning what promotes or conserves health; in theory new forms of medical treatment are accepted into practice and old ones discarded primarily on the basis of their fitness to serve the purpose of health. It is on this basis alone that physicians, in the course of their daily practice, "may, unquestioned and with impunity, slice, puncture, bind, grind, inject, and extract various organic and inorganic substances into and from" their patients (Freedman 1984, 5).

As health is the organizing principle and rule of demarcation for medical practice, it is natural to assume that this concept should apply as well to that system which funds medical practice. That is, it seems natural to assume that problems of demarcation in health care funding cannot be decided unless prior agreement has been arrived at concerning the definition of health, so that the nature of "medically necessary" services may be ascertained. By extension, a government-funded health insurance program may be purposively understood as an institution designed to secure health, although it is constrained by economic and political factors.

If the purpose of the government-funded insurance system is to promote health, and if that purpose is to serve as its rule of demarcation, a definition of health must be presented. However, the definition of health and related concepts (such as illness and disease) has resisted numerous scholarly efforts. Those definitions which have gained favorable attention have succeeded by stipulating a definition which could then be explicated or operationalized (Boorse 1975). But this approach will not serve the purposes of a government-funded health insurance scheme, since these purposes require a definition or an understanding of health with a basis in social consensus and usage.

The most widely known and most frequently criticized definition of health is found in the Preamble to the Constitution of the World Health Organization: "Health is a state of complete physical, mental and social well-being and not merely the absence of disease or infirmity" (WHO 1976). Daniel Callahan, a relatively sympathetic commentator on the WHO definition, notes nonetheless that this definition fosters "the cultural tendency to define all social problems, from war to crime on the streets, as 'health' problems" (Callahan 1973, 78). It "makes the medical profession the gate-keeper for happiness and social well-being ... the final magic-healer of human misery" (p. 81).

These eloquent criticisms relate to the one point that makes the WHO definition of health inadequate for the purposes of our discussion: it provides a government-funded health insurance scheme with no rule of demarcation whatsoever. Because of the wide currency the WHO definition enjoys, this criticism has been voiced in the world of practice as well as in the dusty pages of journals. For example, in Canada abortions are not illegal, provided that (among other conditions) they have been approved by a committee of physicians that finds the abortion necessary to preserve the life or health of the applicant.[1] Some abortion committees have adopted the WHO understanding as their working definition of health. According to many critics, this indicates that the committees have abandoned the effort at demarcating therapeutic abortions from those sought for nontherapeutic reasons.

Mindful of the need for demarcation, Callahan offered the following definition of health as a counterproposal: "Health is a state of physical well-being," a state which need not be "complete" but must be "at least adequate, i.e., without significant impairment of function" (Callahan 1973, 87). With this narrow definition of health, mental illness would qualify as "ill health," if at all, only if it substantially interfered with functioning.

Would Callahan's definition, or one equally narrow, represent a satisfactory rule of demarcation for government-funded health insurance schemes? It is important to examine this question at some length, because the narrowness of the definition as well as its common-sense roots make it attractive to economically pressed governments. Therefore, even if Callahan would not use his definition of health as a rule of demarcation, governments faced with competing priorities might be tempted to do so.

In judging the adequacy of any proposed rule of demarcation, two different kinds of questions may be asked. First, *could* the rule serve (i.e., would it clearly distinguish between those services to be included and those to be excluded from the funding system)? Second, *should* the rule serve (i.e., if applied, would it yield satisfactory results)? The first question concerns the formal adequacy of the rule; the second, its substantive adequacy.

The notions of "well-being" and of "impairment of function" are two crucial elements of Callahan's definition which are unavoidably ambiguous; these ambiguities speak to the issue of formal adequacy. To revert to the example introduced earlier, consider a patient suffering from exercise-onset angina pectoris. Two types of treatment are available. One option is medical management, which requires of the patient a commitment to control of diet, a modification of activity, and the tolerance of some degree of continued pain. The alternative is surgical intervention, which avoids the above problems at the expense of discrete surgical risk and substantial surgical and hospitalization costs. An appeal to "well-being" and "functioning" fails to indicate which of these forms of treatment should appropriately be funded. The problem is further complicated when one considers that the judgments of the patient and of the physician may differ; and, whereas people tend to think of "health" or "therapy" as technical concepts whose application is in the hands of professionals, they tend to define other concepts like "well-being" and "functioning" for themselves. The formal adequacy of Callahan's definition is therefore in question.

What about the substantive adequacy of the definition as a demarcation rule? This may seem to beg the question. We need a demarcation rule because we don't know what should and what should not be funded; therefore, how can we question such a rule by saying that it includes or excludes the wrong items? But this point presumes a false dichotomy, as often occurs when applying deductive approaches to social questions. We may (we almost certainly do) have some idea of the results desired from a rule of demarcation. We likely wish to develop a demarcation rule to sharpen an initially hazy understanding, rather than to fill a total vacuum.

Substantively, a rule may be faulty because it is either overinclusive, underinclusive, or both. Callahan's definition of health, if used as a demarcation rule, would be both. It would be overinclusive because it fails to account for the quantity of resources expended in marginal improvements in well-being or functioning. It does not tell us when the game is no longer worth the candle; and, as was noted at the outset, it is because medicine continues to yield improvements in these parameters, albeit at ever-increasing expense, that the problem we are discussing arises.

Callahan's definition would be underinclusive as well, because if it were applied rigorously benign and worthwhile services would be excluded from coverage. In his concern to combat the view that medicine should be held responsible to deliver perfect happiness, Callahan eliminates any role medicine might legitimately satisfy in this direction. Sometimes medical expertise is necessary to provide a modicum of happiness; if the costs thereby incurred are trivial enough, and the benefits (even in mere happiness) great enough, why should the required service not be funded?

Consider the following. The removal of tattoos is not usually necessary to restore function; nor, strictly speaking, is it a necessary component of well-being. Yet, the safe eradication of tattoos may require medical expertise. In Ontario, in most cases the provincial health insurance scheme does not cover the cost of tattoo removal. However, an exception is made for the eradication of prisoner-of-war or concentration camp tattoos. In some isolated instances well-being or functioning might require the removal of such tattoos, and to these cases Callahan's principle would extend. But in the usual case physical well-being and functioning are not impaired by these offensive tattoos. Is it wrong to fund this service simply out of consideration for the victims' feelings, in a situation where practical concern for these feelings requires medical expertise?

Evidently a definition of health from either end of the continuum — the relatively inclusive WHO definition, and the rather exclusive definition proposed by Callahan — will not serve as a satisfactory demarcation principle. However, quite apart from the specific problems arising from any particular definition of health, a further obstacle confronts the definitional approach to health care funding in that no definition of health has garnered general agreement. This lack of consensus is no mere accident. While on the surface the debate concerning the definition of health is technical in nature, it is clear in the writings of Szasz (1961), Kass (1975), and others that this debate serves an ideological role as well. Often the definitions advocated reflect broad views concerning such disparate issues as technocracy, nature versus nurture, and the allowable limits of eccentricity in liberal societies. Unhappily, therefore, it may be the case that consensus regarding the definition of health will have to wait for prior consensus on political and social ideology.

Also, the economic facts of health care may be another source of dissent regarding the definition of health and disease. Consider a study by Campbell, Scadding, and Roberts (1979), in which subjects were presented with a number of conditions and asked whether these represented "disease." The conditions ranged from malaria and tuberculosis to drowning and starvation. Physicians, and especially general practitioners, were more likely to characterize a condition as "disease" than were lay respondents. The authors suggest that the operational equivalents of "disease" are different in the two groups. For the layman, "disease" means "Do I need a doctor?" For the physician, it means "Is it useful for me to use this label?" An alternative suggestion compatible with the observed differences is that physicians, especially family practitioners, have a vested economic interest in broadening the scope of the term "disease."

We have been arguing that reliance upon the definition of health for the purposive elucidation of a government-funded insurance program is unlikely to result in a consensual, usable, and fair system. To this one might object that the preceding argument has erred in identifying the purpose of a government-funded health insurance system as the provision of "health." A health insurance system cannot provide *health*, but at best can only provide *health care.*

This amended purposive description is not, however, immune from the criticisms noted above. The objection purports to take a realistic look at what the government-funded insurance system actually does: it funds "health care." This is presumed to be a less ambiguous concept than "health." However, the definition of health care itself is crucially dependent upon prior agreement on the definition of health, so the objection only succeeds in pushing the problems we have noted one step back.

Others will object that the health care system provides neither "health" nor "health care" but "medical care" *tout court.* This, however, is no more serious an objection, for although the term "medical care" is perhaps even less ambiguous than the term "health care," the problem remains in that "medical care" is commonly understood to require that a physician's expertise be applied on behalf of restoring or preserving the health of patients. Furthermore, if we were to be fully realistic, we would have to admit that government-funded health insurance systems do not fund medical care or health care any more than they fund health. Rather, they fund health care providers, as public monies are made available precisely to pay for medical services rendered.

STRUCTURAL DEFICIENCIES OF THE PURPOSIVE APPROACH

As noted above, the two definitions of health drawn from either end of the continuum fail to adequately demarcate insurable services. It does not necessarily follow from this, however, that a definition in between these extremes would not serve.

Allowing for the remote possibility that a consensual definition of health were to be adopted, some important structural problems would remain to confront any purposive system of government-funded health insurance. These problems derive from the approach's top-down, deductive fashion of reasoning, and therefore would not be solved by any improvement in the formulation of the premises. In particular, they would persist despite changes in the definition of health or health care.

An inherent problem with the purposive-deductive approach is its rationalization of the issue of demarcation. In principle, once the premises have been adopted, all of the solutions are present; as logicians say, deductive reasoning produces no new knowledge not already embedded in the premises. Two difficulties follow from this. The purposive approach does not in principle allow for an incremental solution to the issues, within which some procedures might be funded on a trial basis while other relevantly similar procedures await the lessons of experience. Furthermore, this rationalized approach does not permit any wisdom of quantification, a problem noted earlier in reference to Callahan. It does not allow us by its premises to say that some procedure does not fall on the "fundable" side of the demarcation line, but that it is still worthy of funding (e.g., tattoo removal), or alternatively that some procedure might fall on the "fundable" side of the demarcation line, but that it is nonetheless too expensive a proposition to fund (e.g., heart transplants).

A further problem is who decides whether some service is fundable under the definition consensually adopted. He almost certainly will be some professional: possibly the individual health care provider, but more likely some government official. Thus, control of the health insurance system passes into the hands of the technocracy, and the patient is lost in the shuffle, as is indeed lay input in general (which currently may be provided through political representation and control). How is the technocracy to resolve these problems? In the deductive mode of reasoning, issues of application are reduced to a search for semantic clarity and consensus. Practical issues of whether it is useful, fair, or right to cover a given treatment for a given condition are converted into an obsessive contemplation of the definition of health.

PROBLEMS OF THE PURPOSIVE APPROACH IN PRACTICE

The purposive-deductive approach is necessarily obsessed with determining whether a condition is "really" an illness. Two representative cases illustrate this point, though many other examples could be cited if space permitted. Jane Smith (a real case, though not her real name) approached an endocrinologist with a presenting complaint of excessive growth of facial and body hair. After an extensive workup (covered, incidentally, by the provincial health plan) in which no endocrinological disorder was established, she was diagnosed as suffering from "essential hirsutism." Mrs. Smith then requested of the physician a referral to an electrolysist, in the belief that the health care plan would then cover the cost of treatment. This request was refused. She was told that if the condition was causing her acute discomfort or embarrassment, she could be referred to a psychiatrist, who could then make the referral for hair removal. The kinds of questions the psychiatrist would be likely to ask could equally well have been asked by the endocrinologist. However, he felt constrained by the purposive nature of the system to validate the electrolytic referral by means of special expertise (into mental illness) which he did not feel he possessed. Thus, inappropriate gate-keeping mechanisms which are both costly and inefficient were introduced. This case illustrates one way in which the technocratic and logomachistic tendencies of the purposive approach reinforce one another.

To further illustrate this point, consider the treatment of infertility, which might include hormonal therapy or surgery as well as counseling. These therapies ordinarily are thought to fall within the boundaries of medical care. But the purposive approach must question whether infertility itself is really a "disease." If we look to an American example, Great Southern Life of Houston, a private insurance company, is reported as having denied coverage for *in vitro* fertilization on the grounds that it is "not a treatment of an illness" *(Surrogate Parenting News* 1983*)*. Presumably a government-funded health care system similarly concerned with purposive considerations might apply the same reasoning.

Another distinction covertly used is that of the internal versus the external. There is a vague feeling that health care is a concept that relates to the individual rather than to the environment, and that fundable, fee-for-service health care interventions may be demarcated in part as those which represent internal adjustments to the human organism rather than modifications of the organism's environment. When a malnourished patient is nursed back to health through intravenous infusions, that is health care; when he or she is given money or remunerative employment supplying the wherewithal for self-nourishment, that is not health care.

The distinction makes less sense in other contexts. What of a patient suffering from a definable illness whose comprehensive treatment would include environmental modification? A major and growing current example are those patients suffering from pan-allergic syndromes. It is sometimes claimed that the alleviation of the symptoms from this disorder requires a total readjustment of the patient's living arrangements, such as moving into a cabin tiled with ceramics and discarding a wardrobe laced with allergens. Although this is asserted to be the treatment of choice, it is "external" and therefore not a covered benefit under the government health insurance scheme. Similarly, prosthetics that are implanted, like heart pacemakers, are covered benefits under Ontario's health insurance scheme, whereas externally attached prosthetics, like limbs, generally are not paid for by the Ontario Health Insurance Plan (OHIP).

THE FUNCTIONAL APPROACH: AN ALTERNATIVE

Most social institutions are established with a purpose in view. When a government-funded health insurance program is initiated, the purpose is vaguely understood to contribute to the provision of health or health care. This original purpose is in fact critical to the establishment of a government health insurance program, which is often given higher priority than comparable welfare schemes dealing in less critical services and commodities. But once an insurance scheme is in place, it would be foolish to freeze the system in its embryonic state. With the continuing development of a health insurance plan, as it confronts issues of macroallocation and demarcation, there is no need to restrict it to the a priori wisdom that went into its establishment. On these grounds we advocate a functional approach to government health care funding.

In accordance with common usage, we define a "function" as any output of a system which is positively evaluated, whether that output was intentional or not.[2] Purposes are therefore a subset of functions, the latter including happy surprises in addition to anticipated outcomes. To revert to our earlier example, the purpose of a television set is to decode electronic signals. In most homes, however, it will also service a variety of additional functions: conversation piece, plant stand, and so on.

What would be distinctive about a functional approach to a government-funded health insurance plan? Three main differences stand between a purposive and a functional approach. These differences have to do with the characterization of those conditions which the government health insurance program should ameliorate, the demarcation of reimbursable from nonreimbursable services, and the relationship between the health plan and other government services.

With the purposive approach to the question of health care funding, funding decisions turn on whether a condition represents ill health, a disease, an illness. With a functional approach, in contrast, questions outside the realm of health are also considered. For example, has the condition resulted in impaired occupational performance? (In the infamous words of an anonymous Polish public health official, "Tuberculosis slows production.") Does the person afflicted with the condition experience disturbed functioning in other areas as a result? Is he severely distressed or depressed as a result of the condition? Is he experiencing pain? These types of considerations do sometimes appear in the purposive conception, but in a distorted, Procrustean way, as questions concerning "mental health" or "adjustment."

To illustrate this point, consider how the different approaches would deal with a difficult case of demarcation like sex-reassignment surgery. The purposive approach would need to discover whether the surgery represented the treatment of a genuine disease. In this context, the neologism "gender dysphoria" has been introduced, and psychiatrists continue to battle over its propriety and etiology. With a functional approach the questions considered in reaching a funding decision on a macro level (by bureaucrats) and in implementing the decision at the micro level (by physicians) are more straightforward. How seriously has the applicant's life been affected? How likely is it that he/she will improve with the treatment? Is the cost justified by these benefits? Admittedly, similar questions might be asked by psychiatrists in the gender dysphoria debate. We suggest, however, that such questions are both clearer and more realistic when not filtered through the prism of a definition of disease.

The second contrast between the purposive and the functional approach is evident when deciding about the funding of discrete services. Whereas with the purposive approach one asks whether some service represents health care, with the functional approach one would ask if the service or procedure is good, worthwhile, and desired.

Consider fertility interventions. For the vast majority of women, tubal ligation per se has almost no discrete medical justification (although it certainly will "cure" the "disorder" of fecundity). On these grounds, Kass (1975) has suggested that tubal ligation or vasectomy not be included within the medical orbit. But clearly, tubal ligation is a much-desired intervention; it has recently become the most popular form of female contraception in Canada. And clearly, medical expertise is necessary to provide ligations. Also, from the economic point of view of the insurance plan, sterilization is one of the most efficient interventions available, obviating both medical costs or parturition and costs of care of the (forever-to-remain) unborn. Whereas the purposive conception forces government health care officials to conceptualize health matters in futile and disingenuous ways, the functional conception allows one to examine the real underlying concerns. Does a requested procedure — for example, tubal ligation — represent a treatment whose cost is rationally proportionate to the need it serves?

When the issue is phrased in this way, we are required to confront questions which are never raised by the purposive approach. For example: Does the procedure in question address a human want or need, or perhaps something people *ought* to want or need? As difficult as these questions are, they seem to us to be the right ones to address. Among their advantages is the fact that their solution demands of us that we understand and respect the patient's perceptions of health care.

A recent study (Freedman 1983) yielded some suggestive data on this very point. The study included interviews of Canadian women applying for microsurgical attempts at reversing a prior ligation (tubal reanatomosis). During the interviews, the women were asked "Do you see the reversal of the sterilization as a health procedure (like an appendectomy) or as a social procedure requiring medical assistance (like cosmetic surgery)?" Most of these women, both in questionnaires and during the subsequent interviews, classified the procedure they requested as medical, but the interview responses of some of the women revealed ambivalence stemming from a variety of considerations. The following representative statements are worthy of careful consideration as they encapsulate a lay response to the issue of demarcation: "I think for my mental and emotional well-being it is necessary. It is not like cosmetic surgery, like something I could do. It is something that is inside of me. I never thought I'd feel as strongly about [it]." "No [it's not a social procedure] ... I don't feel that having a tubal done is the same thing as having a reversal done. I'm having it [the reversal] done so that we can have children ... So I really don't see it as being something that you do just to fit in. It's hard to explain but that's the way I feel about it."

How did these laypeople go about resolving this critical question of demarcation? What themes emerge from their responses? Hints are found of a variety of approaches, including the "internal/external" approach. However, their major point of consensus was the belief that because the procedure was so important to them personally, and because a doctor was needed to perform it, the procedure *must* be medical.

The population from which these responses were drawn would be expected to provide tendentious replies. It is in these women's interest to argue that the procedure they are requesting is medical in nature, and hence reimbursable. However, this fact only sharpens the point, because we would expect that they would be choosing the most persuasive demarcation principle available to support their claim.

The third divergence between the two approaches concerns the relationship between the health care system (and its public funding agent) and other elements of society. The purposive approach makes of the health care system a hermetically sealed enterprise, self-directed in terms of its original purpose and resistant to other legitimate social concerns and institutionalized values. On the other hand, with the functional approach, other social interests and resources are taken into account in deciding whether to supply a particular benefit when its request is justified in terms of health.

A functionalist perspective also allows one to consider whether the health care system is the best institution to respond to demands for particular needs. Needs (or wants) and the associated goods and services that have traditionally been seen as medical in nature may be better served by some other social institution. Alcoholism, obesity, and other diseases of lifestyle are notoriously resistant to treatment by the medical model. For the purposive approach, however, provided that these conditions are diseases and that a physician is prepared to "treat" them, such treatments would be insured. The fact that other social institutions could better deal with these conditions is irrelevant from a purposive perspective. With a functional approach one questions whether we might not be better served by "divestiture" of these conditions from medicine, at least at this point in time. Conversely, the health care system may be better suited to providing some needs which traditionally have been served outside the medical model. One such possibility might be the care of the families of dying patients by physicians, nurses, or medical social workers, a role traditionally relegated to pastors and family support systems. The funding of such a service should not wait upon the discovery of a new "disease" ("impending grief syndrome"), but should proceed immediately upon the recognition that these forms of care are valid, useful, and best accomplished within the institutions of the health care system.

QUESTIONS FOR THE FUNCTIONAL APPROACH

It might seem that the functional approach is necessarily heir to all of the criticisms presented above concerning the WHO definition of health. Under a functional approach, as under the WHO definition, the full range of human suffering and discontent become potential targets of a government-supported health care system. In fact, some might even argue that the functional approach is even more latitudinous than WHO, although it is hard to imagine what has been left out once "a complete state of physical, mental and social well-being" has been included.

This criticism, however, dissolves in the face of a critical distinction. The problem with the WHO definition, which is that it fails to exclude anything from coverage, arises in the context of a purposive system. In contrast, with a functional approach to health care funding, demarcation does not *end* with the recognition of a need or demand for services, but rather only *begins* at this point. It must then be determined whether the health care system, with its particular expertise and modalities of intervention, may redress that need efficiently; whether another social program or practice would better serve; or whether the need is so difficult to satisfy or so at odds with other values that it should not be served at all.

The whole point of the functional approach is the recognition that decisions regarding coverage involve more than semantics. In a purposive approach, once we know that a procedure serves health, we have an argument (which, to be sure, might need to be tempered by political or economic realities) that it should be funded. In a functional approach, when we know that a procedure satisfies a demand, we simply know that it is *potentially* fundable — not that it should be funded, let alone that it should be funded by the health care system.

A further point worth noting is that since functionalism contains no single decision rule for demarcation, it must address new problems which do not trouble a purposive system. However, the fact that a theory raises new questions does not necessarily count as a strike against it, provided that the questions are ones which are worth confronting. In fact, a theory might be deficient precisely because it fails to raise questions which should be answered, as at times the purposive approach slurs over the complications faced by the functional approach. In general the new problems which the functional approach must address are actually complications which arise due to the fact that patient choice is allowed, and that services traditionally considered nonmedical may be included within the boundaries of health care; therefore, a greater range of alternatives must be considered. For example, a possible negative consequence of allowing patient choice is that the costs involved might be greater. This criticism, however, also applies to the purposive approach, as the following examples will serve to illustrate.

Under the Ontario Health Insurance Plan postmastectomy breast reconstruction surgery is a covered service. This type of procedure fits comfortably within the naïve notion of health services, since it involves a direct "internal" procedure on a patient's behalf. On the other hand, prosthetic devices, being "external," have not been a covered benefit for adults and have represented a repeated source of political contention. A system which proceeds under the strong purposive principle of demarcation does not recognize the need to fund environmental adjustments, since these would fall under the rubric of social welfare rather than health care. Ontario, therefore, has long refused to cover the costs of breast prostheses and surgical brassieres for victims of breast cancer, while still funding surgical breast reconstruction for those interested in pursuing that course.

A complicated situation arose in Ontario when a woman eligible for a breast reconstruction procedure offered to exchange this service for a Tucker valve set (a prosthetic device needed for "normal" speech after she had undergone a tracheotomy). The trade would have been cost-effective for the Ministry of Health, and might have saved $1000 or more. The insurance plan declined the offer as there was no apt bureaucratic means of accepting it, given that the health insurance plan funds "services" and not "goods" *(London Free Press 1982)*.

Another Ontario woman suffering from a lung condition lived at home, using a mobile oxygen cart. Eventually her monthly oxygen bills — which the public health insurance program would not cover — rose to over $700. At this point, entering the hospital became, for her, the only practical economic move, because then the insurance plan would supply her with oxygen gratis. The average cost of inpatient hospital care was estimated at approximately ten times the cost of the oxygen alone *(London Free Press 1984)*. This situation similarly indicates the unreasoning prejudice a purposive system may have against environmental adjustment.

A functional approach would deal with such situations differently since patient choice would be independently relevant (if not necessarily decisive) in determining fundability. The implications of this are obviously quite serious, particularly as patients persist in expressing individual preferences on this issue, a fact which must be taken seriously by a system concerned with lay input. Honoring the choice of patients will at times be far more expensive than acceding to the choice dictated by a purposive demarcation rule. Patient autonomy in relation to funding decisions has not been an issue; but, without presuming any particular resolution, we suggest that it should be.

A functional conception would need to reexamine funding of the diverse forms of health care practice. In Ontario's quasi-purposive system, all reimbursements flow directly to, or indirectly from, physicians. Doctors may perform a service directly, or engage another professional (e.g., psychologist, physiotherapist) on a salaried basis to work under their direction, with the physician billing the government insurance program. Since physicians are certified specialists in "health," this arrangement is acceptable (although certainly not inevitable) under a purposive system. Similarly, although a physician may bill for consultation with a patient, parent, or other physician, he or she may not bill for consultation with nonphysician providers of health care. If a child is experiencing behavioral problems in school which have concerned the school psychologist, the physician may charge the government insurance plan for consultation with the parents, who may serve as middlemen between the school psychologist and the physician; but if the physician wishes to discuss the matter with the psychologist directly, he must do so on his own account. A functional system would necessarily call such arrangements into question.

As a result, in implementing a functional approach, a comprehensive government health plan would face bureaucratic dislocation. How serious would this be? To this, three points can be made: some dislocation has already occurred; some dislocation is good; and remaining dislocations need not all be faced at once.

Some dislocation has already occurred. In Ontario, a system of psychiatric hospitals is run by the Ministry of Health. A system of facilities for the developmentally disabled is run by the Ministry of Community and Social Services (COMSOC). This kind of division would be preserved if a consistently functional approach were adopted. The facilities for the developmentally handicapped require a high level of expertise in development and programming, but the specific forms required — training of various sorts, behavioral techniques, and custodial care — are not specifically medical or nursing in nature (although both of these disciplines perform an important ancillary function). Indeed, because developmental handicap constitutes an "illness" under almost any definition, the division that currently exists between psychiatric and COMSOC facilities is inexplicable under a purposive conception.

Some dislocation is good. Many of the decisions noted above (e.g., concerning prostheses and oxygen) would be inappropriate given a functionalist perspective. Their reversal involves dislocation in itself; but in the cases noted, that seems to be all to the good. Also, some bureaucratic awkwardness, intrinsic to a purposive system, would be resolved under a functional approach. While a physician may recover from the Ontario Health Insurance Plan on behalf of the examination of a patient carried out for investigation, confirmation, or documentation of an alleged sexual assault, a portion of its outlays on this behalf are then recovered from the Ministries of the Attorney General and the Solicitor General. Similar cumbersome paper shuffling may be involved in other instances which require medical expertise, albeit outside of medical treatment (e.g., in assessments for insurance or for the purpose of establishing workmen's compensation). It would seem that the only reason the money needs to be shuffled at present is to keep the accounts clear on behalf of a system that is purposively designed to fund health care.

Not all dislocations need be funded at once. The saving grace of the functional approach is that it may, consistent with its own logic, be activated in an incrementalist fashion. The facts of bureaucratic life are, as are the facts of economic, political and medical life, all to be included within the calculation that should precede a decision on inclusion of a service within coverage.

In general, then, new questions of the division between medical and social services and of the cost-effectiveness of different modes of health care would directly arise under a functional system. Quantitative concerns would also need to be directly confronted: How serious is the need or desire? What value should be assigned to the honoring of the preferences of the patient? These questions need not be raised at all in a purposive system, which deals instead with questions concerning the nuances of the definitions of "health" and "health care." We will leave to others the task of parsing the seriousness of these questions. In choosing between these two approaches, however, we ought to consider which kinds of questions we want to contemplate, as well as which results we wish to achieve.

NOTES

1. *Criminal Code of Canada*, R.S.C. 1970, c. C-34, §251.
2. "... functional analysis seeks to understand a behavior pattern or a sociocultural institution by determining the role it plays in keeping the given system in proper working order or maintaining it as a going concern" (Hempel 1985). For a general discussion of the functional approach see the chapter "The Logic of Functional Analysis," pp. 297-330, in Hempel (1985).

REFERENCES

Boorse, C.
1975 "On The Distinction Between Disease and Illness." *Philosophy and Public Affairs* 5 (Fall): 49-68.
Callahan, D.
1973 "The WHO Definition of 'Health.'" *The Hastings Center Studies* 1: 77-87.
Campbell, E. J. M., J. G. Scadding, and R. S. Roberts
1979 "The Concept of Disease." *British Medical Journal* 2 (September): 757-62.
Freedman, B.
1983-85 "Study of Ethical Issues In Infertility" (unpublished material).
1985 "Ethical Issues in Clinical Obstetrics and Gynecology." *Current Problems in Obstetrics, Gynecology and Fertility* 7 (March): 1-47.

Hempel, C. G.
1985 *Aspects of Scientific Explanation*. New York: The Free Press.
Kass, L. R.
1975 "Regarding the End of Medicine and the Pursuit of Health." *The Public Interest* 40 (Summer): 11-42.
London Free Press
1982 "OHIP won't pay for vocal device it calls luxury." 5 June: 2.
1984 "Woman needing pure oxygen may be forced into hospital." 3 August: 12.
Ontario Health Insurance Plan
1983 *Schedule of Benefits: Physician Services.* 1 January. Ministry of Health of the Province of Ontario.
Surrogate Parenting News
1983 "Insurance Coverage of In Vitro." 1 (October/November): 71-72.
Szasz, T.
1961 *The Myth of Mental Illness.* New York: Dell Publishing Co.
Taylor, F. K.
1971 "A Logical Analysis of the Medico-Psychological Concepts of Disease." *Psychological Medicine* 1:356-64.
Turkel, Sherry
1984 *The Second Self.* New York: Simon and Schuster.
Wasserman, J.
1983 "How DRGs Work." *The Hastings Center Report* 13 (October): 24.
World Health Organization
1976 "Constitution of the World Health Organization." In *World Health Organization: Basic Documents,* ed. 26. Geneva: WHO.

Competition and Function:

The Canada — US Free Trade Agreement and the Philosophy of Health Care

Eike-Henner W. Kluge

EQUITY AND JUSTICE

…

Another philosophical difference between the US competition/co-operation approach and the Canadian functional model centres in the notion of health care itself. The US approach sees health care as a commodity: as something to be bought and sold like all other commodities, and where it is essentially the marketplace that determines its availability and distribution.

From E.-H.W. Kluge, "The Canada/US Free Trade Agreement," *Business and Professional Ethics Journal* 10:3 (Fall, 1991)29-52.

The Canadian perspective sees health care not primarily as a commodity but as a right. Therefore while market forces undoubtedly have an impact on the availability of health care services, a much greater role is played by societal values and the commitment to equity and justice on distribution.

It is interesting to note that like Oregon, the Canadian perspective is slowly coming to the realization that equity and justice for all does not mean having a health care system that will provide everything and anything that anyone might want. In fact, it implies quite the opposite. It means that although everyone has an equal right to health care, what health care would actually be available would be functionally determined in terms that involve the individuals and society as a whole. More specifically, it means that the social health care provider must reconcile:

1. the socio-economic capabilities of the society at that time,
2. the prevailing state of medical sophistication,
3. the average health profile of members of society, and
4. competing areas of social endeavour.

What follows is a brief sketch of how this would proceed if the Canadian functional approach were to be developed to its conclusion. It focuses on the operational allocation parameters, not the information-dissemination question. Whether this development will actually occur in light of the pressures resulting from the Free Trade Agreement is, of course, another question. As a sidelight, it could be argued that in a sense, the Oregon experiment, which is attempting to come to grips with some of these issues, is really an attempt to import into the competition/co-operation approach some of the features of the Canadian functional perspective.

FUNCTIONAL PARAMETERS OF MACRO-ALLOCATION FOR HEALTH CARE *PER SE*

1. The Socio-Economic Capabilities of Society

The functional approach, in order to be fully developed, would have to begin with a baseline determination of the socio-economic capabilities of society as a whole. This does not require much comment. Although the process would be complicated, there are enough economic indicators and calculators around to allow the derivation of usable parameters. These parameters would constitute the overall resource framework of society as a whole within which policies of resource allocation would then be developed.

2. The Prevailing State of Medical Sophistication

The next step would be to determine the prevailing state of medical sophistication in general. That also presents no real problems — at least not in principle. It simply involves developing an analytical view of what is and what is not medically feasible at the present time. It should be added that this does not mean what is medically feasible *in a particular society* at this time. It means just what it says: what is medically feasible *tout court*. The adjustment to what is medically feasible within a given society enters only when one takes a look at the resources that are going to be allocated to medical services. So the question of what is feasible can really be decided only after one have determined what amount of resources should be allocated to health care as opposed to other sectors of social endeavour.

3. Average Health Profile of Members of Society

Once the available resource framework has been delineated, and once it has been determined what is medically feasible, the next step would be to develop a statistically valid average health profile of members of society: the average health status, the sorts of conditions someone is likely to develop, and so on. Again, in principle that should present no problem. Medical sociology and above all epidemiology would here be of invaluable assistance.

4. Competing Areas of Social Endeavour

The integration of these parameters into a whole and their weighting in terms of other areas of social endeavour would probably be the most difficult task. (Interestingly enough, even at the present time it is also the area of allocation policy determination that is the least well developed.) It would involve several tasks. First, it would require the development of a multidimensional matrix that correlates service-types within epidemiological groups with each other and with levels of expenditure devoted to the various areas of health services that have been identified on the basis of the health profile of the society as a whole. This would provide the fiscally responsible social party with a variable scale which would allow it to determine at what level of expenditure a particular statistically average level of health care would be available at what cost.

The next step would to identify the other areas of socially mandated expenditure and do something similar for them. With this in hand, it would be possible to develop a comparative matrix that could identify what an expenditure in one area will mean for society in terms of expenditure in other areas: For instance, education vs. health care vs. defense vs. transportation, and so on. With this, one would have what might be called an *expenditure impact analysis* for varying levels of expenditure in the various areas of social endeavour.

THE PLACE OF SOCIAL VALUES

A lot of what has been suggested so far does not really differ very much from what a properly planned outcome-oriented approach to health care resource allocation would do. It would therefore be compatible with a US competition/co-operation perspective — except for two things: The first involves the depth of the expenditure impact analysis. Most outcome-oriented approaches to health care resource allocation would not go as far as would be required by the functional approach as sketched.

The second difference goes much deeper. It is important to remember that a functional approach does not see the various stakeholders in health care delivery as distinct parties. It sees them as different functional components of an overall whole. The material aspects of that functional unity will have been expressed by the expenditure impact analysis sketched a moment ago. However, on its own this provides no means for deciding at which point in the multi-parameter matrix an allocation decision should be made. It provides no means for doing this because this is not a material question. It is a question of values. The material facts carry no values in and by themselves. They are decision-theoretically neutral. Another way of putting that is to say that they lack action-potentials. They are not surrounded by action-gradients. These have to be superimposed on or added to the matrix. The only place from which they can be imposed is from the outside: by people who look at the facts, who bring their values to the facts and who see them in terms of more or less strongly weighted action-potentials.

All of this is merely a theoretical way of saying that from a granular, competition/co-operation perspective, the material facts and their fiscal implication determine availability and distribution. Values enter the availability equation only at the level of individual purchaser and manifest themselves only in terms of her or his willingness to pay.

On the other hand, from a functional perspective, it is not the market forces as such that determine availability and distribution; nor do values enter only at the individual level. It is societal values that determine availability and distribution. Material and economic facts acquire action-related significance only when they are correlated with the values and value-strengths of society as a whole. That is why the societal values referred to above become crucial. It would be sanguine to suggest that the Canadian system as it stands operates according to the implications that flow from this. The system is still influenced by its granular past. However, it has made a beginning towards implementing the implications in the arena of policy formulation. If one were to project current developments in this regard, the completed policy formulation process would look something like this:

(i) Identification

First, those who make allocation decisions would attempt to determine what the fundamental values of society are. Does health figure here? Does security? Mobility? Education? In other words, what has to be determined with accuracy is the valuational playing field.

(ii) Strength

The next step would to find out the strengths of these values: How strongly are they espoused by society as a whole?

(iii) Correlation

The strengths then would have to be compared to each other. The outcome of that exercise would be a series of relative value-strength coefficients. These relative value-strength coefficients would be numerical expressions of the weighted action-potentials mentioned a moment ago. When these relative value-strength coefficients are superimposed in the expenditure impact matrix, this would provide an idea of how much the society would be willing to allocate to what area of social endeavour, given its fundamental values.

With this, one would have a reasonable idea of what society would consider to be the basic minimum level of health care service to which everyone is entitled as a matter of fundamental right. In other words, with this one would have a primary and global health care budget. Nothing here assumes that there are absolutely distinct groups within society whose interests and concerns have to be balanced in terms of conflict and co-operation. In fact, talk of conflict and co-operation would be premature because, as was said before, it would presuppose that one had already identified the parties to such conflict and co-operation and that one had already legitimated the nature and strengths of their values. So far, there is functional unity. Furthermore, this approach does not assume that values are constant. The Canada of today might well hold different values from that of tomorrow. However, that is one of the strengths of the functional approach. In terms of the current vernacular, it is "real."

MACRO-ALLOCATION WITHIN HEALTH CARE BUDGETS[1]

All of the preceding would merely provide for a health care budget as such: a budget determined by the overall values of society. It would still leave the problem of allocation within the health care budget itself. This is sometimes called macro-allocation, once the budget has been set.[2]

At this point there arises one of the greatest dangers to the integrity of the Canadian functional approach: a danger that stems directly from the US model and its market orientation. It is tempting to turn to cost/benefit, cost/effectiveness and related allocatory approaches to decide the pattern and extent of macro-allocation. This is what is frequently done from the granular perspective of the competition/co-operation orientation, and the temptation to do so will be strengthened by the promise of cost-savings that will allow a greater variety of services to become available over a greater range. The ease of interaction between the two countries mandated by the Free Trade Agreement would increase pressures in this regard.

A functional health care perspective cannot consistently adopt such an approach. It would be to sacrifice values to efficiency, and to allow economic considerations to rule on matters of justice and right. If the Canadian approach is to maintain its integrity, it has to resist the pressures that arise from the US perspective and be true to its functional orientation. It would be inappropriate here to go into detail, but a taste of what a functional approach would here look like would probably be useful.

To begin with, it would proceed from the thesis that:

1. Everyone has a *prima facie* right to the same basic minimum of health care services as everyone else, where the level of this minimum is functionally determined by the total amount of resources accorded to health care, the medical sophistication of society and the average health profile of its members.

This may be called primary macro-allocation.

However, this would insufficient because it would ignore the variations in health status (and therefore in the health care needs) of individual members of society. A functional perspective requires that the members of society be treated not the same — because that would ignore their differences and the different relations in which they stand to the rest of society because of those differences — but equitably. That means that appropriate allowances would have to be made for people who have special needs.

The principle of this could be expressed in terms of the notion of a secondary macro-allocation, like this:

2. If the health status of an identifiable group of individuals is lower than the statistical norm for society, then a secondary macro-allocation is *prima facie* mandated.

The Canadian health care system accepts this principle as a matter of course and requires that special health care services be provided for those with special needs. By contrast, the competition/co-operation approach of the US does not need deal with this except insofar as following this principle produces a competitive advantage for one as opposed to another provider.

At this point it becomes clear that the Canadian approach is not yet completely functional. The problem is that while it accepts the principle, and therefore accepts the legitimacy of special allocation for those in need, it does not realize that the principle itself provides no metric. The Canadian model still needs to introduce some way to determine which special needs under what circumstances should receive how much. Without that, the system would assume that a lower-than-average health status in itself is a mandate for preferential allocation. But that would be to focus on what mathematicians might call the absolute nature of the material condition of the individual in isolation from and independently of the context. In other words, it would be to adopt a granular outlook and commit the fallacy of isolation. By the same token, it would be to make the system open-ended — as indeed is the case in Canada at the present time.

If the functional approach were to be developed consistently, it would move differently. It would develop a metric based on the very notion of functionality itself. The key point is that from a functional perspective, equitable health care does not translate into access to the same health services. The value of health services is context-dependent. Therefore sameness of access may be inequitable in practice. Instead, society treats people equitably from a *functional* perspective if it expends the same *effort* in relation to the condition of the individual.

There are measures of expenditure of effort; there are no measures of expenditure of effort-in-relation. Financial or similar measures are unacceptable because they are too closely tied to the vagaries of economic interests. However, one can construct an approximation of an appropriate measure by looking at the standard kinds of health care provided under primary macro-allocation. These fall within a certain range. One can then look at the kind of care that is appropriate for those who have special needs, and measure the effectiveness of this care in terms of quality, degree of improvement of the condition, and so on. All of this can be expressed mathematically in terms of act/effectiveness coefficients. One can then provide a metric for Principle 2 by saying that secondary macro-allocation is mandated when the act/effectiveness coefficients of the relevant services are within the range defined by primary macro-allocation services.

3. A *prima facie* obligation of secondary macro-allocation becomes an actual obligation if and only if the act/effectiveness coefficients of the relevant acts on this secondary macro-allocation fall within the act/effectiveness coefficient range allowed for other acts under primary macro-allocation

That would give the functional approach an indication of where and when to provide special health allocation. It does not yet provide a limit. But again the functional notion of equity — of equality-in-context — would provide an answer.

4. If the health status of the disadvantaged group after secondary macro-allocation is not equal to or better than it was before — where this maintenance or improvement in status is traceable to the fact of secondary macro-allocation — then the obligation to continue to provide secondary macro-allocation ceases.

Some players in the Canadian health care system have already realized the importance of this clause. It was clearly expressed by the Canadian Medical Association when it said that a physician does not have a duty to provide medically useless care; and by the Canadian Hospital Association and the various Canadian provincial ministries of health in general when they adopted the philosophy of quality assurance.

The Canadian system would need one more clause to deal with the situation when the health status of the initially disadvantaged is better than the average health status even though the act/effectiveness coefficient of the relevant acts still falls within the average range.

5. The health status of the initially disadvantaged group must not be better than the health status of the average individual as a result of the secondary macro-allocation.

Clause 5. prevents a can-do/must-do mentality from asserting itself.

The preceding is a brief sketch of how the current Canadian functionally based approach to health care could be completed. Allocation would be based on correlating the statistical determination of improvement of health status in identifiable areas to act-effectiveness coefficients in those areas. Of course to be completely fair, one would also have to introduce weighted parameters in terms of a distinction between conditions that are essentially self-induced and those that are not. These would influence allocation patterns in either a negative or a positive sense, depending on the case. The question of course remains, to what extent the system will be allowed to complete itself in light of the influences resulting from presence of external commercial health care providers from the US: providers whose corporate philosophy does not reflect the functional Canadian perspective. It will also be interesting to see to what extent this functional perspective will be able to penetrate the US perspective itself. From a political perspective, the attractiveness of many of the functional considerations in terms of voter appeal is certainly there.

RIGHT TO HEALTH CARE vs. RIGHT TO HEALTH

One of the considerations that might deter politically motivated acceptance of the functional approach is of course the cost of health care. One of the claims made at the beginning of this discussion was that the Canadian functional perspective maintains that everyone has a right to the same minimum of health care service as everyone else. For those in the political process, it is easy to slide from this claim about health care services to the claim that everyone has a right to the same minimum level of health. It is important to note that this slide would be illegitimate — even for the Canadian setting. The expressions "right to the same minimum of health care services" and "right to the same minimum level of health" mean fundamentally distinct things, and the difference is important. It goes to the very heart of the functional approach to health care as it is applied to the level of the individual health care consumer. To see why, one has to take a brief look at the notion of health itself.

The usual definition of "health" is that of the WHO:[3]

> Health is a state of complete physical, mental and social well being and not merely the absence of disease or infirmity.

This definition is not functional. It is absolutist. The right to health care is then asserted as follows:[4]

> The enjoyment of the highest attainable standard of health is one of the fundamental rights of every human being without distinction of race, religion, political belief, and economic or social condition.

This definition sets the stage for disaster from a functional perspective, because it makes the attainment of this state of complete well-being the hallmark of an appropriate, and above all ethical, health care delivery.[5] That means that any such service which does not meet this goal will be an ethical failure. However, there are certain kinds of health states, certain conditions of the human organism which, by their very natures, cannot yield to any sort of intervention that would lead to a state of complete physical, mental and social well-being: not even in principle. Death is one of them. The various trisomies are another; and one could go on. Furthermore, to identify this goal as a matter of right is to say that society has an obligation to pursue that goal for each individual; otherwise society will be unethical in its delivery of health service.

The fact is that no one can guarantee that a particular level of health will ever be attained by anyone. It may be impossible either because the resources are not there, or because the individuals themselves cannot attain any level of health in principle because of the nature of their conditions. One cannot have a right to something that one in principle cannot provide; correspondingly, one cannot have a duty to provide it. Therefore from a functional perspective, to talk about having to fulfil a right to a certain level of *health* is irrational. What can be provided is a certain level of *health care*. As was argued, that is not an outcome-oriented notion tied to success. It is a functional notion tied the performance of a certain level of activity, irrespective of whether that activity will result in complete health for the individuals themselves. This does not mean that success is an irrelevant factor in calculating allocation. It merely means that it cannot be the determining factor.

The Canadian health care system has realized the importance of the considerations just sketched; certainly so far as medicine is concerned. There has been considerable disquiet about the WHO definition of health for years, and recently the Canadian Medical Association said the following:[6]

> ... the concept of health cannot usefully be defined in absolute terms. The Association believes that a functional perspective would be more appropriate. Put differently, the Association believes that the notion *health* involves the ability to function. It centres in capacity of an organism to be in a state of homeostatic balance with its environment. [More precisely, the organism must exhibit internal homeostasis as well as functional adjustment to the environment in which it is embedded.] [This] ... allows for a dynamic perspective on health that avoids the pitfalls of the traditional WHO definition while at the same time being useful in most health care settings.

Therefore the Canadian health care scene is well on the way to solving the difficult problem of deriving a definition of "health" that is appropriate to its philosophy of health care but without at the same time begging any important social questions.

The US approach still functions essentially with the WHO definition. In a way, this is not surprising. From a competition/co-operation perspective, which sees health care as a commodity and not a right, the very commodification itself (being teleological in nature) will objectify the notion. Again, from a strictly sociological point of view, it will be interesting to see whether the Free Trade Agreement will produce a change in the functional perception of health that is beginning to emerge in Canada. It will be all the more interesting, since even within the US itself, a holistic approach to health care is beginning to be developed. The reasons for this development in the US is of course quite different from the one that is operative in the Canadian setting. It is economic in nature. According to one school of thought, a holistic approach to health care may be cheaper and more cost-effective. However, even if a functional and holistic approach were to be accepted in the US, it is not clear whether the difference in fundamental orientation of the two approaches will not undermine whatever beneficial effect the development of a functional definition would have for the viability of the Canadian system.

SOCIETY AND THE HEALTH CARE PROFESSIONS

Health care services are not generally directly available to the consumer. They require the intermediate agency of health care professionals. The attitudes and perspectives of these professionals in turn shape the delivery of the health care. Therefore, before concluding, it may be appropriate to take a brief look at the relationship between the health care professions and society as a whole, as seen from the perspective of the competition/co-operation as opposed to the functional approach.

The competition/co-operation model suggests that the relationship should be seen as involving two identifiable parties whose interests overlap in some areas but diverge in others. From this perspective, game-theoretical calculations would then be appropriate in order to resolve any conflicts that arise.

However, the functional approach would argue that what the competition/co-operation model ignores is the fact that the health care professions are themselves embedded in a social context, just like anyone else. Pragmatically speaking, the health care professions need a social context to be able to operate. No one practises medicine, nursing or the other health care professions independently and in isolation.

Also, the knowledge and expertise of these professions — their very stock-in-trade — are the result of societal co-operation and participation. They have been developed over millennia through practice and experimentation. Members of society — ordinary people — benefited from these developments and sometimes suffered. However, they were always ineluctable participants in the advancement of the art and science of the professions.

Furthermore, this advancement would not have been possible but for the knowledge that has been developed in such varied sciences as chemistry, physics, engineering, anthropology and psychology: even mathematics — to mention but a few disciplines. Without them, modern health care would simply no exist.

Finally, the conditions under which the health care professions are generally allowed to practise in our society can only be described as monopolistic. However, society does not confer a monopoly for the benefit of the monopoly-holder. It confers the monopoly in the expectation of benefit for society as a whole. In fact, the reasoning that underlies such a conferral is that society is best served in this way. Society therefore attaches certain conditions to a monopoly. In the present context these include the condition that the health care professions and medicine in particular bind themselves to providing quality service in an equitable fashion.

The functional approach accepts this embedding of health care professions within society. It accepts that neither the interests of society nor the interests of the health care professions can be considered or pursued in isolation. In fact, they cannot even be defined independently of each other. Just as the modern health care professions find their existence and *modi operandi* conditioned by the fact of their social existence, so the very nature of contemporary society is itself shaped by the existence and operation of the health care professions. Expectations in terms of social services, allocation of societal resources, possibilities of professional activities — all these play an important role in structuring the fabric of social interaction itself. To a large degree, these are what define Canadian society as opposed to US society, British vs. Brazilian, and Swedish as opposed to Japanese. Therefore the interests of the two — of society and the health care professionals — can only be defined together.

The Canadian health care professions — and in particular the profession of medicine — accepted this functional perspective recently when it took a momentous step. It withdrew its challenge to the Canada Health Act on one condition: that any dispute between the funding agency (which means the provincial governments) and the profession be sent to binding arbitration. This action was recently tested in practice when Manitoba physicians accepted binding arbitration in their dispute with the provincial government. I cannot imagine anything like this happening in a society that has adopted a granular perspective.

CONCLUSION

The Canada-US Free Trade Agreement sets up some rules to regulate the interaction between the two countries in the area of health care delivery. As such, it assumes a level playing field between the two parties. If the preceding analysis is cogent, that assumption may not be quite correct. The Canadian health care perspective is based on the assumption that a functional approach will allow society to preserve an equitable and acceptable standard of health care. This functional approach does not assume that one can never distinguish between identifiable parties in society. It does, however, assume that this difference has to be seen as difference-in-context. The US perspective appears to be based on the assumption that health care is a commodity like all others, and that therefore it should be subject to the economics of the competition/co-operation model as it has been sketched.

There is an analogy that describes the Canadian functional approach. It is that of a fishing net. The knots of a net are distinct from each other and from the strings that bind them together. Nevertheless, the knots are defined by the net itself, just as the net is defined by the knots. Without each other, they would not exist — nor would the knots have the positions which they hold in the net as a whole. The functional approach assumes that health care consumers, health care professionals and the health care industry are like knots in the net: in a sense they are clearly distinct — but in a much deeper sense they are one. The supposedly distinct parties are members of the same society. Therefore their identities and their interests are socially interdependent and inter-defined. Consequently the legitimacy of their endeavours should be evaluated from that perspective.

The analogy that describes the US competition/co-operation approach is that of a heap of sand. In a heap of sand, each grain is distinct from the other, and each grain can be defined independently of the position it has in the heap relative to all other grains. The co-operation/competition perspective assumes that society is like a heap of sand; and that health care consumers, health care professionals and the health care industry are like grains of sand: clearly and fundamentally distinct, even though on occasion, and for certain purposes, they may form an aggregate.

If the difference between the two approaches is as fundamental as I have suggested, then implementation of the Free Trade Agreement may pose problems for the Canadian approach. One of the potential problem areas lies in the extended care sector. As is the case in most other industrialized countries, the percentage of Canadian society over 65 years of age is increasing. Therefore if current social trends with respect to domicile and treatment patterns of the elderly are any indication, it is reasonable to expect that an increasing proportion of Canadian will require the services of extended care facilities. The health care industry in the US has had a long commercial experience in this area. Under the Free Trade Agreement it may not be denied access to this expanding Canadian market. Co-operation is written into the Agreement itself.

However, with this, the Agreement allows the entry of a differently oriented commercial presence into the Canadian health service sector: a presence whose perspective and identity are non-functionally determined. Given its philosophical orientation, this presence will be able to compete in a way which is foreign to the Canadian scene — and it may well gain the advantage, to the detriment and ultimate loss of the functional perspective that is characteristic of the Canadian approach. This speculation is supported by the fact that several provinces have moved to encourage the establishment of privately managed and owned HSOs and HMOs, rather than of not-for-profit institutions. With these, the way is opened for entry by a health industry which has considerable experience in that area — and a considerable measure of success. In the worst-case scenario, nothing would prevent members of that industry from inserting their presence through what commercially are known as loss leaders, and driving the Canadian competitor out of the marketplace. It is not clear that the Canadian perspective can prevail against that.

Before the Canada-US Free Trade Agreement is implemented any further, it may be worthwhile to investigate the functional approach a little more fully, especially in view of the fact that the competition/co-operation approach has resulted in a health care system which leaves almost 40 million citizens without appropriate health care insurance and with a correspondingly depressed standard of health care.

NOTES

1. For an application of some of initial allocation formulae derivable under this approach, see E.-H. W. Kluge "Once and Future Persons: Discriminatory Health Care Resource Allocation to the Elderly," in Thornton and Winkler, *Ethics and Aging* (Vancouver: University of British Columbia Press, 1989). For an expansion, see E.W. Kluge, *Biomedical Ethics in a Canadian Context* (Toronto and New York: Prentice Hall, 1991) chapter nine, "Health Policy and the Allocation of Resources: The Ethics of Discrimination."
2. Here different aspects of health care delivery would become important. Preventive vs. acute vs. long-term; hospitals vs. professional fees vs. research; and so on would be played off against each other.
3. Preamble to the Constitution of the World Health Organization, adopted by the International Health Conference, New York, 1946. *The First Ten Years* WHO (Geneva, 1958).
4. WHO, *The First Ten Years* (Geneva, 1958).
5. For various approaches to the definition of "health," see C. Boorse, "Health as a

Theoretical Concept," *Philosophy of Science* 44 (1977) 542-573; W. Miller Brown, "On Defining 'Disease' " *Journal of Medicine and Philosophy* 10:4(1985) 311-328; W. Goosens, "Values in Health and Medicine," *Philosophy of Science* 47(1980) 100-115; Chester R. Burns, "The Nonnaturals: A Paradox in the Western Concept of Health," *The Journal of Medicine and Philosophy* 1:3(1976) 202-211; Gerald L. Klerman, "Mental Illness, the Medical Model, and Psychiatry," *The Journal of Medicine and Philosophy* 2:3(1977) 222-243; Lennart Nordenfelt, *On the Nature of Health* (Dordrecht and Boston: D. Reidel Pub. Co., 1987); Joel Feinberg, "Disease and Values," in Joel Feinberg, *Doing and Deserving: Essays in the Theory of Responsibility* (Princeton University Press, 1974), pp. 253-55. A somewhat more theoretical and developed analysis is offered by Ellen Idler, ("Definition of Mental Health and Illness and Medical Sociology," *Society, Science and Medicine* 3A, pp. 723-31). She claims that these and other definitions are based on a Parsonian model of illness and disease: one that defines it as "an abstract, biomedical conception of pathological abnormality in people's bodies, where this is indicated by certain abnormal signs and symptoms which can be measured, recorded, classified and analyzed." She argues the concept should be modified so that "subjective reality plays a role in determining whether an individual becomes ill in the first place."

6. Canadian Medical Association, *New Human Reproductive Technologies: Preliminary Perspective of the Canadian Medical Association,* submission to the Royal Commission on New Reproductive Technologies; principal authors, Eike-Henner Kluge and Carol Lucock; (Ottawa, February 1991); pp. 19-20.

FURTHER READINGS:

Bell, Nora K.
"The Scarcity of Medical Resources: Are There Rights to Health Care?" *Journal of Medicine and Philosophy* 4: 2(1979) 158–169.
Daniels, Norman
Just Health Care. (Cambridge and London: Cambridge University Press, 1985).
Drummond, M.F.
Principles of Economic Appraisal in Health Care. (Oxford: Oxford Medical Publications, 1980).
Feeny, David; Gordon Guyatt and Peter Tugwell, eds.
Health Care Technology: Effectiveness, Efficiency and Public Policy. (Montréal: Institute for Research on Public Policy, 1986).
Hall, Mr. Justice Emmett
Report of the Royal Commission on Health Services. (Ottawa: Queen's Printer, 1964).
Health Care for the Elderly in the Year 2000: Symposium Proceedings. (British Columbia Ministry of Health: Victoria, 1986).
Ingelfinger, Franz
"Haves and Have-Nots in the World of Disease," *The New England Journal of Medicine* 287 (Dec. 7, 1972) 1198–1199.

Kawachi, I.
"QUALY's and Justice," *Health Policy* 13:2 (1989) 115-120.
Kilner, John
"The Ethical Legitimacy of Excluding the Elderly When Medical Resources Are Limited," in D. Yeagar, ed., *Annual of the Society of Christian Ethics* (Washington: Georgetown University Press, 1988).
Klarman, H.E., J.O. Francis and G.D. Rosenthal
"Cost-Effectiveness and Analysis Applied to the Treatment of Chronic Renal Disease," *Medical Care* 6 (1968) 48–54.
La Puma, John and E. Lawlor
"Quality-Adjusted Life Years: Ethical Implications for Physicians and Policy Makers," *Journal of the American Medical Association* 263:21 (1990) 2917-1921.
McKeown, Thomas and C.R. Lowe
An Introduction to Social Medicine, 2d ed. (Oxford: Blackwell, 1974).
McKeown, Thomas
The Role of Medicine: Dream, Mirage or Nemesis? 2d ed. (Oxford: Blackwell, 1979).
Millis, J.S.
"Wisdom? Health? Can Society Guarantee Them?" *New England Journal of Medicine*, 283 (July 30, 1970), 260–61.
Mooney, Gavin and Alistair McGuire, eds.
Medical Ethics and Economics in Health Care. (Oxford and New York: Oxford University Press, 1988).
Rosenthal, G.D.
"Cost-Effectiveness and Analysis Applied to the Treatment of Chronic Renal Disease," *Medical Care* 6 (1968) 48–54; Norman Daniels, *Just Health Care*. (Cambridge and London: Cambridge University Press, 1985).
Siegler, Mark
"A Right to Health Care: Ambiguity, Professional Responsibility and Patient Liberties," *Journal of Medicine and Philosophy* 4: 2 (1979), 148–57.
Veatch, Robert
"Just Social Institutions and the Right to Health Care," *Journal of Medicine and Philosophy*, 4: 2 (1979).

CHAPTER 3 MESO- AND MICRO-ALLOCATION

INTRODUCTION

The allocation of resources presents difficult problems when we are dealing with global budgets and groups of population. The problems acquire a wholly new dimension when we know that if we give a certain amount of resources to one person, a whole group of people may be deprived.

An example may bring the issue into focus. Monica Urgele is an elderly person occupying an acute care hospital bed. Her condition does not warrant her being there. However, she has been there for some time, and she does not want to move to an extended care facility that would be more appropriate for her needs. To move her against her will is virtually to guarantee that she will die within a very short period of time. At the same time, to leave her is to deprive a whole series of patients whose condition warrants that they be in an acute care facility, but who cannot be admitted because no bed is available. Does Monica Urgele take priority over the others? Should the hospital administrator discharge her to a more suitable facility and help the many, at the (possible) cost of Monica Urgele's life expectancy? The issue is real, and only one of many that health care professionals face more and more frequently. The nurse on the floor who has to decide how much time to spent with a specific patient, at the expense of all other patients, faces the very same difficulty: what is the strength of the claims of the one against those of the many?

The problem of allocation becomes psychologically still more difficult when a specific person competes with another for what only one can have. This is one of the most difficult issues that a health care professional can face. And yet, sometimes a choice has to be made. Only one person can have the heart that has just become available: but which person? Or, who shall have the only liver? Issues like this become especially difficult when one of the patients has led an immoderate lifestyle — has drunk too much, smoked, was quite sedentary, followed an imprudent diet, etc. — whereas another patient was the model of a responsible health care consumer. The triage nurse in the emergency room faces a similar situation. S/he must decide who is to be taken care of first. On a more mundane level, the same problem faces the long term care nurse in the rural setting who has to make a service plan for seeing her clients, where each of her clients lives some distance away. Which client should she see first? For how long?

Freedman and the McGill/Boston Research Group essentially focus on issues of meso-allocation. They ask the question: under what circumstances should scarce resources be used to provide therapies for specific individuals when these therapies have not (yet) been shown to be effective; and when, moreover, the funding for these therapies will take away from funding for established therapies that are otherwise available?

The article by Moss and Siegler introduces the notion of desert: should the imprudent and immoderate person really have the same chance as the careful and responsible patient? Moss and Siegler suggest that patients who develop end-stage liver disease through no fault of their own should have higher priority to receive a liver transplant than patients whose end-stage liver disease is the result of a failure to obtain treatment for their alcoholism. This approach has been adopted by some transplant centres in Ontario. If it were adopted as a matter of general health care policy, it could have tremendous implications.

Nonvalidated Therapies and HIV Disease

Benjamin Freedman and the McGill / Boston Research Group

The introduction of potential treatments for HIV disease has, in almost every instance, engendered controversy. The speedy approval of AZT (Zidovudine) has led to charges that FDA was inappropriately influenced by political considerations, and the current extensive studies on AZT are pointed out as evidence that the drug was granted approval before adequate testing had been completed.[1] The initial tests of ribavirin were criticized by some for their supposed inappropriate and unethical use of a placebo control group. Organized demonstrations have been held and legal action taken to rectify perceived delays in providing aerosolized pentamidine as prophylaxis against *pneumocystis carinii* pneumonia (PCP).[2]

The controversies that have swirled about nonvalidated treatments (NTs) for HIV disease touch upon crucial questions of ethics and public policy. These questions are unresolved within the communities professionally concerned—physicians, researchers, and government officials — as they are unresolved among patients and in society at large.

Benjamin Freedman and the McGill/Boston Research Group, "Nonvalidated Therapies and HIV Disease," *Hastings Center Report 19:3* (June 1989)14-20.

SCOPE AND CONTEXT OF THE PROBLEM

The definition of nonvalidated therapies has been itself a matter of some controversy in the literature.[3] In what follows, I shall mean by nonvalidated therapies those drugs, medical and surgical interventions, and regimens that are offered to and accepted by a patient on the basis of potential benefit, and that have neither been accepted nor discredited by the expert clinical community. Nonvalidated therapies are distinct from, on the one hand, customary and accepted treatments; and, on the other, quack remedies. Because of the uncertainty surrounding them, the ethics of practice in providing nonvalidated therapies cannot be subsumed under the general ethics of clinical practice; nor are such therapies uniformly provided pursuant to an approved protocol, and in those instances are not subjected to the moral canons of clinical research. What treatments currently fall within this rubric? And what are the characteristics of the population seeking NTs?

Discussions of policy and ethics regarding NTs tend to focus on investigational new drugs (INDs), which are novel pharmacologically active substances under testing for anti-viral, immunomodulating, or other beneficial effect.[4] AZT stands as the paradigm case, a drug whose only previous presumed use, as an anti-cancer agent, had been discredited in early trials.

Investigational new drugs are under the close control of regulatory bodies, such as FDA (in the United States) or Health Protection Branch (in Canada). The view that equates nonvalidated treatments with INDs, therefore, leads naturally to the presumption that reform of the policy and rules governing NTs must focus upon the conduct of such regulatory bodies. The scope of NTs is, however, much broader than that; and the power of regulatory agencies correspondingly limited.

Nonvalidated therapies without IND status fall into several categories; each shares the qualities of uncertainty, therapeutic intention, and immunity from regulatory control:

Licensed drugs offered for an unapproved use.

Whereas a drug receives marketing approval after demonstrated safety and effectiveness under defined conditions of use, once approved, a licensed drug may be prescribed by a physician, exercising his or her clinical discretion, for other conditions.[5] U.S. regulations, for example, state that "the physician may, as part of the practice of medicine, lawfully prescribe a different dosage for his patient or may otherwise vary the conditions of use from those approved in the package insert without informing or obtaining the approval of the Food and Drug Administration."[6] Antabuse is an example of a drug licensed for one condition that is currently taken by many persons infected with HIV. Regulatory agencies have taken the stance that enforcing the restriction of licensed drugs to approved uses is beyond their jurisdiction. The point is not always appreciated. The expert panel FDA assembled on AZT, for example, had recommended that the drug be approved only as a treatment for AIDS patients who had had an episode of PCP.[7] In licensing the drug for marketing, however, FDA cannot enforce such a restriction.

Non-drugs and not-necessarily-drugs

Among the treatments touted for HIV are dietary and life-style changes, which are obviously beyond regulatory control. One interesting case is AL-721. This substance, with suspected anti-viral properties, is a special preparation of common foodstuffs. It is being marketed as a prescription drug in Great Britain, but because of the cost and delay involved in receiving U.S. regulatory approval, and under pressure from generic competitors, its manufacturer now plans to market it as a "food supplement" in the United States.[8] Other possible inclusions within this category would be substances such as dextran sulfate or DTC (Imuthiol), which are under clinical investigation but may be obtained by the public from nonpharmaceutical sources such as chemical supply houses and which the patient may then self-administer.

New combinations of treatments

As with the first category of unapproved use of licensed substances, attempting new combinations of treatments reproduces the combination of therapeutic intent and scientific uncertainty. Current AIDS research is largely preoccupied with testing new combinations of drugs and other treatments (for example, AZT in combination with interferon or acyclovir), and this category will necessarily grow as new drugs are included within the validated AIDS pharmacopoeia.

Smuggled substances

The growing use of drugs smuggled from Europe and Mexico by AIDS patients or their doctors has been widely noted; FDA has in fact recently informed its agents in writing to ignore the importation of unapproved drugs by patients for their own use.[9]

In the light of these categories of nonvalidated therapies, it is clear that the role of regulators, though crucial, is limited. By the same token, the central importance of the doctor-patient relationship in confronting these issues is brought to the fore. Only in the clinical setting can much use of NTs in HIV be monitored (if indeed it can be done there); only in that setting can such use be influenced by informed judgment. At the same time, it must be acknowledged that the controversies to date have largely swirled about IND treatments, and that IND policy is the element most given to rapid reform.

Previous experience with treatments for other conditions, notably tuberculosis, indicates that unproven therapy remains popular until such point as an effective therapy is developed; thus, the issue in HIV treatment is likely to persist for some time to come. Current research on those being treated for cancer by unorthodox means also has some lessons to teach us. Among cancer patients, there is a strong direct relationship between experienced toxicity from standard treatment and the subsequent use of unorthodox treatments. In addition, contrary to the stereotype of the uneducated, credulous patient victimized by the unscrupulous practitioner, "[t]he evidence seems overwhelming that socioeconomic status is either independent of the use of such therapies or that higher status and better educated individuals are overrepresented among the patients of unorthodox practitioners."[10]

These characteristics have expressed themselves in our context of HIV disease in a way that raises an urgent ethical problem of equity.[11] In the United States, the bulk of the infected population is increasingly bifurcated, being composed of gay men on the one hand, and, on the other, intravenous drug users and their sexual partners. The latter group has little in the way of education, information, or resources to deploy toward novel therapies. Gay infected men, on the other hand — particularly as their illness progresses — have voted with their feet, vigorously gathering information about potential therapies and aggressively pursuing access to them. Within this group, motivated by desperation, the use of nonvalidated therapies with or without a physician's assistance may yet become the rule rather than the exception. At one meeting of Body Positive in 1987, for example, more than three quarters of the audience of 400 raised their hands when asked how many were taking experimental or alternative drug treatment.[12]

In part their efforts are expressed in unprecedented activity providing information about current clinical trials directly to infected persons. The American Foundation for AIDS Research publishes a pamphlet with regular updates listing the protocols of clinical trials currently underway, together with their operative criteria of inclusion and exclusion.[13] This publication is distributed gratis upon request to persons who have tested positive for HIV antibodies. Groups such as Project Inform in San Francisco and Treatment AIDS in Toronto gather information about the clinical use of NTs and distribute it to persons with AIDS via newsletters. Some sources will inform persons about means of preparation and self-administration of experimental substances, and how they may be smuggled into the country.

These facts raise some clear challenges to any proposal for reform of the process regarding NTs. Overall, the number of persons prepared to take the risks involved in receiving nonvalidated treatment far outnumber those who may be admitted to controlled scientific trials. The regulatory authorities are increasingly in danger of becoming irrelevant; as I will suggest below, the response to this adopted by FDA — strategic retreat in the form of the treatment IND exemption — only hastens this mounting irrelevancy, with added unfortunate precedential value for other conditions. In turn, the gay male community is left to self-help resources; without a counterbalance, this leaves it potential prey to rumor fostered by hope and nourished by companies who see a profit opportunity in the manufacture of nonvalidated therapies. Finally, the other major group of infected persons — inner-city IV drug users and their sexual partners — has no entrée to the system. Often excluded from trials because of supposed unreliability, or dropping out because of actual unreliability, and lacking the knowledge or resources to pursue NTs on an off-protocol basis, they are denied any potential benefits that may accrue to those receiving drugs prior to conclusion of the validating process.

SOME POLICY OPTIONS

Proposals for reforming the process for dealing with NTs fall along a continuum of change. The least radical changes involve reform of the manner in which the drug agencies operate under current regulations and statutory authority. Much remains to be done along these lines. "Compassionate use" exemptions, for example, could be interpreted broadly rather than narrowly; queuing and consequent delays in reviewing could be managed better than in noncrisis times; traditional cautious practices, such as requiring the replication of well-designed double blind randomized trials, could be amended. However, most attention has been focused upon radical proposed changes to the process altering the underlying philosophy of drug regulation.

An early proposal by Mathilde Krim may be the most familiar.[14] She had proposed maintaining the bureaucratic *status quo* with respect to asymptomatic infected persons, or those in the early stages of HIV disease (AIDS-Related Complex), but eliminating all restrictions to free access, via their physician, to any substance proposed for treatment of a person with full-blown AIDS. In exempting an entire class of patients from regulatory restraints on the basis of the severity of their illness, Krim's proposal represents a radical departure from traditional drug regulation philosophy, which held the critically ill to be in at least as great need of protection through regulation as any other patient.

Were Krim's proposal to be implemented, it might become impossible to conduct controlled trials on AIDS patients since they would all have unrestricted access to experimental substances. This consequence does not concern her, for in her view "[t]he most valuable proof of the efficacy of the drugs will be studies conducted on patients in the earlier stages of illness." The ravages involved in the progression to AIDS make it unlikely in her view that treatment would help, but nevertheless she believes that offering such treatment is ethically imperative:

> Permitting physicians to use experimental drugs to treat patients whose lives are in immediate jeopardy should not be done out of a wishful belief that the treatment would work. It should be done out of respect for the patient's right to fight for life with whatever tools we can offer.

AZT itself demonstrates several problems with her proposal. As AZT shows, AIDS patients can receive significant therapeutic benefit; meaningful controlled results can be obtained in tests upon a population with full-blown AIDS; and, the harm-benefit ratio associated with a drug changes over the course of disease, rendering drug toxicity that may be excessive early on acceptable as the patient's options shrink. Moreover, persons with AIDS die of opportunistic infections, not HIV, and treatments specific to these infections cannot be tested before they occur, whether early or late in the progressive breakdown of the immune system. In general, our growing knowledge of the erratic continuum of HIV disease makes a hard division between AIDS itself and everything up to it medically inappropriate.

One final point is most troubling. Even were it the case that an AIDS patient is beyond help, it does not follow that he or she is beyond being hurt as well — and both must be true if drugs are to be made available that have satisfied neither norms of safety or of efficacy. For example, the early experimental treatment suramin proved in tests to be both toxic and, in some instances, to contribute itself to worsening immune disorders. The death of an AIDS patient is not so imminent that it cannot be hastened by misguided treatment, nor is the disease so dreadful that the quality of life of its sufferers cannot be worsened by inappropriate treatment. As Oliver Wendell Holmes, Sr., once said, if all of the unproven remedies doctors carry in their saddle bags were to be dumped in to the ocean, it would be so much the better for their patients and so much the worse for the fish.

A second radical proposal that has been implemented by FDA, the introduction of the category of the treatment IND, responds to some of these points.[15] The new category was adopted under the obvious impetus and avowed influence of the AIDS crisis, although since its recent adoption its most frequent use has been for non-AIDS drugs. The treatment IND category is intended to weaken substantially, without abandoning altogether, the requirement that a drug be demonstrably effective before being allowed into clinical practice. In brief, it requires that a drug for an immediately life-threatening condition be approved provided FDA is satisfied that it "may be effective" and the risk of its use is not "unreasonable and significant"; if a drug is intended for use on a serious but not immediately life-threatening condition, it shall be approved for clinical use upon demonstration of safety and preliminary evidence of effectiveness.[16]

It is still uncertain how this amended regulation will be interpreted and work out in practice. For example, a broad reading of the regulation would include asymptomatic

HIV infection under the "immediately life-threatening" rubric, defined as "a stage of a disease in which there is a reasonable likelihood that death will occur within a matter of months *or in which premature death is likely without early treatment*" (emphasis added). The financial implications for drug companies are also unclear at this point. It appears that while the preparation of applications for treatment IND status will be fairly expensive, they will nonetheless still be much cheaper than the ordinary cost of drug development is currently;[17] and treatment IND status is granted prior to completion of Phase III trials, which represent by far the most expensive phase of drug testing for companies. Until the treatment IND category was introduced, drug companies were not permitted to charge for drugs in clinical trials without special approval. Supplying drugs for trials was considered part of the normal costs of doing business. Drug companies by contrast are automatically permitted to charge for the use of drugs with treatment IND status, at a rate that permits them "to recover costs of manufacture, research, development, and handling" of the drug. The companies are nonetheless forbidden to "commercialize" treatment INDs, a prohibition whose force and meaning remains uncertain.

The Pharmaceutical Manufacturers Association has warned that a company that can charge for its drug will have no incentive to complete the expensive testing necessary to achieve regular marketing approval.[18] In response, the regulations require that the companies whose product has been granted this status be vigorously engaged concurrently in completing testing and the approval process. As a matter of structural public policy, however, this seems an inadequate response. Heretofore, the drug companies' vigorous pursuit of testing was motivated by the pull toward potential drug profits, which could not be realized without FDA approval. Henceforward, rather than being pulled by natural market forces, testing will be pushed by FDA pressure. It is economically wasteful to substitute artificial regulatory pressure for natural market forces, and it is particularly doubtful that in the current context of scarce regulatory resources the money needed will be found — money that must be carved out of the same budget that is already failing to keep up with IND and other new drug (NDA) applications.

Other practical concerns stated by university researchers and the American Medical Association express fear that controlled clinical trials of drugs granted this status will become impossible due to a failure of enrollment of subjects. Patients may not agree to be randomized into treatment or placebo control groups if they have guaranteed access to the treatment by clinical prescription. Clamor to receive the "new treatment" may prove to be intensified by a now-unjustified reliance by patients upon regulators, for patients have become accustomed to the idea that a drug cannot be legally sold unless it is safe and effective. But the failure to complete these trials will serve neither those patients themselves — who serve as guinea pigs for treatments of unproved efficacy, and pay for the privilege — nor future patients, who are denied the advantage of prior validation of treatments.

One final conceptual difficulty of the regulations should be noted. It treats safety and efficacy as two separate categories. As long as a drug is shown to be safe (more precisely, not unreasonably risky) its treatment use may be authorized pending a finding of efficacy. But safety and efficacy must nearly always be judged in relative rather than absolute terms, and nearly always as a balance rather than as independent factors — a function rather than a conjunction. The bottom line — Is this drug worth prescribing or not? — is affected by knowledge concerning systemic or symptomatic benefit, side effects, and other factors, and safety and efficacy may only be understood as elements within this function. To make the same point in other words, a drug's pharmacologic activity is the basis of both positive and negative effects (that is, "efficacy" as well as "risk"). The only perfectly safe drug is a perfectly inert — hence, perfectly useless — drug. A regulation presuming the contrary will yield either limited or distorted application.

Libertarians have seen in AIDS an opportunity to further their anti-regulationist agenda. Dale Gieringer, on behalf of the Cato Institute, has suggested that the informed consent of the patient, rather than regulation, be the determinant of access to investigational drugs.[19] Any patient who, being fully informed about any new substance, chooses to risk his life and health by taking it, should be granted that option.

Confidence in consent is misplaced in this instance. By definition of nonvalidated therapies, the consent would be minimally informed at best. It would be consent granted under desperation, and consent that is likely fostered by drug company promotion. Adherence to such a consent in the form of administering such a drug also professionally impugns the responsible physician, who is trained to use his or her own educated judgment rather than simply complying with patients' requests. The testing and medical research upon which this professional judgment relies would be entirely undercut by Gieringer's proposal.

WHAT CONSTITUTES A DESIRABLE POLICY?

The elements of desirable changes in policy toward nonvalidated treatments used for HIV disease have emerged from the above critique. The central points of the current philosophy of drug regulation should be conserved. In particular, drugs should not be licensed for marketing until they have been proved safe and effective under proposed conditions of use, a judgment that should be arrived at by a panel with comprehensive expertise rather than by private practitioners and their patients alone. (It may, however, be argued that "comprehensive expertise" requires representation from the points of view of patients and private physicians.) Finally, it is critically important that drug companies should not be permitted to reap any economic benefit from a drug until this process has been completed.

One additional desideratum is implicit in the above discussion: Any change in the process must be at least consistent with, if not positively enhancing of, the ability to speedily conclude sound scientific evaluations of any new treatments. Because of the ever-growing numbers of infected persons, practices and procedures within the context of the regulations should be streamlined to the maximum extent. Equally, however, the growing number of cases argues for the early resolution of the question of safety and effectiveness.

This double-edged character of the epidemic factor in AIDS may be illustrated by a simple analogy. A large boulder is rolling down a cliff, toward a populated area. An early nudge will achieve the largest alteration of its path with the minimum effort. But you want to be sure that you're nudging it in the right direction: because you don't want to waste your effort; because there may not be time to mount a second effort; because a misguided nudge might endanger a still-more-populated region. For AIDS, as for the boulder, the message is: Hurry up — carefully. More lives will be saved, in the end, by aiming accurately than by aiming early. Applied to the specific issue of drug licensure, the metaphor cautions us not to jeopardize the conclusion of needed clinical trials in the interest of satisfying patient demands for access to an NT.

This point requires some further discussion. It entails that, when conflict between a patient or treating physician's desire for access to a nonvalidated treatment and the pursuit and early conclusion of a sound, ethical trial is unavoidable, the latter may be allowed to take precedence. If, for example, it is only possible to recruit sufficient subjects by restricting access to the drug to those eligible persons who agree to enroll, we would be expressing such a preference. Yet seemingly, to do this would grant the progress of science priority over patient rights.

The justification depends upon establishing that the patient's right to medical treatment is unimpaired by denying the patient access to an unvalidated intervention. The ethics of a controlled clinical trial require that throughout its conduct a state of clinical equipoise exist between the experimental and control arm(s) (including placebo control, if any); in other words, that the relative therapeutic merit of the proposed innovation remains a genuinely undecided question amongst the community of expert practitioners.[20] It is this state of equipoise, of clinical uncertainty, that serves to justify the withholding of the innovation from the control population, because as long as this state of uncertainty persists, the innovation cannot be classified for normative purposes as a medical treatment. Once the uncertainty has been resolved, however, the trial must ethically be terminated, and the now-validated treatment offered to all eligible patients.

The same ethical analysis concerning the right to treatment that applies to the control population applies to the patient population outside of the trial as well. A patient, within a trial as without, is unconditionally entitled to receive medical treatment. "Medical treatment" as a normative concept, however, must be defined and delimited by medical expertise rather than by a patient's beliefs. The right to medical treatment does not encompass every drug or intervention that a patient considers therapeutically worthwhile, on whatever evidence he or she has found convincing. Until the therapeutic advantage of an innovation has been demonstrated to the satisfaction of the community of expert practitioners, an innovation is no medical treatment, and so is not covered by a patient's right to access to medical treatments. Consistent with the above, however, we may add that to the extent that a patient's desire to receive an innovation may be satisfied without jeopardizing the conduct of a clinical trial, then, consistent with good clinical judgment, the desire of the patient should be allowed to prevail.

A reform that might satisfy these various desiderata would focus upon the factor missing from other proposals, the physician-researcher treating persons with HIV infection. The proposal builds upon the growing development of specialized research and treatment units for AIDS — for example, AIDS Clinical Trial Units (ACTUs) — which combine substantial expertise in AIDS diagnosis, treatment, and research, together with sophisticated laboratory support. Clinicians in these units are active collaborators in treatment protocols granted high priority by the AIDS Clinical Drug Development Committee, and play an important role in developing treatment protocols and in their accelerated evaluation.[21] They have not yet been assigned any formal role, however, in expediting the evaluation of NTs, nor have other similarly designated expert units.[22]

The proposal is to institute similar units (or specified investigators), in the United States and Canada, which are formally granted the authority to utilize restricted investigational drugs on a compassionate use basis.[23] The regulatory authorities would be notified about such use, and would be able to monitor these Authorized Investigational Units (AIUs) and provide retrospective control, but their prior approval for individual use would not be needed. In effect, any drug having IND status would be available for the testing and clinical use of the designated AIDS facilities; something resembling "treatment IND" status would be granted at the (monitored) discretion of the expert practitioners of these units. Consistent with previous practice, drug companies would not be permitted to charge for drugs employed within protocols. For those drugs used on an "off-protocol" basis, they would be permitted to recover the direct marginal cost of production and handling only. Charges allowing amortization of other costs of research and development would not be permitted until the drug had completed the approval process, so that the natural incentives for completion of testing would be retained.

How would this improve upon the current system, and over the U.S. treatment IND modification? A number of points can be noted:

Regulatory expense and delay is minimized — or moved to after-the-fact review, when delay is not bought at the patient's expense.

Current practice on compassionate and other exemptions to access to investigational drugs would be formalized and regularized. Currently, such exemptions are said to rely upon the regulator's judgment that the practitioner in question possesses the needed expertise; under this proposal, a formal determination to this effect would be made of the unit as a whole, in advance of a request commonly made when a patient is *in extremis.*

The conflict of interest of drug companies in concluding trials would be eliminated. The personnel of the authorized unit, active researchers as well as clinicians, already possess and would retain a natural incentive vigorously to pursue to conclusion scientifically sound protocols. Even while ostensibly seeking the same goal — for example, approval of the drug regulatory authority — the incentive system governing the clinical investigator radically differs from that of a drug company. The researcher's incentives (publication, recognition, etc.) are themselves contingent upon satisfying norms of value and validity of clinical research. For the investigator, FDA approval is the by-product of sound, cautious research into a drug's safety and efficacy, and at most, from that point of view, serves to ratify the choices and findings of the investigator. FDA approval plays a different role in the rational economic calculations of a drug company; rather than a by-product, it is significant in itself as the major necessary step to licensure and marketing of a drug. Neither undue naïveté about the motivations of researchers nor excessive cynicism about the intentions of drug companies is required to conclude that it is safer to relax the regulatory harness upon the former than the latter.

Authorized units could be set up in such a way as to enhance the possibility of pooling uncontrolled data as well. For those receiving a drug outside of an approved protocol, there has always been difficulty in monitoring and assessing the significance of drug incidents and misadventures, which can be important clues, especially to low-probability adverse side effects. The uniformity of laboratory support and expertise of authorized centres that are the only ones accumulating experience with these substances would go some way toward satisfying the need for pooled uncontrolled data.

Optimal information could be provided to patients seeking access to nonvalidated treatments. At present, the local practitioner without an AIDS specialty is likely to be confronted with demands by the patient for some experimental treatment spoken of on the AIDS grapevine but of which the practitioner knows nothing. He faces an impossible dilemma in deciding whether to accede to or resist the request. Under the AIU system, for those nonvalidated treatments only available at authorized units or by practitioners under their aegis and guidance the dilemma would not occur. In addition, the formal role held by AIUs in the provision of NTs would foster a tendency for these units to act as clearing houses for the entire range of novel therapies, and as magnets for that segment of the patient population interested in access to NTs.

The proposal could ameliorate the relative lack of access to nonvalidated therapies on the part of intravenous drug users (IVDUs) and their sexual partners. First, by formalizing and extending the provision of nonvalidated therapies within specialized units, all patients treated within these units would have easier access to NTs. Second, the provision of NTs in these settings would not depend, as is often now the case, upon the informed and determined efforts of patients themselves, calling for resources beyond those possessed by IVDUs. Third and most importantly, nonvalidated treatments could be made available to IVDUs who are ineligible for participation within a protocol. (The major inequity suffered by this population in the U.S. — access to health care itself — would of course remain. However, it would not be compounded at the level of NTs.)

This proposal may be administered in a manner fully compatible with the need to complete testing on new agents, a concern that many other proposals to enhance access to NTs do not satisfy. One suggestion would be that the Authorized Investigational Unit only offer a nonvalidated therapy off-protocol to those persons ineligible for participation in the study. When a patient is ineligible for participation in research, or when enrollment in the protocol is complete (or closed), for example, the conduct of the trial is not affected by allowing a patient access to an investigational agent; and, as was argued above, until that point it is not unethical to so restrict access. These factors are better determined at a local level (the AIU) than by an outside agency.

Consideration of a final set of advantages afforded by this proposal requires some more fundamental consideration of the effect drug regulation has on medical research.[24] The process of regulatory review itself creates a large gulf between mandated clinical trials and clinical practice. For example, the regulatory focus upon new molecular entities artificially dichotomizes medical research which is, of its nature, a continuous phenomenon. The spectrum of nonvalidated therapies described above — unapproved uses for licensed drugs, new drug combinations, drugs illegally imported, and non-drug substances (foodstuffs, chemicals, and lifestyle alterations) — implicate uncertainties equivalent to those associated with investigational new drugs, but remain "research orphans," beyond the reach and concern of regulated investigations.

The clinical trials conducted on an investigational new drug are a powerful focusing lens, providing the most rapid reliable assessment of the agent in question. However, a medical analogue of Heisenberg's Uncertainty Principle obtains: a trial's power and precision are bought at some expense to our capacity to generalize its conclusions to common clinical practice. Studies are designed with rigorous criteria of inclusion and exclusion that define an atypical patient population (one that is, for example, homogeneous in age and gender and free from common intercurrent diseases) being treated in an atypical way (to exclude confounding synergistic and antagonistic effects of other common treatments). Yet upon approval for marketing, the practitioner is permitted (and perhaps required) to extrapolate these results toward a treatment recommendation in his or her variegated clinical practice. This extrapolation is difficult when the conduct of the trial has rigidly adhered to the focused protocol; regulation has provided no bridge between the world of the trial and that of the clinic.

In the real world, further complicating factors intrude. One such is the problem of relying upon the integrity and compliance of the enrolled patient/subject, who might be motivated to conceal facts that would threaten his continued participation in the trial. Nor is the problem one of patients alone: when a patient falls outside the trial's scope, physician and patient alike may chafe under this constraint; and when the nonvalidated therapy is only available within the protocol, sometimes, perhaps often, the inclusion criteria are fudged.[25] This clandestine practice, when discovered, renders results uninterpretable; and even when merely suspected, dubious.

Some of these differences between mandated clinical trials and clinical practice are necessary, and reflect diverse contexts and purposes. Yet the need to narrow these gaps has become increasingly apparent, and the present proposed AIUs could help. Their exemption from the need for prospective regulatory approval would enable the units to do coordinated research across the spectrum of nonvalidated therapies. Experience with patients on and off protocol will provide an important comparative perspective within the unit, and a firmer basis for the extrapolation of results to diverse patient populations. The ability to provide NTs to ineligible patients off protocol will take some pressure off physicians to evade rigid criteria of inclusion. The knowledge that the nonvalidated treatment is not confined to those satisfying criteria of inclusion will remove one motivation of patient deception. We might expect that in general, the natural trust existing between patient and physician will be bolstered by the patient's knowledge that his or her physician's clinical and ethical judgment is not subject to being countermanded by some distant bureaucracy. And finally, this renewed focus upon the role of the treating unit in providing nonvalidated treatments would allow a reevaluation of the process for non-IND innovations.

To recapitulate: The reform of designated units for investigational drugs would combine maximum flexibility with minimum delay, expense, and intrusion in the conduct of clinical trials. By giving AIDS researcher-practitioners more authority, it would undoubtedly add to their burden of moral responsibility (including the potential for an ethical conflict of interest between the roles of clinician and investigator). The reform should nonetheless be welcomed by them, for this increment of responsibility in effect amounts to granting them the ability to make effective decisions regarding the medical care of their patients without seeking prior bureaucratic permission. The combination of rapid access to new treatments consistent with sound evaluation and advancement of clinical practice should be welcomed by associations representing persons with AIDS as well. Finally, while regulators will have lost some prospective control over access to INDs, they would retain a monitoring retrospective function, as a check against eccentric enthusiasm that could develop at one or more designated centres. As such, they would be fulfilling their protective mandate vis-à-vis the public.

If the above is persuasive, it would seem that a compelling logical case could be made on behalf of utilizing the AIU model for other conditions, for example, cancer and its treatment. However, logic in advance of experience is unreliable. Indeed, prior to the recent AIDS challenge, the common response of FDA in the face of controversy was to yield in the individual case on an ad hoc basis, rather than modify the entire system to accommodate one exceptional circumstance. The more cautious approach is appropriate here: Try the AIU system out on AIDS on an experimental basis, and evaluate the results before considering whether the model merits broad application.

Numerous questions remain. For example, should the designated units approach be added to the current system of compassionate exemption, or substituted for it? (The former approach would avoid problems of access arising from the centralization of care embedded within this proposal.) Should units have authority limited to drugs currently being tested at those same units? Is coordination between on-protocol and off-protocol decisions of AIUs in a given geographical region required, to ensure satisfactory trial enrollment? What government controls or incentives might be needed to cause drug companies to supply drugs to those centres employing them off of protocol, on a pure cost-recovery basis?

Many more may be added. If the approach is promising, however, these questions should be pursued with the same appropriate urgency as attaches to scientific work on AIDS.

ACKNOWLEDGMENTS

The ideas in this paper were discussed at workshops of the McGill University/Boston University Cooperative Research Group on Ethics, Law and Policy on HIV. Major support for this work was provided by Grant #6605-2897, National Health Research and Development Program, Ministry of Health, Government of Canada. While it is not possible to acknowledge all who contributed, special thanks must be given to Margaret Sommerville, George J. Annas, Norbert Gilmore, and Julie Hamblin.

NOTES

1. "Are Experimental Drugs Moving Through System Too Slowly?" *AIDS Alert* 3:1 (1988), 1-6.
2. George J. Annas, "AIDS, Judges, and the Right to Medical Care," *Hastings Center Report* 18:4 (1988), 20-22.
3. Dale H. Cowan and Eva Bertch, "Innovative Therapy: The Responsibility of Hospitals," *Journal of Legal Medicine* 5:2 (1984), 219-51.
4. Mathilde Krim, "Making Experimental Drugs Available for AIDS Treatment," *AIDS and Public Policy Journal* 2:2 (1987), 1-5.
5. Lynn McMonagle, "Private Rights to Adulterated/Misbranded Articles," *AIDS and Public Policy Journal* 2:2 (1987), 33-49.
6. 37 *Fed. Reg.* 16,503 (1972).
7. David J. Rothman, "Ethical and Social Issues in the Development of New Drugs and Vaccines," *Bulletin of the New York Academy of Medicine* 63:6 (1987), 557-68.
8. "Makers of AL-721 to Market Compound as Food Supplement," *AIDS and Policy Law* 3:6 (1988), 6.

9. "In Brief: Unapproved Drugs," *Rx Ipsa Loquitur* 15:8 (1988), 3.
10. B.R. Cassileth and H. Brown, "Unorthodox Cancer Medicine," *CA-Cancer Journal for Clinicians* 38:3 (1988), 176-86.
11. I am grateful to Gary Freedman for raising this important point.
12. J.A. Revson, "HIV Positive: Living Under the Shadow," *Newsday,* 18 Feb. 1988, Part II, 4-5, 11.
13. American Foundation for AIDS Research, *AIDS/HIV Experimental Treatment Directory,* (NY: AmFAR).
14. Mathilde Krim, "A Chance at Life for AIDS Sufferers," *New York Times,* 8 August 1986, A-27.
15. Frank E. Young *et al.,* "The FDA's New Procedures for the Use of Investigational Drugs in Treatment," *Journal of the American Medical Association* 259:15 (1988), 2267-70.
16. 52 *Fed. Reg.* no. 99, May 22, 1987, 19467-77.
17. Robert E. Wittes, "Noninvestigational Uses of Investigational Drugs: Some Implications of FDA's Revised Regulations," *Journal of the National Cancer Institute* 80:5 (1988), 301-304.
18. "Proposal to Make Investigational New Drugs Available Without Clinical Trial Participation in Certain Cases is Receiving Mixed Responses," *Journal of the American Medical Association* 257:22 (1987), 3020.
19. Dale Gieringer, "Twice Wrong on AIDS," *New York Times,* 12 January 1987, A-21.
20. Benjamin Freedman, "Equipoise and the Ethics of Clinical Research," *New England Journal of Medicine* 317 (1987), 141-45.
21. *Dateline: NIAID,* November 1987 (AIDS Research Issue), 7 ff.
22. I. Feldman *et al.,* "AIDS Center Designation/AIDS Intervention Management System," *AIDS and Public Policy Journal* 3:1 (1988), 29-31.
23. Currently, the open trial of long-term effects of AZT run by Burroughs-Wellcome in selected Canadian centres bears some resemblance to the system described herein, but differs in the degree of control granted to the drug company, in conformity with Canadian regulations on the control of investigational drugs. The designated centre approach has also been utilized in the introductory period of some medical devices and surgical procedures (for example, major organ transplants), but this has commonly been under the direction of insurers, governmental or private.
24. Dr. Norbert Gilmore cogently and forcefully presented these points.
25. Harold Vanderpool and Gary Weiss, "False Data and Last Hopes: Enrolling Ineligible Patients in Clinical Trials," *Hastings Center Report* 17:2 (1987), 16-19.

Should Alcoholics Compete Equally for Liver Transplantation?

Alvin H. Moss and Mark Siegler

The circumstances of liver transplantation are unique among organ transplantation because of the dire, absolute scarcity of donor livers and the predominance of one disease — alcohol-related end-stage liver disease — as the principal cause of liver failure. We propose that patients who develop end-stage liver disease through no fault of their own should have higher priority for receiving a liver transplant than those whose end-stage liver disease results from failure to obtain treatment for alcoholism. We base our proposal on considerations of fairness and on whether public support for liver transplantation can be maintained if, as a result of a first-come, first-served approach, patients with alcohol-related end-stage liver disease receive more than half the available donor livers. We conclude that since not all can live, priorities must be established for the use of scarce health care resources.

Until recently, liver transplantation for patients with alcohol-related end-stage liver disease (ARESLD) was not considered a treatment o ption. Most physicians in the transplant community did not recommend it because of initial poor results in this population[1] and because of a predicted high recidivism rate that would preclude long-term survival.[2] In 1988, however, Starzl and colleagues[3] reported 1-year survival rates for patients with ARESLD comparable to results in patients with other causes of end-stage liver disease (ESLD). Although the patients in the Pittsburgh series may represent a carefully selected population,[3,4] the question is no longer Can we perform transplants in patients with alcoholic liver disease and obtain acceptable results? but Should we? This question is particularly timely since the Health Care Financing Administration (HCFA) has recommended that Medicare coverage for liver transplantation be offered to patients with alcoholic cirrhosis who are abstinent. The HCFA proposes that the same eligibility criteria be used for patients with ARESLD as are used for patients with other causes of ESLD, such as primary biliary cirrhosis and sclerosing cholangitis.[5]

SHOULD PATIENTS WITH ARESLD RECEIVE TRANSPLANTS?

At first glance, this question seems simple to answer. Generally, in medicine, a therapy is used if it works and saves lives. But the circumstances of liver transplantation differ from those of most other lifesaving

Alvin H. Moss and Mark Siegler, "Should Alcoholics Compete Equally for Liver Transplantation? *JAMA 265*:(March 13, 1991) 1295-1298.

therapies, including long-term mechanical ventilation and dialysis, in three important respects:

Nonrenewable Resource

First, although most lifesaving therapies are expensive, liver transplantation uses a nonrenewable, absolutely scarce resource — a donor liver. In contrast to patients with end-stage renal disease, who may receive either a transplant or dialysis therapy, every patient with ESLD who does not receive a liver transplant will die. This dire, absolute scarcity of donor livers would be greatly exacerbated by including patients with ARESLD as potential candidates for liver transplantation. In 1985, 63 737 deaths due to hepatic disease occurred in the United States, at least 36 000 of which were related to alcoholism, but fewer than 1000 liver transplants were performed.[6] Although patients with ARESLD represent more than 50% of the patients with ESLD, patients with ARESLD account for less than 10% of those receiving transplants (*New York Times*. April 3, 1990:B6[col 1]). If patients with ARESLD were accepted for liver transplantation on an equal basis, as suggested by the HCFA, there would potentially be more than 30 000 additional candidates each year. (No data exist to indicate how many patients in the late stages of ARESLD would meet transplantation eligibility criteria.) In 1987, only 1182 liver transplants were performed; in 1989, fewer than 2000 were done.[6] Even if all donor livers available were given to patients with ARESLD, it would not be feasible to provide transplants for even a small fraction of them. Thus, the dire, absolute nature of donor liver scarcity mandates that distribution be based on unusually rigorous standards — standards not required for the allocation of most other resources such as dialysis machines and ventilators, both of which are only *relatively* scarce.

Comparison With Cardiac Transplantation

Second, although a similar dire, absolute scarcity of donor hearts exists for cardiac transplantation, the allocational decisions for cardiac transplantation differ from those for liver transplantation. In liver transplantation, ARESLD causes more than 50% of the cases of ESLD; in cardiac transplantation, however, no one predominant disease or contributory factor is responsible. Even for patients with end-stage ischemic heart disease who smoked or who failed to adhere to dietary regimens, it is rarely clear that one particular behavior caused the disease. Also, unlike our proposed consideration for liver transplantation, a history of alcohol abuse is considered a contraindication and is a common reason for a patient with heart disease to be denied cardiac transplantation.[7,8] Thus, the allocational decisions for heart transplantation differ from those for liver transplantation in two ways: determining a cause for end-stage heart disease is less certain, and patients with a history of alcoholism are usually rejected from heart transplant programs.

Expensive Technology

Third, a unique aspect of liver transplantation is that it is an expensive technology that has become a target of cost containment in health care.[9] It is, therefore, essential to maintain the approbation and support of the public so that organs continue to be donated under appropriate clinical circumstances — even in spite of the high cost of transplantation.

General Guideline Proposed

In view of the distinctive circumstances surrounding liver transplantation, we propose as a general guideline that patients with ARESLD should not compete equally with other candidates for liver transplantation. We are *not* suggesting that patients with ARESLD should *never* receive liver transplants. Rather, we propose that a priority ranking be established for the use of this dire, absolutely scarce societal resource and that patients with ARESLD be lower on the list than others with ESLD.

OBJECTIONS TO PROPOSAL

We realize that our proposal may meet with two immediate objections: (1) Some may argue that since alcoholism is a disease, patients with ARESLD should be considered equally for liver transplantation.[10] (2) Some will question why patients with ARESLD should be singled out for discrimination, when the medical profession treats many patients who engage in behavior that causes their diseases.[11] We will discuss these objections in turn.

Alcoholism: How Is It Similar to and Different From Other Diseases?

We do not dispute the reclassification of alcoholism as a disease.[12] Both hereditary and environmental factors contribute to alcoholism, and physiological, biochemical, and genetic markers have been associated with increased susceptibility.[13] Identifying alcoholism as a disease enables physicians to approach it as they do other medical problems and to differentiate it from bad habits, crimes, or moral weaknesses. More important, identifying alcoholism as a disease also legitimizes medical interventions to treat it.[14]

Alcoholism is a chronic disease,[12,15] for which treatment is available and effective. More than 1.43 million patients were treated in 5586 alcohol treatment units in the 12-month period ending October 30, 1987.[16] One comprehensive review concluded that more than two thirds of patients who accept therapy improve.[17] Another cited four studies in which at least 54% of patients were abstinent a minimum of 1 year after treatment.[18] A recent study of alcohol-impaired physicians reported a 100% abstinence rate an average of 33.4 months after therapy was initiated. In this study, physician-patients rated Alcoholics Anonymous, the largest organization of recovering alcoholics in the world, as the most important component of their therapy.[19]

Like other chronic diseases — such as type I diabetes mellitus, which requires the patient to administer insulin over a lifetime — alcoholism requires the patient to assume responsibility for participating in continuous treatment. Two key elements are required to successfully treat alcoholism: the patient must accept his or her diagnosis and must assume responsibility for treatment.[20,21] The high success rates of some alcoholism treatment programs indicate that many patients can accept responsibility for their treatment. ARESLD, one of the sequelae of alcoholism, results from 10 to 20 years of heavy alcohol consumption. The risk of ARESLD increases with the amount of alcohol consumed and with the duration of heavy consumption.[22] In view of the quantity of alcohol consumed, the years, even decades, required to develop ARESLD, and the availability of effective alcohol treatment, attributing personal responsibility for ARESLD to the patient seems all the more justified. We believe, therefore, that even though alcoholism is a chronic disease, alcoholics should be held responsible for seeking and obtaining treatment that could prevent the development of late-stage complications such as ARESLD. Our view is consistent with that of Alcoholics Anonymous: alcoholics are responsible for undertaking a program for recovery that will keep their disease of alcoholism in remission.[23]

Are We Discriminating Against Alcoholics?

Why should patients with ARESLD be singled out when a large number of patients have health problems that can be attributed to so-called voluntary health-risk behavior? Such patients include smokers with chronic lung disease; obese people who develop type II diabetes; some individuals who test positive for the human immunodeficiency virus; individuals with multiple behavioral risk factors (inattention to blood pressure, cholesterol, diet, and exercise) who develop coronary artery disease; and people such as skiers, motorcyclists, and football players who sustain activity-related injuries. We believe that the health care system should respond based on the actual medical needs of patients rather than on the factors (eg, genetic, infectious, or behavioral) that cause the problem. We also believe that individuals should bear some responsibility — such as increased insurance premiums — for medical problems associated with voluntary choices. The critical distinguishing factor for treatment of ARESLD is the scarcity of the resource needed to treat it. The resources needed to treat most of these other conditions are only moderately or relatively scarce, and patients with these diseases or injuries can receive a share of the resources (ie, money, personnel, and medication) roughly equivalent to their need. In contrast, there are insufficient donor livers to sustain the lives of all with ESLD who are in need.[24] This difference permits us to make some discriminating choices — or to establish priorities — in selecting candidates for liver transplantation based on notions of fairness. In addition, this reasoning enables us to offer patients with alcohol-related medical and surgical problems their fair share of relatively scarce resources, such as blood products, surgical care, and intensive care beds, while still maintaining that their claim on donor livers is less compelling than the claims of others.

REASONS PATIENTS WITH ARESLD SHOULD HAVE A LOWER PRIORITY ON TRANSPLANT WAITING LISTS

Two arguments support our proposal. The first argument is a moral one based on considerations of fairness. The second one is based on policy considerations and examines whether public support of liver transplantation can be maintained if, as a result of a first-come, first-served approach, patients with ARESLD receive more than half the available donor livers. Finally, we will consider further research necessary to determine which patients with ARESLD should be candidates for transplantation, albeit with a lower priority.

Fairness

Given a tragic shortage of donor livers, what is the fair or just way to allocate them? We suggest that patients who develop ESLD through no fault of their own (eg, those with congenital biliary atresia or primary biliary cirrhosis) should have a higher priority in receiving a liver transplant than those whose liver disease results from failure to obtain treatment for alcoholism. In view of the dire, absolute scarcity of donor livers, we believe it is fair to hold people responsible for their choices, including decisions to refuse alcoholism treatment, and to allocate organs on this basis.

It is unfortunate but not unfair to make this distinction.[25] When not enough donor livers are available for all who need one, choices have to be made, and they should be founded on one or more proposed principles of fairness for distributing scarce resources.[26,27] We shall consider four that are particularly relevant:

- *To each, an equal share of treatment.*
- *To each, similar treatment for similar cases.*
- *To each, treatment according to personal effort.*
- *To each, treatment according to ability to pay.*

It is not possible to give each patient with ESLD an *equal share*, or, in this case, a functioning liver. The problem created by the absolute scarcity of donor livers is that of inequality; some receive livers while others do not. But what is fair, need not be equal. Although a first-come, first-served approach has been suggested to provide each patient with an equal chance, we believe it is fairer to give a child dying of biliary atresia an opportunity for a *first* normal liver than it is to give a patient with ARESLD who was born with a normal liver a *second* one.

Because the goal of providing each person with an equal share of health care sometimes collides with the realities of finite medical resources, the principle of *similar treatment for similar cases* has been found to be helpful. Outka[26] stated it this way: "If we accept the case for equal access, but if we simply cannot, physically cannot, treat all who are in need, it seems more just to discriminate by virtue of categories of illness, rather than between rich ill and poor ill." This principle is derived from the principle of formal justice, which, roughly stated, says that people who are equal in relevant respects should be treated equally and that people who are unequal in relevant respects should be treated differently.[27] We believe that patients with ARESLD are unequal in a relevant respect to others with ESLD, since their liver failure was preventable; therefore, it is acceptable to treat them differently.

Our view also relies on the principle of *To each, treatment according to personal effort*. Although alcoholics cannot be held responsible for their disease, once their condition has been diagnosed they can be held responsible for seeking treatment and for preventing the complication of ARESLD. The standard of personal effort and responsibility we propose for alcoholics is the same as that held by Alcoholics Anonymous. We are not suggesting that some lives and behaviors have greater value than others — an approach used and appropriately repudiated when dialysis machines were in short supply.[26-30] But we are holding people responsible for their personal effort.

Health policymakers have predicted that this principle will assume greater importance in the future. In the context of scarce health care resources, Blank[31] foresees a reevaluation of our health care priorities, with a shift toward individual responsibility and a renewed emphasis on the individual's obligation to society to maximize one's health. Similarly, more than a decade ago, Knowles[32] observed that prevention of disease requires effort. He envisioned that the next major advances in the health of the American people would be determined by what individuals are willing to do for themselves.

To each, treatment according to ability to pay has also been used as a principle of distributive justice. Since alcoholism is prevalent in all socioeconomic strata, it is not discrimination against the poor to deny liver transplantation to patients with alcoholic liver disease.[33] In fact, we believe that poor patients with ARESLD have a stronger claim for a donor liver than rich patients, precisely because many alcohol treatment programs are not available to patients lacking in substantial private resources or health insurance. Ironically, it is precisely this group of poor and uninsured patients who are most likely not to be eligible to receive a liver transplant because of their inability to pay. We agree with Outka's view of fairness that would discriminate according to categories of illness rather than according to wealth.

Policy Considerations Regarding Public Support for Liver Transplantation

Today, the main health policy concerns involve issues of financing, distributive justice, and rationing medical care.[34-37] Because of the many deficiencies in the US health care system — in maternal and child health, in the unmet needs of the elderly, and in the millions of Americans without health insurance — an increasing number of commentators are drawing attention to the trade-offs between basic health care for the many and expensive, albeit lifesaving care for the few.[9,25,38,39]

Because of its high unit cost, liver transplantation is often at the center of these discussions, as it has been in Oregon, where the legislature voted to eliminate Medicaid reimbursement for all transplants except kidneys and corneas.[9] In this era of health care cost containment, a sense of limits is emerging and allocational choices are being made. Oregon has already shown that elected officials and the public are prepared to face these issues.

In our democracy, it is appropriate that community mores and values be regarded seriously when deciding the most appropriate use of a scarce and nonrenewable organ symbolized as a "Gift of Life." As if to underscore this point, the report of the Task Force on Organ Transplantation recommended that each donated organ be considered a national resource for the public good and that the public must participate in decisions on how to use this resource to best serve the public's interests.[40]

Much of the initial success in securing public and political approval for liver transplantation was achieved by focusing media and political attention not on adults but on children dying of ESLD. The public may not support transplantation for patients with ARESLD in the same way that they have endorsed this procedure for babies born with biliary atresia. This assertion is bolstered not only by the events in Oregon but also by the results of a Louis Harris and Associates[41] national survey, which showed that lifesaving therapy for premature infants or for patients with cancer was given the highest health care priority by the public and that lifesaving therapy for patients with alcoholic liver disease was given the lowest. In this poll, the public's view of health care priorities was shared by leadership groups also polled: physicians, nurses, employers, and politicians.

Just because a majority of the public holds these views does not mean that they are right, but the moral intuition of the public, which is also shared by its leaders, reflects community values that must be seriously considered. Also indicative of community values are organizations such as Mothers Against Drunk Driving, Students Against Drunk Driving, corporate employee assistance programs, and school student assistance programs. Their existence signals that many believe that a person's behavior can be modified so that the consequences of behavior such as alcoholism can be prevented.[42] Thus, giving donor livers to patients with ARESLD on an equal basis with other patients who have ESLD might lead to a decline in public support for liver transplantation.

Should any Alcoholics Be Considered for Transplantation? Need for Further Research

Our proposal for giving lower priority for liver transplantation to patients with ARESLD does not completely rule out transplantation for this group. Patients with ARESLD who had not previously been offered therapy and who are now abstinent could be acceptable candidates. In addition, patients lower on the waiting list, such as patients with ARESLD who have been treated and are now abstinent, might be eligible for a donor liver in some regions because of the increased availability of donor organs there. Even if only because of these possible conditions for transplantation, further research is needed to determine which patients with ARESLD would have the best outcomes after liver transplantation.

Transplant programs have been reluctant to provide transplants to alcoholics because of concern about one unfavorable outcome: a high recidivism rate. Although the overall recidivism rate for the Pittsburgh patients was only 11.5%, in the patients who had been abstinent less than 6 months it was 43%.[2] Also, compared with the entire group in which 1-year survival was 74%, the survival rate in this subgroup was lower, at 64%.[2]

In the recently proposed Medicare criteria for coverage of liver transplantation, the HCFA acknowledged that the decision to insure patients with alcoholic cirrhosis "may be considered controversial by some."[5] As if to counter possible objections, the HCFA listed requirements for patients with alcoholic cirrhosis: patients must meet the transplant center's requirement for abstinence prior to liver transplantation and have documented evidence of sufficient social support to ensure both recovery from alcoholism and compliance with the regimen of immunosuppressive medication.

Further research should answer lingering questions about liver transplantation for ARESLD patients: Which characteristics of a patient with ARESLD can predict a successful outcome? How long is abstinence necessary to qualify for transplantation? What type of a social support system must a patient have to ensure good results? These questions are being addressed.[43] Until the answers are known, we propose that further transplantation for patients with ARESLD be limited to abstinent patients who had not previously been offered alcoholism treatment and to abstinent treated patients in regions of increased donor liver availability and that it be carried out as part of prospective research protocols at a few centers skilled in transplantation and alcohol research.

COMMENT

Should patients with ARESLD compete equally for liver transplants? In a setting in which there is a dire, absolute scarcity of donor livers, we believe the answer is no. Considerations of fairness suggest that a first-come, first-served approach for liver transplantation is not the most just approach. Although this decision is difficult, it is only fair that patients who have not assumed equal responsibility for maintaining their health or for accepting treatment for a chronic disease should be treated differently. Considerations of public values and mores suggest that the public may not support liver transplantation if patients with ARESLD routinely receive more than half of the available donor livers. We conclude that since not all can live, priorities must be established and that patients with ARESLD should be given a lower priority for liver transplantation than others with ESLD.

NOTES

The Center for Clinical Medical Ethics and Alvin H. Moss, MD, are supported by grants from the Henry J. Kaiser Family Foundation and the Pew Charitable Trusts. The opinions expressed are those of the authors and should not be taken to represent those of the foundation or trust.

The authors thank Abe Kaplan for assistance in literature review; Rolly Sullivan, MD, for information on alcoholism treatment programs; and Michael D. Swenson, MD, PhD, for review of an earlier draft of the manuscript.

1. Scharschmidt, B.F. "Human liver transplantation: analysis of data on 540 patients from four centers." *Hepatology.* 1984;4:95S-101S.
2. Kumar, S., Stauber, R.E., Gavaler, J.S., et al. "Orthotopic liver transplantation for alcoholic liver disease." *Hepatology.* 1990;11:159-164.
3. Starzl, T.E., Van Thiel, D., Tzakis, A.G., et al. "Orthotopic liver transplantation for alcoholic cirrhosis." *JAMA.* 1988;260:2542-2544.
4. Olbrisch, M.E., Levenson, J.L. "Liver transplantation for alcoholic cirrhosis." *JAMA.* 1989;261:2958.
5. Health Care Financing Administration. "Medicare program: criteria for Medicare coverage of adult liver transplants." *Federal Register.* 1990;55:3545-3553.
6. Office of Health Technology Assessment, Agency for Health Care Policy Research. *Assessment of Liver Transplantation.* Rockville, Md: US Dept of Health and Human Services; 1990:3,25.
7. Schroeder, J.S., Hunt, S. "Cardiac transplantation update 1987." *JAMA.* 1987;258:3142-3145.
8. Surman, O.S. "Psychiatric aspects of organ transplantation." *Am J Psychiatry.* 1989;146:972-982.
9. Welch, H.G., Larson, E.B. "Dealing with limited resources: the Oregon decision to curtail funding for organ transplantation." *N Engl J Med.* 1988;319:171-173.
10. Flavin, D.K., Niven, R.G., Kelsey, J.E. "Alcoholism and orthotopic liver transplantation." *JAMA.* 1988;259:1546-1547.
11. Atterbury, C.E. "The alcoholic in the lifeboat: should drinkers be candidates for liver transplantation?" *J Clin Gastroenterol.* 1986;8:1-4.
12. Mendelson, J.H., Mello, N.K. *The Diagnosis and Treatment of Alcoholism.* 2nd ed. New York, NY: McGraw-Hill International Book Co; 1985:1-20.
13. Blum, K., Noble, E.P., Sheridan, P.J., et al. "Allelic association of human dopamine D_2 receptor gene in alcoholism." *JAMA.* 1990;263:2055-2060.
14. Aronson, M.D. "Definition of alcoholism." In: Barnes, H.N., Aronson, M.D., Delbanco, T.L., eds. *Alcoholism: A Guide for the Primary Care Physician.* New York, NY: Springer-Verlag NY Inc; 1987:9-15.
15. Klerman, G.L. "Treatment of alcoholism." *N Engl J Med.* 1989;320:394-395.
16. *Seventh Special Report to the US Congress on Alcohol and Health.* Washington, DC: US Dept of Health and Human Services; 1990. Publication 90-1656.

17. Saxe, L. *The Effectiveness and Costs of Alcoholism Treatment: Health Technology Case Study No. 22.* Washington, DC: Congress of the United States, Office of Technology Assessment;1983:3-6.

18. Nace, E.P. *The Treatment of Alcoholism.* New York, NY: Brunner/Mazel Publishers; 1987:43-46.

19. Galanter, M., Talbott, D., Gallegos, K., Rubenstone, E. "Combined Alcoholics Anonymous and professional care for addicted physicians." *Am J Psychiatry.* 1990;147:64-68.

20. Johnson, B., Clark, W. "Alcoholism: a challenging physician-patient encounter." *J Gen Intern Med.* 1989;4:445-452.

21. Bigby, J.A. "Negotiating treatment and monitoring recovery." In: Barnes, H.N., Aronson, M.D., Delbanco, T.L., eds. *Alcoholism: A Guide for the Primary Care Physician.* New York, NY: Springer-Verlag NY Inc; 1987:66-72.

22. Grant, B.F., Dufour, M.C., Harford, T.C. "Epidemiology of alcoholic liver disease." *Sem Liver Dis.* 1988;8:12-25.

23. Thoreson, R.W., Budd, F.C. "Self-help groups and other group procedures for treating alcohol problems." In: Cox, W.M., ed. *Treatment and Prevention of Alcohol Problems: A Resource Manual.* Orlando, Fla: Academic Press Inc; 1987:157-181.

24. Winslow, G.R. *Triage and Justice.* Berkeley: University of California Press; 1982:39-44, 133-150.

25. Engelhardt, H.T. Jr. "Shattuck Lecture: allocating scarce medical resources and the availability of organ transplantation." *N Engl J Med.* 1984;311:66-71.

26. Outka, G. "Social justice and equal access to health care." *J Religious Ethics.* 1974;2:11-32.

27. Beauchamp, T.L., Childress, J.F. *Principles of Biomedical Ethics.* 3rd ed. New York, NY: Oxford University Press; 1989:256-306.

28. Ramsey, P. *The Patient as Person.* New Haven, Conn: Yale University Press; 1970:242-252.

29. Fox, R.C., Swazey, J.P. *The Courage to Fail.* 2nd ed. Chicago, Ill: University of Chicago Press; 1978:226-265.

30. Annas, G.J. "The prostitute, the playboy, and the poet: rationing schemes for organ transplantation." *Am J Public Health.* 1985;75:187-189.

31. Blank, R.H. *Rationing Medicine.* New York, NY: Columbia University Press; 1988:1-37, 189-252.

32. Knowles, J.H. "Responsibility for health." *Science.* 1977;198:1103.

33. Moore, R.D., Bone, L.R., Geller, G., Marmon, J.A., Stokes, E.J., Levine, D.M. "Prevalence, detection, and treatment of alcoholism in hospitalized patients." *JAMA.* 1989;261:403-407.

34. Fuchs, V.R. "The 'rationing' of medical care." *N Engl J Med.* 1984;311:1572-1573.

35. Daniels, N. "Why saying no to patients in the United States is so hard: cost containment, justice, and provider autonomy." *N Engl J Med.* 1986;314:1380-1383.

36. Callahan, D. "Allocating health resources." *Hastings Cent Rep.* 1988;18:14-20.
37. Evans, R.W. "Health care technology and the inevitability of resource allocation and rationing decisions." *JAMA.* 1983;249:2047-2053, 2208-2219.
38. Thurow, L.C. "Learning to say no." *N Engl J Med.* 1984;311:1569-1572.
39. Caper, P. "Solving the medical care dilemma." *N Engl J Med.* 1988;318:1535-1536.
40. Task Force on Organ Transplantation. *Organ Transplantation: Issues and Recommendations.* Washington, DC: US Dept of Health and Human Services; 1986:9.
41. Louis Harris and Associates. *Making Difficult Health Care Decisions.* Boston, Mass: The Loran Commission; 1987:73-89.
42. Fishman, R. *Alcohol and Alcoholism.* New York, NY: Chelsea House Publishers; 1986:27-34.
43. Beresford, T.P., Turcotte, J.G., Merion, R., et al. "A rational approach to liver transplantation for the alcoholic patient." *Psychosomatics.* 1990;31:241-254.

FURTHER READINGS

Anscombe, Elizabeth
"Who Is Wronged?" *The Oxford Review* 5 (1967) 16–17.
Atterbury, C.E.
"The Alcoholic in the Lifeboat: Should Drinkers be Candidates for Liver Transplantation?" *Journal of Clinical Gastroenterology.* 1986; 8:1-4.
Cassel, Christine et al, eds.
Geriatric Medicine (New York: Springer Verlag, 1990).
Kluge, E.-H.W.
"Designated Organ Donation: Private Choice in Social Context," *Hastings Center Report* September/October 1989, 10–15.
Kluge, E.-H.W.
"Health Policy and the Allocation of Resources: The Ethics of Discrimination" in J.E. Thornton and E.R.Winkler, *Ethics and Aging: The Right to Live and the Right to Die.* (Vancouver: The University of British Columbia Press, 1988)
Magnet, J.E. and E.-H.W. Kluge
Withholding Treatment from Defective Newborn Children. (Cowansville: Brown Legal Publ., 1985), chapters 1 and 2
Rachels, James F.
"Who Shall Live when Not All Can Live?" *Soundings: An Interdisciplinary Journal* 53 (Winter, 1970) 339–355.
Report of the Council on Scientific Affairs of the American Medical Association
"Societal Effects and Other Factors Affecting Health Care for the Elderly," *Archives of Internal Medicine* 150: 6 (June 1990) 1184–1189.
Report of the Council on Ethical and Judicial Affairs of the American Medical Association
Ethical Implications of Age-Based Rationing of Health Care. (Chicago, Ill.: American Medical Association, 1988) I–88.

Rescher, Nicholas
"The Allocation of Exotic Medical Lifesaving Therapy," *Ethics* 79 (1969) 173–180.
Singer, P.
"A Review of Public Policies to Procure and Distribute Kidneys for Transplantation," *Archives of Internal Medicine* 150: 3 (March 1990) 523–527, 525–6.
Storch, Janet
Patients' Rights, Ethical and Legal Issues in Health Care and Nursing. (Toronto: McGraw-Hill, 1984), 122.
Sugden, R. and A. Williams
The Principles of Practical Cost-Benefit Analysis (Oxford: Oxford University Press, 1978).
Thornton, James E. and Earl R. Winkler, eds.
Ethics and Aging: The Right to Live, the Right to Die (Vancouver: The University of British Columbia Press, 1988).
Veatch, Robert
"Who Should Pay for Smokers' Medical Care?" *Hastings Center Report,* 4 (Nov. 1974), 8–9.
Veatch, R.M.
"Voluntary Risk to Health: The Ethical Issues," *Journal of the American Medical Association* 243 (Jan. 4, 1980) 50–55.
Young, Robert
"Some Criteria for Making Decisions Concerning the Distribution of Scarce Medical Resources," *Theory and Decision* 6 (1975) 439–455.
H. Moss, MD, Mark Siegler, MD

PART 2 THE PATIENT AND THE PROFESSIONAL

CHAPTER 4 THE HEALTH CARE PROFESSIONAL-PATIENT RELATIONSHIP

INTRODUCTION

In human terms, the most important thing in the delivery of health care is the relationship between the health care professional and the patient. This is not to say that no other factors have to be taken into account, or that no other relationships are important. For instance, the availability of health care resources plays a crucial role, because it defines the limits within which the delivery of care can take place. Likewise the relationship between the professional and next-of-kin of the patient, or with other health care professionals and society are also important, because they define the extended setting in which the delivery of care actually takes place.

However, the relationship between the professional and the patient is central, because it is the basis of the health care professional's interaction with all the other parties. It is also the *raison d'être* of health care itself. Therefore it is logically primary. How this relationship is structured sets the tone for everything else.

It could be argued that the relationship between a public health professional and society as a whole is different. But even here similar ethical problems arise and similar ethical considerations apply. Issues such as those of authority, compliance, informed consent and above all trust are also implicated. The only difference is that in the case of public health, society itself has taken the place of the individual patient.

Of course the fact that society is composed of many individuals does introduce issues that do not exist in the usual health care professional-patient relationship. The question of aggregate, as opposed to individual, rights constitutes a particular thorny — and distinctive — issue. However, even here the relationship between the health care professional and the individual patient remains important; because in the end, activities that are directed towards the public good must be translated into actions that affect individual patients. With this, the professional-patient relationship once again comes to the fore.

The traditional view held by *physicians themselves* was that the physician is the captain of the ship, and that the patient has to follow orders. We find this expressed in the writings of Hippocrates — himself a physician — and those of later medical writers like Galen, Razes, Maimonides and so on. For the English-speaking world, this found its classic statement in Thomas Percival's *Medical Ethics*. (Incidentally, Percival also had a similar view of nurses and other health care workers.)

While for centuries this was the outlook of physicians themselves, for a long time society did not entirely share this perspective. Until well into the nineteenth century, the physician was seen as a figure of last resort — and even then, as someone who gave advice, but whose advice could be ignored by the patient. It was not until the nineteenth century, and even more in the twentieth when medicine became a legally recognized service-provider monopoly, that the physician came to be seen as the primary decision-maker: as the person who knew best, and who therefore had not only the right but also the duty to make the decision.

Nowadays, such a physician-centred perspective is no longer in vogue. In fact, this sort of approach to physician authority would be characterized as being extremely paternalistic in nature. The selections that follow present an examination of how the relationship between the health care professional and the patient should be structured from a contemporary perspective.

In an article that has become a classic, Robert Veatch identified four models of the physician-patient relationship. He distinguished between what he called the engineering model, the priestly model, the collegial and the contractual model.

According to the engineering model, the physician is nothing more than an "applied scientist," who simply presents the patient with diagnosis, prognosis and treatment options, but leaves the decision-making completely up to the patient. Questions of ethics and values do not enter into the relationship so far as the physician is concerned. "The physician becomes a plumber without any moral integrity."

What Veatch called the priestly model is what is also often called the paternalistic model. This model is exactly the reverse of the engineering model. The physician here acts on the basis of the principle, "Benefit and do not harm the patient," but it is the physician who decides what constitutes benefit and harm. "The moral authority [of the physician] so dominates ... that the patient's freedom and dignity are extinguished."

According to the collegial model, both physician and patient are connected by common bonds of mutual loyalty, common interests and goals. It is also characterized by the assumption that physician and patient come together as independent equals.

Finally, the contractual model questions this assumption of equality. It recognizes the differences in knowledge and power between physician and patient, and tries to compensate for this in terms of an assumed — and sometimes even explicit — contractual perspective that leaves both parties their own dignity and moral authority. There have been various modifications and improvements on Veatch's account. Some of them are listed in the *Further Readings* at the end of this chapter. However, Veatch's account has remained most influential.

Christie and Hoffmaster focus on the physician-patient relationship in the context of family medicine, rather than of medicine in general. They look at several different models — that of Veatch included — and argue that not only are these models generally too idealistic, they are also unrealistic. Christie and Hoffmaster contend that "the sharp distinction between clinical decision and value or moral decisions is untenable."

Christie and Hoffmaster identify four roles played by physicians: (1) dispensing information, (2) dispensing information, and giving advice as well, (3) giving information and advice, but at the same time trying to persuade, and (4) simply acting as the ultimate decision-maker. Christie and Hoffmaster argue that all four roles have their appropriate place, and that an analysis of the physician-patient relationship that is not alive to this "is not sensitive to the realities and intricacies of clinical encounters."

Finally, there is a branch of health care that is frequently overlooked in discussion of patient-professional relationships: psychiatry. Yet the relationship between psychiatrist and patient is in some ways unique. In no other health care context is the opportunity for shaping the personal life of the patient so great — and in no other branch of health care is there so much opportunity for abuse of the trust and the dependence that the patient brings to the interaction. Lakin, who is himself a practising psychiatrist, explores some of the ethical aspects of the relationship, and indicates some dangers inherent in it. It might be useful to compare what he says on the nature of the psychiatrist-patient relationship with what Hoffmaster and Christie have to say about the specialized relationship between family physicians and their patients.

Models for Ethical Medicine in a Revolutionary Age

Robert M. Veatch

Most of the ethical problems in the practice of medicine come up in cases where the medical condition or desired procedure itself presents no moral problem. Most day-to-day patient contacts are just not cases which are ethically exotic. For the woman who spends five hours in the clinic waiting room with two screaming children waiting to be seen for the flu, the flu is not a special moral problem; her wait is. When medical students practice drawing bloods from clinic patients in the cardiac care unit — when teaching material is treated as material — the moral problem is not really related to the patient's heart in the way it might be in a more exotic heart transplant. Many more blood samples are drawn, however, than hearts transplanted. It is only by moving beyond the specific issues to more basic underlying ethical themes that the real ethical problems in medicine can be dealt with.

Most fundamental of the underlying themes of the new medical ethics is that health care must be a human right, no longer a privilege limited to those who can afford it. It has not always been that way, and, of course, is not anything near that in practice today. But the norm, the moral claim, is becoming increasingly recognized. Both of the twin revolutions have made their contribution to this change. Until this century health care could be treated as a luxury, no matter how offensive this might be now. The amount of real healing that went on was minimal anyway. But now, with the biological revolution, health care really is essential to "life, liberty, and the pursuit of happiness." And health care is a right for everyone because of the social revolution which is really a revolution in our conception of justice. If the obscure phrase "all men are created equal" means anything in the medical context where biologically it is clear that they are not equal, it means that they are equal in the legitimacy of their moral claim. They must be treated equally in what is essential to their humanity: dignity, freedom, individuality. The sign in front of the prestigious, modern hospital, "Methadone patients use side door" is morally offensive even if it means nothing more than that the Methadone Unit is located near that door. It is strikingly similar to "Coloreds to the back of the bus." With this affirmation of the right to health care, what are the models of professional-lay relationships which permit this and other basic ethical theme to be conveyed?

1. THE ENGINEERING MODEL

One of the impacts of the biological revolution is to make the physician scientific. All too often he behaves like an applied scientist. The rhetoric of the scientific tradition in the modern world is that the scientist must be "pure." He must be factual, divorcing himself from all considerations of value. It has taken atomic bombs and Nazi medical research to let us see the foolishness and danger of such a stance. In the first place the scientist, and certainly the applied scientist, just cannot logically be

Robert M. Veatch, "Models for Ethical Medicine in a Revolutionary Age," from *The Hastings Center Report* vol 2 (June 1972).

value-free. Choices must be made daily — in research design, in significance levels of statistical tests, and in perception of the "significant" observations from an infinite perceptual field, and each of these choices requires a frame of values on which it is based. Even more so in an applied science like medicine choices based upon what is "significant," what is "valuable," must be made constantly. The physician who thinks he can just present all the facts and let the patient make the choices is fooling himself even if it is morally sound and responsible to do this at all the critical points where decisive choices are to be made. Furthermore, even if the physician logically could eliminate all ethical and other value considerations from his decision-making and even if he could in practice conform to the impossible value-free ideal, it would be morally outrageous for him to do so. It would make him an engineer, a plumber making repairs, connecting tubes and flushing out clogged systems, with no questions asked. Even though I strongly favor abortion reform, I am deeply troubled by a physician who really believes abortion is murder *in the full sense* if he agrees to either perform one or refer to another physician. Hopefully no physician would do so when confronted with a request for technical advice about murdering a postnatal human.

2. THE PRIESTLY MODEL

In proper moral revulsion to the model which makes the physician into a plumber for whom his own ethical judgments are completely excluded, some move to the opposite extreme, making the physician a new priest. Establishment sociologist of medicine Robert N. Wilson describes the physician-patient relationship as religious. "The doctor's office or the hospital room, for example," he says, "have somewhat the aura of a sanctuary, ... the patient must view his doctor in a manner far removed from the prosaic and the mundane."

The priestly model leads to what I call the "As-a syndrome." The symptoms are verbal, but the disease is moral. The chief diagnostic sign is the phrase "speaking-as-a ..." In counseling a pregnant woman who has taken Thalidomide, a physician says, "The odds are against a normal baby and 'speaking-as-a-physician' that is a risk you shouldn't take." One must ask what it is about medical training that lets this be said "as-a-physician" rather than as a friend or as a moral man or as a priest. The problem is one of generalization of expertise: transferring of expertise in the technical aspects of a subject to expertise in moral advice.

The main ethical principle which summarizes this priestly tradition is "Benefit and do no harm to the patient." Now attacking the principle of doing no harm to the patient is a bit like attacking fatherhood. (Motherhood has not dominated the profession in the Western tradition.) But Fatherhood has long been an alternative symbol for the priestly model; "Father" has traditionally been a personalistic metaphor for God and for the priest. Likewise, the classical medical sociology literature (the same literature using the religious images) always uses the parent-child image as an analogy for the physician-patient relationship. It is this paternalism in the realm of values which is represented in the moral slogan "Benefit and do no harm to the patient." It takes the locus of decision-making away from the patient and places it in the hands of the professional. In doing so it destroys or at least minimizes the other moral themes essential to a more balanced ethical system. While a professional group may affirm this principle as adequate for a professional ethic, it is clear that society, more generally, has a much broader set of ethical norms. If the professional group is affirming one norm while society affirms another for the same circumstances, then the physician is placed in the uncomfortable position of having to decide whether his loyalty is to the norms of his professional group or to those of the broader society. What would this larger set of norms include?

Producing Good and Not Harm

Outside of the narrowest Kantian tradition, no one excludes the moral duty of producing good and avoiding harm entirely. Let this be said from the start. Some separate producing good and avoiding evil into two different principles placing greater moral weight on the latter, but this is also true within the tradition of professional medical ethics. The real difference is that in a set of ethical norms used more universally in the broader society producing good and avoiding harm is set in a much broader context and becomes just one of a much larger set of moral obligations.

Protecting Individual Freedom

Personal freedom is a fundamental value in society. It is essential to being truly human. Individual freedom for both physician and patient must be protected even if it looks like some harm is going to be done in the process. This is why legally competent patients are permitted by society to refuse blood transfusions or other types of medical care even when to the vast majority of us the price seems to be one of great harm. Authority about what constitutes harm and what constitutes good (as opposed to procedures required to obtain a particular predetermined good or harm) cannot be vested in any one particular group of individuals. To do so would be to make the error of generalizing expertise.

Preserving Individual Dignity

Equality of moral significance of all persons means that each is given fundamental dignity. Individual freedom of choice and control over one's own life and body contribute to that dignity. We might say that this more universal, societal ethic of freedom and dignity is one which moves beyond B. F. Skinner.

Many of the steps in the hospitalization, care, and maintenance of the patient, particularly seriously ill patients, are currently an assault on that dignity. The emaciated, senile man connected to life by IV tubes, tracheotomy, and colostomy has difficulty retaining his sense of dignity. Small wonder that many prefer to return to their own homes to die. It is there on their own turf that they have a sense of power and dignity.

Truth-Telling and Promise-Keeping

As traditional as they sound, the ethical obligations of truth-telling and promise-keeping have retained their place in ethics because they are seen as essential to the quality of human relationships. It is disturbing to see these fundamental elements of human interaction compromised, minimized, and even eliminated supposedly in order to keep from harming the patient. This is a much broader problem than the issue of what to tell the terminal carcinoma patient or the patient for whom there has been an unanticipated discovery of an XYY chromosome pattern when doing an amniocentesis for mongolism. It arises when the young boy getting his measles shot is told "Now this won't hurt a bit" and when a medical student is introduced on the hospital floor as "Doctor." And these all may be defended as ways of keeping from harming the patient. It is clear that in each case, also, especially if one takes into account the long range threat to trust and confidence, that in the long run these violations of truth-telling and promise-keeping may do more harm than good. Both the young boy getting the shot and the medical student are being taught what to expect from the medical profession in the future. But even if that were not the case, each is an assault on patient dignity and freedom and humanity. Such actions may be justifiable sometimes, but the case must be awfully strong.

Maintaining and Restoring Justice

Another way in which the ethical norms of the broader society move beyond concern for helping and not harming the patient is by insisting on a fair distribution of health services. What we have been calling the social revolution, as prefigurative as it may be, has heightened our concern for equality in the distribution of basic health services. If health care is a right then it is a right for all. It is not enough to produce individual cases of good health or even the best aggregate health statistics. Even if the United States had the best health statistics in the world (which it does not have), if this were attained at the expense of inferior health care for certain groups within the society it would be ethically unacceptable.

At this point in history with our current record of discriminatory delivery of health services there is a special concern for restoring justice. Justice must also be compensatory. The health of those who have been discriminated against must be maintained and restored as a special priority.

3. THE COLLEGIAL MODEL

With the engineering model the physician becomes a plumber without any moral integrity. With the priestly model his moral authority so dominates the patient that the patient's freedom and dignity are extinguished. In the effort to develop a more proper balance which would permit the other fundamental values and obligations to be preserved, some have suggested that the physician and the patient should see themselves as colleagues pursuing the common goal of eliminating the illness and preserving the health of the patient. The physician is the patient's "pal." It is in the collegial model that the themes of trust and confidence play the most crucial role. When two individuals or groups are truly committed to common goals then trust and confidence are justified and the collegial model is appropriate. It is a very pleasant, harmonious way to interact with one's fellow human beings. There is an equality of dignity and respect, an equality of value contributions, lacking in the earlier models.

But social realism makes us ask the embarrassing question. Is there, in fact, any real basis for the assumption of mutual loyalty and goals, of common interest which would permit the unregulated community of colleagues model to apply to the physician-patient relationship?

There is some proleptic sign of a community of real common interests in some elements of the radical health movement and free clinics, but for the most part we have to admit that ethnic, class, economic, and value differences make the assumption of common interest which is necessary for the collegial model to function are a mere pipedream. What is needed is a more provisional model which permits equality in the realm of moral significance between patient and physician without making the utopian assumption of collegiality.

4 THE CONTRACTUAL MODEL

The model of social relationship which fits these conditions is that of the contract or covenant. The notion of contract should not be loaded with legalistic implications, but taken in its more symbolic form as in the traditional religious or marriage "contract" or "covenant." Here two individuals or groups are interacting in a way where there are obligations and expected benefits for both parties. The obligations and benefits are limited in scope, though, even if they are expressed in somewhat vague terms. The basic norms of freedom, dignity, truth-telling, promise-keeping, and justice are essential to a contractual relationship. The premise is trust and confidence even though it is recognized that there is not a full mutuality of interests. Social sanctions institutionalize and stand behind the relationship, in case there is a violation of the contract, but for the most part the assumption is that there will be a faithful fulfillment of the obligations.

Only in the contractual model can there be a true sharing of ethical authority and responsibility. This avoids the moral abdication on the part of the physician in the engineering model and the moral abdication on the part of the patient in the priestly model. It also avoids the uncontrolled and false sense of equality in the collegial model. With the contractual relationship there is a sharing in which the physician recognizes that the patient must maintain freedom of control over his own life and destiny when significant choices are to be made. Should the physician not be able to live with his conscience under those terms the contract is not made or is broken. This means that there will have to be relatively greater open discussion of the moral premises hiding in medical decisions before and as they are made.

With the contractual model there is a sharing in which the patient has legitimate grounds for trusting that once the basic value framework for medical decision-making is established on the basis of the patient's own values, the myriads of minute medical decisions which must be made day in and day out in the care of the patient will be made by the physician within that frame of reference.

In the contractual model, then, there is a real sharing of decision-making in a way that there is realistic assurance that both patient and physician will retain their moral integrity. In this contractual context patient control of decision-making in the individual level is assured without the necessity of insisting that the patient participate in every trivial decision. On the social level community control of health care is made possible in the same way. The lay community is given and should be given the status of contractor. The locus of decision-making is thus in the lay community, but the day-to-day medical decisions can, with trust and confidence, rest with the medical community. If trust and confidence are broken the contract is broken.

Medical ethics in the midst of the biological and social revolutions is dealing with a great number of new and difficult ethical cases: in vitro fertilization, psychosurgery, happiness pills, brain death, and the military use of medical technology. But the real day-to-day ethical crises may not be nearly so exotic. Whether the issue is in an exotic context or one which is nothing more complicated medically than a routine physical exam, the ethos of ethical responsibility established by the appropriate selection of a model for the moral relationship between the professional and the lay communities will be decisive. This is the real framework for medical ethics in a revolutionary age.

The Physician-Patient Relationship

Ronald J. Christie and C. Barry Hoffmaster

> Clinical medicine should be regarded neither as an art nor as a science in itself, but as a special kind of relationship between two persons, a doctor and a patient...
>
> – Ashley Montagu[1]

The physician-patient relationship is the core and "basic tool"[2] of family medicine. Family physicians should seek to develop and maintain a rapport with patients because good relationships have both intrinsic and instrumental value. Personal relationships between human beings, whether inside or outside medicine, are valuable in themselves. But a close, friendly relationship between physician and patient also can improve the quality of care a patient receives. Peabody recognized long ago that "the practice of medicine in its broadest sense includes the whole relationship of the physician with his patient."[3]

The importance of good relationships with patients helps to explain why continuity of care is central to family practice.[4] Harmonious, trusting relationships require time to develop, and continuous care provided over an extended period makes that time available. Sharing meaningful and challenging experiences, such as pregnancy and childbirth, the raising of children, and acute, chronic, and terminal illnesses, contributes to the strength of the relationship. From the perspective of a family physician, the value of close relationships with patients is difficult to underestimate. McWhinney even suggests that such relationships can be the chief reward of a family physician's career.[5]

The physician-patient relationship can be examined in many ways.[6] Of direct relevance to family physicians is an understanding of its therapeutic dimensions. How does a good physician-patient relationship enhance the quality of care given to a patient? Again, the classic statement, emphasizing the clinical value of a personal physician-patient relationship and anticipating much of what has been incorporated into family medicine, comes from Peabody:

> Now the essence of the practice of medicine is that it is an intensely personal matter, and one of the chief differences between private practice and hospital practice is that the latter always tends to become impersonal.... The treatment of a disease may be entirely impersonal; the care of a patient must be completely personal. The significance of the intimate personal relationship between physician and patient cannot be too strongly emphasized, for in an extraordinarily large number of cases both diagnosis and treatment are directly dependent on it, and the failure of the young physician to establish this relationship accounts for much of his ineffectiveness in the care of patients.[7]

...Peabody recognizes the extent to which psychological and emotional causes of diseases and problems of living are part

Ronald J. Christie and C. Barry Hoffmaster, "The Physician-Patient Relationship," from Christie and Hoffmaster, *Ethical Issues in Family Medicine*. (New York and Oxford: Oxford University Press, 1986) chapter 2. (pp.19-31).

of family practice.[8] In this large group of patients, it is not the disease but rather the person who requires treatment. Successful diagnosis and treatment of these patients depend upon a close personal relationship. Without such a relationship, it is difficult for a physician to discover the underlying emotional and psychological roots of their problems. Peabody's article could be a handbook for family physicians, because it directs physicians to get to know their patients as persons. This entails learning about their families and friends, their work, and their play. Peabody advises physicians to practice various nursing techniques, because during the performance of these friendly services, the physician will find that "the patient suddenly starts to unburden himself, and a flood of light is thrown on the situation."[9]

In summary, knowing the character and personal life of a patient is important for both the management of functional problems and the treatment of organic diseases and is best achieved through a friendly, personal physician-patient relationship, which in itself has considerable therapeutic potential. For this reason family physicians will appreciate Peabody's oft-quoted aphorism that "the secret of the care of the patient is in caring for the patient."[10]

Because a good physician-patient relationship can have therapeutic benefits for a patient, family physicians should strive to foster such relationships. There is another perspective on the physician-patient relationship that is important from an ethical point of view, however. Who should be making what decisions in the context of this relationship? This question is most evident with respect to the selection of treatment plans, but it also arises for diagnostic tests. What should a physician do, for example, when a patient refuses a diagnostic x-ray? In the past, patients used to request or demand x-rays; today, physicians frequently hear, "I don't want an x-ray, Doctor: it's too dangerous."[11] This is a value decision because it involves a judgment about competing risks and benefits. Should the physician or the patient make this decision? Advocates of patient autonomy contend that it should be left to the patient. Physicians are likely to resist such a proposal and argue that this is a matter for a clinician's professional judgment:

> What should the doctor's attitude be when a patient refuses roentgenography? Some socially conscious individuals argue that it is up to the patient to make the decision once the physician properly informs him. In my opinion asking a patient to make his own decision is unethical. The attending physician cannot communicate his years of training and experience to the patient. No matter how well the problem is explained, the decision will have to be made by the physician. The patient just does not have enough knowledge of the risk of a wrong or absent diagnosis, and he will be unduly influenced by what is essentially distorted information in the news media.[12]

A common strategy for addressing the question "Who should decide?" consists of formulating models of where the locus of decision-making in the physician-patient relationship ought to reside.

Three such models are provided by Szasz and Hollender: the "activity-passivity" model, the "guidance-cooperation" model, and the "mutual participation" model.[13] In the activity-passivity model, a physician acts on a patient who remains passive. The patient is in no position to participate and, for all practical purposes, can be regarded as inanimate. Clinical applications of this model include the treatment of patients under anesthesia or during emergencies when a patient is severely injured, delirious, or in a coma. A nonmedical analogue is the relationship between a parent and an infant.

The model of guidance-cooperation applies when a patient is ill and comes to a physician seeking help. Because the patient takes the initiative of coming to a physician, it is assumed that the patient is willing to cooperate with the physician and accepts the physician's position of power. In this situation both parties can contribute and therefore are active. The main difference is the inequality in power. The patient is expected to cooperate, to "look up to" and to "obey" the doctor. This model is used in the treatment of acute diseases. It is analogous to the relationship between a parent and an adolescent.

The model of mutual participation assumes equality among individuals. In this model the participants must have approximately equal power, must be mutually interdependent, and must engage in an activity that is satisfying to both. It is preferred by patients who want to assume responsibility for their own care. Clinically it is used in the treatment of chronic illnesses, for example, diabetes mellitus and chronic heart disease. A relationship between two adults is the analogue of this model.

These three models are primarily descriptive, in that they depict the different relationships or interactions that actually occur between physicians and patients. But there are also normative dimensions to the models. Szasz and Hollender use the models normatively when they make claims about their appropriateness. They view the activity-passivity model, for example, as entirely appropriate for emergencies and the mutual participation model as rarely appropriate for children or for persons who are mentally deficient, poorly educated, or profoundly immature. Moreover, in their view, the greater the similarity between the intellectual, educational, and general experiences of physician and patient, the more appropriate the model of mutual participation becomes. They claim the model of guidance-cooperation underlies much of medical practice and imply that this is as it should be. Patient preferences for the models are considered, but not in a way that accords them ethical significance. Rather, the ethical force of patient preferences sometimes is dismissed. A patient who favors the mutual participation model, they suggest, might be exhibiting "an overcompensatory attempt at mastering anxieties associated with helplessness and passivity."[14] They recognize that a discrepancy between the preferences of physician and patient often is resolved by the patient seeking a new physician. Szasz and Hollender avoid direct claims about whether one model is better than another. They feel that "each of the three types of therapeutic relationship is entirely appropriate under certain circumstances and each is inappropriate under others."[15]

The main virtue of Szasz and Hollender's account is their appreciation that different models suit different circumstances. The status and condition of the patient and the nature and seriousness of the patient's problem are particularly important in determining which model fits. No single model is applicable to the diverse array of clinical situations. The main flaw in their account is their failure to grasp the extent to which claims about the appropriateness of the models are founded on normative considerations. When the appropriateness of one model depends on the impossibility of using the other models, no value judgment is involved. But when the appropriateness of a model rests on a comparison of the intellectual, educational, and general experiences of physician and patient, for example, a value judgment is involved. Likewise, the extent to which patient preferences are relevant is a key normative issue. With Szasz and Hollender, the normative foundations of their views remain largely covert.

By way of contrast, Veatch's models of the physician-patient relationship are unabashedly normative.[16] His four models — the "engineering" model, the "priestly" model, the "collegial" model, and the "contractual" model — concern where the locus of decision-making *ought* to be in the physician-patient relationship. In the engineering model, a physician is viewed as an engineer or a plumber hired by the patient. Because decisions are assumed to be value-free, the job of the physician is merely to present the facts to the patient and allow the patient to make decisions. The priestly model is the opposite of the engineering model. A physician is seen as a priest who has the authority to make moral decisions on behalf of patients. According to Veatch, this model is paternalistic, because it takes decision-making responsibility away from the patient and puts it in the hands of the physician. The collegial model regards physician and patient as colleagues pursuing the common goal of eliminating illness and preserving the health of the patient. In Veatch's words, the physician is the patient's "pal." In the contractual model, the contract is not to be understood as a formal legal contract but rather more symbolically as a covenant or undertaking. Obligations are imposed on both parties, and both parties derive benefits. The terms of the "contract," even when expressed vaguely, restrict these obligations and benefits. Indeterminacy should not be a significant problem, Veatch contends, because the contract is founded upon mutual trust and confidence.

Veatch argues that the contractual model should be adopted by physicians and patients:

> Only in the contractual model can there be a true sharing of ethical authority and responsibility. This avoids the moral abdication on the part of the physician in the engineering model and the moral abdication on the part of the patient in the priestly model. It also avoids the uncontrolled and false sense of equality in the collegial model. With the contractual relationship there is a sharing in which the physician recognizes that the patient must maintain freedom of control over his own life and destiny when significant choices are to be made.[17]

In this view, patient and physician "share" decision-making. This means that they should hold an open discussion of moral and value issues. The resulting, mutually accepted framework within which subsequent decisions are to be made must be based *exclusively* upon the patient's values, however. The patient retains the authority to make major or "significant" decisions, while the physician is trusted to make inconsequential "medical" decisions. Thus, in the contractual model, "patient control of decision-making in the individual level is assured without the necessity of insisting that the patient participate in every trivial decision."[18] Veatch takes this model to be universally applicable. The contractual model should structure all encounters between physician and patient.

There are two theoretical problems with Veatch's view. The first concerns the "fallacy of the generalization of expertise," which Veatch introduces as an objection to the priestly model. The fallacy of the generalization of expertise is defined as the "transferring of expertise in the technical aspects of a subject to expertise in moral advice."[19] The illicit nature of this move frequently is used as an argument against allowing physicians to make *any* moral or value decisions on behalf of patients. As the recapitulation of the argument by a doctor reveals, this line of reasoning appeals to physicians as well as philosophers:

> Part of being a patient is admitting that a physician has more knowledge about certain malfunctions than you have. An implication of this is that you follow his instructions because he is a doctor and you trust him. In moral matters, the physician has no reason to have the special knowledge he has in physiologic matters. Indeed, some have argued that in moral matters no one but the person making the decision has any special knowledge or should have a special position. For a physician to suggest a moral decision to his patient is for him to lay aside his professional expertise and act as a friend and counsellor. Physicians may play this part well or badly, but it is not part of medicine's role as such. To make it part of that role would be to coerce patients in a way inimical to our free system. A man must be allowed to choose what he thinks is right; to set up a professional who has expertise in one field as an expert in moral decision-making is to use illegitimately the respect garnered in one capacity for influence that may have no relation to that capacity.[20]

While this is an influential argument,[21] one should avoid being seduced by it. The argument is valid only insofar as it shows that expertise in one area does not confer expertise in another area, in particular, that medical expertise does not confer moral expertise. One can legitimately conclude that physicians are not moral experts by virtue of their medical training. But that is a weak conclusion. What is commonly taken to follow from the argument, but what does not follow, is the stronger conclusion that physicians are not allowed to make value or moral decisions on behalf of their patients *simpliciter*. To defend this stronger claim, one would need to produce independent arguments. In other words, the argument merely points to one bad reason for thinking that doctors should be allowed to make value or moral decisions for their patients. The argument does not establish that there can never be a good reason for this claim. The so-called "fallacy" of the generalization of expertise does not, by itself, entail that physicians may not make *any* value or moral decisions on behalf of their patients.[22]

Another problem with the "fallacy" of the generalization of expertise is that the sharp distinction between clinical decisions and value or moral decisions it presupposes is untenable. The argument grants that physicians have expertise to make clinical decisions by virtue of their medical training, but insists that this expertise does not extend to a different category of decisions, namely, those that involve value or moral issues. What the argument fails to recognize is that many clinical decisions are value decisions. Clinical decisions involve the playing of odds, the weighing of risks and benefits.[23] Case 2-1 illustrates this point with a deliberately mundane example.

Case 2-1

Mr. D, who is 27 years old, sees Dr. G, his family physician, because of a cough and fever which have been present for the past three days. Mr. D's sleep is disturbed by his coughing, and he generally feels unwell. Dr. G examines Mr. D and concludes that the diagnosis is acute bronchitis. After inquiring about a history of allergic reaction, Dr. G prescribes penicillin.

On the one hand, penicillin may kill the organisms that are causing the bronchitis. On the other hand, Mr. D may have an allergic reaction to the penicillin and even die. A physician will naturally ask a patient about penicillin allergy, but even if the patient has never had an allergic reaction, it is possible for one to occur. A physician must weigh the values of alternative outcomes and the probabilities associated with them in deciding whether to use penicillin to treat bronchitis. This is a value decision, yet many people would regard it as a paradigm of a clinical decision that falls within a physician's expertise. Thus, one cannot draw a rigid distinction between clinical decisions and value or moral decisions and hold that while the former fall within a physician's purview, the latter do not.

Even if many treatment decisions are value decisions, not all treatment decisions should be made by physicians. Some treatment decisions should be made by the patient, as in the following case.

Case 2-2

Ms. S, a 38-year-old lawyer, is found at a routine examination by Dr. W, her family physician, to have a nodule in her right breast. Dr. W refers her to a surgeon for assessment and management. A biopsy reveals that the lesion is malignant, and a modified radical mastectomy is recommended by the surgeon.

Ms. S is aware that other forms of therapy are possible. Several of her friends advise her to undergo only local excision of the lump so that her appearance will not be significantly altered and she will not experience the psychological trauma of mastectomy. The surgeon, however, continues to argue that the best treatment would be a modified radical mastectomy.

A decision about the "best" treatment in this case extends beyond the clinical judgments of either Ms. S's surgeon or family physician. What is the difference between Cases 2-1 and 2-2? The two cases cannot be differentiated on the basis of a simplistic appeal to the "fallacy" of the generalization of expertise or a rigid distinction between clinical and value decisions. Other considerations must be adduced, and these must involve more than the potential seriousness of the outcome, for the management of both bronchitis and breast cancer raises the possibility of the patient's death. One important difference is that the probability of death is higher in Case 2-2. But how much significance should be attached to varying probabilities? That is a crucial value decision as well. The question of what value decisions a physician may make on behalf of patients is more complicated than people have recognized. One could start to construct an answer by analyzing all the relevant differences between Cases 2-1 and 2-2. At this point, however, we are concerned only with refuting the extreme claim that doctors are never permitted to make value or moral decisions for their patients.

The second problem with Veatch's view concerns his endorsement of the contractual model. His primary argument is that the contractual model avoids the moral abdication inherent in the engineering and priestly models by allowing for "a true sharing of ethical authority and responsibility." But given the way in which Veatch describes the decision-making process, how does a physician participate in this "sharing"? All decisions, whether trivial or significant, are to be made within the framework of the patient's values. The patient makes significant decisions himself, presumably through the mechanism of informed consent. A physician is granted discretion to make trivial "medical" decisions within the limits imposed by the patient's values. It would be surprising if the question of responsibility for these trivial decisions arose at all. If it did, however, who would be responsible for them? A physician could be held responsible, and thus blameworthy, if he made a decision inconsistent with the patient's values. But as long as the decision is consistent with those values, ultimate responsibility resides with the patient. The physician is merely an agent of the patient. Veatch concedes this point when he says that the contractual model assures patient control of decision-making at the individual level. Likewise, at the level of social or community control of health care, the contractual model puts the locus of decision-making in the lay community. Thus, Veatch's key notion of "sharing" is a facade. A physician does not "share" in decision-making — he is simply an instrument of the patient. Ultimate control of, and therefore ultimate responsibility for, decision-making rests with the patient. In other words, the contractual model collapses into the engineering model, the only significant difference being that a physician can explicitly "opt out" in the contractual model. But the conditions for "opting out" also are unsatisfactory. The alternatives Veatch offers a physician when the obligations of a contract violate his conscience are unpalatable. A physician either acquiesces to the patient's demands and does something he believes is morally wrong, or breaks the contract, presumably by "firing" the patient. No middle ground or compromise solution is allowed.[24]

Despite its ultimate incoherence, this notion of a physician and patient "sharing" decision-making is popular, presumably because it offers an easy answer to the hard question of who should decide. David Brody, for example, also advocates "mutual" participation in clinical decision-making.[25] But again it is difficult to understand the sense in which participation in the actual making of a decision is mutual. On the one hand, Brody, like Veatch, wants the patient's values to be the basis for treatment decisions. On the other hand, when Brody enumerates the steps that lead to mutual participation, one gets the distinct impression that it is still the physician's decision. These steps include establishing a conducive atmosphere, ascertaining the patient's goals and expectations, educating the patient about the problem and the advantages and disadvantages of alternative treatment plans, and eliciting suggestions and preferences from patients and negotiating disagreements. Throughout these steps it is the physician who plays the active role in decision-making. Yet Brody recognizes that informed consent requirements give patients a veto over any interventions proposed by physicians. Because this veto puts final decision-making in the hands of the patient — the patient eventually must say yea or nay — the ultimate decision cannot be "shared" or "mutual." The only respect in which genuine "sharing" of decision-making exists is when disagreements are negotiated and a compromise solution is reached. If both physician and patient make concessions and adopt a course of action that is not the first choice of either, the decision is, in some sense, "shared" or "mutual." Otherwise, the claim that decision-making can be "shared" or "mutual" is simply confused.

Those who have observed or participated in team decision-making, in family medicine, psychiatry, or elsewhere, will understand this point about the impossibility of shared decision-making. Members of such teams can provide facts, assess evidence, offer advice, and make recommendations. In the absence of a consensus, however, the head of the team, usually the physician, makes the decision. This is as it should be, because responsibility for decisions accompanies the authority to make them. If decision-making authority were spread over a group, responsibility for the resulting decisions would be diffuse. The *appearance* of shared or diffuse responsibility may be psychologically comforting to those involved in the decision-making process, especially when the decision is a major one, but in the context of patient management decisions, the notion of shared responsibility is illusory. Actual decision-making cannot be shared. Ultimately, one person, either physician or patient, must take a stand and say, "This is what we will do." That is the end of the decision-making process. From then on, it is a matter of implementing the decision.

Although the act of making a decision, and the responsibility that accompanies this act, cannot be shared, the process leading to the making of a decision can be shared. A physician can participate in this process by providing information to a patient, pointing out important considerations that have been overlooked, and providing emotional support. What remains incoherent is the suggestion that patient and physician can "share" the final act of decision-making.

Appearances can be deceptive when one is trying to identify the real decision-maker in the physician-patient relationship. It might seem that physicians make decisions on behalf of patients when they prescribe medications. But by deciding whether to have the prescriptions filled, patients make the ultimate decision about their own care. Even that might not be the end of the matter. A patient could have a prescription filled but then decide not to take the medication for countless reasons. The illusion can work the other way as well. A patient may demand a particular form of treatment, and a physician may appear to acquiesce yet deceive the patient by substituting a placebo. One must be sensitive to these realities in discussions of where the locus of decision-making resides. It is easy to talk theoretically about the power of a physician. But the substantial, perhaps less conspicuous, power of a patient should not be underestimated.

Despite these criticisms of the contractual model, family physicians nevertheless may be drawn to it because they frequently talk about the "contracts" they have with patients. The notion of a contract in family medicine is ambiguous, and unfortunately there is little discussion of it in the literature.[26] Some family physicians even refer to the "implicit" contract they have with patients, but the idea of an implicit contract makes no sense. If the terms of a contract have not been discussed and agreed upon in advance by a patient and a family physician, and if the terms of a contract are not clear and precise, an "implicit" contract becomes nothing more than a rationalization for whatever action a family physician thinks is in a patient's best interest. The notion of an "implicit" contract should have no place in family medicine.[27]

Explicit contracts are only marginally more helpful. A patient and a family physician could never anticipate all the issues that might arise in their relationship and try to cover them in a contract. The terms of a contract would have to remain general, vague, and ambiguous and therefore would be subject to divergent and self-serving interpretations on the part of patient and family physician.[28]

In addition to the unavoidable problem of indeterminacy, what would be the content of a family medicine contract? When patients are willing to bargain about the terms of a contract and to be precise, family physicians are unlikely to be happy with the results. One patient sent a letter to a family physician setting out the terms under which he and his family would accept a relationship with that physician. The terms included:

- That the physician provide a home phone number which, the patient assured the physician, would not be abused.
- That the physician make house calls at any time they were requested.

- That all medical records be given to the patient upon his request.
- That all lab work and other tests be done quickly and the results given to the patient immediately.
- That the physician be honest and straightforward with the patient and not hold back any information.
- That the patient and his wife be allowed in the consulting room with any family member at any time.
- That waiting time be no longer than ten minutes for any appointment. If the physician is running late, he should have his secretary advise the patient, or the patient would charge the physician back for his own time.

No family physician could be likely to sign a contract with such inordinate patient demands. While this is an extreme example, it is further evidence that contracts are of limited value in understanding and improving the physician-patient relationship. They may be of some use with respect to narrow, well-defined issues, but they cannot provide a comprehensive moral foundation for the dealings between doctor and patient.

Two general lessons can be drawn from this discussion of the physician-patient relationship. The first is that one must not become too general or abstract in trying to understand the relationship. No single model will apply, either descriptively or prescriptively, to all patients and all problems at all times.[29] A plausible analysis must take account of relevant differences in the multifarious encounters between physician and patient. Szasz and Hollender recognize two of these differences, but three others need to be mentioned. The distinction between acute and chronic illnesses is one. Howard Brody suggests that a "physician-control approach" works best for acute illnesses, in which it is important that a patient adhere to a treatment plan; but for chronic illnesses, in which a patient must establish some mastery over the illness and integrate it into his life, a "patient-control approach" is preferable.[30]

A second variable is the reason why a person consults a physician.[31] Is the person ill and in need of treatment? If so, the person assumes the traditional status of patient, and the ensuing relationship is drastically unequal. In addition to lacking a physician's knowledge and power, patients are rendered vulnerable by their illness. The physician-patient relationship must be sensitive to what Pellegrino has called the "fact of illness."[32] Or is the person consulting a physician for a reason related to public health and health promotion? If so, the person more appropriately assumes the status of client. In this case, he still lacks a physician's knowledge and power, and therefore must seek the services of a physician, but is not additionally disadvantaged by his illness. He simply desires a service that can be provided only by a physician, for example, a vasectomy. In this situation, the relationship can be more balanced. A client is in a stronger position to assert his own views and desires and to resist the persuasion or coercion of a physician. It also is more feasible for a client to change physicians if a disagreement is intractable.

A third factor is the degree of certainty a physician brings to a decision. Every decision in medicine is surrounded by some uncertainty, yet some decisions are more uncertain than others. A physician using a new diagnostic procedure or prescribing a new drug, for instance, is less "certain" of the outcome than when the procedure or medication is one with which he has extensive experience. Sorenson recognizes how uncertainty affects the general nature of physician-patient encounters, and more specifically, how it can structure the relationship between genetic counsellor and counsellee.[33] He suggests that as the degree of uncertainty surrounding a health issue increases, so should the responsibility of a patient for making a decision regarding that issue.

Thus it is wrong to assume that one model of decision-making fits every patient, every physician, and every physician-patient encounter. At least five variables are relevant to determining the kind of relationship that should exist between physician and patient: (1) the reason that a person consults a physician; (2) the patient's condition; (3) the type and severity of the patient's illness; (4) the patient's desires; and (5) the degree of certainty attached to a decision.

The second lesson to be learned is that none of the proposed models accurately depicts the various roles that physician and patient can play in the decision-making process. If one focuses on how active a physician should be, there are four different roles a physician can play. First, a physician can be a dispenser of information. This role is consistent with the doctrines of informed consent and the promotion of patient self-determination. When a decision concerns the choice of a treatment plan, for example, the job of a physician is to explain to the patient the alternative forms of treatment available; the likely benefits and probability of success of each; the risks and side effects associated with each, as well as the likelihood that these will occur; and the prognosis if no treatment is instituted. The decision then is left entirely to the patient. A physician may not offer advice or make a recommendation.[34] If the decision concerns a diagnostic test, a physician must explain the nature of the test, the reasons for performing it, its risks and side effects, and the consequences of not performing it. The patient then decides whether he will have the test. A physician puts the patient in a position to make an informed, rational decision, but plays no part in the assessment of alternatives or the final choice.

The second and third roles allow a physician to be more active. In the second role a physician provides all of the information required by the first role, but in addition he offers advice or makes a recommendation. The patient still must be left entirely free to accept or reject this advice. A physician should not try to influence the patient's decision in any way. Once the patient has made a decision, the physician must accept it, even if he disagrees. The physician may not try to persuade the patient, but must merely carry out the patient's decision.

The third role goes a step beyond the second in that it allows a physician to try to change the patient's mind when the physician believes the patient has made a bad decision. The physician may supply additional information, reason with the patient, wheedle, coddle, or cajole, or enlist the patient's relatives or friends as supporters. In short, the physician may use his full persuasive powers. If the patient nevertheless resists, the physician must accept the decision.

The fourth role allows a physician to impose his view of what is in the best interest of the patient on the patient. If all attempts at persuasion have failed, a physician may resort to coercion.[35] For example, the physician may threaten to "fire" the patient or discharge the patient from the hospital if he does not acquiesce. Or, as in the case of involuntary civil commitment, the physician may invoke the coercive powers of the state to compel treatment. In this approach, the ultimate decision rests with the physician. A physician will give a patient every opportunity to make the decision the physician believes is best, and will try less objectionable methods to overcome resistance before resorting to coercion. But a physician will not allow a patient to make a decision that the physician believes jeopardizes the patient's overall welfare.

No single model of decision-making can account for the different circumstances in which these four roles might be appropriate. A simple, a priori model of the physician-patient relationship is not sensitive to the realities and intricacies of clinical encounters.

Two ethical aspects of the physician-patient relationship have been considered in this chapter. First, knowing that the relationship itself can be a therapeutic tool makes it morally incumbent on family physicians to try to cultivate close, caring, trusting relationships with their patients. Family physicians always should deliver the best care they can. Second, constructing models of where decision-making authority ought to reside in the physician-patient relationship is a familiar approach to moral problems in medicine. Attempts to provide theoretical answers to the question "Who should decide?" fail, however. An influential argument designed to show that physicians are not permitted to make any moral or value decisions on behalf of patients is inconclusive. The attractive notion of "shared" decision-making is incoherent. Contracts are of limited help. The physician-patient relationship ultimately is too rich, diverse, and complex to be captured by one model. Moreover, appeals to the notions of protecting patient welfare and promoting patient autonomy do not yield straightforward answers to the question of where the locus of decision-making ought to be. One therefore needs to transcend this popular approach to develop a helpful applied ethics for family medicine.

Viewing the question of who should decide as the central ethical issue in medicine is dangerous as well because it can result in a failure to characterize the respective duties of physicians and patients adequately.[36] Making therapeutic decisions is only one of the responsibilities that must be allocated within the physician-patient relationship. A family physician might have a duty to provide emotional support to an anxious or depressed patient, for instance. Focusing exclusively on decision-making is the primary reason there is not a richer description of a physician's role in the literature of biomedical ethics. One of our aims is to provide a more comprehensive understanding of family physicians' relationship with their patients.

NOTES

1. Montagu, A. "Anthropology and medical education." *JAMA,* 1963, 183, 579.
2. Williams, J. I. and Leaman, T. L. "Family structure and function." In Conn, H. F., et al., eds., *Family Practice.* Philadelphia: W. B. Saunders Co., 1973, p. 3.
3. Peabody, F. W. "The care of the patient." *Journal of the American Medical Association,* 1927, 88, 877.
4. The points in this paragraph are taken from McWhinney, I. R., "Continuity of care." *Journal of Family Practice,* 1982, 15, 847.
5. *Ibid.*
6. For a good summary of social-science investigations of the physician-patient relationship, see Bloom, S. W. and Wilson, R. N., "Patient-practitioner relationships." In Freedman, H., et al., eds., *Handbook of Medical Sociology,* 3rd ed. Englewood Cliffs, N.J.: Prentice Hall, 1979, p. 275.

7. Peabody, note 3 supra, 877.
8. The influence of these factors has been developed in the writings of Michael Balint.
9. Peabody, note 3 supra, 881.
10. *Ibid.*, p. 882.
11. Létourneau, E. G. "I don't want an x-ray, Doctor: it's too dangerous." *CMA Journal,* 1982, 127, 1158.
12. *Ibid.*, p. 1159.
13. Szasz, T. S., and Hollender, M. H. "The basic models of the doctor-patient relationship." *A.M.A. Archives of Internal Medicine,* 1956, 97, 585.
14. *Ibid.*, p. 587.
15. *Ibid.*, p. 591.
16. Veatch, R. "Models for ethical medicine in a revolutionary age." *Hastings Center Report,* June, 1972, 2, 5.
17. *Ibid.*, p. 7.
18. *Ibid.*
19. *Ibid.*, p. 6. For a longer discussion, see Veatch, R. "Generalization of expertise." *Hastings Center Studies,* 1973, 1, 2, 29.
20. Black, P. McL. "Must physicians treat the 'whole man' for proper medical care?" *The Pharos,* 1976, 39, 9.
21. For two other invocations of it, see Buchanan, A. "Medical paternalism." *Philosophy and Public Affairs,* 1978, 7, 383, and Ladd, J. "Medical ethics: Who knows best?" *The Lancet,* November 22, 1980, 1128.
22. See Hoffmaster, B. "Physicians, patients, and paternalism." *Man and Medicine,* 1980, 5, 194.
23. For a similar view, see Cassell, E. J. "Autonomy and ethics in action." *New England Journal of Medicine,* 1977, 297, 333.
24. Veatch's single contract subsequently has proliferated into a triple contract in his "Professional medical ethics: The grounding of its principles." *Journal of Medicine and Philosophy,* 1979, 4, 1, and *A Theory Of Medical Ethics.* New York: Basic Books, 1981. Although in these later works Veatch clearly allows physicians discretion in setting the terms of contracts with patients, he does not appear to offer them any better alternatives for dealing with moral conflicts that might arise afterward. He seems to assume that all such problems would be resolved in the initial process of negotiation. Even when Veatch discusses this problem explicitly — in the context of a disagreement about the treatment of an infant with spina bifida — his view remains ambiguous. He unquestionably grants a physician the right to refuse to participate in a course of action the physician believes is wrong, but the moral basis of this right is obscure. There is the continuing suggestion that it rests on a refusal to enter into a contract, not opt out of a contract. See his "Abnormal newborns and the physician's role: Models of physician decision making." In Swinyard, C. A., ed., *Decision Making and the Defective Newborn.* Springfield, Illinois: Charles C. Thomas, 1978, pp. 183-184.

25. Brody, D. S. "The patient's role in clinical decision-making." *Annals of Internal Medicine,* 1980, 93, 718.

26. A "family continuity of care contract" and an "attitudinal contract" have been discussed, but it is difficult to understand what these "contracts" are supposed to involve. See Driggers, D., et al. "The family continuity of care contract." *Journal of Family Practice,* 1982, 15, 471. McWhinney says an *explicit* doctor-patient contract is useful, but by "contract" he means a mutual understanding of the patient's and physician's respective commitments, rights, and responsibilities, not necessarily a written contract. He then, confusingly, goes on to attribute many of the recent problems in physician-patient relationships to misunderstandings of the *implied* contract. See McWhinney, I. R. *An Introduction to Family Medicine.* New York: Oxford University Press, 1981, p. 59.

27. It might be countered that courts frequently rely upon "implicit" contracts, so the notion must make some sense. Implicit contracts in the law make sense, however, only because a neutral third party, a judge, is allowed to make authoritative, final decisions about what vague, ambiguous, or "implicit" contractual terms mean after a dispute arises. No analogous third party exists for resolving disputes about family medicine "contracts." Moreover, judicial dispute resolution is a means of ending disagreements, not preventing them, which presumably is the aim of "contracts" in family medicine. Finally, the extent to which judicial decisions interpreting indeterminate or implicit contractual terms are rational or objectively justifiable remains a controversial issue.

28. For an apt example of this failing of written contracts and of how such a failing can be exploited (on this occasion by the patient), see Bursztajn, H., et al. *Medical Choices, Medical Chances.* New York: Dell Publishing Co., 1981, p. 299.

29. At least one philosopher has resisted this temptation. See Bayles, M. D. "Physicians as body mechanics." In Davis, J. W., et al., eds., *Contemporary Issues in Biomedical Ethics.* Clifton, N.J.: Humana Press, 1978, p. 167.

30. Brody, H. *Placebos and the Philosophy of Medicine.* Chicago: University of Chicago Press, 1977, p. 126.

31. Bradley, P.A. "A response to the March 1979 issue of the *Journal of Medicine and Philosophy.*" *Journal of Medicine and Philosophy,* 1980, 5, 213.

32. Pellegrino, E. D. "Toward a reconstruction of medical morality: The primacy of the act of profession and the fact of illness." *Journal of Medicine and Philosophy,* 1979, 4, 44.

33. Sorenson, J. R. "Biomedical innovation, uncertainty, and doctor-patient interaction." *Journal of Health and Social Behavior,* 1974, 15, 366.

34. For a parody of this approach, see Donaldson, R. M., Jr. "Advice for the patient with 'silent' gallstones." *New England Journal of Medicine,* 1982, 307, 815.

35. For a discussion of the notion of coercion in medicine, see Brody, H. "Empirical studies of ethics in family medicine." *Journal of Family Practice,* 1983, 6, 1061.

36. We want to thank Terrence Ackerman for help with this point.

Whose Agent is the Therapist?

Martin Lakin

The clearest picture of agency would seem to be a therapy in which a single therapist treats a mentally competent adult. However, even then the question of agency arises, because it is a rare case where others — spouse, children, colleagues, and friends — are unaffected by what happens to the client. The therapist is, of course, mainly responsive to the needs of the client or group of clients seeking help, but effects on others involved, such as a divorce or a job change, can be profoundly negative.

The problem of agency is most dramatically manifested in family treatments or in counseling couples. As many family therapists point out, a decision to see one of two spouses, or both together, may initiate a course of events leading either to divorce or to reconciliation. Too, dealing with a family is rarely a neutral experience. Therapists find themselves siding with one or the other spouse or with one of the children; moreover, they may become enmeshed in the family's conflicts. Even the most fair-minded and objective therapists must weigh decisions about whether and how impartial to appear on a moment-to-moment basis. The psychiatrist Larry Gerson acknowledges, for example, that therapy with married couples is especially taxing and ethically complex because of the participants' conflicting goals.

> For me, the most common problem has to do with seeing a patient who is going through a separation. And one of them wants to separate, the other doesn't. What's best for your patient may not be good for the couple. This woman is getting physically abused, but this was her fourth husband who was doing this to her. So I began to push her about this crazy pattern. I asked, "Why are you staying with this guy?" But then the husband began to call me on the phone. It turns out he was very dependent on her despite the physical abuse. So I had the two of them in together. And we began to do some joint work which has the two of them back together. Now I could have referred him to someone else, but I thought, no, that other therapist wouldn't have all the pieces of the puzzle.

Dr. Gerson believes that he should anticipate the conflicts in a marriage that are likely to ensue when a married individual seeks his help. He outlines his attitude as follows.

> I'll forecast it to the patient if I think that things are likely to go in a direction that will affect the marriage. Maybe they don't want to go that way. This woman had pretty much let her husband dominate her, and she wanted to be more assertive. I told her that it might be very good for her to do that, but if she went into therapy without her husband, she'd probably end up getting a divorce. After we talked about it for a while, she decided that her marriage was more important than the change and she got out of therapy.

Martin Lakin, "Whose Agent is the Therapist?" from Martin Lakin, *Ethical Issues in Psychotherapy*. (New York: Oxford University Press, 1988) pp. 8-13 and 21-25.

Another therapist, Carol Jessup, who specializes in sex therapy and in couple counseling, describes one result of a "successful" treatment program.

> According to this guy's story, she was cold and asexual. They had been married for twenty-some years. Now I warned them that there was only a low probability for a good outcome because of their long-standing pattern of mutual avoidance, but I would do it if they wanted. Well, the situation became just awful. She became much more sensuous, but he couldn't stand it. He not only became bored with sex; he would say awful things to her about her body. Now they really fight all the time and I don't know that they can stay together.

Do therapists have an obligation to be concerned about the effects of treatment on intimates of the treated person? Is the therapist supposed to maintain neutrality in the conflicts among the clients? As we see, the problem is especially visible when dealing with couples or families. In the following instance, Carol Singer worries about a natural tendency of the participants to side with one or another.

> I invariably do like one member of a family better than another. I've found that I have to be especially careful that I don't undercut the woman by being sort of flirtatious with the man. I usually do feel more of a kinship with the guy. Maybe it's their sense of humor or something like that. You know, to try to be balanced and available to both of them — or in families, to all of them — it's a hell of a job!

Issues of agency and confidentiality become intermixed in multiperson therapies. Irving Ratner, an experienced practitioner, has had to face the ethical dilemmas involved in dealing with couples many times. A typical problem is exemplified in the following case.

> Even when I am seeing one patient, there are others involved, and I often wonder what my responsibilities are to those people. Of course, I try to keep it limited to the patient. But when I see couples it's really unclear. It often happens that one of them is having an affair. It's just as clear as can be, but the other one doesn't realize it. So what do I do? I figure it's a "no-no" to disclose the facts. Sometimes I am asked, "Well, is she? ... Is he?" So I say something like, "I don't feel licensed to discuss these things with you." I guess I see my role as a sort of interpreter to each about the other, to try to make each one sort of more sympathetic to the other.

The therapist who deals primarily with children often faces the problem of how to balance needs for confidentiality and trust in the relationship with the child in treatment against the legitimate concerns of the parents. Helen Eland describes how she approaches this situation.

> The big issue is how much to open up with the parents when it is a child or adolescent. I mean when you have to be clinically effective and not transgress on the relationship which you are trying to build with the patient. If I know that the child has had an abortion and doesn't want me to share the information with the parent, I would try to bring the situation — I mean the child — to the point where the information could be shared. To simply tell the parents would be to ruin the therapeutic trust. So I always have a dilemma about keeping everybody's needs in mind.

What kinds of conflicts of agency arise regarding the conduct of group therapies? In the interest of effective and responsible care, group therapists would wish to be equally accessible to all participants and to facilitate positive outcomes for each. However, therapists who conduct groups may experience likes and dislikes, countertransferential attitudes toward specific individuals that may "leak out," just as in other forms of therapy. There is also another reason for the emergence of "favorites" in group treatments — group therapists are naturally inclined to enlist the aid of other members in addressing a particular individual's problem. Although group therapy certainly is not a classroom situation, its members may be favored or disfavored in ways reminiscent of early school experiences, with similar consequences.

Social comparison is inescapably as much a part of group therapy experience as of earlier groups, and so comparative self-esteem is a perennial issue. Using members to amplify one's message inevitably affects the self-esteem of those targeted by that message. Who may become the voice of the group and who will be its target become clear only as a group develops, but the constant question for members is: "How do they [he/she] choose to talk about me? How do I stand in comparison to them?" The ethical challenge for the therapist is to be aware of the likelihood of such tendencies and avoid cultivating favorites.

Ethical problems also arise in connection with the widespread practice of treating individual patients in groups led by the therapist. No doubt, most therapists who use this method do so in the belief that they are providing an important therapeutic supplement to individual treatment; familiarity and convenience are also advantages, as are financial considerations. However, one must decide what consequences may ensue from being treated by one's therapist privately and then in a group together with other patients of the same therapist. Are not jealousies and sibling rivalries unnecessarily stimulated? Since proprietary feelings are intrinsic to any therapy (e.g., *my* therapist, *my* session, *our* group), doesn't the question of whose agent become confusing or even burdensome when the group's leader is also the individual therapist for its members?

The problem of agency is especially ambiguous in organization consulting and in the interventions launched to resolve interpersonal problems in the organization. It is generally recognized that the workplace can become an arena of abrasive and demoralizing interactions. Resultant symptoms may be excessive competitiveness, debilitating anxiety, inner conflicts, apathy, and diminished self-esteem.

Walton and Warwick (1973) pointed out a number of ethical issues raised by psychological interventions in organizations; chief among them was that the personal interests of targets of the intervention may not be identical with those of the employers who pay for the consultant's services. As a consequence, such interventions are often profoundly distrusted by workers who feel that the consultant is management's agent, not theirs. An example of this problem is shown in the attitude of the organization consultant, Aaron Todd.

> Who is my client? The director will hire me and say, "I'd like you to do some team building with such and such a group," but then he'll add, "Incidentally, that manager of the division has some shortcomings, so look it over." So what's the message? I think that he doesn't like this guy, but he wants me to check him out through this team-building business. I have a really tough decision. Who needs my help and what am I going to do about it? I don't want to do the director's dirty work.

Who pays the piper calls the tune is an old maxim that would seem to apply in such cases. This consultant is faced with a difficult situation, yet his stance is probably not a common one in the corporate world. Awareness of ethical issues may be increasing among managers just as it is among therapists. Is it possible that greater latitude can be allowed organization consultants in determining the needs of their client systems? An optimistic view is reflected in the statement by Albert Grobart.

> I feel I can open the door for any employee to set his agenda or his problem on somebody's agenda, I mean somebody who can really do something about it for him. I act as a facilitator around here. I can get guarantees against the possibility of reprisals so that anybody can go and complain about anything or anybody he needs or wants to.

Managers may dictate the kinds and the limits of permissible interventions, regardless of the consultant's diagnosis of the problems, as in the following experience of Timothy Jeffries.

> I was consulting in the outfit and they asked me to work with this unit that had had the trauma of their section head drinking himself to death. This group was really upset because they had all been very involved with him. Nobody felt good and they were all beating themselves up about it. After I had worked with them five days, they felt they needed to continue, and so did I. But the CEO wouldn't permit it, and he was paying the bill.

CONFIDENTIALITY

The secrecy in which therapy is conducted is one of the most sensitive issues in any psychotherapy. Clients are of course concerned that their disclosures should not become public, nor revealed to their detriment or shame. Confidentiality is at risk, however, especially in group therapies.

Another important aspect involves the protective environment almost all psychotherapies foster. A half century of public education and promotion of the idea that mental illness is like any other and that personal growth and emotional development could be positive outgrowths of therapy has not really altered the popular conception that being in therapy is a sign of fundamental weakness or moral infirmity. It's as if there were still something to be ashamed of. Consider the problem facing the counseling psychologist Roger Rycroft.

> Lots of the information, if it gets out, could be damaging to the student's future. Sometimes they ask you to send out documentation about them, apparently not mindful of what they're asking for in terms of its possible consequences for them. I just don't know what to do when that occurs. One kid is now a high official and I guess he needed the documentation, so he asked for it, and I had no choice. Maybe I could have alerted him by asking, "You want to specify what you want released and what you want kept back?"

The debate within the mental health professions about the range and the limitations of confidentiality has become increasingly complicated. Should assurances of confidentiality cover minor children with respect to their parents or guardians? What about instances where self-destructive acts are reported or when the individual seems likely to harm others? Some state rulings (e.g., Tarasoff, 1976) have made therapists quite uneasy about their own liability if a patient commits a crime. Martin Thomas, the therapist who provided the following material, works in a student mental health center. He describes his concerns about the confidentiality of records, the release of information and "judgment calls" about what is in the patient's best interest.

> I guess for me this issue of confidentiality and the release of information is about the most troubling question and one that arises frequently. Now it is fairly easy if you get a consent form, but what about parents who have legitimate concerns with how their son or daughter is doing? I mean you have to maintain some kind of alliance with parents when you treat the kid. You have hospitalization or other problems and you'll surely want their cooperation *[How do you resolve it?]* Well, with difficulty! *[Laugh.]* I respond to parents to try to reassure them, but avoiding giving them details of what the kid has said.

Children and adolescents in psychotherapy pose delicate problems in maintaining or breaching confidentiality. Those who work with children and their families have reason to be concerned about conflicts of interests and whose agent they try to be but also about what to tell parents or guardians. The following child-family therapist (David Bently) discusses historical sources of the ethical dilemmas involved and the viewpoint he now adopts.

> For over thirty years I have been working mostly with children and their families. I've got to say that the question of strict confidentiality that many others consider to be a big ethical issue, I don't. I think it's a misconstrual of an original psychoanalytic premise with adults, that the material of the therapeutic hour is private property for the client, and under no circumstances should it be shared with others. Sure, I think it's important with children and adolescents that what they say and deal with is their private, personal thing, but it will be shared with others — family and parents — when that seems clearly needed. What I say to them is something like, "Whatever we talk about here is mostly just between the two of us. Now if anything comes up that seems to me as though it ought to be talked about with your folks, then I will raise it with you and we will decide together how to do that."

When working in a public agency one faces a different set of problems regarding confidentiality. The psychiatrist Ted Engle explains why such problems are more complex in his work for a mental health center than in his own private practice.

> Over there, you are put in a situation of representing the agency. I can't really promise confidentiality because the administrators may change the policy about what goes in records. But if I get a call about one of my private patients where they want to review my notes about his treatment, I say, "I'll give you a summary." The other day I got such a request about a guy I had treated for homosexuality who's got a top-notch job as a government scientist. Apparently, he wanted to do "top secret" stuff. So I get the call from Captain So-and-So who wants to come down and see the records. Well, I was evasive and I told the captain that I would agree only to reading him my summary based on old notes; that is, if I ever could decipher them. But I was polite and of course I was telling half-truths through my teeth.

Confidentiality is difficult, if not impossible to maintain in group therapy. As suggested by Lillian Townsend, the problem is exacerbated when patients are seen by the same therapist in both group and individual therapy.

> Sometimes people tell me things in individual therapy they don't want discussed in the group. My way of handling it is to go along with the contract. But my colleague who works with me says to the patient, "Look, nothing you tell me individually is sacrosanct; anything goes in the group." For me it is a struggle, you might say a dilemma, because I see beneficial aspects of both positions. If they tell me something and then work it through to a point where they can eventually bring it to the group, that is useful. But what if they tell me something, say they are having sex with another member (which is against our group guidelines by the way), and that would be cause for kicking them both out of the group? It would also necessitate an intervention to help the other person involved. Now I have the issue of needing to help the other person involved as well as this person. So I have that kind of difficulty.

...

THE IMPOSITION OF VALUES: THERAPISTS AS MORAL ARBITERS AND AGENTS OF SOCIAL CHANGE

The few studies that have explored the question of the role of psychotherapists' values in their practices have found that therapists consciously or unwittingly communicate their own values to their clients (Murray, 1956; Parloff, Goldstein, and Iflund, 1960; Parloff, Iflund, and Goldstein, 1957; Truax, 1966; Wolfe, 1977). London (1986) points out that an extreme form of such value communication occurs when a therapist threatens sanctions against a client, such as warning that therapy may be terminated if the client does not comply with the therapist's advice. The therapist Hans Hobart recalls when he was confronted by his own therapist's heavy-handed proscription of his behavior; it is clearly a case of value imposition.

> I went to see this therapist because I had had anxiety attacks. I had the feeling, even back then, that I was really bisexual and I told him so in an early session. He waited until I was really hooked and quite dependent on him. Then he tells me that if I ever had sex with a man, he would refuse to see me for six months! There was no exploration of my problem, no explanation, nothing! He was in this power position because at the time I really needed his help. Even back in those days it was an unethical thing to do.

Such values, whether related to one's activities or one's relationships, can be decisive in the lives of the clients. If a therapist approves of the individual's behavior, it is reinforced; if the therapist disapproves, it may be changed. Therapists' probes, comments, and interpretations are frequently concerned with value questions involving attitudes about relationships, social obligations, work, and the whole range of human activity. If a client experiences guilt, for instance, the therapist must inquire into the infractions or impulses that cause the guilt. Inevitably the question of standards of conduct — the therapist's as well as the client's — become focal issues in their interactions. Value-neutral therapy has been critiqued by Bergin (1985) who says that contemporary therapists have not been sufficiently cognizant of the role of traditional values in fostering and maintaining mental health. He emphasizes values inherent in traditional family life, such as monogamy and fidelity. Vitz (1985) similarly stresses traditional values, particularly religious affiliation and feelings, and charges therapists with ignoring their importance. But, as we will see, many therapists argue the contrary, believing that most therapists are too traditional because they impose the sexist and role-restrictive standards of conduct they have absorbed on the individuals and families they treat.

In this section, we confront the fact that therapists are often in the position of acting as moral guides for their patients, and that ethical dilemmas will result from such a stance. The first ethical responsibility of therapists, regardless of what values they espouse, is to be fully aware of what they communicate to their clients. Equally important is to be respectful toward the clients' values and not to impose their own on them.

The accusation of value imposition has assumed increased significance with the emergence of the women's movement. Female patients have legitimate grounds for objecting to the patronizing manner in which their problems are viewed in some therapies and for the ways in which they have been treated by some male therapists. The therapies themselves may be informed by stereotypical notions of sex roles that are obstacles to equal treatment; charges of sexism leveled at certain forms of therapy have not been without foundation.

Psychotherapists are sometimes criticized for psychoengineering, that is, manipulating clients not for their own welfare but for what is thought to be good role adjustment. Family therapists are usually singled out in particular for such manipulation. A case of how a depressed woman was dealt with that appears in texts of abnormal psychology is described by Liberman and Raskin (1971).

> Whenever mother did the expected household jobs of cooking, cleaning, and so forth, without complaint, the children and the father were instructed to applaud and comment proudly. But when she acted depressed, she was to be ignored. [After inducing changes] as an experiment, they were instructed to go back to noting and responding to her depressed state, with the consequence that she rapidly returned to being depressed. Then the therapeutic reversal was once more — this time permanently — engineered.

Focusing as they do on many aspects of marital and family relationships, family therapists have increasingly come to reflect the divisions along value lines about gender roles and relationships between the sexes. Although many espouse the values of society as a whole, there are those who would use their positions as therapists to push for changes in line with a different ideal. Thus, Hare-Mustin (1978) advocated a more feminist approach to family therapy, claiming that such therapy provides unique and unparalleled opportunities for facilitating desired changes in male-female relations. Margolin (1982) similarly suggests utilizing family therapies to change the "oppressive consequences" of stereotyped roles and expectations in the family (pp. 798-99) and both these authors warn male therapists against imposing sexist values on their clients.

Not all family therapists agree with this position, and Wendorf and Wendorf (1985) challenge it. Although they accept Margolin's right to object to the imposition of sexist (wrong) values, they question the ethicality of trying to influence clients to accept their own nonsexist (right) values. Even though Hare-Mustin and Margolin recognize harmful effects of value imposition, they don't seem to question pushing their own.

Wendorf and Wendorf (1985) wonder, "Are we beginning to see ourselves as the moral judges of our society with answers for every question? Are we too sure of ourselves and becoming rigid, dogmatic, or arrogant?"

Behavioral and dynamic family therapists disagree about the ways therapies should be carried out; both systems are characterized by "school" values as well as the values of the particular therapist. As behaviorists O'Leary and Turkewitz (1978) acknowledge, "While we strive not to have our values unduly influence our clients, it seems clear that we do influence them by the questions we ask ... and by the therapeutic targets we help establish ... [This can lead to a] bias left unsaid which may result in a more subtle or insidious influence process which can be counterproductive." Gurman, Knudson, and Kniskern (1978) suggest that the prescriptive "pleases" and "displeases" to be reinforced per instruction by behavior therapists are equated by patients with "goodness" and "badness." But behavior therapists counter that all models of family therapy must state a conception of a "good" successful marriage. If one cannot define a successful marriage, how can one judge the outcome of a marital therapy? The rejoinder by Gurman et al. is that they object to the quid pro quo contacting by behavioral family therapists as furthering the practice of mutual controlling by the spouses.

What are the values influencing the typical family therapeutic encounter? Most therapists who work with families are committed to ideals of benign family interactions and to autonomy for each member, within reasonable limits, so that family members can develop and live as independently as possible. But a family therapist may come into conflict with more traditional, perhaps even authoritarian values with which he disagrees, as in the following case reported by Arthur Jackson.

> I had been after her to give her two boys a little living space. She really rides hard on them. Her husband split and she's had no word from him. She's trying to bring them up right and works eight to ten hours a day outside the house. Maybe she is right when she bawls me out. She gives me a look and wades right in: "What the hell do you know about raising teenage boys? They don't have a father to keep them in line. It's all up to me! I'll bet you're not even married!" I had no comeback at all.

Values concerning extramarital sex, modes of child-rearing, candor in interpersonal relations, and levels of emotional expressiveness differ according to one's own background and beliefs. They also differ for psychotherapists. But these are not the only, or necessarily the most ethically significant values in therapies. Several therapies are based on certain moral principles. Mowrer's is actively concerned with "sin" in the sense of moral wrongdoing and its expiation through confession followed by redemptive good works and social involvement. There are also psychopolitical therapies such as Dr. Huber's psychotherapy group, "The Socialists' Patients Collective" in Heidelberg, Germany, which spawned a considerable amount of terrorist activity on the premise that society, not the participants, was sick (Baeyer-Katte, 1982). A recent example of politically oriented therapies is that of the consciousness-raising groups so popular in our own society.

Lately there has been a revived interest in meeting the needs of religiously inclined patients. However, it has also happened that born-again therapists have tried to influence their secular patients to accept a religious answer to their problems, as illustrated in the following example given by John Summer.

> My patient tells me that she was altogether shocked and disbelieving when this guy says, "Well, I'm sure that if we pray together, it's going to be helpful for you" and then he gets on his knees and expects her to do the same! Of course, she didn't know what to do or where to turn. Her best friend suggested she come to see me.

A more benign approach is typical of therapists who want religiously inclined persons to feel they may avail themselves of therapy services without compromising their religious faith or beliefs. The following example by Abraham Lorber, describes one therapist's strategy to get around the biblical injunction "Honor thy father and thy mother."

> You know of course, that a great deal is said about parents in therapy. Often one cries about them and complains, but one also curses them for the miseries they brought on your head. The problem for Orthodox Jews is in that commandment. How can you be obeying it if you are yelling about how horrible, how awful they were? But you see, there is another commandment — Pikuach Nefesh — which means, figuratively, that when a person is ill, he or she can do almost anything necessary — break just about every commandment — to get well. So I tell them that this gives them God's own permission to be mad with their folks, or at least to talk about them.

In the wake of various kinds of social militancy — ethnic, racial, and gender — some therapists are beginning to question how they can help those of different cultural backgrounds, gender, or social class. Psychotherapy is administered mainly by white middle-class professionals whose knowledge and experience of other subcultures is often limited. It is also true that a number of therapy or therapy-like procedures have been designated as alternatives to mainstream treatments. Thus, consciousness-raising for women's groups has given way to therapies intended to foster feminist pride and self-esteem. Gay therapists are turned to by homosexuals who feel they will not be understood by "straight" therapists. Ethnotherapies have been proposed for members of oppressed or discriminated ethnic groups as a way of replacing their debilitating self-contempt with ethnic pride. Veterans of the unpopular Vietnam War suffering from Post Traumatic Stress Disorder have been treated in rap groups composed of similarly troubled individuals that are frequently led by someone with experience of that war.

Therapists are also becoming aware of their own ethnocentric proclivities as a result of the surge of ethnic and minority issues. Sometimes the problem is reflective of the civil rights issues in the streets and schools and businesses. Often it involves unfamiliarity with the cultural and socioeconomic background of the client, as suggested in the case provided by Larry Phillips.

> When I began therapy with Angela and Tim, I could smell trouble because they were so different. He was "el Waspo," passive, quiet, not a drop of revealed feelings, and she was a real Italian girl, yelling and screaming. She described her family as warm and expressive, and of course very vocal. But as we worked, I began to sympathize with Tim. She even yelled at *me*. So I tried to tone her down. She got just livid and said to me, "You are just like him, you hate Italians and so does he!"

Although black individuals and families have been successfully treated in psychotherapy, their relative number is small.

A great part of their reluctance to enter therapy is a shared perception of its social class values. Jerome Costner illustrates the problem as he describes his (and their) frustration in trying to establish a workable therapeutic relationship.

> You see, they often don't come at the appointed times, and when I try to remonstrate with them, it's like I'm insulting them. They give me this look ... "Well, OK Mr. Whitey. ..." So I feel like I'm walking on eggs through a different world. When I tried to get them to turn off the TV when the kids were supposed to be doing homework, they say they do, but it turns out that they don't. I think maybe a black therapist wouldn't be quite so tender about it as I feel I am being.

FURTHER READINGS

Bayles, Michael D.
"The Professional Client Relationship," from Michael D. Bayles, *Professional Ethics.* (Belmont,Calif: Wadsworth, 1981).
Beauchamp, T.L.
"The Promise of the Beneficence Model for Medical Ethics," *Journal of Contemporary Health Law and Policy* 6:(199) 145-155.
Becker, M. and L. Maiman
"Strategies for Enhancing Patient Compliance," *Journal of Community Health* 6 (1980) 113-132.
Buchanan, Allan
"Medical Paternalism," *Philosophy and Public Affairs* 7(1978) 370-390.
Callahan, Joan C.
"Paternalism and Voluntariness," *Canadian Journal of Philosophy* 16: 2 (1986) 199-220.
Childress, James I. and Mark S. Siegler
"Metaphors and Models of Doctor-Patient Relationships: Their Implication for Autonomy," *Theoretical Medicine* 5 (1984) 17-30.
Chinen, A.
"Modes of Understanding and Mindfulness of Clinical Medicine," *Theoretical Medicine* 9: 1(February 1988) 45-72.
Dworkin, Gerald
"Paternalism," *The Monist* 56 (Jan. 1972).
Gert, Bernard and Charles M. Culver
"Paternalistic Behaviour," *Philosophy and Public Affairs* 6 (1976) 45-47.
Gordon, Harry H.
"The Doctor-Patient Relationship: A Judaic Perspective," *The Journal of Medicine and Philosophy*, vol. 8 (1983) 243-255.
Graber, Glenn C.
"On Paternalism in Health Care," in John W. Davis, Barry Hoffmaster and Sarah Shorten, eds., *Contemporary Issues in Biomedical Ethics* (Humana Press: Clifton, N.J., 1981).
Ingelfinger, Franz
"Arrogance," *New England Journal of Medicine* 303(1980) 1509.

Katz, Jay
The Silent World of Doctor and Patient. (Free Press: New York, 1984) I and II.
Masters, Roger
"Is Contract an Adequate Basis for Medical Ethics?" *Hastings Center Report* 5(Dec. 1975) 24-28.
O'Hair, Dan
"Patient Preference for Persuasion," *Theoretical Medicine* 7(1986)147-164.
Percival, Thomas
Medical Ethics.
Roach, M.S.
The Human Act of Caring: A Blueprint for the Health Professions (Ottawa: Canadian Hospital Association, 1987).
Smith, David H. and Lloyd S. Pettegrew
"Mutual Persuasion as a Model for Doctor-Patient Communication," *Theoretical Medicine* 7(1986) 127-146.
Staum, Martin S. and Donald E. Larson, eds.
Doctors, Patients and Society: Power and Authority in Medical Care. (Wilfrid Laurier University Press: Waterloo 1981).
Storch, J.
Patients' Rights. (Toronto: McGraw Hill, 1982).
Szaz, Thomas and Marc H. Hollender
"A Contribution to the Philosophy of Medicine: The Basic Models of the Doctor-Patient Relationship," *Archives of Internal Medicine* 97(1956) 585-592.
Thomasma, D.C.
"Beyond Medical Paternalism and Patient Autonomy: A Model of Physician Conscience for the Physician-Patient Relationship," *Annals of Internal Medicine* 98: 3 (February, 1983) 243-247.
Veatch, R.
"Generalization of Expertise," *Hastings Center Studies* 1: 2 (1973), 29-40.

CHAPTER 5 INFORMED CONSENT AND THE COMPETENT PATIENT

INTRODUCTION

It is a fundamental principle of Canadian health care theory and law that, all other things being equal, competent patients have the right to accept or reject any treatment and any diagnostic or other intervention. The only limitation on this freedom is that the health of other people should not be threatened and that the rights of others should not be interfered with. As the old adage has it, "Your right to swing your fist stops where my face begins!"

However, someone who makes a decision without having appropriate or sufficient information is not in fact choosing freely. The very lack of information acts as a constraint on the choice of the decision-maker. Therefore, in order to be able to exercise their right of choice in a meaningful way, patients have to be informed. Canadian bioethics tries to capture this insight in the phrase "informed consent." Competent patients have the right to informed consent. Of course the phrase refers to more than just accepting a procedure, course of action or intervention. It also refers to refusal. The two are but different sides of the same coin.

The precise nature of informed decision-making — and who should act as decision-maker when the patient is unable to do so — has been a matter of some controversy and uncertainty.

The focus of the readings in this chapter is the question of what informed consent really amounts to, and what must happen in order for a proper informed consent to exist.

The UK accepts what is called a professional standard of disclosure. A physician has to disclose to the patient all and only what another physician, similarly placed, would normally disclose. The US accepts an objective reasonable-person standard. A physician need only disclose what the ordinary reasonable person would want to know before agreeing to or rejecting the procedure that is being offered.

The Canadian approach is different. *Reibl v. Hughes* is the classic Canadian legal case in this regard. It is a decision by the Supreme Court of Canada. It sets the standards that Canadian health care professionals must legally follow in order to have an informed consent from their patients.

The case puts more emphasis on patient autonomy than the US cases.[1] It begins by recognizing that to be told something and to actually understand it are not necessarily the same thing. It therefore distinguishes between what the patient should be told — this has become known as the *standard of disclosure* — and the level at which the information must be pitched so that the patient can actually understand the information that is being provided. This has become known as the *standard of comprehension*.

It then says — and again this is somewhat different from the US — that the appropriate standard of disclosure is not what the ordinary reasonable person would want to know, but what an objective reasonable person *in the patient's particular position* would want to know. As for the level at which the information must be pitched, it says that it must be geared to the level of the particular patient. It must not be assumed that just because people would normally understand the information the way it is being provided, therefore *this* patient actually understands it.

The two standards have become known as the *objective reasonable person standard of disclosure, geared to the particular patient*; and the *subjective standard of comprehension*. *Reibl v. Hughes* is important not only from a legal perspective. It also captures what would be expected from a deontologically oriented ethical perspective that places primary emphasis on the autonomy of persons.

The selection from the Royal College of Physicians and Surgeons gives some indication of how the medical profession has understood both the law and the ethics in this regard.

Benjamin Freedman's discussion is philosophical in orientation. It is conceptually much deeper than the other selections. Freedman raises questions such as: Where does the right to informed consent come from? How far does it extend? How much information — and what sort of information — should be revealed? Freedman maintains that there are two requirements for informed consent to be present: the consent must be voluntary and it must be informed. He also touches on the question of whether consent is invalidated by reward in the experimental setting.

Both selections make it very clear that informed consent is not something that takes place by having a patient sign a form. They agree that informed consent is a process that involves information transfer and agreement. The signed form is merely an indication that this process has taken place.

NOTE:

1. See *Canterbury v. Spence* (1972), 464 F.2d; *Cobbs v. Grant*, 502 P.2d 1.

Reibl v. Hughes

Supreme Court of Canada, Laskin, C.J.C., Martland, Dickson, Beetz, Estey, McIntyre and Chouinard J.J. October 7, 1980.

LASKIN, C.J.C.: — The plaintiff appellant, then 44 years of age, underwent serious surgery on March 18, 1970, for the removal of an occlusion in the left internal carotid artery, which had prevented more than a 15% flow of blood through the vessel. The operation was competently performed by the defendant respondent, a qualified neurosurgeon. However, during or immediately following the surgery the plaintiff suffered a massive stroke which left him paralyzed on the right side of his body and also impotent. The plaintiff had, of course, formally consented to the operation. Alleging, however, that his was not an "informed consent", he sued for damages and recovered on this ground in both battery and negligence. The trial Judge, Haines J., awarded a global sum of $225,000 [78 D.L.R. (3d) 35, 16 O.R. (2d) 306].

A majority of the Ontario Court of Appeal ordered a new trial on both liability and damages [89 D.L.R. (3d) 112, 21 O.R. (2d) 14, 6 C.C.L.T. 227]. Speaking through Brooke J.A. (Blair J.A. concurring) the Court ruled out battery as a possible ground of liability on the facts of the case. Jessup J.A., dissenting in part, would have ordered a new trial on damages alone, accepting the judgment at trial on liability.

On the hearing of the appeal by this Court, leave to come here having been obtained by the plaintiff, counsel for the defendant respondent agreed to accept the award of damages and limited his contestation to liability, seeking not only to hold the judgment in appeal but a "variation" thereof by way of dismissal of the action. Although, strictly speaking, the claim for a variation should have been made the subject of a cross-appeal, counsel for the appellant took no objection and I see no reason why I should not regularize the claim for dismissal *nunc pro tunc*. Indeed, neither counsel wished to have a new trial, an understandable position when the physical damage suffered took place more than ten years ago. Unless, therefore, there are good reasons to support the order for a new trial on liability alone, the proper course is to determine whether to restore the judgment at trial on either or both grounds upon which it proceeded or whether the defendant should be relieved of liability.

It is now undoubted that the relationship between surgeon and patient gives rise to a duty of the surgeon to make disclosure to the patient of what I would call all material risks attending the surgery which is recommended. The scope of the duty of disclosure was considered in *Hopp v. Lepp*, a judgment of this Court, delivered on May 20, 1980, ... [112 D.L.R. (3d) 67, 22 A.R. 361, [1980] 4 W.W.R. 645], where it was generalized as follows [at p. 81]:

Reibl v. Hughes, 16 O.R. (2d)306, 78 D.L.R. (3d)35, reversed 21 O.R.(2d) 14,6 C.C.L.T.,227, 89 D.L.R.(3d)112; reverse [1980] 2 S.C.R. 880, 14 C.C.C.T.I., 114 D.L.R.(3d)1, 33 N.R., 17.

> In summary, the decided cases appear to indicate that, in obtaining the consent of a patient for the performance upon him of a surgical operation, a surgeon, generally, should answer any specific questions posed by the patient as to the risks involved and should, without being questioned, disclose to him the nature of the proposed operation, its gravity, any material risks and any special or unusual risks attendant upon the performance of the operation. However, having said that, it should be added that the scope of the duty of disclosure and whether or not it has been breached are matters which must be decided in relation to the circumstances of each particular case.

The Court in *Hopp v. Lepp* also pointed out that even if a certain risk is a mere possibility which ordinarily need not be disclosed, yet if its occurrence carries serious consequences, as for example, paralysis or even death, it should be regarded as a material risk requiring disclosure.

In the present case, the risk attending the surgery or its immediate aftermath was the risk of a stroke, of paralysis and, indeed, of death. This was, without question, a material risk. At the same time, the evidence made it clear that there was also a risk of a stroke and of resulting death if surgery for the removal of the occlusion was refused by the patient. The delicacy of the surgery is beyond question, and its execution is no longer in any way faulted. (I would note here that in this Court no issue was raised as to the adequacy of post-operative care.) How specific, therefore, must the information to the patient be, in a case such as this, to enable him to make an "informed" choice between surgery and no surgery? One of the considerations weighing upon the plaintiff was the fact that he was about a year and a half away from earning a life-time retirement pension as a Ford Motor Company employee. The trial Judge noted (to use his words) ... that "Due to this tragedy befalling him at the time it did, he was not eligible for certain extended disability benefits available under the collective agreement between the Ford Motor Company of Canada Limited and its hourly employees of 10 years' standing." At the time of the operation, the plaintiff had 8.4 years' service with his employer. He stated in his evidence that if he had been properly informed of the magnitude of the risk involved in the surgery he would have elected to forego it, at least until his pension had vested and, further, he would have opted for a shorter normal life than a longer one as a cripple because of the surgery. Although elective surgery was indicated for the condition from which the plaintiff suffered, there was (as the trial Judge found) no emergency in the sense that immediate surgical treatment was imperative.

This brings me back to the question of the nature of the information provided by the respondent surgeon to the plaintiff and its adequacy in the circumstances. I will deal, in turn, with: (1) the findings and conclusion of the trial Judge on this issue; (2) whether, even on his findings, there was a basis for imposing liability for battery; (3) the assessment made by the Court of Appeal in ordering a new trial; (4) the evidence in the case, which consisted, in support of the plaintiff's case, mainly of the testimony of the plaintiff and of two neurosurgeons, Dr. Irving Schacter and Dr. Robert Elgie, and portions of the examination for discovery of the defendant and, in support of the defendant's case, the testimony of the defendant and of a neurosurgeon, Dr. William Lougheed, who were the only two witnesses called for the defendant; (5) the duty of disclosure and review of the findings below; and (6) whether causation was established.

...The well-known statement of Cardozo J. in *Schloendorff v. Society of New York Hospital* (1914), 211 N.Y. 125 at p. 129, 105 N.E. 92 at p. 93, that "every human being of adult years and sound mind has a right to determine what shall be done with his own body; and a surgeon who performs an operation without his patient's consent commits an assault, for which he is liable in damages" cannot be taken beyond the compass of its words to support an action of battery where there has been consent to the very surgical procedure carried out upon a patient but there has been a breach of the duty of disclosure of attendant risks. In my opinion, actions of battery in respect of surgical or other medical treatment should be confined to cases where surgery or treatment has been performed or given to which there has been no consent at all or where, emergency situations aside, surgery or treatment has been performed or given beyond that to which there was consent.

This standard would comprehend cases where there was misrepresentation of the surgery or treatment for which consent was elicited and a different surgical procedure or treatment was carried out. See, for example, *Marshall v. Curry,* [1933] 3 D.L.R. 260, 60 C.C.C. 136 (consent given to operation to cure hernia; doctor removes patient's testicle; action in battery); *Murray v. McMurchy,* [1949] 2 D.L.R. 442, [1949] 1 W.W.R. 989 (consent given to a caesarian operation; doctor goes on and sterilizes the patient; doctor liable for trespass to the person); *Mulloy v. Hop Sang,* [1935] 1 W.W.R. 714 (doctor told to repair hand and not to amputate; performs amputation; held liable in trespass); *Winn et al. v. Alexander et al.,* [1940] 3 D.L.R. 778, [1940] O.W.N. 238 (consent given to caesarian; doctor goes further and sterilizes the patient); *Schweizer v. Central Hospital et al.* (1974), 53 D.L.R. (3d) 494, 6 O.R. (2d) 606 (patient consented to operation on his toe; doctor operated on back instead [spinal fusion]; doctor liable for trespass to the person).

In situations where the allegation is that attendant risks which should have been disclosed were not communicated to the patient and yet the surgery or other medical treatment carried out was that to which the plaintiff consented (there being no negligence basis of liability for the recommended surgery or treatment to deal with the patient's condition), I do not understand how it can be said that the consent was vitiated by the failure of disclosure so as to make the surgery or other treatment an unprivileged, inconsented to and intentional invasion of the patient's bodily integrity. I can appreciate the temptation to say that the genuineness of consent to medical treatment depends on proper disclosure of the risks which it entails, but in my view, unless there has been misrepresentation or fraud to secure consent to the treatment, a failure to disclose the attendant risks, however serious, should go to negligence rather than to battery. Although such a failure relates to an informed choice of submitting to or refusing recommended and appropriate treatment, it arises as the breach of an anterior duty of due care, comparable in legal obligation to the duty of due care in carrying out the particular treatment to which the patient has consented. It is not a test of the validity of the consent.

3. THE ASSESSMENT OF THE COURT OF APPEAL

Brooke J.A., speaking for the majority of the Court of Appeal, noted, ...quite properly, that:

> The duty [of disclosure] to the patient is determined by the Court and the evidence of the expert witnesses, if accepted, is relevant to determining whether or not the defendant has dis-

> charged that duty. To be actionable [in negligence] the defendant's failure in his duty of care must cause the plaintiff loss and damage.

He went on to examine the reasons of Haines J. and made the following observations upon that trial Judge's determination: ...

> In finding that the plaintiff was left with the impression that the surgery carried no risk of consequence other than those in any surgical procedure I think it must be assumed that the learned trial Judge has rejected the defendant's explanation that the plaintiff was aware of the risk of a stroke as a risk of the surgery. Of some importance, the learned trial Judge makes no specific finding of credibility and indeed does not disbelieve the defendant's evidence that he thought the plaintiff understood the risk. However, the learned trial Judge did not put his judgment simply on the failure to warn, but also on the failure to take sufficient care to discuss the degree of risk. He relied upon the evidence of Dr. Elgie and Dr. Schacter and it is my respectful view that, having regard for the emphasis which the learned trial Judge places upon the statistical details, he has misunderstood the real significance of the evidence of these two doctors. Drs. Schacter and Elgie appear to have taken a similar approach to the question of explaining the risks of the surgery, but the emphasis is not on statistical detail. Dr. Elgie alone made reference to statistics in discussing the manner in which he would advise his patient when seeking a consent to perform this operation and in this respect his answer was different from that of Dr. Schacter.

Brooke J.A. was highly critical of the use of unexplained statistics which appeared to be directed to the degree of risk involved in the particular surgery. This is what he said in that respect: ...

> One need only look at the contrast in the evidence of the statistics quoted by Dr. Hughes and Dr. Elgie to demonstrate the confusion that could arise from their use. When asked in cross-examination, Dr. Hughes' figure as to the incidence of death because of surgery was 4%, which was equal to Dr. Elgie's highest figure where he put the range between 2% and 4%, and with respect to the incidence of stroke causing paralysis or transient weakness, Dr. Hughes put the figure at 10% which was five times Dr. Elgie's lowest figure and almost two and one-half times his highest figure. Taken cumulatively, Dr. Hughes' figure at 14% is more than three times Dr. Elgie's lowest estimate and almost twice his highest. They were really very different. The reason for the difference went unexplained. No one asked the doctors. And yet the trial Judge referred principally in his reasons, and particularly in testing the defendant's conduct, to the statistics recounted by Dr. Hughes, which there was no suggestion the doctor attempted to use. If the difference is based solely or partly on the personal experience of the surgeons, and there is in the evidence some reason suggested that this may be so, then perhaps the explanation lies in the nature of the cases that each has dealt with and that the chance of survivorship of those undertaken by one was less than the other. If this is so, there may have been good reason not to mention sta-

> tistics to the patient, but rather to simply contrast his position if he undertakes the surgery with that of not undertaking it and urge him to proceed because of his youth and strength giving some assurance of survivorship. I do not think the evidence justifies the statement made by the learned trial Judge and I would hesitate to lay down any such requirements, for in my view, statistics can be very misleading. The manner in which the nature and degree of risk is explained to a particular patient is better left to the judgment of the doctor in dealing with the man before him. Its adequacy can be simply tested.

I think the Ontario Court of Appeal went too far, when dealing with the standard of disclosure of risks, in saying, as it did in the passage of its reasons just quoted, that "the manner in which the nature and degree of risk is explained to a particular patient is better left to the judgment of the doctor in dealing with the man before him". Of course, it can be tested by expert medical evidence but that too is not determinative. The patient may have expressed certain concerns to the doctor and the latter is obliged to meet them in a reasonable way. What the doctor knows or should know that the particular patient deems relevant to a decision whether to undergo prescribed treatment goes equally to his duty of disclosure as do the material risks recognized as a matter of required medical knowledge.

It is important to examine this issue in greater detail. The Ontario Court of Appeal appears to have adopted a professional medical standard, not only for determining what are the material risks that should be disclosed but also, and concurrently, for determining whether there has been a breach of the duty of disclosure. This was also the approach of the trial Judge, notwithstanding that on the facts he found against the defendant. (Indeed, the trial Judge seems also to have overstated the duty of disclosure. The Court of Appeal, in contrast, seems to have understated it. Generally, the failure to mention statistics should not affect the duty to inform nor be a factor in deciding whether the duty has been breached.) To allow expert medical evidence to determine what risks are material and, hence, should be disclosed and, correlatively, what risks are not material is to hand over to the medical profession the entire question of the scope of the duty of disclosure, including the question whether there has been a breach of that duty. Expert medical evidence is, of course, relevant to findings as to the risks that reside in or are a result of recommended surgery or other treatment. It will also have a bearing on their materiality but this is not a question that is to be concluded on the basis of the expert medical evidence alone. The issue under consideration is a different issue from that involved where the question is whether the doctor carried out his professional activities by applicable professional standards. What is under consideration here is the patient's right to know what risks are involved in undergoing or foregoing certain surgery or other treatment.

The materiality of non-disclosure of certain risks to an informed decision is a matter for the trier of fact, a matter on which there would, in all likelihood, be medical evidence but also other evidence, including evidence from the patient or from members of his family. It is, of course, possible that a particular patient may waive aside any question of risks and be quite prepared to submit to the surgery or treatment, whatever they be. Such a situation presents no difficulty. Again, it may be the case that a particular patient may, because of emotional factors, be unable to cope with facts relevant to recommended surgery or treatment and the doctor may, in such a case, be justified in withholding or generalizing information as to which he would otherwise be required to be more specific.

...

If Canadian case law has so far proceeded on a subjective test of causation, it is in Courts other than this one that such an approach has been taken: see *Koehler v. Cook* (1975), 65 D.L.R. (3d) 766 at p. 767, [1976] W.W.D. 71, and *Kelly v. Hazlett* (1976), 75 D.L.R. (3d) 536 at pp. 565-6, 15 O.R. (2d) 290 at p. 320. The matter is *res integra* here. An alternative to the subjective test is an objective one, that is, what would a reasonable person in the patient's position have done if there had been proper disclosure of attendant risks. The case for the objective standard has been tersely put in the following passage from a comment in 48 N.Y.U.L. Rev. 548 (1973), at p. 550, entitled "Informed Consent — A Proposed Standard for Medical Disclosure":

> Since proximate causation exists only if disclosure would have resulted in the patient's foregoing the proposed treatment, a standard must be developed to determine whether the patient would have decided against the treatment had he been informed of its risks. Two possible standards exist: whether, if informed, the particular patient would have foregone treatment (subjective view); or whether the average prudent person in plaintiff's position, informed of all material risks, would have foregone treatment (objective view). The objective standard is preferable, since the subjective standard has a gross defect: it depends on the plaintiff's testimony as to his state of mind, thereby exposing the physician to the patient's hindsight and bitterness.

However, a vexing problem raised by the objective standard is whether causation could ever be established if the surgeon has recommended surgery which is warranted by the patient's condition. Can it be said that a reasonable person in the patient's position, to whom proper disclosure of attendant risks has been made, would decide against the surgery, that is, against the surgeon's recommendation that it be undergone? The objective standard of what a reasonable person in the patient's position would do would seem to put a premium on the surgeon's assessment of the relative need for the surgery and on supporting medical evidence of that need. Could it be reasonably refused? Brooke J.A. appeared to be sensitive to this problem by suggesting a combined objective-subjective test.

I doubt that this will solve the problem. It could hardly be expected that the patient who is suing would admit that he would have agreed to have the surgery, even knowing all the accompanying risks. His suit would indicate that, having suffered serious disablement because of the surgery, he is convinced that he would not have permitted it if there had been proper disclosure of the risks, balanced by the risks of refusing the surgery. Yet, to apply a subjective test to causation would, correlatively, put a premium on hindsight, even more of a premium than would be put on medical evidence in assessing causation by an objective standard.

I think it is the safer course on the issue of causation to consider objectively how far the balance in the risks of surgery or no surgery is in favour of undergoing surgery. The failure of proper disclosure pro and con becomes therefore very material. And so too are any special considerations affecting the particular patient. For example, the patient may have asked specific questions which were either brushed aside or were not fully answered or were answered wrongly. In the present case, the anticipation of a full pension would be a special consideration, and, while it would have to be viewed objectively, it emerges from the patient's particular circumstances. So too, other aspects of the objective standard would have to be geared to what the average prudent person, the reasonable person in the patient's particular position, would agree to or not agree to, if all material and special risks of going ahead with the surgery or foregoing it were made known to him. Far from making the patient's own testimony irrelevant, it is essential to his case that he put his own position forward.

The adoption of an objective standard does not mean that the issue of causation is completely in the hands of the surgeon. Merely because medical evidence establishes the reasonableness of a recommended operation does not mean that a reasonable person in the patient's position would necessarily agree to it, if proper disclosure had been made of the risks attendant upon it, balanced by those against it. The patient's particular situation and the degree to which the risks of surgery or no surgery are balanced would reduce the force, on an objective appraisal, of the surgeon's recommendation. Admittedly, if the risk of foregoing the surgery would be considerably graver to a patient than the risks attendant upon it, the objective standard would favour exoneration of the surgeon who has not made the required disclosure. Since liability rests only in negligence, in a failure to disclose material risks, the issue of causation would be in the patient's hands on a subjective test, and would, if his evidence was accepted, result inevitably in liability unless, of course, there was a finding that there was no breach of the duty of disclosure. In my view, therefore, the objective standard is the preferable one on the issue of causation.

In saying that the test is based on the decision that a reasonable person in the patient's position would have made, I should make it clear that the patient's particular concerns must also be reasonably based; otherwise, there would be more subjectivity than would be warranted under an objective test. Thus, for example, fears which are not related to the material risks which should have been but were not disclosed would not be causative factors. However, economic considerations could reasonably go to causation where, for example, the loss of an eye as a result of nondisclosure of a material risk brings about the loss of a job for which good eyesight is required. In short, although account must be taken of a patient's particular position, a position which will vary with the patient, it must be objectively assessed in terms of reasonableness.

...

5. BREACH OF DUTY OF DISCLOSURE: THE FINDINGS BELOW REVIEWED

In my opinion, the record of evidence amply justifies the trial Judge's findings that the plaintiff was told no more or understood no more than that he would be better off to have the operation than not to have it. This was not an adequate, not a sufficient disclosure of the risk attendant upon the operation itself, a risk well appreciated by the defendant in view of his own experience that of the 60 to 70 such operations that he had previously performed, 8 to 10 resulted in the death of the patients. Although the mortality rate was falling by 1970, the morbidity (the sickness or disease) rate, according to Dr. Hughes, was still about 10%. The trial Judge was also justified in finding that the plaintiff, who was concerned about his continuing headaches and who was found to be suffering from hypertension, had the impression that the surgery would alleviate his headaches and hypertension so that he could carry on with his job. Dr. Hughes made it plain in his evidence that the surgery would not cure the headaches but did not, as the trial Judge found, make this plain to the plaintiff.

The foregoing findings have a basis in the evidence independent of any reliance on so-called statistics which was criticized by the majority of the Court of Appeal. Although Brooke J.A., speaking for the majority, appeared to discount the trial Judge's determinations because the latter made no specific finding on credibility, it is patent to me that the trial Judge's conclusions involved a weighing of the evidence and, hence, a measuring of its relative worth on the issues that he had to decide. There were inconsistencies in the defendant's evidence, as the trial Judge noted in his reasons, and it was for him to reconcile them in arriving at his findings. For example, the defendant said in-chief that he had told the plaintiff of the risk of a stroke during surgery and then said on cross-examination that the risks of the surgery were quite minimal. Again, on cross-examination, he said that he did not tell the patient that there was a risk of a stroke as a result of the surgery at any specific time thereafter, and he returned to an oft repeated statement that the chances of paralysis were greater without an operation than with it. (This was also the only reference by Dr. Lougheed, who testified for the defence, as to the risk involved in submitting to or foregoing the surgery. His evidence was almost exclusively related to post-operative care and whether a re-operation was feasible. He said it was not. However, as I noted earlier, post-operative care was not an issue in this Court.) Moreover, the defendant placed this risk as one within a few years and not within any immediate time. Indeed, when asked in cross-examination whether he told the patient that the surgery carried the risk of a stroke, he answered, "I didn't say that specifically." This was certainly a case in which a trial Judge, here an experienced Judge, was in a better position than an appellate Court or this Court to determine what evidence to accept and what conclusions to draw from it.

In the ... reasons of Brooke J.A., speaking for the majority of the Court of Appeal, there are two approaches on the crucial issue whether the defendant apprised the plaintiff of the risk of a stroke from the very operation. In the first ... passage, the learned Justice of Appeal appears to have viewed the trial Judge's finding on this question as a finding that the plaintiff was not made aware of that risk. This is clearly a correct assessment of the trial Judge's conclusion. However, Brooke J.A. went on to deal with the case and with the evidence as if there was a partial albeit not a sufficient disclosure of the particular risk, and he proceeded from there into an appraisal of the statistics to which the trial Judge referred and found fault in their use. In the second ... passage ... Brooke J.A. ... ignores the finding of the trial Judge that there was no disclosure of the risks inherent in the surgery itself. In my opinion, there was a failure by the Court of Appeal to address this point directly. In the light of the defendant's own evidence that there was a failure on his part to disclose the risk, even though the plaintiff himself raised the question of the risks he faced on the operating table, I do not see how there could be any doubt of a breach in this respect of the duty of disclosure.

Indeed, the reasons of the Court of Appeal ... appear to support the trial Judge's finding that there was no proper disclosure by the defendant of the risk of the surgery itself. Brooke J.A. said this on the question [at p. 119]:

> He [the defendant] did not specifically discuss the questions of death or paralysis as risks of the surgery,

> his explanation being that he believed the patient was aware of the risk because of questions that he asked when the surgery was being discussed. It was his view that no further detail was necessary.

In this respect then, there would seem to be concurrent findings of fact against the defendant on a central point in case.

There were a number of relevant considerations informing the findings of the trial Judge, about which there was no dispute. First, there was no emergency making surgery imperative. There was no noticeable neurological deficit. The defendant himself placed the risk of a stroke as one off in the future, four to five years. Any immediate risk would be from the surgery and not from foregoing it. Moreover, it must have been obvious to the defendant that the plaintiff had some difficulty with the English language and that he should, therefore, have made certain that he was understood. Finally, there was no evidence that the plaintiff was emotionally taut or unable to accept disclosure of the grave risk to which he would be exposed by submitting to surgery. I do not see in the reasons of the majority of the Court of Appeal any evidentiary basis for challenging the findings of the trial Judge on the defendant's breach of the duty of disclosure. Of course, the medical evidence was relevant to what that duty entailed but, that said, it was for the trier of fact to determine the scope of the duty and to decide whether there had been a breach of the duty. As I have already said, the so-called statistical data used by the trial Judge did not affect the grounds upon which he made his critical findings. The Court of Appeal held, however, that the trial Judge did not examine the issue of causation with the necessary care that this issue required. He did not ignore it, even if he might have gone into it at greater length. The question that remains, therefore, is whether this was a sufficient basis upon which to direct a new trial.

6. CAUSATION

Relevant in this case to the issue whether a reasonable person in the plaintiff's position would have declined surgery at the particular time is the fact that he was within about one and one-half years of earning pension benefits if he continued at his job; that there was no neurological deficit then apparent; that there was no immediate emergency making the surgery imperative; that there was a grave risk of a stroke or worse during or as a result of the operation, while the risk of a stroke without it was in the future, with no precise time fixed or which could be fixed except as a guess of three or more years ahead. Since, on the trial Judge's finding, the plaintiff was under the mistaken impression, as a result of the defendant's breach of the duty of disclosure, that the surgery would relieve his continuing headaches, this would in the opinion of a reasonable person in the plaintiff's position, also weigh against submitting to the surgery at the particular time.

In my opinion, a reasonable person in the plaintiff's position would, on a balance of probabilities, have opted against the surgery rather than undergoing it at the particular time.

CONCLUSION

I would, accordingly, allow the appeal, set aside the order of the Court of Appeal and restore the judgment at trial. The appellant is entitled to costs throughout.

Informed Consent
Ethical Considerations for Physicians and Surgeons

The Royal College of Physicians and Surgeons of Canada

PREMISES

In the medical context, informed consent refers to the prerogative of patients to make decisions about their medical treatment. The nature of this prerogative is a matter of dispute in both law and ethics.

Physicians should learn about the legal requirements for informed consent (for example, the 1980 Supreme Court of Canada judgement in the Reibl versus Hughes case). However, adherence to the law does not guarantee acceptable ethical behavior. Whether in the Code of Ethics of the Canadian Medical Association/Royal College or in specific physician-patient relationships, higher standards of informed consent than those required by law may be appropriate.

There is a range of positions on decision-making authority in the physician-patient relationship. One extreme option, commonly called paternalism, would vest absolute authority in the physician. The other extreme would require the physician to do whatever the patient demands. Between these two poles are various forms of shared responsibility.

Medical paternalism has been found inappropriate for contemporary medical practice. It is considered to be at odds with the principle of individual autonomy, which has emerged as a paramount value in Western nations.

With the decline of paternalism there has arisen a great emphasis on patients' rights to decision-making authority in health care. Although this represents a necessary corrective to paternalism, there is a danger of exaggerating these rights at the expense of both the duties of patients to co-operate with physicians, and the rights of physicians and other health care professionals, which may conflict with those of patients.

Informed consent, however conceived, should not be an end, but a means of optimal medical care for all patients. Patients and physicians should strive for agreement about the treatment to be undertaken, but this is not always possible. Procedures need to be established to deal with situations in which the patient is not competent to participate in the decision-making process, or where physician and patient cannot agree on what should be done.

PRINCIPLES

An essential condition for the exercise of informed consent is good communication between physician and patients (or their surrogates). The physician has primary responsibility for ensuring that such communication occurs. Patients have an obligation to provide the physician with all relevant information about their conditions,

"Informed Consent: Ethical Considerations for Physicians and Surgeons," *Annals of the Royal College of Physicians and Surgeons of Canada, 21:1*(1988).

to enable him or her to offer the best diagnosis and treatment.

Competent patients (those who can make rational decisions about their medical care), have the right to make such decisions. The physician is morally obliged to respect this right by providing patients with all reasonable data about diagnostic and therapeutic procedures, and possible alternatives and risks, and by allowing patients to make their decisions without coercion. Competent patients may waive this right to informed consent in full or in part, in which case the physician should provide whatever treatment he or she believes to be in the patients' best interests.

Incompetent patients should be treated in their best interests, as determined by the physician on the basis of the patients' expressed wishes while competent. For patients who have not indicated how they want to be treated, the physician should make the decision about treatment in consultation with the patients' families or guardians, other medical staff, and other persons he or she may wish to consult (for example, close friends, clergy) as time and circumstances permit.

PROCEDURES

The physician should encourage his or her patients to exercise their right to make their own decisions about their medical treatment. If he or she detects unusual hesitation on their part regarding their willingness or ability to make such decisions, he or she should ascertain whether they are competent and act accordingly.

If the patients are competent and wish to make their own decisions, the physician should provide all the information that they need to make adequately informed decisions. If the decisions involve treatment or refusal of treatment in which the physician cannot, in good conscience, participate, he or she should try to refer the patients to another physician or institution which can fulfill the patients' wishes.

If the patients are competent but cannot decide among treatment options, the physician might suggest that they seek a second opinion from another physician.

If the patients are competent but prefer to let the physician make the decisions, he or she should attempt to determine their reasons for so acting. If they seem reasonable (for example, uncertainty about treatment options or trust in the physician's judgement), he or she should act according to his or her estimation of the patients' best interests.

If the patients are obviously incompetent (infants, the unconscious, the severely retarded), the physician should consult, where possible, the families or guardians, and other medical staff before deciding on a course of treatment. Where parents or guardians request treatment that, in the physician's opinion, are contrary to the best interests of the patients, or refuse treatments that he or she believes are in their best interests, the physician should take whatever action is necessary to prevent harm to the patients; this may include recourse to the courts.

If the patients' competence is uncertain, the physician should attempt to minimize the uncertainty by seeking medical consultation before trying to secure informed consent. If the patients' decisions or refusal to decide seem unreasonable and are likely to result in serious harm to them, the physician should consult with the families, colleagues, and hospital authorities about the advisability of acting against, or in the absence of the patients' expressed wishes, at least until their competence is no longer in doubt.

In emergency situations where the patient is incompetent, the physician should provide whatever treatment he or she believes to be in the patient's best interests.

Where there is more than one physician dealing with a patient, each one should deal directly with the patient in securing informed consent for medical treatment. Physicians should not rely on medical students, nurses or other physicians to secure this consent.

Before undergoing exploratory surgery or other temporarily incapacitating treatment, patients should be adequately informed about the possible interventions which may be necessary while they are incompetent. They should be given the opportunity to indicate in advance which types of procedures they would be willing to undergo and which they would refuse.

MAXIMS

— Tell your patients all they want and need to know about their medical care.

— Know your own expertise as a physician and do not hesitate to refer patients to more qualified colleagues.

— Listen closely to your patients and, if necessary, their families and acquaintances in order to determine what is in their best interests.

— Aim for agreement with your patients as to the best medical treatment for them.

— Where agreement is absent, defer to your patients' judgement except where their competence is doubtful or lacking.

— In any circumstances involving apparently contentious issues of informed consent, record in the patient's clinical file all relevant information concerning the acquisition of such consent.

A Moral Theory of Consent

Benjamin Freedman

Most medical codes of ethics, and most physicians, agree that the physician ought to obtain the "free and informed consent" of his subject or patient before attempting any serious medical procedures, experimental or therapeutic in nature. They agree, moreover, that a proxy consent ought to be obtained on behalf of the incompetent subject. And informed consent is seen as not merely a legal requirement, and not merely a formality: it is a substantial requirement of morality.

Acceptance of this doctrine, however, requires the solution of a number of problems. How much information need be imparted? At what age is a person mature enough to consent on his own behalf? Can prisoners give a "free and informed consent" to be experimented upon? Lurking behind these and similar questions there are more fundamental difficulties. What are the functions of consent for the competent and the incompetent? What is the sense in which the patient/subject must be

Benjamin Freedman, "A Moral Theory of Consent," *Hastings Center Report 5:4* (August 1975); 32-39.

"free," "informed," and "competent?" It is by way of an approach to these latter questions that I shall attempt to respond to the more specific questions.[1]

I. CONSENT AND THE COMPETENT

The negative aspects of the doctrine of informed consent have ordinarily been the focus of attention; difficulties in obtaining the informed consent of the subject/patient render the ethics of experimentation and therapeutic measures questionable. Our common view of informed consent is that, when at all relevant, it represents a minimum condition which ethics imposes upon the physician. It is seen as a necessary condition for medical manipulation, but hardly as a sufficient condition.

The reasons why this is so — why it is not sufficient that an experimenter, for instance, have received informed consent from his subject before proceeding — are quite obvious. The scarcity of medical resources (which includes a scarcity of qualified physician-investigators) forbids us from wasting time upon poorly-designed experiments, or upon experiments which merely replicate well-established conclusions. There seems to be, as well, a limit to the dangers which we (ordinarily) allow subjects to face. We do not, as a matter of policy, think it wise to allow would-be suicides to accomplish their end with the aid of a scientific investigator. Many other reasons could be given for the proposition that a person does not have a right to be experimented upon, even when he has given valid consent to the procedure.

The Right to Consent

But there does seem to exist a positive right of informed consent, which exists in both therapeutic and experimental settings. A person who has the capacity to give valid consent, and who has in fact consented to the procedure in question, has a right to have that fact recognized by us. We all have a duty to recognize a valid consent when confronted with it.

From whence derives this right? It arises from the right which each of us possesses to be treated as a person, and in the duty which all of us have, to have respect for persons, to treat a person as such, and not as an object. For this entails that our capacities for personhood ought to be recognized by all — these capacities including the capacity for rational decision, and for action consequent upon rational decision. Perhaps the worst which we may do to a man is to deny him his humanity, for example, by classifying him as mentally incompetent when he is, in fact, sane. It is a terrible thing to be hated or persecuted; it is far worse to be ignored, to be notified that you "don't count."

If an individual is capable of and has given valid consent, I would argue that he has a right, as against the world but more particularly as against his physician, to have it recognized that valid consent has been given. (The same applies, of course, with still greater force, with regard to *refusals* to consent to medical procedures.) The limited force of this claim must be emphasized: it does not entail a right to be treated, or to be experimented upon. It is a most innocuous right, one which most of us would have little hesitation about granting.

It is, therefore, curious that the literature on informed consent has failed to recognize this right — has, in fact, tacitly denied this right, at least as regards experimentation. In writings on informed consent it seems to have been assumed that if, under certain conditions, it is *doubtful* that valid consent to an experiment has been granted, it is best to "play it safe" ethically. In cases of doubt, we prefer not to take chances: in this case, we will not take a chance upon violating the canons of ethics by experimenting without being certain that the subject has validly consented to the experiment. Since we do not at present know whether a prisoner can give a valid consent, let us not take chances: we call for a moratorium on prison experimentation. Since we do not know at what age a person has the capacity to give a valid consent, we avoid the problem by setting the age of majority at a point where it is beyond doubt that maturity has been attained. If we must err, we shall ensure that we err in being overly ethical.

The establishment of the innocuous right to have valid consent recognized as such eliminates this expedient. Other writers have conceptualized the conflict as one between a right and, at best, a mere liberty. From the patient's point of view, he has a right to have his health protected by the physician, and a mere liberty to be experimented upon. From the physician-investigator's point of view, he has a duty to protect the subject's health, and a mere liberty to experiment upon the subject (contingent, of course, upon obtaining the subject's consent). A recognition of the claims of personhood and autonomy, however, reveals this to be a conflict between rights and duties. The physician-investigator has a duty to recognize consent when validly offered. When the consent is of doubtful validity, therefore, the physician experiences a conflict between two duties. He will not be ethically well-protected by choosing not to experiment, for there exists the possibility — which, as cases are multiplied, becomes a probability — that he is violating a duty in so choosing. Problems in informed consent present us with a dilemma. It is no longer the case that the burden of proof devolves upon the would-be experimenter. The would-be abstainer-from-experiments may have to prove his case as well.

These considerations give us a new point of departure in investigating problems of informed consent. They show us that there is no "fail-safe" procedure which we can fall back upon in cases of doubt. Rather, what is required is an exhaustive examination of each case and issue, to see whether or not a valid consent has in fact been obtained.

When we fail to recognize a valid consent, of course, more is involved than a denial of personhood. Other benefits may be denied as well. Dr. Vernon Mark, for example, maintains that psychosurgery should not be done on prisoners with epilepsy because of the problem in obtaining a voluntary consent from prisoners.[2] But a resolution of this problem has not been shown to be impossible. Surely, the proper thing to do here would be to see whether prisoners can or cannot give valid consent to such a procedure. To remain satisfied with doubts, to fail to investigate this question, complex though it be, results in a denial of medical treatment for the prisoner, as well as representing a negation of the prisoner's human capacities. In depriving prisoners of the opportunity to serve as subjects in medical experiments, there are losses other than those of human respect.[3] Not the least of these is the loss of an opportunity to be of altruistic service to mankind.[4] Even a child feels at times a need to be useful; in promoting a moratorium on prison experimentation we deny prisoners the satisfaction of this psychic need. We should not need a reminder from John Stuart Mill that there are "higher" as well as "lower" pleasures and needs.

The right to have valid consent recognized as such does not indicate that we must experiment on prisoners. What it does indicate is that we have a moral responsibility to investigate in detail the question of whether prisoners can, under certain conditions, validly consent to experimentation. It also requires that we not prevent a researcher from experimenting on the basis of over-scrupulousness. If prisoners *can* give valid consent, we wrong not only the researcher but the prisoner as well by forbidding prison experimentation.

The Requirement of Information

The most common locution for the requirement which I am discussing is "informed consent" — we require "informed consent" to protect a doctor from legal liability resultant from his therapeutic endeavors, or to ensure the "ethicacy" of an experiment. But I believe "informed consent" to be a serious misnomer for what we do, in fact, want medical practice to conform to.

No lengthy rehearsal of the absurdities consequent upon taking the term "informed consent" at face value is necessary. The claim has been made, and repeated with approval, that "fully informed consent" is a goal which we can never achieve, but toward which we must strive. In order to ensure that fully informed consent has been given, it has seriously been suggested that only medical students or graduate students in the life sciences ought to be accepted as subjects for experimentation. *Reductio ad absurdum* examples of "fully informed consent" have been elaborated, in forms which list all the minutiae of the proposed medical procedure, together with all of its conceivable sequelae. With such a view of "informed consent" and its requirements, it is not surprising to find doctors who claim that since they cannot fully inform patients, they will tell them nothing, but instead will personally assume the responsibility for assuring the subject's safety.

In truth, a *reductio ad absurdum* of this view of "informed consent" need not be constructed; it serves as its own *reductio ad absurdum*. For there is no end to "fully informing" patients. When the doctor wishes to insert a catheter, must he commend to the subject's attention a textbook of anatomy? Although this, of course, would not suffice: he must ensure that the patient understands the text as well. Must he tell the patient the story of Dr. X, that bogey of first-year medical students, who, in a state of inebriation, inserted ("by mistake") his pen-refill instead of the catheter? With, of course, the assurance that *this* physician never gets drunk ("Well, rarely, anyway"). Must the patient be informed of the chemical formula of the catheter? Its melting point?

The basic mistake which is committed by those who harp upon the difficulties in obtaining informed consent (and by critics of the doctrine) is in believing that we can talk about information in the abstract, without reference to any human purpose. It is very likely impossible to talk about "information" in this way; but impossible or not, when we do in fact talk about, or request, information, we do not mean "information in the abstract." If I ask someone to "tell me about those clouds" he will, ordinarily, know what I mean; and he will answer me, in the spirit in which he was asked, by virtue of his professional expertise as an artist, meteorologist, astronomer, soothsayer, or what-have-you. The meteorologist will not object that he cannot tell you the optical refraction index of the clouds, and therefore that he cannot "fully answer" your question. He knows that you are asking him with a given end in mind, and that much information about the cloud is irrelevant *relative to that purpose*.

That this "abstract information" requirement is not in question in obtaining valid consent is hardly an original point, but it is worth repeating. One of the leading court opinions on human experimentation puts it like this: "...the patient's interest in information does not extend to a lengthy polysyllabic discourse on all possible complications. A mini-course in medical science is not required...."[5]

The proper question to ask, then, is not "What information must be given?" That would be premature: we must first know for what purpose information is needed. *Why* must the patient be informed? Put that way, the answer is immediately forthcoming. The patient must be informed so that he will know what he is getting into, what he may expect from the procedure, what his likely alternatives are — in short, what the procedure (and forbearance from it) will mean, so that a responsible decision on the matter may be made. This is the legal stance, as well as, I think, a "common-sensical" stance; as Alexander Capron writes, the information component in valid consent derives in law from the recognition that information is "necessary to make meaningful the power to decide."[6] The proper test of whether a given piece of information needs to be given is, then, whether the physician, knowing what he does about the patient/subject, feels that that patient/subject would want to know this before making up his mind. Outré, improbable consequences would not ordinarily, therefore, be relevant information. Exceptionally, they will be: for example, when there is a small risk of impotence consequent upon the procedure which the physician proposes to perform upon a man with a great stake in his sexual prowess. This is only sensible.

Our main conclusion, then, is that valid consent entails only the imparting of that information which the patient/subject requires in order to make a responsible decision. This entails, I think, the possibility of a valid yet ignorant consent.

Consider, first, the therapeutic context. It is, I believe, not unusual for a patient to give his doctor *carte blanche* to perform any medical procedure which the physician deems proper in order to effect a cure. He is telling the doctor to act as his agent in choosing which procedure to follow. This decision is neither unwise nor (in any serious sense) an abdication of responsibility and an unwarranted burden upon the physician. We each of us choose to delegate our power of choice in this way in dealing with our auto mechanic or stockbroker.

It may be harder to accept an ignorant consent as valid in the purely experimental context. I think, however, that much of this difficulty is due to our paucity of imagination, our failure to imagine circumstances in which a person might choose to proceed in this way. We might approach such a case, for example, by imagining a Quaker who chooses to serve society by acting as a research subject, but who has a morbid fear of knives and pointed instruments. The Quaker might say to the physician-investigator that he wants to serve science but is afraid that his phobia would overcome his better judgment. He might consequently request that any experiment which would involve use of scalpels, hypodermic needles, and such, be performed without informing him: while, say, he is asleep or unconscious. He might further ask the doctor not to proceed should the experiment involve considerable risk. In such a case, or one similar, we would find an instance of a valid yet ignorant consent to experimentation.

The ostensible differences between the therapeutic and experimental contexts may be resolved into two components: in the therapeutic context it is supposed that the physician knows what the sequelae to treatment will be, which information, by definition, is not available in the experimental situation; and in the therapeutic context the doctor may be said to be seeking his patient's good, in contrast to the experimental context where some other good is being sought. On the basis of these differences it may be claimed that a valid yet ignorant consent is enough permission for therapy, but not for experimentation.

Closer examination, however, reveals that these differences do not necessarily obtain. First, because I believe it would be granted that a valid yet ignorant consent can be given in the "therapeutic-experimental" situation, where a new drug or procedure is being attempted to aid the patient (in the absence of any traditional available therapy). In the therapeutic-experimental situation, as in the purely experimental situation, the sequelae are not known (although of course in both cases some definite result is expected or anticipated). If a valid yet ignorant consent is acceptable in the one, therefore, it must be acceptable in the other.

Secondly, because it is patently not the case that we can expect there to be no good accruing to the subject of an experiment by reason of his participation. There are, commonly, financial and other "tangible" benefits forthcoming (laboratory training, and so on). And it must once again be said that the pleasures of altruism are not negligible. The proposed differences between experimentation and therapy do not stand up, and so we must say that if a valid yet ignorant consent is acceptable in the one it must be acceptable in the other. It must be remembered that this statement only concerns itself with one part of the consent doctrine, which is, itself, only one of the requirements which the ethical experiment must satisfy.

To mention — without claiming totally to resolve — two problems which may be raised at this point: First, it is said that a doctor often does not know what will happen as a consequence of a recommended procedure, and so cannot tell the patient what the patient wants to know. The obvious response to this seems to be right: the physician should, in that case, tell the patient/subject that he does not know what will happen (which does not exclude an explanation of what the doctor expects to happen, and on what he bases this expectation).

Second, it will be objected that the adoption of a requirement such as I propose would forbid the use of placebos and blind experiments. I am not sure that this is so; sometimes it must be the case that the subjects in an experiment may be asked (without introducing artifacts into the results) to consent to an experiment knowing that some will, and some will not, be receiving placebos. Another alternative would be to inform the subjects that the experiment may or may not involve some subjects receiving placebos.[7] I am aware, however, that these remarks are less than adequate responses to these problems.

Our conclusion, then, is that the informing of the patient/subject is not a fundamental requirement of valid consent. It is, rather, derivative from the requirement that the consent be the expression of a responsible choice. The two requirements which I do see as fundamental in this doctrine are that the choice be responsible and that it be voluntary.

The Requirement of Responsibility

What is meant by saying that the choice must be "responsible"? Does this entail that the physician may at any time override a patient's judgment on the basis that, in the physician's view, the patient has not chosen responsibly? Surely not; to adopt such a criterion would defeat the purpose embodied in the doctrine of consent. It would mean that a person's exercise of autonomy is always subject to review.

Still, some such requirement would appear to be necessary. A small child can certainly make choices.[8] Small children can also be intelligent enough to understand the necessary information. Yet surely we would not want to say that a small child can give valid consent to a serious medical procedure.[9] The reason for this is that the child cannot choose *responsibly*.

We are faced with a dilemma. On the one hand, it appears that we must require that the choice be responsible. To require only that the choice be free would yield counter-intuitive results. On the other hand, if we do require that the choice made be a responsible one, we seem to presuppose some body which shall judge the reasonableness of choices; this represents a paternalism which is antithetical to the doctrine of consent. An elderly patient chooses to forgo further life-saving measures. How are we to judge whether or not this choice is a responsible one?

The path between the horns of this dilemma involves saying that the "responsibility" which we require is to be predicated not on the nature of the particular choice, but on the nature of the patient/subject. What we need to know is whether *he* is a responsible man ("in general," so to speak), not whether the choice which has been made is responsible. In this way, we avoid the danger of upholding as "responsible" only those choices which we ourselves feel are good choices. We can and do admit into the community of responsible persons individuals who make choices with which we do not agree.

In this sense, responsibility is a dispositional characteristic. To say that someone is a responsible individual means that he makes choices, typically, on the basis of reasons, arguments, or beliefs — and that he remains open to the claims of reason, so that further rational argument might lead him to change his mind. It is to say that a person is capable of making and carrying through a life-plan — that he is prepared to act on the basis of his choices. It is to say that a person is capable of living with his life-plan; he can live with the consequences of his choices, he *takes responsibility* for his choices.[10] Of course, none of these are absolutes: all responsible people are at times pigheaded, at times short-sighted, at times flighty. That is to say, all responsible men at times act irresponsibly. Should the lack of responsibility persist, of course, to an extreme degree, we may say that the person has left the community of responsible folk.

Voluntarism and Reward

The other requirement of valid consent is that it be given voluntarily. The choice which the consent expresses must be freely made.

We all know some conditions which, if satisfied, make us say that a consent has been given involuntarily. The case which immediately springs to mind occurs when an individual succumbs under a threat: we call this duress or coercion. But the threat need not be overt; and perhaps there need not be a threat at all to render consent involuntary.

Hence, the major problem currently engendered by the requirement of voluntariness. It is typified by the prisoner who "volunteers" for an experiment in the hope or expectation of a reward: significantly higher wages, an opportunity for job training, better health care while involved in the experiment, a favorable report to his parole board. Is the consent which the prisoner offers a voluntary consent? The problem may be stated more generally thus: At what point does reward render consent involuntary?

The problem of reward is particularly difficult, since it involves questions of degree. Is a prisoner's consent involuntary if the reward for his participation in the experiment is a three-month reduction of sentence? Is it relevant here that the prisoner is serving a twenty-year sentence, rather than a one-to-five-year sentence? Does a possible increase in wages from twenty-five cents per hour to one dollar per hour constitute duress? Should we consider the percentage increase, or the increase in absolute value, or the increase in actual value which the seventy-five cent disparity represents in the prison environment?

To some, of course, questions like these have little meaning. They have little meaning to those who are indifferent to the demands of justice and autonomy which the consent doctrine represents, to those who are willing to buy guinea pigs, rather than to reward human beings. And they have little meaning for those who are convinced that prisoners are inherently unfree, and who thus would call for a total cessation of prison experimentation. Each of these positions denies, in an a *priori* fashion, freedom to prisoners; each must be rejected. A recognition of the fact that decisions about consent may be over- as well as under-protective forces us to deal with this sort of question, complex though it may be.

As is so often the case, posing the question in a different way may facilitate response. We have been considering the question of how much reward nullifies the validity of consent, how much reward renders the subject unfree. But is it in fact the case that *reward* is the disruptive factor here?

This problem may be clarified by the following examples. Imagine an upper-middle-class individual, who can provide for his family all of their needs and most of the amenities of civilized life. Let us say that this person is offered one hundred dollars to cross the street — if you like, make it one thousand or ten thousand dollars? He chooses to cross the street. Is his choice *involuntary?* Despite the substantial reward, I think most of us would agree that the consent was freely offered (and would that we should have such problems!).

Consider a person who deeply wants to be an astronaut. He is told that as part of the program he must participate in experiments to determine resistance to high-G conditions. Is his consent to this invalid, involuntary? I think not. We would say, this is part of his job; he should have expected it; and if he can't stand the heat, he should get out of the kitchen. In this vein, consider Evel Knievel, a financially prosperous man, who is offered millions of dollars to perform daredevil stunts. His choice may be bizarre, even crazy: but has his reward rendered it unfree?

Finally, consider a man who is informed by his doctor that he will most likely die unless he has open-heart surgery. His "reward" for consenting is his life; the penalty for not consenting is death. Does this mean this man cannot give the doctor valid consent — morally valid consent — to proceed?

There are two distinctions which, I think, go a long way towards dispelling these problems. First, I think it must be granted that natural contingencies ("acts of God," things which come to pass naturally, those contingencies which we cannot hold anyone responsible for) do not render a person unfree, nor do they render unfree the choices which a person makes in light of those contingencies.[11]

That natural contingencies do not render a man unfree is a point which is apt to be forgotten in the present context. I am not — in the morally relevant sense — lacking in freedom because I cannot, unaided, fly through the air, or live on grass. Nor am I unfree because my heart is about to give out. Nor am I unfree when, recognizing that my heart may give out, I choose to undergo surgery. I may, of course, be so crazed by knowing that I am near death's door that I am in a state of general impotence, and hence must have the choice made for me; but general incompetence is not in question here. The distinction between choices forced by man, and choices forced by nature, is, then, of importance.

The second distinction is between those pressures which are, and those which are not, in Daube's words, "consonant with the dignity and responsibility of free life."[12] I would explain this as follows: there are certain basic freedoms and rights which we possess which *entitle* us (morally) to certain things (or states of affairs). We would all, no doubt, draw up different lists of these rights and freedoms; but included in them would be safety of person, freedom of conscience and religion, a right to a certain level of education, and, for some of us, a right to some level of health care. When the "reward" is such as only to give us the necessary conditions of these rights and freedoms — when all that the reward does is to bring us up to a level of living to which we are entitled, and of which we have been deprived by man — then the "reward," I think, constitutes duress. A reward which accrues to one who has achieved this level, or who can easily achieve it (other than by taking the reward-option), and which hence serves only to grant us "luxury" items, does not constitute duress, and hence does not render choice unfree, no matter how great this reward may be.

The rewards above the moral subsistence level are true rewards. In contrast, we may say (with some touch of metaphor) that the "rewards" which only bring us up to the level to which we were in any event entitled are properly viewed as functioning as *threats*: "Do this, or stay where you are:" — when you should not have been "where you are" in the first place.

The astronaut, Evel Knievel, and the upper-middle-class street-crosser are being granted "luxury" items, and hence are capable of giving free consent. But consider a man who will not be admitted to the hospital for treatment unless he agrees to be a subject in an experiment (unrelated to his treatment). Those who feel, as I do, that we are, here and now, morally entitled to medical treatment would agree, I trust, that this illegitimate option coerces the man into agreeing. Or consider a man who has religious scruples against donating blood, who takes his daughter to a hospital for treatment. He is told that the doctors will not treat her unless the family donates a certain amount of blood. His freedom has been nullified: his "consent" to donating blood is morally invalid. Similarly, the college student whose grade is contingent upon his participation in the instructor's psychological experiments is not validly consenting to serve. He is entitled to have his grade based upon his classroom work.

It yet remains to apply this distinction to our original problem, prison experimentation. The application will not be attempted here, for we would first need to be clear in our minds what rights and freedoms a prisoner is entitled to. I would not hesitate to say, though, that when a situation is created whereby a prisoner can only receive decent health care by participating in an experiment, he is being coerced into that experiment. I would have little hesitation in claiming that if subjecting himself to experimentation is the only way in which a prisoner could learn a trade which may be used "outside," then that prisoner is being coerced, his consent is not free. When we take into account the condition of our society, these would seem to be reasonable entitlements for the prisoner. Other rewards — for example, higher pay — may or may not constitute rewards above the moral subsistence level; if they are, then consent in light of these rewards could be freely offered. Perhaps too much has been said already; judgments like these must be made in an individualized fashion, one which is sensitive to the realities of prison life.

NOTES

The research for this paper was begun during an internship at the Institute of Society, Ethics and the Life Sciences in the month of June, 1973. I gratefully acknowledge the help of Drs. Daniel Callahan, Marc Lappé, Peter Steinfels, and Robert Veatch, of the Institute, who helped make my internship profitable and enjoyable. My wife Barbara read the manuscript and suggested a number of needed changes.

1. For examples of a similar method applied to different problems, see Thomas I. Emerson, *Toward A General Theory of the First Amendment* (New York: Vintage Books, 1967).
2. "Brain Surgery in Aggressive Epileptics," in *Hastings Center Report,* February 1973.
3. See the insert to Alexander M. Capron's call for a moratorium on prison experimentation, "Medical Research in Prisons," *Hastings Center Report,* June 1973. The insert is a report from *The New York Times,* April 15, 1973, and reads in part: "Ninety-six of the 175 inmates at Lancaster County prison have written to a newspaper here protesting a recent decision by the state to halt all medical experiments on state prisoners. In their letter to the *Lancaster New Era,* they urged that state to allow the research [which] did not harm them and enabled them to pay off their fines and court costs."
4. See Henry K. Beecher, *Research and the Individual: Human Studies* (Boston: Little, Brown, 1970), p. 56. Professor Beecher notes a study of prison inmates, who, for participation in an experiment involving malaria, received pay but no reduction of sentence. Half of the volunteers cited "altruism" rather than money as their motive for volunteering. Those inmates who did not volunteer "expressed or implied respect for those who did volunteer."
5. *Cobbs* v. *Grant,* 502 P. 2d 1, 11.
6. Alexander M. Capron, "Legal Rights and Moral Rights," in Hilton, *et al.,* eds., *Ethical Issues in Human Genetics* (Plenum Press, 1973), 228.
7. If this sort of explanation were given as a matter of course in *all* experiments, this might still further reduce the problem of artifacts. The remarks, it should be noted, are directed towards medical experiments. By and large, they are inapplicable to, say, experiments in social psychology.
8. The counter-suggestion may be made that children cannot *really* make choices. This would, I think, put too great a weight upon the requirement of voluntarism. We would be recruiting the concepts of choice and volition to do a job which they have not been designed for.
9. I am speaking of course in the moral, not the legal, context. It may be that in an emergency a child may, in the absence of his parents, give legally valid consent.
10. This gives us the link between "responsible" in the dispositional sense explained here, and "responsible" in the blame-sense of the word ("I'll hold you responsible for that.").
11. The *caveat* must be added: natural contingencies do not have, as their *sole* result, the rendering of a person unfree, in the sense which vitiates consent: a man's

brain tumor can make the man an idiot, schizophrenia can make a man insane, but these do not so much affect a person's volition as they do disturb his entire psychic structure.

12. David Daube, quoted in Beecher, p. 146.
13. *In re Gault,* 387 U.S. 1 (1967).

FURTHER READINGS

Donagan, Alan
"Informed Consent in Therapy and Experimentation," *The Journal of Medicine and Philosophy* 2:4 (December 1977) 319.

Faden, Ruth R. and Tom L. Beauchamp
A History and Theory of Informed Consent. (New York and Oxford: Oxford University Press, 1986).

Ingelfinger, Franz J.
"Informed (But Uneducated) Consent," *The New England Journal of Medicine* 287 (August 31, 1972) 465–466.

Kelly v. Hazlett, (1976), 15 O.R. (2d) 290, 1 C.C.L.T.1, 75 D.L.R. (3d) 536 (H.C.)

Kluge, E.-H. W.
Biomedical Ethics in the Canadian Context. (Prentice Hall: Scarborough, Ont., 1991), Chapter 7.

Law Reform Commission of Canada
Working Paper 26, *Medical Treatment and the Criminal Law.* (Ottawa: Queen's Printer, 1980).

Mallary, S.D., B. Gert and C.M. Culver
"Family Coercion and Valid Consent," *Theoretical Medicine* 7:2 (1986) 123-126.

Mulloy v. HopSang,(1935)W.W.R. 714 (Alberta Supreme Court, App.Div).

Patenaude, Andrea Farkas, Joel M. Rappeport and Brian R. Smith
"Physician's Influence on Informed Consent for Bone Marrow Transplantation," *Theoretical Medicine* 7(1986) 165–179.

Picard, E.
Legal Liability of Doctors and Hospitality in Canada (Toronto: Carswell, 1984), Chapter 3, "Consent".

Salgo v. Leyland Stanford, Jr. University Board of Trustees (1957), 317 p. 2d., 270.

Somerville, M.
Consent to Medical Care. Study Paper for the Law Reform Commission of Canada (Ottawa, 1980).

CHAPTER 6 INFORMED CONSENT IN THE EXPERIMENTAL CONTEXT

INTRODUCTION

The usual view of health care is that when patients go to see their physicians, the physicians will prescribes therapies, investigative procedures or other types of intervention that are well-established as treatment options and that are of known efficacy.

However, there are times when there is no established or validated treatment for a specific condition; when there is no proven way of investigating, or no well-established way of proceeding. Sometimes the only thing that physicians can do is recommend something that in the end is really unproven or experimental. This raises several issues. One is that of decision-making: who should make the decision in this sort of context? And on what basis?

The Medical Research Council of Canada has spent years trying to develop guidelines for informed consent in the experimental and research setting. They are reproduced in part below. These guidelines have important implications for Canadian researchers. Any experiment or research that is funded by the federal government or by a federal agency must, at a minimum, meet the guidelines set out by the Medical Research Council. Therefore, these guidelines may be seen as setting a minimal national standard.

Barry Hoffmaster's piece is a reaction to the Medical Research Council's guidelines. It is written from the perspective of someone who, as a consulting ethicist, is intimately familiar with family practice. Hoffmaster points to what he thinks are some of the more serious flaws of the guidelines. Other Canadian commentators have had similar concerns.[1]

NOTE

1. For instance, see E.- H.W. Kluge, *Biomedical Ethics in the Canadian Context.* (Scarborough, Ont: Prentice Hall, 1991) Chapter 8.

Guidelines On Research Involving Human Subjects

Medical Research Council of Canada

PRINCIPLES OF CONSENT

The law of consent has been much debated and has recently undergone a good degree of development. The law is technical, and a measure of forensic precision is required in addressing this aspect of the Guidelines.

A. Informed Decision-Making

The cardinal principle of research on human subjects is that, to the extent that it is possible, a subject's involvement should be informed and voluntary. Ideally, subjects should be fully informed, and should make their decision on whether to participate at leisure and in complete freedom from any pressure. Practically speaking, this is rarely, if ever, possible.

Potential research subjects seldom have the knowledge needed to evaluate fully the scientific information on which the research is based. Much research involves people who are under care, and thus feel themselves under pressure to participate. Some potential subjects may be mentally incapable of the discussions or comprehension needed for consent, through reasons of mental illness, trauma or age. Decisions may have to be taken too rapidly to allow transfer of information or reflection on information, because delays might be against the therapeutic interests of the patient. However, research is necessary if the care of people in these situations is to improve.

The obtaining of informed consent is only one step in a continuing process. The educative effort commences before and continues after the signing of a document, and continuing consent must be elicited during the progress of the research.

Put simply, prospective subjects must receive, in a language which they understand, enough information about the proposed study and their prospective role, to enable them to decide whether or not to participate. Investigators must anticipate what information may be important. They can be guided by tailoring the disclosure to a reasonable person in the circumstances of the prospective subject.

The research protocol must outline what information is to be given to prospective subjects. Copies of information sheets should be submitted to the REB as well.

A protocol will normally be expected to state what prospective subjects will be told; these points may include:

a) the reasons for the study;
b) research techniques which will involve the prospective subject,

Medical Research Council of Canada, *Guidelines on Research Involving Human Subjects 1987.* (Ottawa: Minister of Supply and Services, 1987), Chapter V.

such as randomization of treatments;

c) the reason why the prospective subject is being invited to take part;
d) the reasonably anticipated benefits and consequences of the study itself;
e) the reasonably anticipated benefits and consequences of the study for the prospective subject and society (if none, this should be stated);
f) the foreseeable risks, including discomforts and inconveniences, to the prospective subject;
g) the foreseeable risks of the study itself;
h) complete details regarding confidentiality of prospective subjects;
i) the anticipated time commitment for subjects;
j) the intent to conduct a follow-up study in the future and the retention of data;
k) the rules for stopping the study and withdrawing the subject; and
l) the right of the subject to withdraw from the study at any time and without penalty.

Additional information requirements must be met for potential subjects who are also patients and whose care may be directly affected by participation in the study. Information would include:

a) the patient's prognosis without intervention;
b) alternative interventions available;
c) experimental aspects of interventions proposed;
d) interventions to be unavailable to a patient who becomes a subject, for the sake of the research;
e) an estimate of the likely success and failure of all the interventions which may be offered and withheld;
f) an estimate of the risks and possible adverse effects of interventions offered; and
g) a clear distinction between procedures in the research protocol and those that would be part of usual patient care.

The level of disclosure should be proportionate to the likelihood and the scale of possible harm, but even the remote possibility of injury should be disclosed.

B. Free Consent

The invitation to a prospective research subject must be made in a way that allows the individual freedom of choice. Sufficient time to reflect is important. It need scarcely be said that undue influence must not be employed. Prospective subjects, for example patients who are asked by those responsible for their care to serve as subjects, may feel pressure which investigators do not at first perceive.

The law recognizes unequal relationships as inherently suspect. In such relationships, the law presumes that any agreement between a weaker and stronger party, from which the stronger party gains unusual advantage, is tainted. There is little doubt that such a relationship exists when patients are asked by those treating them to serve as their research subjects.

In such cases, physician-investigators must do their utmost to ensure and maintain their patient's independence. The invitation to participate in a research project must always be proffered in a manner that fully describes the objectives of the study, and outlines the reasons underlying the selection of suitable patient participants. In general, the clinician who is to be responsible for the research study is in the best scientific position to implement this early phase of subject enrollment. Notwithstanding the fact that patients almost invariably bear a sense of dependency on their personal physicians, often coupled with a sense of allegiance and at times with a degree of anxiety about their future health care, care must be taken to avoid coercion or undue influence, both of which can reduce independently arrived at consent.

Communication of the final decision, to participate or decline, may be difficult for the patient if the question is posed directly by the physician who will be responsible for continuing care. Under these circumstances, it may well be desirable to delegate the ultimate decision-seeking question to another member of the health care team, possibly another health professional who has no direct link to the patient's future medical management.

A single consent and information form provides a useful permanent record of the essential information given, and records consent. The subject must be given a copy of this document, which should also provide other information, such as a name and telephone number to allow the subject to ask questions about the project later, and to remind the subject that he or she can decline to participate or withdraw from the project at any time without any prejudice to future rights. The subject must receive information about remuneration, if any. If the investigator or institution is not insured, the subject must be informed.

Evidence of consent is almost invariably obtained in writing. In the province of Québec, this is legally required (see art. 20, *Civil Code)*. Outside Québec, consent may occasionally be allowed to be taken orally, but, whether in written or oral form, there should generally be an independent witness to the consent. In very minor cases, consent may be implied by the subject's freely entering into the research project; a subject voluntarily completing an anonymous questionnaire would be an example.

C. Induced Consent and Payment

Improperly induced consent like pressured consent is unacceptable. Particular populations, such as students, laboratory staff and technicians, to name but a few, may consider it advantageous to volunteer for participation in a study.

Such groups are readily identified and often accessible. It may be convenient to use them when knowledge applicable to the general population is sought. As a result, certain groups may be asked repeatedly to serve as research subjects. While they may be happy to participate, there are reasons in justice to distribute the risks as well as the benefits of the research more widely throughout society.

Beyond the advantage of career progress or security is the inducement of money or the offer of free medical or dental care for subjects or members of their families. Such inducements must be treated as rewards and be assessed under the same principles. Remuneration limited to compensation for expenses actually incurred and losses reasonably assessed, including loss of wages, is ethically acceptable, provided that it does not distort freedom of choice but facilitates collaboration by indemnifying subjects for their direct and indirect expenditures. Payments for time and inconvenience, if nominal, are similarly acceptable. Excessive remuneration, or other advantages or benefits, however, are an improper inducement to participate in a research project. The REB must have information about remuneration and determine whether it is reasonable.

D. Continuing Consent

Consent to participate in research as a human subject arises in a collaborative relationship between investigators and subjects; it is not a contractually binding commitment. Subjects are informed that, even though their consent is in writing, they may leave the study at any time without prejudice to their rights, and they must be free to do so. Research must not become dependent upon the continued participation of any particular subject in order to maintain the statistical validity of data. Subjects should not be offered such rewards for participation as will constrict their freedom to leave a study. Reimbursement should therefore be as expenses are incurred.

Prospective subjects must be informed of the duration of their involvement in a study. This includes the duration of any procedures involving them, such as physical or psychological testing, and also the duration of retention of identifiable data. If such identifiable records are to be kept, prospective subjects have a right to know that their consent to involvement in the study includes continuing consent to retention of data.

E. Non-Consensual Research

Epidemiological research has greatly advanced medical science and should be fostered.

Research on identifiable human subjects, without their prior informed and free consent, has been seen to be contrary to principle, but it may be ethically permissible in limited circumstances. Research upon subjects incapable of consenting is considered in a following section. Other research may be ethically conducted, however, to which the competent human subjects do not consent. In cases such as epidemiological research where records of patients may be reviewed, the potential benefit and the degree of compromise of the patient's confidentiality must be carefully weighed by the REB. In these studies, often human subjects' medical conditions are reviewed, but identifiable individual cases may not be. Confidentiality must not be unduly compromised. If identifiable data are used in epidemiological research, and prior consent is not to be sought, the prospective investigators bear the responsibility of showing in the protocol that it is ethical for the requirement of consent to be waived, and that adequate means exist to ensure the confidentiality of the data.

This holds even if the records concern people who are now dead. The essential issue is the possibility of harm from indignity felt by the patients or their relatives resulting from use or release of information.

If a study involves the public conduct of subjects, their consent may be waived if the conduct is purely spontaneous and not conditioned or influenced by any act of the investigator and the subjects are neither identified nor identifiable. The behaviour will be available to an investigator's scrutiny by reason of its being voluntarily undertaken in public, even though subjects do not expect the purposeful and systematic scrutiny of their acts. Even where confidentiality is not at stake, care must always be taken to protect subjects' identities, and they must be treated with dignity and respect.

Consent is generally unnecessary for research undertaken, for example, upon surplus blood, urine, tissue, and similar samples obtained for diagnostic or treatment purposes if the patient is not identifiable, and the requirements of the research do not influence the procedures used for obtaining the samples.

F. Deception

The MRC is committed to both openness and accountability. In view of the critical importance of informed and free consent, consideration of deception seems incongruous.

Although deception is not used in the vast majority of medical research, the Standing Committee was advised that some areas of behavioural or psychological research can only be carried out if the research subject is not aware of the reasons for the research.

Deception involves the intentional misleading of prospective subjects or withholding information from them, so that subjects believe that the procedures or the objectives of the research are different from what they actually are. Deception may include deliberate presentation of false information, suppression of material information, or selection of revealed truths in a way designed to mislead.[1]

Because the concept of deliberately misleading research subjects runs so much counter to the principle of respect for the individual, the Committee had great difficulty accepting that deception could ever be ethically justified. However, should research situations arise where it is essential to scientific integrity that the subjects remain unaware of the nature of the research, the following rules should be applied. Such situations warrant particular scrutiny by the REB.

1) Deception should not be used where any other methodology would accomplish the research objective. The investigator should demonstrate in the protocol that no other method is feasible.
2) Research involving deception should not be carried out where there is any reasonably anticipated risk to subjects; it is impossible to justify exposing subjects to risk when they have not consented to incur that risk.
3) The REB should be satisfied that nothing is withheld from the subjects which might, if divulged, cause them to refuse to participate.
4) The REB should be satisfied that significant scientific advance can be expected from the research, in order to justify even minimal deception.
5) Deception should be permitted only when it is possible to inform and "debrief" subjects afterwards and to obtain subsequent consent to use the data obtained. Debriefing procedures should be written into the research protocol and should take place immediately following participation in the research, while the data remain identifiable. It must be recognized that debriefing does not remedy deception. Data obtained from subjects who subsequently decline to participate should be destroyed or surrendered to the subjects. This in itself, we think, will discourage the use of deception.

NOTE

1. Placebos. The use of placebos which amounts to deception should be distinguished from the situation where the subject knows that an inactive substance may be used and agrees to its possible use. Placebos are defined as medicines given to humour rather than cure (*Concise Oxford Dictionary*, 7th ed., 1982).

The Medical Research Council's New Guidelines on Research Involving Human Subjects: Too Much Law, Too Little Ethics

Barry Hoffmaster

The main difference between the Medical Research Council's (MRC) 1978 guidelines on research involving human subjects and its revised guidelines can be seen by comparing their titles. The earlier document is called MRC Report No. 6, *Ethics in Human Experimentation*:[1] the name of the new document is *Guidelines on Research Involving Human Subject 1987* ("1987 Guidelines)[2]. What has happened to "ethics" between 1978 and 1987? The answer is simple. Ethics has been displaced by law. When the voice of the new guidelines is firm and clear, it is because the MRC is confident about what the law says and is comfortable applying these legal requirements to medical research. Ethics is offstage in the chorus. But when the voice of the guidelines becomes tremulous — as it frequently does — because the law is uncertain or because the implications of applying a favoured interpretation of the law to medical research are disquieting, ethics is allowed on stage as a bit player. It becomes part of the action, but it contributes nothing significant to the performance.

Why has law supplanted ethics? Again, the answer is simple. The MRC feels it needs a philosophy to justify its guidelines. It has to reject the "philosophy of *laissez-faire* in medical research" because that philosophy has countenanced research that would not be tolerated today (1987 Guidelines, p. 3). Where, then to turn? To the philosophy of liberalism, of course. But why liberalism? Because liberalism is firmly embedded in the western political and legal tradition. What about ethics, though? What do politics and law have to do with ethics? A good question, one that is not easy to answer. The MRC's "initial" reply is that "an ethical obligation exists to act in accordance with legal requirements" (1987 Guidelines, p. 11). What that claim means and in what respects it might be correct have generated extensive philosophical controversy.[3] The immediate point, however, is merely that morality has been quickly and thoroughly subjugated to law.[4] Law provides guidance; ethics is consigned to the more menial task of producing reasons or motivation for acting as the law requires.

Having established the pre-eminence of law, the MRC then takes a legal paradigm that fits the vast majority of research protocols involving human subjects, namely, that of an adult who is legally competent to consent to participate, and applies this paradigm to all research protocols, without considering whether its assumptions and its requirements are appropriate for persons who are legally incompetent to consent. The result is a discussion that is, in general, badly skewed and that is, for the particular problems raised by incompetent subjects, confusing to the point of incoherence. It is skewed because it is oblivious to other relevant considerations, and it is con-

Barry Hoffmaster, "The Medical Research Council's New Guidelines on Research Involving Human Subjects: Too Much Law, Too Little Ethics," *Health Law In Canada* 10:1(1989) 146-155.

fusing because the MRC, quite rightly, has difficulty applying this paradigm in situations it does not fit. Such an unfortunate outcome is the result of three failings: 1) a constricted, forced reading of the theoretical underpinnings of the Western democratic and legal tradition; 2) an erroneous understanding of a central concept in medical ethics; and 3) a superficial account of the relationship between law and morality. The first two will be considered next; the third will surface when the MRC's own ambivalence about the implications of the law for research involving incompetent subjects is discussed.

The MRC's theorizing about law and morality has, I think, three components. First, the MRC sees Western law, from the time of the Romans to the present, as reflecting and manifesting the philosophy of liberal individualism. Second, the MRC regards law and morality as intertwined and explains their intimate connection in terms of the incorporation of the morality of liberalism into the law.[5] Third, the MRC views liberalism as exhaustive of morality or at least as exhaustive of the morality that is relevant to medical research. All three claims are, I believe, false. Whatever superficial plausibility they possess is a function of the MRC's vague and abstruse rendition of liberalism. Exactly what is this liberalism that supposedly forms the moral core of Western law?

The foremost principle of liberalism is, according to the MRC, "the primacy of individuals, their freedoms and their right to be left alone" (1987 Guidelines, p. 3). That individual freedom is and has been a longstanding concern in the occidental world is supported by quotations from political and legal documents as old as the *Institutes of Justinian.* The MRC needs more than the claim that freedom is an important value in Western culture, however. To support its global, legally-inspired position that research is permissible only if subjects have voluntarily consented on their own behalf, it needs the much stronger claim that, of all the values relevant to medical research, the freedom of potential subjects is always the most important.

Do the materials cited by the MRC support such a strong normative stance? The excerpt from the *Institutes of Justinian*, offered to establish liberalism's antiquarian roots, reads: "Freedom, from which we get the description of men as free, is a man's natural capacity of *doing what he pleases* unless he is prevented by force or law ..." (1987 Guidelines, pp. 3-4, emphasis provided by MRC). That is simply a definition of freedom; it acknowledges that freedom can be circumscribed by force or law, but says nothing about when force or law may legitimately delimit freedom, which, of course, is precisely the issue.

The passage from the *Magna Carta* is: "No Freeman shall be taken or imprisoned ... *or in any way destroyed* ... except by the legal Judgment of his peers, or by the laws of the land" (1987 Guidelines, p. 4, emphasis provided by MRC). One wonders whether an investigation of the historical and cultural milieu of the *Magna Carta* would support the MRC's capacious view of freedom. Who, in 1215, counted as a "freeman," for example, and are we really to believe that the limits of individual freedom were the same in a feudal society as they are today? Moreover, does the MRC want to accept the apparent consequence that research on incompetent subjects may proceed only with explicit endorsement by the "legal judgment of peers" or the "laws of the land"? As we shall see, the MRC vacillates on this issue.

The American *Declaration of Independence* is cited for the proposition that people possess the "unalienable rights" of *"Life, Liberty and the pursuit of Happiness"* (1987 Guidelines, p. 4, emphasis provided by MRC). It is unclear how such vague and abstract rights as the right to life and the right to liberty apply to the concrete moral problems posed by medical research. No right is absolute. The crucial moral task, therefore, is determining the boundaries of a right, and bare appeals to the existence of a right have no implications for where those boundaries should be set. Moreover, the right to liberty and the right to life could easily conflict in the context of medical research. Suppose research on infants, who obviously cannot give legal consent on their own behalf, provides the only hope for dealing with a life-threatening childhood disease. What authority does the American *Declaration of Independence* provide for the claim that the right to liberty prevails over the right to life here, that is, that the liberty of infants not to participate in research is more important than the lives of infants stricken with this disease?[6] A moral argument is needed to defend this preference, but none is forthcoming.

The MRC then invokes the French *Declaration of the Rights of Man and the Citizen:* "Liberty consists in the freedom to do everything *which injures no one else*" (1987 Guidelines, p. 4, emphasis provided by MRC). This is simultaneously a definition of liberty and an account of the appropriate limits of liberty. It introduces the MRC's only paradigmatic moral authority, Mill's famous statement of the liberal principle in *On Liberty* (1987 Guidelines, p. 4):

> ... the only purpose for which power can be rightfully exercised over any member of a civilized community, against his will, is to prevent harm to others. *His own good, either physical or moral, is not a sufficient warrant.* He cannot rightfully be compelled to do or forebear because it will be better for him to do so, because it will make him happier, because, *in the opinions of others, to do so would be wise or even right.* (emphasis provided by MRC).

Unfortunately, Mill's anti-paternalistic principle has nothing to do with the moral problems of medical research. Person A acts paternalistically towards person B when A gets B to do or to refrain from doing something because A believes that he or she knows B's interests better than B himself or herself does and because A believes that B's behaving in this way will make B better off. That is a cumbersome definition; the point is that paternalistic acts are always directed at the good of the person towards whom one acts paternalistically, not at the good of some third party. Thus an issue that bothers the MRC greatly, using incompetent persons in research designed to bring about benefits for others, is not an issue of paternalism. Nor is using competent adults without their consent when the research is intended to benefit others an instance of paternalism. The revised guidelines nevertheless open with the claim that "[b]enevolent paternalism was without doubt a dominant force ... in the early ethics of experimentation...." (1987 Guidelines, p. 3). Yet the example the MRC provides, "the Ptolemies' consent to the vivisection of criminals in the third century B.C." (1987 Guidelines, p. 3), completely undermines this claim. How can the MRC possibly regard the vivisection of criminals as paternalistic, let alone benevolent? The vivisections were not designed to benefit the criminals upon whom they were performed. Important moral issues about not treating people as means alone do arise here, but these are not issues of paternalism.

How could such a grievous misunderstanding have occurred? An uncharitable answer is that the MRC was blinded by its zealotry for individual freedom. One could reason as follows: paternalism and individual freedom are contradictory; paternalism is always wrong; therefore, individual freedom must always be respected. This argument could, of course, be invoked in contexts in which paternalism is a possibility.[7] But medical research is not one of those contexts. An experimental procedure could be performed on a legally incompetent person either for that person's potential benefit or for the potential benefit of others. In the latter case it is, by definition, not paternalism. In the former case it might be regarded as innovative therapy and thus fall outside the purview of guidelines for research on human subjects. Alternatively, it might be deemed research, but it still would not qualify as paternalism because one can act paternalistically only towards those individuals who possess a conception of their own good, and incompetent persons lack such a conception.[8] That this component of the definition of paternalism is not arbitrary can be seen by considering the moral objection of paternalism. Why is paternalism taken to be morally wrong? The usual answer is that paternalism is wrong because it violates autonomy, that is, it overrides an individual's conception of his or her own good. One cannot act paternalistically, therefore, towards individuals who lack autonomy. In the eyes of the MRC, legally incompetent subjects are, by definition, not autonomous (1987 Guidelines, p. 28) so researchers cannot act paternalistically towards them, even if an experimental procedure is intended to benefit them.

The issue of paternalism simply does not arise here. Because individual freedom and paternalism are regarded as antinomies, the MRC might have found the rhetorical ploy of defending freedom by castigating paternalism irresistible. But in a setting in which paternalism is not an issue, that would be sophistry. Thus whatever force or authority Mill's statement possesses is beside the point in this context.

There is a more charitable interpretation. As we have seen, most of the quotations on which the MRC relies merely define freedom or assert a right to freedom. On what grounds, then, is the freedom of potential subjects to be preferred to the freedom of researchers? Why, in other words, is the philosophy of *laissez-faire* in medical research, abjured by the MRC, not an equally legitimate part of the liberal tradition? The MRC realizes it has no answer to this question, so it is forced to fall back on the notion of paternalism. In areas of medical ethics in which it is relevant, the critique of paternalism gives the wishes of patients moral priority over the wishes of physicians. The MRC likewise wants the wishes of potential subjects to prevail over the wishes of researchers. But that outcome cannot be achieved in the research context by rejecting paternalism. The theoretical support for the MRC's guidelines consequently vanishes.

The quotation from Mill's *On Liberty* illustrates how selective is the MRC's reading of its chosen texts. The MRC has no compunctions about emphasizing particular phrases to make absolutely sure we understand just how overridingly important individual freedom is. But even with this orientation, how can the MRC ignore the first sentence in Mill's remark: "... the only purpose for which power can be rightfully exercised over any member of a civilized community, *against his will,* is *to prevent harm to others*" (my emphasis now). Don't disease and illness do harm to others? Why, then, can't individuals, even in the MRC's enlightened liberal state, be used as research subjects without their consent? How does the mere invocation of Mill's principle preclude this?

The MRC's choice of texts is equally selective. Why are we given Mill's *On Liberty,* for example, but not Mill's *Utilitarianism*? The individualism of *Utilitarianism* belongs to the Western liberal tradition in that it treats persons as equals by counting each person equally in the calculation of utility. It also falls within the liberal tradition insofar as it is neutral among persons' competing conceptions of the good. Because utilitarianism allows the interests of an individual to be sacrificed to the interests of a group, however, it could countenance research on incompetent subjects or research without consent that is designed to benefit others. Individual freedom is not the paramount value for utilitarianism, so either it must be purged from the canon of liberalism or liberalism must be narrowly construed to exclude it. Either alternative makes the MRC's concept of liberalism appear wispy.

The vital lesson here is the importance of definition. How an issue is treated is a function of how that issue is posed. What considerations are deemed relevant, how much weight is attached to various considerations and how resolutions are extracted from a welter of conflicting considerations depend crucially upon how issues are conceived. As the MRC recognizes, its emphasis on individual freedom leads directly to a concern for consent: "The elements of consent, so important now in law and ethics, flow in great part from this [liberal] philosophy" (1987 Guidelines, p. 4). In contrast, for the 1978 guidelines the central moral problem in medical research is the allocation of benefits and burdens. When the burden of accepting the potential risks of research and the potential benefit of being bettered by that research would devolve upon the same person, the key issues are whether the risks and benefits are proportional and whether the subject understands those benefits and burdens and gives a voluntary, informed consent to participate. An emphasis on consent is, in this situation, appropriate and proper. But when the potential risks would fall exclusively upon one group and the potential benefits would accrue to a different group, an issue of justice arises. Is it fair to impose risks on one person so that someone else might benefit? There are, that is, two distinct categories of moral problems here. By transforming every problem into one of protecting freedom through consent, the MRC conflates these two categories.[9] Every issue is couched as a problem of consent. That might be acceptable when subjects are competent, but it is a perversion when subjects are incompetent. The rationale behind consent is the protection of individual autonomy, yet, as the MRC itself points out, "[b]y definition, a legally incompetent subject is not autonomous, and cannot give a legally or ethically valid consent" (1987 Guidelines, p. 28). The MRC nevertheless addresses the problem of research involving incompetent subjects in Chapter V, "Principles of Consent." The result can be nothing but confusion and incoherence when a theoretical approach is imposed upon an area in which the rationale for that approach is missing. With respect to incompetent subjects, the MRC's preoccupation with consent strips away relevant considerations and bludgeons distinctions to death, so that issues become truncated and distorted. The 1978 guidelines are vastly superior in their sensitivity to the different kinds of moral problems posed by research with human subjects as well as the plethora of considerations relevant to these problems.

Lest these remarks so far sound like animadversions, let me quickly add that the importance of protecting individuals both from medical research and in medical research is indisputable. The MRC justifies this concern by reminding us of celebrated abuses of research subjects, including the notorious Canadian case of *Halushka v. The University of Saskatchewan*[10] To its list might have been added another distinctive Canadian contribution, the CIA-sponsored research of Dr. Ewen Cameron at McGill University. Insisting on voluntary, informed consent is a crucial safeguard against such abuses. The point, however, is that consent is not the *only* issue in medical research and that there are situations in which the paradigm of consent does not make sense. In these situations alternative approaches must be pursued.

Despite the overwhelming and overweening influence of the law on the MRC, ethics cannot be banished from a discussion of research with human subjects, and an unresolved tension between morality and law recurs uneasily throughout the revised guidelines. The disappearance of "ethics" from the title of the new guidelines is, for instance, compensated by the name the MRC adopts for the institutional committees that review research proposals involving human subjects. The MRC dubs them "Research Ethics Boards" in order, it says, "to indicate its emphasis on the ethics of research, in contrast to the previous MRC (Canada) use of 'Ethics Review Committee,' and the US title, 'Institutional Review Board'" (1987 Guidelines, p. 12, note 10)[11] To cite another example, the MRC holds that in general there should be an independent witness to the process of obtaining consent (1987 Guidelines, p. 24), but at the same time insists that consent to participate in research "is not a contractually-binding commitment" (1987 Guidelines, p. 25). The ethics committee on which I served for nine years used to delete witness signatures routinely from consent forms precisely because it did not want to create in subjects the impression that, by signing a consent form and having it witnessed, they were undertaking a legally binding obligation. The procedural requirement of a witness appears to be an artifact of the MRC's deference to law and, I think, gets in the way of good ethics here. What is the point of having an independent witness to the consent? Is the witness simply supposed to observe the process by which consent is obtained, or is the witness supposed to sign the consent form as well? The MRC is silent.

The problem runs deeper, however, as the discussion of cross-cultural studies reveals. The MRC recognizes that some cultural groups do not share its liberalism and might even regard its exaltation of the individual as subversive of their communities and hence immoral. Should the MRC nevertheless impose its liberal (moral? legal? both?) principles on these groups? Its answer is unclear. The MRC says that the approval of tribal leaders (so the criterion for a distinctive ethnic or cultural group is membership in a tribe?) may be a necessary but not a sufficient condition for studying individual subjects and then adds (1987 Guidelines, p. 28):

> concepts of privacy and confidentiality may also differ among cultures. Such concepts must always be viewed from the perspective of the culture studied, as well as from that of the investigator.

This remark suggests that, in deference to the moral views of certain cultural groups, exceptions to the requirements of individual consent might be warranted. But the MRC immediately renounces this tolerance (1987 Guidelines, p. 28):

> In meeting these needs, an investigator involved in cross-cultural studies should be expected to meet all of the requirements normally expected in ethical review, as well as the additional requirements necessitated by the use of the distinct cultural group.

The impression that a waiver of requirements might be the appropriate response to moral pluralism is replaced by the imposition of "additional requirements." What are these "additional requirements," though, and how is respect for a moral ethos at odds with liberalism achieved by supplementing, rather than modifying, guidelines devoted to the rigorous protection of individual freedom, privacy, and confidentiality? the MRC's "add-on" solution is paradoxical because one of the principles commonly associated with liberalism is tolerance. Is tolerance not part of the MRC's vision of liberalism, or are there other (moral? legal? both?) considerations that override a deferential posture towards alternative moral visions, and, if so, what are they?

The dissonance between morality and law is greatest however, in the discussion of research on incompetent subjects. The MRC is, at times, sensitive to both the procedural and substantive dimensions of morality. In its discussion of why it prefers guidelines to legislation, for example, the MRC recognizes that "the truly ethical quality of the assessments to be made may atrophy when judgments are directed by law" (1987 Guidelines, p. 11). It is aware that the control of the *Criminal Code*[12] can be "heavy-handed"; that "decisions in medical ethics depend on striking a balance between competing ethical claims" and that "the ethical assessment of a research proposal may raise a wide range of interests and values, some novel, and may require risk-to-benefit determinations which cannot easily be prescribed or standardized" (1987 Guidelines, p. 10). As well, it acknowledges the problem of justice "in allocating the anticipated risks and the hoped-for benefits" of medical research (1987 Guidelines, p. 12), a problem that is particularly acute when subjects are incompetent. At one point, the MRC displays a discerning ethical sensibility (1987 Guidelines, p. 13):

> The ethical challenge then is to decide in the light of principle what risks are justifiable and for whom, in relation to presumed gain. These dilemmas are the central focus of the Guidelines.

While these dilemmas may remain the central focus of the new guidelines, ethics does not. When the issue of incompetent subjects is considered, ethics becomes no more than prolegomenon. The problem of justice is forgotten, and recognizing and balancing a wide range of interests and values is abandoned. As mentioned, the organization of the revised guidelines reveals this clearly, for the discussion of incompetent subjects occurs in the chapter devoted to the law of consent. The "ethical challenge" of appraising the nature and distribution of risks and benefits vanishes, replaced by "the cardinal principle of research on human subjects, "namely, "that, to the extent that it is possible, a subject's involvement should be informed and voluntary" (1987 Guidelines, p. 21).

Why the MRC persists in its legalistic approach, especially in the face of difficulties it openly recognizes, is puzzling. The MRC is aware that the point of consent is to protect autonomy, and the MRC also is aware that incompetent persons, by the very nature of their incompetency, have no autonomy to protect, so why not abandon an approach that clearly does not fit the issue and address the novel interests and values that are relevant? The MRC is obviously uneasy with its legalism here because it points out that the law of assault and common law principles about autonomy and consent, *"strictly interpreted"* (1987 Guidelines, p. 28, my emphasis), would prohibit non-therapeutic research on incompetent persons and thus destroy virtually any hope for progress on the diseases that incapacitate these persons. When applying the law to medical research has implications that are morally unsettling, the refuge of the MRC is that this application rests on a "strict interpretation" of the law. But on what grounds does the MRC decide when the law is being strictly interpreted and when it is not? And what does this distinction between a strict and a non-strict interpretation of the law do for the MRC's claims about the relationship between law and morality? If law represents "a minimum ethic," why do not strict interpretations of the law reflect this minimum ethic?

And if there is "an ethical obligation ... to act in accordance with legal requirements," why is this ethical obligation missing from strict interpretations of the law?

The entire discussion of incompetent subjects is convoluted because issues are artificially circumscribed and contorted into shapes that fit the framework of consent.[13] The incoherence that results is especially prominent in the section on research involving children. The section begins promisingly with the statement, "The ethical challenge is to determine the conditions and limits under which children may be involved in medical research" (1987 Guidelines, p. 29). Unfortunately, the MRC does not rise to the challenge. Rather than adopting the ethical method it described earlier, the MRC jumbles legal concepts of assault, competency, consent, and assent with notions gleaned from the U.S. regulations on research involving children. Positions that appear to be plucked from the air are assembled into a confusing series of *non sequiturs*.

Following the encouraging opening of this section, the second paragraph notes that parents control the extent to which their children are exposed to the risks of everyday life, and the third paragraph applies this consideration to research. Parents may consent to inspection of their children's medical records and collection of excreted materials, as long as the method of collection causes no pain or embarrassment. Why the restriction to inspection of records and collection of excreted materials? Why is parental discretion not extended to all kinds of research? The answer is, as one would expect, legal. Inspecting records and collected excreta can be done without touching a child. To touch a child without that child's consent is assault, and one must remember one's moral obligation to obey the law. Why the other restriction, that the method of collection cause no pain or embarrassment? That, I think, will remain a mystery to parents, who will be surprised to learn that pain and embarrassment are not among the risks of everyday life to which their children are exposed.

When the MRC moves to research that involves touching a child, the intrusion of the law again causes it discomfort. Such research could be innocuous, for example, measuring a child's height, but it still constitutes an assault and there is still that moral obligation. Thus such an assault is quickly denominated a "technical and minor legal assault" (1987 Guidelines, p. 29). Because it is technical and minor, parents may consent to such touching, seemingly without having to agonize about violating their moral obligation. There is a restriction, however: "but not where pain or discomfort beyond carefully defined limits would be liable to occur" (1987 Guidelines, p. 29). Unfortunately, the MRC finds it unnecessary to suggest what these "carefully defined limits" might be.

The fourth paragraph discusses when children may volunteer for non-therapeutic research. Does this mean the second and third paragraphs pertain to only therapeutic research? If so, does touching a child for the purposes of therapeutic research constitute a legal assault, however minor and technical? And if the second and third paragraphs are about only therapeutic research, the MRC's position on non-therapeutic research remains opaque. Does the MRC mean to suggest that only children themselves, and not their parents, may consent to non-therapeutic research? The fifth paragraph introduces the notion of a child's "assent" to participate in research. Does this mean parents may consent to non-therapeutic research on their children as long as their children also "assent" to it? Or does the decision about non-therapeutic research remain exclusively with the child, but with the concept of assent replacing the concept of consent in certain circumstances? The fifth paragraph also introduces the notion of "invasive" research, but without defining that term or clarifying how it relates to the limits on pain and discomfort mentioned previously.

The sixth paragraph takes up research on older children and adolescents. Presumably this discussion is legally motivated as well, an attempt to incorporate the "mature minor" rule about consent into the guidelines. "Mature" adolescents are said to have a "claim to respect for privacy and to freedom of participation" (1987 Guidelines, p. 30), but the preceding sentence suggests that "their parents' approval will be necessary" (1987 Guidelines, p. 29) if they want to participate. If these adolescents are "mature," and therefore legally competent to consent, why is their parents' consent needed at all? And does this position apply only to non-therapeutic research or to all research?

The section on research involving children is irretrievably muddled. Relevantly different categories of research are not distinguished and discussed separately; crucial terms are not explicated; and reasons for positions are not articulated. Rather than providing even "some guidance" (1987 Guidelines, p. 28), this section serves only to bewilder.

The MRC's declared approach to research involving incompetent adults is similar to that for children: "Where intellectually-impaired adults are assessed to establish their mental capacity, the principles outlined above regarding children and adolescents may be applicable in principle" (1987 Guidelines, p. 30). But in discussing research on elderly persons, for example, into Alzheimer's disease, the MRC turns to a different branch of the law:

> ... mentally and physically-disabled persons' legal protections are strengthened under the *Canadian Charter of Rights and Freedoms,* reducing the likelihood that provincial public hospital, mental-health or mental incompetency legislation would be construed to allow ... research not related to therapy. Rights to integrity of the mentally-disabled protected by law and the Charter cannot be reduced or compromised simply upon the basis of decisions of REBs; only courts have authority to approve invasive forms of management, and to say what consent process will be adequate for invasive non-therapeutic procedures. The points that we have outlined in regards to the limits of the use of children in research will apply equally here.

How can the MRC say that the points made with respect to children "apply equally here" when the application of the Charter to children was never discussed and when the MRC did not stipulate that only a court could approve invasive non-therapeutic procedures on children? There is a glaring difference between the MRC's positions on incompetent children and incompetent adults, yet the MRC paints it over. Moreover, what justifies this difference? Doesn't s.15 of the Charter prohibit discrimination on the basis of age, as well as discrimination on the basis of mental and physical handicap? Why, then, don't its legal protections extend to children in the way in which they extend to the mentally and physically disabled? Why is the MRC selective in its appeal to the Charter?

Overall the MRC's stand on research involving incompetent adults has a slight edge in clarity over its discussion of research with children. Non-therapeutic research on incompetent adults that involves "uncomfortable," "above-minimum-risk," or "invasive" procedures may be conducted only with the approval of the courts. What the MRC's position is on non-therapeutic research involving children is impossible to fathom. Nevertheless, the inconsistency in its treatment of incompetent children and adults raises serious worries about the justification for this difference. A non-charitable interpretation is that elderly people are going to die soon anyway, so it is not as important to conduct research on the diseases that afflict them as it is on the diseases that afflict children. Consequently, it is easier to insist on Charter-based restrictions designed to protect the incompetent elderly from research. But wouldn't this constitute legal discrimination on the basis of age as well as mental and physical handicap? And what about the right to life of these elderly persons? What is the charitable interpretation here?

Two aspects of the MRC's discussion of incompetent children and adults are valuable, however. One is the advice to seek help from third parties, the child's physician or family physician in the former case and community groups concerned with the mentally disabled in the latter. The other is the recognition that competency is not a global property but depends upon the nature of the issue about which a decision must be made. The clearest, most helpful attempt to elucidate and apply the factors that enter into such specific determinations of competency are contained in the *Consent Handbook* published by the American Association on Mental Deficiency. It is unfortunate that this work escaped the attention of the MRC.

The *reductio ad absurdum* of the MRC's fixation on consent comes in the section dealing with research on fetuses and embryos, which opens with this hesitant but nevertheless startling inference: "At this time, the legal status of embryos and fetuses is not well defined, nor is the social consensus ... [I]ssues of consent and autonomy may not therefore apply" (1987 Guidelines, p. 32). What can it possibly mean to say "issues of consent and autonomy may not therefore apply" to fetuses and embryos? How could a fetus or an embryo ever be thought to possess autonomy or to be in a position to give consent? Could an act of Parliament bestow this capacity upon them, or perhaps a changing social consensus? What could the MRC possibly have had in mind in discussing fetuses and embryos in the section on "Research Involving Legally Incompetent Subjects"? The suggestion that issues of consent and autonomy ever could be relevant to research on fetuses and embryos shows how fundamentally warped the theoretical approach of the revised guidelines is.

At least with respect to research on embryos, the MRC concedes that the law does not settle the ethical questions. Research directed at improving infertility management is permissible using embryos up to 17 days of development, an extension of the 14-day limitation more commonly adopted. Unfortunately, this position is simply conveyed as representing the opinion of the Committee that wrote the guidelines. The Committee understands the potential for abuse in research on embryos, but it "sees a broad prohibition of all research on embryos, as neither justified nor wise" (1987 Guidelines, p. 34). No reasons are offered to support this conclusion. When the discussion moves beyond liberalism and freedom, law and consent, as it clearly must do here despite a valiant attempt to rein it in, all one gets is a report of opinion and beliefs. There is no sojourn into ethics, only an expression of the Committee's belief that "the purpose of intended research is a critical element in deciding whether embryo research is acceptable" (1987 Guidelines, p. 34). Once again, one wonders about consistency. Why doesn't the purpose of the research carry comparable weight for children and incompetent adults, those other categories of legally incompetent subjects?

In one important respect the new guidelines are, I think, too weak. The MRC recognizes that "commercially-directed research" is inherently suspect, that such research raises "questions of concern by its very nature" (1987 Guidelines, p. 19), but follows this with an inappropriately sanguine conclusion (p. 19):

> The professional integrity of the principal investigator, the vigilance of the REB, and a critical consideration of all the ethical, medical and scientific aspects of using human subjects for commercial rather than truly scientific purposes will, we believe, lead to proper conclusions should questions arise.

As recent experience in the United States dramatically reveals,[14] the potential for abuse in commercially linked research should be taken more seriously. To its credit, the MRC is now concerned with continuing review and monitoring of research, (1987 Guidelines, pp. 49-51) but the practical ramifications of its proposals are disconcerting. The MRC acknowledges that "[m]onitoring may ... strain professional and personal relationships between colleagues", (1987 Guidelines, p. 50) and given that, who would volunteer to be a monitor? If monitors have to be impressed into service, how good a job are they likely to do? And how effective is the monitoring effort likely to be if the costs are imposed upon the researchers and institutions? The amalgamation of profit and research creates a pressing need for unequivocal guidelines backed up by realistic proposals for continuous monitoring and enforcement of those guidelines.

The MRC should be commended for the extensive effort it made to involve the public in the reformulation of its guidelines. It is hard to disparage the egalitarian, democratic proposal that society should decide difficult ethical issues that can have profound and wide-ranging consequences, and calls for such involvement are frequent. The one I heard most recently was to let society decide whether anencephalic infants should be organ donors. Exactly how is this proposal to be implemented, however? Who or what constitutes "society"? How does "society" get the information it needs to make these decisions, and how does "society" go about making them? A way to begin appraising this recommendation would be to analyze the 120 letters of comment the Standing Committee received on its discussion document to see whether, and if so, how extensively, these contributions from the public affected the final report to the MRC. As well, it would be interesting to see who "the public" was here. Did it consist primarily of groups who will be subject to the guidelines and academics, or was there a broader constituency? A larger project would be an investigation of the consultation process and the submissions that led to the writing of the discussion document. I am not aware of any organization that has tried harder to involve the public in the formulation of ethical policy. How successful was this effort? The MRC's experience provides an opportunity for a case study that could assess the effectiveness, and perhaps the desirability, of such an approach. That would be a significant contribution to an understanding of policy formation on ethical issues.

Two final questions. First, what force do the revised guidelines have? The MRC takes the strong stand of requiring all research which it funds to comply with the new guidelines (1987 Guidelines, p. iii). The Committee that wrote the guidelines is more modest, however. In its view, the guidelines are intended to "stimulate discussion and understanding of human research ethics" and to foster "ethical awareness in both the research community and the broader public" (1987 Guidelines, p. xi). The Committee even seems to disavow the stronger stand of the MRC (1987 Guidelines, p. xi):

> The purpose of the guidelines ... is not to tell those responsible for making the ethical judgments on research proposals what decisions they must reach. Their purpose is rather to sensitize and guide decision makers on the range of perceptions they should bring to bear and to describe the processes of decision making that must be observed.

How successful are the guidelines on the Committee's own terms? The guidelines do a good job of articulating structure and procedure, but they are abysmal in "sensitizing and guiding" decision makers on the range of moral considerations that are relevant to the task of assessing the ethics of research protocols. That failure leads to the second question.

What is, or, perhaps, what should be, the relationship between the revised guidelines and the 1978 guidelines? The MRC suggests that the 1978 guidelines have been "superseded" by the new guidelines (1987 Guidelines, p. xi). That would be unfortunate. The comparatively extensive discussion of consent in the revised guidelines could be helpful to researchers writing protocols for REBs and to members of REBs scrutinizing consent forms and information sheets. The mandate for continuing review of research projects is, in theory, good, but there will be a wide gap between theory and practice here. In virtually every other respect, the 1978 guidelines are decidedly superior. They contain lucid analyses of issues, balanced presentations of alternatives, and judicious recommendations. Don't throw them away.

NOTES

1. Medical Research Council of Canada: Ottawa, 1978.
2. Medical Research Council of Canada: Ottawa, 1987.
3. For a recent discussion, see Kent Greenawalt, *Conflicts of Law and Morality* (New York: Oxford University Press, 1987).
4. A perusal of the footnotes in Chapter I demonstrates this point. Six of the nine references are to legal or political materials. Only one (note 6) is to a work in moral philosophy, and, as we shall see, the moral issue it discusses is not relevant to medical research.
5. I think this is what the MRC means when it says that "the law is a minimum ethic" (1987 Guidelines, p. 10).
6. The MRC itself says that "the basic ethical principle in research, as in health care, is respect for life" and that the concept of autonomy flows from this principle (p. 12). This suggests that life is more fundamental than autonomy and therefore life should have priority over freedom. The MRC does not accept that conclusion, however.
7. See, for example, Allen Buchanan, "Medical Paternalism," (1978) *Philosophy and Public Affairs,* Vol. 7, pp. 370-390.
8. This is the point of the fifth clause in the definition of paternalism provided by Gert and Culver, according to which the person towards whom someone is acting paternalistically "...believes (perhaps falsely) that he ... generally knows

what is for his own good." See Bernard Gert and Charles Culver, "Paternalistic Behaviour," (1976) *Philosophy and Public Affairs,* Vol. 6, p. 50.

9. At one point the MRC does recognize the problem of justice: "Justice must be exercised in allocating the anticipated risks and the hoped-for benefits [of research]" (p. 12). This concern is fleeting, however, because the problem of justice dissolves into the problem of consent.
10. (1965), 53 D.L.R. (2d) 436, 52 W.W.R. 608.
11. The abbreviation of the name for the US committees nevertheless retains a distinct mellifluous advantage.
12. R.S.C. 1985, c. C-46.
13. The same problem arises in the Supreme Court of Canada's decision in the *Re Eve* case, to which the MRC alludes in its section on research involving children (p. 29, note 12). See Barry Hoffmaster, "Judicial Review of the Charter of Rights and Freedoms: What are the Limits of Judging?" in *Legal Theory Meets Legal Practice,* ed. Anne Bayefsky (Edmonton: Academic Printing and Publishing, 1988), pp. 163-186.
14. "Flawed study helps doctors profit on drug," *The Boston Globe,* October 19, 1988, pp. 1, 16-17; "2 universities start probes of research," *The Boston Globe,* October 26, 1988, pp. 1, 14; "US halts 2 scientists' funding," *The Boston Globe,* December 1, 1988, pp. 1, 24; "Scientists grapple with increase in fraud," *The Boston Globe,* December 4, 1988, pp. 1, 28; "Scientists sued over drug firm stock sale," *The Boston Globe,* December 5, 1988, pp. 21-22; and "The system failed in drug research probe," *The Boston Globe,* December 5, 1988, pp. 29, 31.

FURTHER READINGS

Annas, G.J., L.H. Glantz and B.F. Katz
Informed Consent to Human Experimentation: The Subject's Dilemma. (Cambridge, Mass.: Ballinger Publication Co., 1977).

Beecher, H.K.
"Ethics in Clinical Research," *New England Journal of Medicine* 274 (1966), 1354-60.

Beecher, H.K.
Experimentation in Man. (Springfield, Ill.: Charles C. Thomas, 1959).

Cohen, C.
"Medical Experimentation on Prisoners," *Perspectives in Biology and Medicine*. Vol. 21, No. 3 (Spring 1978), 357-372.

Dickens, B.
"What is a Medical Experiment?" *Canadian Medical Association Journal* 113 (Oct. 4, 1975), 635-639.

Donagan, A.
"Informed Consent in Therapy and Experimentation," *The Journal of Medicine and Philosophy*. 2:4 (1977) 307-329.

Frenkel, D.A.
"Human Experimentation: Codes of Ethic," *Legal Medical Quarterly* 1: 1 (1977) 7-14.

Freund, P.A., ed.
Experimentation with Human Subjects. (New York: American Academy of Arts and Sciences, 1970).
Halushka v. The University of Saskatchewan, (1965), 53 D.L.R.(2d) 436.
Katz, Jay
Experimenting With Human Beings. (New York: Russell Sage Foundation, 1972).
Kluge, E.-H. W.
Biomedical Ethics in the Canadian Context. (Scarborough, Ont.: Prentice Hall, 1991), Chapter 7.
Law Reform Commission of Canada
Working Paper 61, *Biomedical Experimentation Involving Human Subjects.* (Ottawa, 1989).
Levine, Robert J.
Ethics and Regulation of Clinical Research. (New Haven and London: Yale University Press, 1988).
Medical Research Council of Canada
Guidelines on Research Involving Human Subjects 1987. (Ottawa: Minister of Supply and Services, 1987).
National Commission for the Protection of Human Subjects of Biomedical and Behavioral Research
The Belmont Report: Ethical Principles for the Protection of Human Subjects of Research. (Washington, DC: US Government Printing Office, 1978) pub. no. 78-0012.
Nuremberg Code
The Trials of War Criminals before the Nuremberg Military Tribunal. (Washington DC: US Government Printing Office, 1948).
Park, *et al.*
"Effects of Informed Consent in Research Patients and Study Results," *Journal of Nervous and Mental Diseases* 195 (1976) 349-357.

CHAPTER 7 INFORMATION AND MEDICAL TREATMENT

INTRODUCTION

When we think of informed consent, we usually think of getting sufficient information about a procedure or undertaking to be able to make an informed and competent choice. We usually don't think about the fact that the choice that we make is really informed if, and only if, we know not only the treatment options but also our own health-status or condition.

However, to know what our health status is, we have to have an overview of our own clinical picture; and in most cases we can get this only from our health care records: that is, from the records that detail the medically relevant findings that health care professionals — and especially physicians — have made about our health. Patient-rights groups have therefore maintained for some time that since informed consent is not really possible if patients do not know their own health care records, patients should have the right to see their records and to have copies made of them if they so wish.

The organizations that represent health care professionals — in particular, the Canadian Medical Association — have tended to resist this. First of all, they have argued that this record was never intended for patients: only for the physician her- or himself, or for other physicians. And following the line that a little knowledge is a dangerous thing, they have gone on to say that patients don't know enough about how to interpret these health care records, and therefore would jump to the wrong conclusions. They have also argued that patients might actually be harmed by finding out what is in their records. Physicians cannot allow this to happen. The primary obligation of physicians is to look out for the welfare of the patient. Finally, they have maintained that the patient record belongs to the physician because it is the physician who originated it.

If the courts are any indication, Canadian society does not agree with this. We find a graphic illustration of this in the New Brunswick case of *McInerney v. MacDonald.* It sets out that under normal circumstances a patient does indeed have the right of access to her or his records. It is simply part of the evolving societal insistence on individual autonomy; an insistence that appears to reflect a deontological ethical perspective. At the same time, it does not address a major issue that has been worrying health care professionals ever since: what if the records contain confidential information about *other* people? Another question is: what about third-party access? For example, what if a patient gives a lawyer or an insurance company authorization to have access to her or his records? Do the patients really understand what this means? Especially in the case of insurance companies? Should health care professionals worry about this? Should health care institutions?

The case of *McInerney* deals only with competent patients. Not all patients are competent. Young children are not — at least not in the sense necessary for giving an informed consent — and neither are people who are mentally disturbed in a clinical sense. Should these people also have access to their records? What if the information in those records disturbs them even more, and makes them worse? Kline, who is a practising physician, addresses this issue.

Howard Brody, who is also a physician, deals with an entirely different subject that also falls under the heading of informed consent. Health care professionals sometimes deliberately mislead their patients. Physicians are the major group who do this. For example, they do it when they lead their patients to believe that the prescriptions they give them or the treatments they recommend are causally effective for the patient's condition, when in actuality this is not the case.

Sometimes there appear to be good practical reasons for doing this. For instance, the patients may not actually have anything physiologically wrong with them at all, yet they *feel* ill. It may also be that there is no known treatment that is causally effective, yet there is a chance that the simple fact of prescribing something or of doing something will have a beneficial effect.

In these and similar cases, the physicians may be banking on what is known as the "placebo" effect to make the patients feel better. That is to say, they may be hoping that the psychosomatic effect of doing *something* will help the patients. Nurses and other health care professionals also deceive the patients when they go along with this.

Of course, not all cases of deliberate deception are like this. There is the case of the addict who is convinced that no method of treatment will help. The physician gradually weakens the injection of morphine with a saline solution — and after a while the patient is completely weaned. Are practices like this unethical? Brody looks at some of the issues that are involved.

The selection by Kline examines some of the implications of giving medical information to people who are mentally incompetent to handle it. Kline's discussion is from a legal perspective. However, it raises a serious ethical concern: precisely where is the line of access to information about ourselves to be drawn? Who should draw the line? Under what circumstances? Should there be any avenue of appeal?

McInerney v. MacDonald (N.B.C.A.)

Reasons for judgment by: Ryan J.A. Concurred in by: Hoyt J.A. Dissenting reasons by: Rice J.A.

RYAN J.A.: — Dr. Elizabeth A. McInerney, a physician, has been ordered by a judge of the Court of Queen's Bench to provide her patient, Margaret R. MacDonald, with copies of certain medical reports in her possession which the doctor had received from other physicians. Dr. McInerney appeals that decision...

Dr. McInerney co-operated with her patient to the extent of providing, for a fee, copies of notes, memoranda and reports prepared by her. She refused to deliver "consultants' reports and records of other physicians" because, she argued, they are the property of those physicians, five in number, and it would not be ethical for her to release their reports and records. She identified the other five physicians but would provide no other information ...

The relationship between the parties in the present case arises from contract where the patient sought and obtained professional medical services from her physician ...

The appellant does not dispute the right of the patient to have access to copies of material and notes generated by the appellant. The issue here is not ownership but the right of the patient to have access to the chart and its contents. Dr. McInerney disputes the patient's right, through her, to have access to "consultants' reports and records of other physicians" whom the respondent had consulted before becoming her patient. The line of reasoning advanced by counsel for the appellant physician is that the other doctors should be given the right to raise any legitimate argument before a court as to why the patient ought not to have access to the contents of the chart. Examples proffered are that it may not be in the best interests of the patient to view certain documents; that the patient may misinterpret the technical information, that the documents may contain information about other persons which is confidential or that the patient's reaction to certain information in the chart may endanger some third person. The appellant, however, does not raise any of these issues.

The arguments against this approach are that refusal is paternalistic and, in any event, the physician has a right to have a court determine whether valid grounds exist to prevent the patient from obtaining a copy of the information in her chart. The patient claims that her right arises out of a contract for treatment and that included with this is an implied contract for information relating to the treatment. The patient says that the physician received the charts containing her personal medical history from the other five doctors so that they could be used by Dr. McInerney in her treatment of the respondent. Because they contain her personal medical history and because the information in them was used by the appellant in order to treat her, she insists that she has a right of access to them arising out of contract.

I agree with the arguments adduced by the respondent patient. I come to this conclusion based on the contractual relationship between the physician and patient. I imply a right in the patient of access to

McInerney v. MacDonald [1990] N.B.J. No. 106 Action No. 74/89/CA all the information in her chart which the physician considered in providing professional services to the patient subject only to regulatory legislation and any superintending role which a court may assume. To my mind, the supervisory responsibility must rest with the courts as guided by the common law or regulations adopted by the state. People must generally have access to all the information in their charts. We live in a mobile society with a growing emphasis on access to information. This claim to information is simply one facet of a many sided repository of rights aimed at self-determination insisted upon by Canadians to-day. To hold otherwise would plunge the judgment-making power of whether or not to grant access into a sea of subjective decisions ...

Subject to the court's supervisory role referred to earlier, if the material contained in the patient's chart relates in any way to the treatment or advice provided by the physician to the patient, the patient has a right of access to it. That was the conclusion of the judge hearing the Notice of Application in this case and I agree with him. Having concluded that the patient has a right to copies of documentation in her chart and would therefore have the same right to material in the files of her other five doctors I can see no purpose in forcing the patient to make individual demands upon the other five doctors or to have to commence similar lawsuits against them in order to obtain access to her records ...

I would dismiss the appeal with costs to the respondent in the sum of $500.00.

RYAN J.A.

I concur: HOYT J.A.

The Lie That Heals: The Ethics of Giving Placebos

Howard Brody

The 170-year-long debate in the medical literature about the ethics of prescribing placebos in medical therapeutics needs to be reevaluated in light of recent placebo research and improved understanding of the placebo effect as an integral part of the doctor-patient relationship. It has traditionally been assumed that deception is an indispensible component of successful placebo use. Therefore, placebos have been attacked because they are deceptive, and defended on the grounds that the deception is illusory or that the beneficent intentions of the physician justify the deception. However, a proper understanding of the placebo effect shows that deception need play no essential role in eliciting this powerful therapeutic modality; physicians can use nondeceptive means to promote a positive placebo response in their patients.

H. Brody, "The Lie that Heals: The Ethics of Giving Placebos," *Annals of Internal Medicine* 97:1(1982).

The debate over whether it is ethical for physicians to prescribe placebos for patients has surfaced at intervals in the medical literature since the 19th century. Because traditional oaths and codes of ethics are silent on this issue, physicians taking a stand on placebo use have been unable to appeal to authority and have been prompted to develop original and often highly creative moral arguments. Although these arguments deserve review simply as an often-neglected feature of medical history, they also require critical reexamination in light of two recent developments. The first is the awakening of experimental interest in the placebo effect, and a gradual reconceptualization of placebo phenomena to recognize their pervasiveness as part of medical practice (1). The second is the emphasis in contemporary medical ethics of individual rights and patient autonomy in the doctor-patient relationship (2-4), leading to the rejection of many paternalistic assumptions previously thought to justify medical deception (5).

PLACEBOS AND THE PLACEBO EFFECT

"An empiric oftentimes, and a silly chirurgeon, doth more strange cures than a rational physician ... because the patient puts his confidence in him," Robert Burton wrote in 1628 (6), showing that at least by Renaissance times physicians appreciated the power of the imagination and expectation to change bodily states and to cure disease. In 1785 Benjamin Franklin led a commission to investigate Mesmer's animal magnetism and, in a series of elegant experiments, showed that the subjects' imagination was the most important factor in explaining the bizarre effects and miraculous cures attributed to that practice (7). Physicians were not reluctant to take advantage of this phenomenon by prescribing medications thought to be pharmacologically inert when no specific remedy was indicated. Thomas Jefferson wrote to Dr. Casper Wistar in 1807, "One of the most successful physicians I have ever known, has assured me, that he used more of bread pills, drops of colored water, and powders of hickory ashes, than of all other medicines put together" (8).

The contemporary era of placebo research began with the adoption of the double-blind controlled trial as the standard experimental method in the 1940s; subsequent findings on the placebo effect have been reviewed extensively (1, 9-13). Whenever a supposedly inert treatment is used in an experimental situation, 30% to 40% of subjects can be expected to show some benefit from the placebo treatment (9). The pattern of the response to placebo typically resembles the pharmacologic findings of active drug responses (14). In one study of the effect of both clofibrate and placebo on cholesterol level and cardiovascular mortality, those control subjects who reliably took their placebos showed lower cholesterol and reduced mortality compared with their less compliant counterparts (15). Placebo response is not limited to the patient's subjective experience; placebos alter laboratory values and other measures of objective physiologic change (16). Although placebos are commonly thought of primarily as pain relievers, virtually all potentially reversible symptoms and diseases that have been investigated in double-blind studies show some response to placebo — including diabetes (17), angina pectoris (18), and malignant neoplasms (19). Placebos can also cause many of the same side effects seen with active medication (20, 21). For all these reasons it is impossible to use placebo response to distinguish between a real, organic symptom and a symptom that is "all in the patient's head," although the myth to the contrary still persists (22).

From an early focus on attempting to elucidate the "personality type" of persons who react to placebos (which failed in part because the same person may respond or fail to respond to placebo in different circumstances [9]), attempts to understand placebo phenomena have shifted to a broader approach to factors in the doctor-patient relationship, in the overall situational context, and in the cultural background (23-29). It has become more clear that whatever happens when a patient gets better after ingesting a sugar pill also happens to some degree whenever the patient receives a pharmacologically potent treatment within a supportive healing relationship; that at least some of the symptom relief that follows administration of the active treatment arises from emotional and symbolic factors. That is, the placebo effect pervades much of medical practice even when no placebo has been used.

For example, when meprobamate, phenobarbital, and placebo were administered blindly to anxious patients, the two pharmacologically active drugs were clearly superior to placebo when administered by a physician who had confidence in the drugs' efficacy and who was viewed by the subjects as supportive; the drugs and placebo showed no difference when administered by a less supportive and more skeptical physician. Subjects of the first physician also showed more overall symptom relief (30). It is reasonable to suspect, then, that when the family physician prescribes decongestants for a viral upper respiratory infection, some of the patient's symptom relief is due to the pharmacologic action of the drug, but some is also due to the emotional support of the doctor-patient relationship, the doctor's confirmation and legitimization of the illness, and the reassurance that the symptoms do not represent something more serious than a bad cold.

DEFINITIONS

The expanded concept of the placebo effect just described makes it undesirable to have the definition of "placebo effect" totally dependent on the definition of "placebo." The following definitions may serve satisfactorily for our purposes: The placebo effect is the change in the patient's condition that is attributable to the symbolic import of the healing intervention rather than to the intervention's specific pharmacologic or physiologic effects; a placebo is a form of medical therapy, or an intervention designed to simulate medical therapy, that is believed to be without specific activity for the condition being treated, and that is used either for its symbolic effect or to eliminate observer bias in a controlled experiment. It is worth recalling here that although the sugar pill is cited as the paradigm case of placebo use, any medical treatment, including such diverse techniques as surgery (31) and biofeedback (32), can function as a placebo.

Another useful distinction uses the terms "pure" and "impure" placebos. A pure placebo, such as a lactose pill or a saline injection, is totally without pharmacologic potency. An impure placebo has some pharmacologic properties, but these are not relevant to the current circumstances and the treatment is used solely for its psychologic effect. Common examples are thyroid, vitamin B12, and penicillin, when used in patients who do not have hypothyroidism, pernicious anemia, or bacterial infections, respectively.

PLACEBOS AND DECEPTION

Jefferson said of the use of bread pills and drops of colored water in 1807, "It was certainly a pious fraud" (8). Subsequent writers, including physicians, philosophers, and scientists, have adopted widely divergent positions on the ethics of giving placebos (33). All authorities, however, are agreed on one point — if there is an ethical problem in therapeutic use of placebos, the problem is that of deception. This agreement in turn arises from a shared assumption about how placebos are typically used in clinical practice, which will be called here the "traditional use" of placebos. In the traditional use, the physician administers a treatment known to him or her to be without pharmacologic potency; but the physician either tells or allows the patient to believe that the treatment has such potency. It is further assumed in the traditional-use model that the patient's false belief in the potency of the treatment is essential for the placebo effect to occur (34-36).

Enough has already been said about the recently expanded concept of the placebo effect to call the traditional-use model into question on several counts. However, the bulk of the medical literature on the ethics of placebos accepts this model as a given. Hence, to do justice to most of the arguments offered by physicians for and against placebo use, the traditional-use model must form the point of departure. In a subsequent section, the ethical position that results from replacing the traditional model with the expanded concept will be considered.

It will be most convenient to survey first the arguments offered against placebo use, as these assume that deception is generally wrong, and that it is just as wrong (if indeed not worse) when encountered in medicine as when encountered elsewhere in life. Next, arguments in favor of placebo use can be investigated to see how successfully they defuse the deception issue.

ARGUMENTS AGAINST PLACEBOS

It is standard in modern writings on medical ethics to oppose placebo use because it represents a specific instance of the more general issue of patient deception (2, 3, 5, 37, 38). The value of avoiding deception is grounded in the more basic values of the autonomy and dignity of the individual patient. The basic idea is that of moral reciprocity. We generally wish that other people treat us in a manner that shows their respect for us as persons; and this entails that they not use manipulation or deception on us, even if they judge the results to be for our own good. If we are to regard our patients as our moral equals and to respect their dignity as persons, we are similarly prohibited from practicing deception or manipulation on them.

This line of reasoning is most at home in the context of a deontologic or duty-based ethical theory. Deception is condemned because it violates an *a priori* moral rule — *a priori* because the rule appeals to the very nature of our beings (that is, persons deserving respect) rather than to the good or bad consequences of our actions. Appeal to duty and to moral rule has always been a popular mode of argument. Thus one medical editor (39) wrote in 1885, "Physicians ... cannot always tell the plain truth to a patient without injuring him. It should be the rule of ... life, however, to be straightforward and candid. Therefore, we say that placebos should be ... rarely, if ever, prescribed." Describing the characteristics of the trustworthy and virtuous physician, the writer concluded, "We venture to say that such a man would not find it necessary to keep a polychromatic assortment of sugar pills in his closet."

This commentator explicitly rejects an argument from consequences — at times, indeed, being truthful may injure patients. But more basic than negative consequences is the a *priori* "rule of ... life," which in the

19th century was closely tied to concepts of virtue and gentlemanly conduct, and hence truthfulness.

Other physicians, however, have been uncomfortable with *a priori* appeals and have preferred a utilitarian mode of argument, demanding to be shown that placebo use, generally applied, would lead to a net increase in unhappiness over happiness for all concerned. Among many adopting a utilitarian stand, the most articulate and forceful was Richard C. Cabot, best known today as originator of the clinicopathologic conferences of the Massachusetts General Hospital, but in his day an innovative writer on medical ethics as well as on medicine, and holder of the Chair of Professor of Social Ethics at Harvard University in addition to his medical appointment (40). Cabot (41) rejected an *a priori* approach to issues of truth and falsehood — "you will notice I am not now arguing that a lie is, in itself and apart from its consequences, a bad thing" — but felt that the negative consequences of placebo use condemned the practice. The obvious short-range consequence occurred when the patient discovered the deception and lost trust in the physician. True, it was probable in any single case that the physician would not be found out; but Cabot (41) rejoined, "Is it good for us as professional men to have our reputations rest on the expectation of not being found out?"

But Cabot (41) was much more concerned about the long range consequences of creating unhealthy public attitudes toward medicine and medications:

> The majority of placebos are given because we believe that the patient will not be satisfied without them. He has learned to expect medicine for every symptom and without it he simply won't get well. True, but who taught him to expect a medicine for every symptom? He was not born with that expectation. He learned it from an ignorant doctor who really believed it.... It is we physicians who are responsible for perpetuating false ideas about disease and its cure ... and with every placebo that we give we do our part in perpetuating error, and harmful error at that.

Cabot elsewhere (42) stated even more bluntly, "Placebo giving is quackery." He concluded (41) that in general the negative consequences of placebo use outweighed the positive; but that placebos could be justified in some rare cases:

> No patient whose language you can speak, whose mind you can approach, needs a placebo. I give placebos now and then ... to Armenians and others with whom I cannot communicate, because to refuse to give them would create more misunderstandings, a falser impression, than to give them. The patient will think that I am refusing to treat him at all; but if I can get hold of an interpreter and explain the matter, I tell him no lies in the shape of placebos.

Another more recent commentator reflected on both the occasional justification for giving placebos, and the rarity with which such a case ought to arise: "Some patients are so unintelligent, neurotic, and inadequate as to be incurable, and life is made easier for them by a placebo." Then, paraphrasing an earlier commentator (43), he concluded: "It has been said that the use of placebos is in inverse ratio to the combined intelligences of patient and doctor" (44).

In assessing the consequences of placebo use as a general policy, one should note the tendency of deception to multiply itself, and the need to cover up for the original lie. Prescribing placebos now involves insuring the complicity of the nurse, the pharmacist, and all other parties to the prescription. There is also the problem of setting a fee for the placebo prescription — if too high, them someone will appear to making an unjustified profit from deception; if too low, the deception may inadvertently be discovered. It may be more for such mundane reasons and not out of any increased ethical insight that the use of totally inert medicines like lactose pills has declined once physicians stopped dispensing their own drugs. In more recent times, fear of lawsuits may also have played a role.

ARGUMENTS FOR PLACEBOS

Deceptive or not, placebos have in fact been widely administered by practicing physicians, and to many the fascinating power of the body to respond to purely symbolic interventions seemed too potent a therapeutic tool to pass up. A number of commentators have tried to give a formal justification for placebo use. Once again, two general moral approaches have been used. For the deontologist, the force of the moral rule against deception cannot be denied; so it must be argued either that the deception rule does not properly apply to the placebo case, or that other moral rules may mitigate it. The utilitarian may calculate all the good consequences attributable to placebos, and argue (or assume) that these outweigh the evils of deception. For each of these attempts at justification, however, the placebo opponents have had a ready and generally persuasive reply.

First, one may forthrightly deny that placebo use need involve deception by the physician. This position, while occasionally alluded to (45), is seldom stated explicitly in the medical literature; but it is frequently encountered in debate and discussion among physicians. It is usually argued that if the physician tells the patient that a sugar pill is morphine or penicillin, he is guilty of an outright and unethical lie. But if he administers the pill with a noncommittal statement, such as, "This pill will make you feel much better," he has not deceived the patient; any false beliefs result from the patient's deceiving himself and are not the moral responsibility of the physician: "should a patient become suspicious ..., the therapist need only give an honest evasion, rather than a lie" (36).

Richard Cabot (41) attacked this and other arguments defending medical practices that mislead the patient by stating, *"a true impression*, not certain words literally true, is what we must try to convey." By way of fleshing out Cabot's objection, it may be acknowledged that what counts as deception may be dependent on the norms and expectations associated with particular social settings. For instance, when we go to the theater and see Mark Twain reading from *Huckleberry Finn,* we do not consider ourselves to have been deceived when we discover he is a cleverly made-up actor. We may then ask whether the clinical setting is one of those special social situations where creating a false impression by deliberate misdirection does not count as deception. Cabot appears to have assumed that a patient may reasonably expect in that setting that, if a drug or other treatment is given, it is selected for its pharmacologic potency for the patient's condition. It also seems reasonable to assume that the patient will not expect that the physician will specifically name the treatment — the patient is accustomed to receiving pills alluded to by the physician merely as "an antibiotic" or "a decongestant," but these remedies are still assumed by the patient to be pharmacologically potent. One may then conclude that if the physician prescribes an inert pill and conceals this from the patient by verbal misdirection, he has violated these legitimate patient expectations and is guilty of deception; the special nature of the clinical setting gives no license for creating a false impression in this manner.

Legal backing (46) for Cabot's argument comes with the characterization of the physician-patient relationship as a fiduciary one, in which one party assumes a special responsibility to look out for the best interests of the other. "Where a person sustains toward others a relation of trust and confidence, his silence when he should speak, or his failure to disclose what he ought to disclose, is as much a fraud in law as an actual affirmative false representation" (47).

Still, the physician is not responsible for false beliefs the patient may bring into the encounter, if the physician has taken no action to cause those beliefs (48, 49); how far the physician's duty extends to dispel those false beliefs, if they do not lead directly to health-threatening behavior, is an interesting ethical question in itself. What is the physician's duty toward the patient who arrives with a firmly entrenched belief in the therapeutic and preventive powers of vitamins, and asks the physician to recommend a good daily vitamin supplement? This patient harbors a false belief, and energetic and prolonged discussion from the physician might mitigate or dispel it. But this reeducation seems hardly worth the effort, given the low probability of harm and the (presumed) low readiness of the patient to assimilate the new information. Thus the postulated duty not to create false beliefs in the patient by one's words or actions need not imply a more onerous duty to seek out and dispel all the false beliefs the patient may have acquired elsewhere.

Second, the placebo advocate may admit that placebos as traditionally used involve deception, but still insist that this use is ethically justified. Social practice recognizes a class of deceptions called white lies, which are felt to be essentially harmless because of their innocuous content and benign motivation (50). Even if the special circumstances of medical practice do not automatically permit out-and-out deception, it still seems to be the case that many partial truths or euphemisms are appropriate. For example, proper supportive care of the cancer patient seeking some hope to mitigate the frightening diagnosis calls for a somewhat slanted presentation emphasizing the potential gains from therapy, not merely for a listing of the 5-year survival statistics.

But a problem in including placebos in the category of white lies is that what counts as a white lie is fairly well demarcated by social convention; otherwise anyone uttering a falsehood, however blatant, could excuse his act by claiming it was "only a white lie." Members of society are thus in effect forewarned about this practice and, if they choose to ask their friends how their new hats or ties look on them, they can be said to have given at least implied consent to any white lie that results. By contrast, the traditional-use model assumes that knowledge of the lie will be restricted to the medical profession, lest placebos lose their effectiveness with wider publicity. Recipients of the so-called white lie are therefore systematically excluded from any knowledge of the existence of this practice, and they have no opportunity to challenge questionable uses of placebo deception by reference to generally accepted social norms and limits. This would make placebo use morally suspect in a way that the usual white lies are not.

Leslie (51) attempted to justify placebo deception in a similar fashion: "There is a fine line of distinction between the words, *deception* and *deceit* ... deceit implies blameworthiness whereas deception does not necessarily do so...." Leslie emphasized the benign intent of the physician and offered as an analogy a magician practicing sleight of hand to entertain an audience. But Bok (50) has emphasized that the supposedly benign intent of the person doing the lying, and the expected value of the resulting benefits, often look very different from the perspective of the person being lied to. The audience choosing voluntarily to witness the magician's performance can weigh for themselves the degree of deception, the intent, and the value of the benefits; the patient in the traditional-use model of placebos is denied this opportunity. (It may in fact be argued that the magic show is not "deception" at all, as any reasonably well informed person knows what goes on at such events and is not fooled in any substantive way.) Thus, Leslie is either merely asserting that some deceptions are justified and others are not, without giving any arguments to prove that placebos belong in the justified category; or else his "fine line" between deception and deceit is so fine as to escape attention altogether.

All this discussion of justified and unjustified deception, however, may seem pointless to the pragmatic physician who adopts the traditional use of placebos merely because it can benefit the patient. By this pragmatic view, either the physician's duty not to deceive is of no moral concern at all, or else it is far outweighed by the much stronger duty to benefit the patient — a duty which, Veatch (38) has argued, has dominated the so-called Hippocratic ethical tradition in medicine to the unwarranted exclusion of other, equally rational moral considerations. This view has gained added impetus since the recent wave of research described above, showing the extent and frequency of placebo responses. The pragmatic approach has been further bolstered by research linking the placebo response to endorphins (52). Because endorphins function primarily in analgesia, and because, as was noted above, the placebo response is not limited to pain, this endorphin research really provides a very limited account of the physiologic means by which placebos may exert their effects. But to the uncritical medical mind, the identified biochemical basis for some placebo responses has somehow made the whole placebo issue suddenly respectable. (Shapiro [53] discovered in an informal survey that negativism toward placebo use among physicians correlated with greater age, private rather than academic practice, and nonparticipation in clinical research.)

In this setting, the placebo advocate may attribute, rightly or wrongly, several false beliefs to the person who argues against placebo use. The opponent of placebos may be thought to believe: that placebos really do not work, or work only for a limited number of medical conditions; that some pharmacologically active remedy exists for all conditions, so that the doctor who prescribes a placebo is automatically withholding the "correct" drug; or that any treatment that works by psychologic mechanisms is thereby inferior to a treatment that works by biochemical means. As we saw, ethical concern over placebos does not depend on any of these false assumptions, yet placebo opponents are still sometimes labeled as if their arguments ran contrary to modern scientific medicine. It may have been a mistaken attribution of these false beliefs that led a distinguished investigator of the placebo response (54) to characterize as "oft-quoted but fatuous" one of the better recent papers (55) offering arguments of the sort first used by Cabot.

One could, of course, offer a utilitarian counter-attack to Cabot (41) and contend that he had miscalculated the likelihood and the severity of the various consequences of placebo use. But any balanced view of the pros and cons makes this a remote possibility. First, if past studies are reliable, only 30% to 40% of patients will respond to placebo positively. Second, even though lactose can be expected to have fewer toxic effects than active drugs, placebo side effects and even addiction do periodically occur. Finally, even if one rejects these considerations, one is still left with the long-range consequences Cabot predicted — a public conditioned to look for the cure for all ills in a bottle of medicine, and to neglect prevention and a healthy life-style in favor of a medical quick fix.

But most pragmatic authors do not even attempt a balanced utilitarian consideration. If anything, they are content with a crude risk-benefit ratio: Anything that benefits the patient is good; placebos have been shown in scientific trials to benefit patients; therefore, placebos should be used, at least in selected sorts of cases. A frequent hidden assumption is that the only harm worth considering in this crude pragmatic calculus is direct physical harm such as that due to a toxic drug reaction. Less tangible harms — risks to doctor-patient trust, unhealthy views about drug-taking, and decreased opportunity for the patient to make choices about his own care — are simply left out of the equation (34, 36, 43, 56-65). The nature of the risk-benefit calculus is further illustrated by those authors who list specific contraindications or limitations for placebo use (33, 34, 51), for instance, the concern that overuse of placebos will lead to diminished diagnostic vigilance (57) or that the placebo-treated patient will be more resistant to definitive psychotherapy (66).

Placebo use may thus be cautiously endorsed because of its success, without raising ethical qualms:

> I knew a surgeon years ago who thought nothing of performing an oblique lower right quadrant incision, then suturing without entering the abdominal cavity in patients who had emotional problems manifested by pain in the abdomen. His results were excellent and as one might expect his operative mortality and morbidity were exceptionally low.... Certainly this is not common and I doubt whether anyone else would have done such procedures. However, I am certain that thousands of appendectomies and hysterectomies are done yearly as placebos. In retrospect, though at the time I was horrified at what he had done, and still am aware of the possible grave consequence, I am inclined to admire his courage (63).

The unnecessary-surgery argument indicates that the less scientifically-inclined physician may inadvertently use therapy that actually can benefit the patient only through the placebo effect. One may then argue that it is better for the physician to use a pure placebo rather than an impure placebo. Prescribing pure placebos at least promotes full knowledge (for the physician, at least) of the approach being taken; impure placebos promote unscientific medicine and expose the patient to increased risk of toxic reactions (43, 57, 60).

> If deception is involved in the case of the pure placebo, it applies to only one person, namely, the patient, for the physician knows that the agent is devoid of all but psychotherapeutic properties. But when we use [an impure placebo] there is the danger of deceiving two people.... The doctor may come to think that the agent has potency when, in fact, it has none. That danger is real ... (67)

Other authors are vaguely concerned about the deception issue but feel it to be merely a semantic problem: "If placebo therapy is regarded as a form of deception, then, of course, an ethical dilemma arises.... What is needed is a redefinition of placebo or nonspecific effects in psychologic or psychotherapeutic terms" (27). "If we give patients a placebo as an honest psychotherapeutic device, we can be considered fulfilling [our] primary responsibility" (63). But just because a substance is used for its symbolic properties does not eliminate the possibility of morally blameworthy deception:

> We like to think that our patients bring us their symptoms and problems for our consideration, expecting thoughtful and honest advice. With ... the declining influence of the Church, the doctor's value to the community as an impartial and educated adviser has become as important as the priest's used to be. The placebo is a form of deception and a betrayal of trust equivalent to the sale of bottles of ditch-water as water of the River Jordan (44).

There is, however, another form of defense for placebos that does not look at a weighing of the good and bad consequences, but rather at the nature of the implied expectations in the doctor-patient relationship. Placebo use is unjustified if the patient's proper expectation is "that the physician will give me the chance to be informed about the treatment"; but not if the expectation is "that the physician will choose on my behalf the treatment most likely to help." Thus it is argued that placebo use "does not amount to deception of the patient who trusts the doctor to order whatever he considers is most likely to be of benefit" (45).

There is nothing illogical about an expectation that gives the physician this extensive a blank check. But it is unlikely that most patients have such an expectation, at least in modern times, and specifically in relation to placebos. On the contrary, the indignation with which most people respond on learning they have received placebo surreptitiously is strong evidence against any widespread acceptance of this much paternalism. An individual patient, of course, may negotiate such an arrangement with his or her physician; but that hardly justifies the blanket attribution of paternalistic expectations to patients generally.

AN ALTERNATIVE POSITION: PLACEBO EFFECT WITHOUT DECEPTION

Of all the positions above, opposition to placebo use unless there are especially strong extenuating circumstances in a specific case is ethically most sound; the other positions either evade the deception issue or fail to disarm its legitimate force. But one must recall that all of these arguments assume the traditional-use model, which holds that the deception is an essential ingredient for successful placebo treatment. The considerations noted at the beginning of this paper, however, based on newer placebo research and appropriate redefinition of the terms "placebo effect" and "placebo," point the way to an effective separation of deception and the placebo effect in clinical practice. Once deception is eliminated (and not merely glossed over) the ethical problem is defused.

One excellent and commonplace example of nondeceptive use of placebos occurs in properly designed double-blind research with informed consent. The research subject is ignorant as to whether he or she is actually receiving placebo or the experimental drug; but he or she has been fully informed of the experimental design, about the use of placebos in the study, and about the risks and benefits associated with the design. If free consent is given based on that information, no deception has occurred and all the criteria for ethical research have been met. Unfortunately there are a few experiments, more commonly occurring in social science research, where deception about the nature of the experimental design is essential if the data are to be valid. Whether and with what consent arrangements such studies may be ethically conducted requires additional analysis (68).

The first empirical rejection of the traditional-use model of the placebo response was a nonblind placebo trial (69). Thirteen of 14 psychiatric outpatients with somatic symptoms who completed a week's trial of sugar pills, having been openly informed that they were sugar pills and that many patients experienced relief with such medication, experienced objective symptom reduction. Such a study, of course, has severe limitations, and this work has not been replicated. But a more recent survey of placebo therapeutics gives several case reports of successful placebo therapy in patients who were openly informed that they were receiving pharmacologically inert substances (70). Furthermore, Norman Cousins (71), in describing the response of his mysterious connective tissue disease to a combination of high-dose ascorbic acid, laughter, and positive thinking, commented, "It is quite possible that this treatment — like everything else I did — was a demonstration of the placebo effect." Here is anecdotal testimony that a well-informed patient may be aware of the mental or symbolic effect of a therapy and still experience major bodily changes.

Whereas possibilities for nondeceptive use of placebos are theoretically intriguing and are of some limited clinical applicability, the nondeceptive use of the placebo effect has much more important practical implications, because some element of the placebo effect exists in every clinical encounter even when no placebo is used (1, 23, 25, 28, 29). An analysis of the symbolic elements of the physician-patient relationship suggests that a clinical approach that makes the illness experience more understandable to the patient, that instills a sense of caring and social support, and that increases a feeling of mastery and control over the course of the illness, will be most likely to create a positive placebo response and to improve symptoms (24, 26, 29). Empirical support for this thesis is provided by a study of the effect of the anesthesiology pre-operative visit on postoperative pain. The control group received a standard visit whereas the experimental group received teaching about the nature of postoperative pain, advice on simple techniques to avoid pain and increase relaxation, and reassurance that back-up medication was available from the nurses. The experimental group required half as much pain medication and were able to be discharged an average of 2 days earlier. These investigators (72) — who used no inert substances and who committed no deceptions on the subjects — described their results as illustrating "a placebo effect without a placebo." Once clinicians realize the extent to which simple information and encouragement can elicit a positive placebo response and thus supplement the pharmacologic effects of any active medication, the perceived need to use deception or inert medication in clinical practice ought to be markedly diminished.

CONCLUSION

The placebo, as traditionally used, could be called the lie that heals. But a satisfactory understanding of the nature of the placebo effect shows that the healing comes not from the lie itself, but rather from the relationship between healer and patient, and the latter's own capacity for self-healing via symbolic and psychological approaches as well as via biological intervention.

For some time medical science has looked almost exclusively at technical means of diagnosis and treatment; the doctor-patient relationship that forms the setting for their application has been naïvely viewed as a noncontributory background factor, relegated to the amorphous realm of the "art of medicine," or simply ignored. In this setting, the placebo effect has inevitably been viewed as a nuisance variable, interfering with our ability to elicit "clean data" from clinical trials; and deception in medicine has been seen either as an unimportant side issue or as a tolerated means toward another end. But, as the doctor-patient relationship is rediscovered as a worthy focus for medical research and medical education, the placebo effect assumes center stage as one approach to a more sophisticated understanding of this relationship (73). Deception is avoided, as ethically inappropriate and as a threat to the long-term stability of the relationship; and clinicians turn to alternative, nondeceptive ways to elicit positive placebo responses in all patient encounters at the same time that they apply the most appropriate medical technology.

REFERENCES

1. Brody, H. *Placebos and the Philosophy of Medicine*. Chicago: University of Chicago Press; 1980.
2. Beauchamp, T.H., Childress, J.F. *Principles of Biomedical Ethics*. New York: Oxford University Press; 1979.
3. Brody, H. *Ethical Decisions in Medicine*, 2nd ed. Boston: Little, Brown & Co.; 1981.
4. Buchanan, A. Medical paternalism. *Philosophy and Public Affairs*. 1978;7:370-90.
5. Reiser, S.J. Words as scalpels: Transmitting evidence in the clinical dialogue. *Ann Intern Med*. 1980;92:837-42.
6. Burton, R. *The Anatomy of Melancholy*. New York: Empire State Book Co.; 1924:168.
7. *Report of Dr. Benjamin Franklin and Other Commissioners Charged by the King of France with the Examination of the Animal Magnetism, as now Practised at Paris*. London: J. Johnson; 1785. (Fabin's Bibliotecha Americana, microcard #25 579).
8. Ford P.L., ed. *The Writings of Thomas Jefferson*. Vol. IX. New York: Putnam; 1898:78-85.
9. Beecher, H.K. The powerful placebo. *JAMA*. 1955;159:1602-6.
10. Kurland, A.A. Placebo effect. In: Uhr, L., Millar, J.G., eds. *Drugs and Behavior*. New York: John Wiley; 1960:156-65.
11. Berg, A.O. Placebos: A brief review for family physicians. *J Fam Pract*. 1977;5:97-100.
12. Shapiro, A.K., Morris, L.A. The placebo effect in medical and psychological therapies. In: Garfield, S.L., Bergin, A.E., eds. *Handbook of Psychotherapy and Behavior Change*. 2nd ed. New York: John Wiley; 1978.
13. Turner, J.L., Gallimore, R., Fox, C. *Placebo: An Annotated Bibliography*. available from: UCLA, Neuropsychiatric Institute, Center for the Health Sciences, 760 Westwood Plaza, Los Angeles, CA 90024.
14. Lasagna, L., Laties, V.G., Dohan, J.L. Further studies on the "pharmacology" of placebo administration. *J Clin Invest*. 1958;37:533-7.
15. The Coronary Drug Project Research Group. Influence of adherence to treatment and response of cholesterol on mortality in the Coronary Drug Project. *N Engl J Med*. 1980;303:1038-41.
16. Wolf, S. Affects of suggestion and conditioning on the action of chemical agents in human subjects — the pharmacology of placebos. *J Clin Invest*. 1950;29:100-9.

17. Singer, D.L., Hurwitz, D. Long-term experience with sulfonylureas and placebo. *N Engl J Med.* 1967;277:450-6.
18. Benson, H., McCallie, D.P. Angina pectoris and the placebo effect. *N Engl J Med.* 1979;300:1424-9.
19. Klopfer, B. Psychological variables in human cancer. *J Projective Techniques.* 1957;21:331-40.
20. Wolf, S., Pinsky, R.H. Effects of placebo administration and occurrence of toxic reactions. *JAMA.* 1954;155:339-41.
21. Honzak, R., Horackova, E., Culik, A. Our experience with the effect of placebo in some functional and psychosomatic disorders. *Activitas Nervosa Superior.* 1972;14:184-5.
22. Goodwin, J.S., Goodwin, J.M., Vogel, A.V. Knowledge and use of placebos by house officers and nurses. *Ann Intern Med.* 1979;91:106-10.
23. Modell, W. *The Relief of Symptoms.* Philadelphia: WB Saunders; 1955.
24. Adler, H.M., Hammett, V.B.O. The doctor-patient relationship revisited. An analysis of the placebo effect. *Ann Intern Med.* 1973;78:595-8.
25. Benson, H., Epstein, M.D. The placebo effect: a neglected asset in the care of patients. *JAMA.* 1975;232:1225-7.
26. Cassell, E.J. The healer's art: A new approach to the doctor-patient relationship. Philadelphia: JB Lippincott; 1976.
27. Gallimore, R., Turner, J.L. Contemporary studies of placebo phenomena. In: Jarvik, M.E., ed. *Psychopharmacology in the Practice of Medicine.* New York: Appleton-Century-Crofts; 1977:45-57.
28. Silber, T.J. Placebo therapy: The ethical dimension. *JAMA.* 1979;242:245-6.
29. Brody, H., Waters, D.B. Diagnosis is treatment. *J Fam Pract.* 1980;10:445-9.
30. Uhlenhuth, E.H., Canter, A., Neustadt, J.O., Payson, H.E. The symptomatic relief of anxiety with meprobamate, phenobarbital, and placebo. *Am J Psychiatry.* 1959;115:905-10.
31. Beecher, H.K.. Surgery as placebo: A quantitative study of bias. *JAMA.* 1961;176:1102-7.
32. Stroebel, E.F., Glueck, B.C. Biofeedback treatment in medicine and psychiatry: An ultimate placebo? *Semin Psychiatry.* 1973;5:379-93.
33. Shapiro, A.K. Attitudes toward the use of placebos in treatment. *J Nerv Ment Dis.* 1960;130:200-9.
34. Abramowitz, E.W. The use of placebos in the local therapy of skin diseases. *NY State J Med.* 1948;48:1927-30.
35. Hofling, C.K. The place of placebos in medical practice. *GP.* 1955;11(6):103-7.
36. Fischer, H.K., Dlin, B.M. The dynamics of placebo therapy: A clinical study. *Am J Med Sci.* 1956;232:504-12.
37. Simmons, B. Problems in deceptive medical procedures: An ethical and legal analysis of the administration of placebos. *J Med Ethics.* 1978;4:172-81.
38. Veatch, R.M. *A Theory of Medical Ethics.* New York: Basic Books; 1981.
39. Placebos. *Med Record.* 1885;27:576-7.
40. Burns, C.R. Richard Clarke Cabot and reformation in American medical ethics. *Bull Hist Med.* 1977;51:353-68.
41. Cabot, R.C. The use of truth and falsehood in medicine: An experimental study. *Am Med.* 1903;5:344-9.

42. Cabot, R.C. The physician's responsibility for the nostrum evil. *JAMA*. 1906;47:982-3.
43. Platt, R. Two essays on the practice of medicine. *Lancet*. 1947;253:305-7.
44. Handfield-Jones, R.P.C. A bottle of medicine from the doctor. *Lancet*. 1953;265:823-5.
45. Placebo therapy. *Practitioner*. 1964;192:590.
46. Brody, H. The physician-patient contract: Ethical and legal aspects. *J Legal Med*. 1976;4:25-30.
47. Perkins v. First National Bank of Atlanta. 143 SE 2d 474: Georgia; 1975.
48. McDermott, J.F. A specific placebo effect encountered in the use of dexedrine in hyperactive child. *Am J Psychiatry*. 1965;121:923-4.
49. Cassel, C., Jameton, A.L. Power of the placebo: a dialog on principles and practice. *Art of Medication*. 1980;1(3):22-7.
50. Bok, S. *Lying: Moral Choice in Public and Private Life*. New York: Pantheon; 1978.
51. Leslie, A. Ethics and the practice of placebo therapy. *Am J Med*. 1954;16:854-62.
52. Levine, J.D., Gordon, N.C., Fields, H.L. The mechanism of placebo analgesia. *Lancet*. 1978;2:654-7.
53. Shapiro, A.K. The use of placebos: A study of ethics and physicians' attitudes. *Psychiatry in Med*. 1973;4:17-29.
54. Lasagna, L. The powerful cipher. *The Sciences*. 1980;20(20):31-2.
55. Bok, S. The ethics of giving placebos. *Sci Am*. 1974;231(5):17-23.
56. Carter, A.B. The placebo: Its use and abuse. *Lancet*. 1953;265:823.
57. The humble humbug [Editorial]. *Lancet*. 1954;267:321.
58. Wayne, E.J. Placebos [Abstract]. *Br Med J*. 1956;2:157.
59. Lasagna, L. Placebos. *Sci Am*. 1956;193:(7)68-71.
60. Koteen, H. Use of a "double-blind" study investigating the clinical merits of a new tranquilizing agent. *Ann Intern Med*. 1957;47:978-89.
61. Atkinson, E.C. Dummy tablets [letter]. *Br Med J*. 1958:1:1478.
62. Branson, H.K., Ward, R. The place of the placebo in geriatric nursing. *Hosp Management*. 1964:98(6):34, 37.
63. Shure, N. The placebo in allergy. *Ann Allergy*. 1965;23:368-76.
64. Thrift, C.B., Traut, E.F. Further studies on placebo management of skeletal disease. *Ill Med J*. 1966;129:683-5.
65. Sicé, J. Evaluating medication [Letter]. *Lancet*. 1972;2:651.
66. Salfield, D.J. The placebo. *Lancet*. 1953;265:940.
67. Wolff, H.G., DuBois, E.F., Cattell, M., et al. Conferences on therapy: The use of placebos in therapy. *NY State J Med*. 1946;46:1718-27.
68. Soble, A. Deception in social science research: Is informed consent possible? *Hastings Cen Rep*. 1978;8(October):40-6.
69. Park, L.C., Covi, L. Nonblind placebo trial: An exploration of neurotic outpatients' response to placebo when its inert content is disclosed. *Arch Gen Psychiatry*. 1965;12:336-45.
70. Vogel, A.V., Goodwin, J.S., Goodwin, J.M. The therapeutics of placebo. *Am Fam Physician*. 1980;22(1):105-9.
71. Cousins, N. Anatomy of an illness (as perceived by the patient). *N Engl J Med*. 1976;295:1458-63.
72. Egbert, L.D., Battit, G.E., Welch, C.E., Bartlett, M.K. Reduction of postoperative pain by encouragement and instruction of patients. *N Engl J Med*. 1964;270:825-7.
73. Jensen, P.S. The doctor-patient relationship: Headed for impasse or improvement? *Ann Intern Med*. 1981;95:769-71.

Release of Information: Mental Competency Considerations

Stephen A. Kline

The common law doctrine of informed consent should ensure both access to and disclosure of information, but in reality, state and provincial statutes or regulations determine the extent to which that right is applied.[1] However, both of these must be considered in a discussion of a patient's mental competency with respect to his or her own medical record.

ACCESS TO RECORDS

In the United States and Canada, although there exists a distinct trend towards permitting patients access to their own records, the choices between jurisdictions vary from little or no access, except through litigation, to virtually unlimited access, excepting extraordinary circumstances.[2]

In most jurisdictions permitting access, portions of the record that may render the patient dangerous to self or others are excluded, subject to judicial or quasijudicial review.

Those persons with strong civil libertarian views maintain that should a patient express a wish to review the chart, that wish alone should stand as the threshold test for mental competency to review one's own record. At the opposing pole, many see access as requiring a high standard of competency similar to that required for medical decision-making, arguing that an appreciation of the importance of the contents of a document such as a medical record is a sufficient standard.

The author's perspective sits midway between these views. A patient should be able to understand the nature of a record. Operationally, the clinician should explain the general nature of the chart to the patient who, in turn, should be able to repeat that basic information, submitting some of his or her own words. Any manifest threats of harm to oneself or others are clearly serious risks to the integrity of the access situation and should be a limiting factor. By closely applying these tests, we can provide access to the vast majority of patients, but exclude those few to whom access is dangerous, meaningless or merely a source of agitation.

Clinical Examples

Partial Access

E. was a large, powerful man with paranoid schizophrenia. On admission and during the first few weeks following admission to hospital, he was intimidating and occasionally violent towards staff and fellow patients alike. Nonetheless, he improved markedly with a vigorous treatment program, including substantial amounts of antipsychotic medication. After about six

Stephen A. Kline, "Release of Information: Mental Competency Considerations," *Health Law in Canada* 10:1(1989)144-145.

weeks in hospital, he demanded to see his chart. He was convinced his relatives were conspiring with the attending physician against him and he made it clear that he intended to avenge himself on those wrongdoers should he find the necessary evidence. He was easily able to understand the nature of his record, but there was obvious concern about the potential effect on him of the notes regarding interviews with his relatives. He was granted limited access to his record, with the exclusion of those portions describing the interviews with relatives. He seemed satisfied with his review and, in the remaining three weeks of his hospitalization, never expressed further wishes to see the chart.

Close Supervision

F. was a young, agitated woman with a lengthy history of explosive behaviour. She was admitted following a violent domestic episode primarily to allow her home situation time to settle down. After a fairly tranquil week in hospital, she requested a look at her chart. Her ability to understand the nature of the chart was well above any reasonable threshold, and she displayed no undue concern about the contents. Nonetheless, when the chart was presented, she began to tear it into pieces. She was restrained momentarily, and after an explanation that destruction of the chart was not allowed she resumed reading it, this time under very close supervision. There were no further incidents.

TRANSMISSION OF RECORD

The release and disclosure of the medical record to persons other than the patient to whom it relates or to institutions demands a more stringent standard for mental competency assessments. It may be difficult to ensure the application of the doctrine of informed consent in these situations because the patient's voluntariness may be challenged by those demanding the information; for example, in the case of receiving financial benefits from an institution, or of an insurance company requesting health data for an application.

Clearly, the patient cannot make a relevant decision about disclosure unless he or she has reviewed the chart in detail and had the opportunity to discuss its contents with a clinician directly involved in the case.

Therefore, the patient should appreciate the nature of the chart and the potential consequences of its receipt by another designated person or institution. Following a reason able explanation, the patient, on testing, should be able to repeat and explain both the information provided as well as the rationale used in making the subsequent decision.

Clinical Examples

Temporary Suspension of Disclosure

G. is a youthful, energetic woman with manic depressive illness. She was a considerable financial success, and made a great deal of money by dabbling in real estate. On this particular occasion, she was hospitalized *during* a period of markedly elevated mood. She had spent a number of days racing around the nursing unit, chattering incessantly, all without the benefit of sleep. A lawyer on the other side of a major real estate transaction sent a request for health care information, ostensibly because of his concern over the patient's capacity to enter into a contract. When presented with this request, G. jubilantly declared that she had nothing to hide, that there were no consequences attached to disclosure and that she was thrilled to provide her own chart information to anyone. On the basis that G. did not appreciate the consequences of her decision, the information was not immediately disclosed. Three days later, G.'s mood returned to normal. She was again presented with the same request for information. This time she was firm and decisive in stating that under no circumstances was the lawyer on the other side to receive information that might compromise her negotiations.

NOTES

1. Arnup, C.J., "Patients' Right of Access to Their Own Records" (1984) 5 *Health L. Can.*, No. 1, p. 15.
2. Meisel, A., "Making Mental Health Care Decisions: Informed Consent and Involuntary Civil Commitment" (1983) 1 *Behavioural Sciences and the Law* (4), p. 73.

ADDITIONAL REFERENCES

1. Burns, R.E., "Casenote on Tarasoff v. Regents of the University of California" (1975) 9 Akron Law Review, p. 191.
2. Smith, D., "Unfinished Business with Informed Consent Procedures" (1981) 36 American Psychologist (1), p. 22.
3. Warren, D.G., "Patient Medical Information and Records in the United States: Disclosure and Access" (1981) 2 Health L. in Canada (2), p. 38.

FURTHER READINGS

Beauchamp, T.L. and J.F.Childress
Principles of Biomedical Ethics. (New York and Oxford: Oxford University Press, 1979).
Emson, H. E.
The Doctor and the Law. (Toronto: Butterworths, 1989).
Engelhardt, Jr., H.T.
Foundations of Bioethics. (New York and Oxford: Oxford University Press, 1986).
Jospe, M.
The Placebo Effect in Healing. (Lexington, Mass: Health, 1978).
Kluge, E.-H.W.
"Placebos: Some Ethical Considerations," *Canadian Medical Association Journal* 1990; 142 (4) 293-295.
Lipkin, M.
"Suggestion and Healing," *Perspectives in Biology and Medicine* 20 (1984) 121–126.
Mallary, S.D., B. Gert and C.M. Culver

"Family Coercion and Valid Consent," *Theoretical Medicine* 7: 2 (June, 1986) 123–126.
Parks, L.C. and L. Covi
"Non-Blind Placebo Trials," *Archives of General Psychiatry*. 124 (1965) 334-45.
Savage, H. and Carla McKague
Mental Health Law in Canada. (Toronto and Vancouver: Butterworths, 1987).
Simmons, Beth
"Problems in Deceptive Medical Procedures: An Ethical and Legal Analysis of the Administration of Placebos," *Journal of Medical Ethics* 4 (1978) 172–181.
Spiro, H.K.
Doctors, Patients and Placebos. (New Haven: Yale University Press, 1986) 33.

CHAPTER 8 PROXY DECISION-MAKING

INTRODUCTION

The last selection in the previous chapter touched on the issue of competence. This notion is very important when it comes to informed consent. The paradigm case of informed consent involves a health care professional and someone who is adult, who can understand what is being said, and who can react appropriately. However, many times the patient is not competent in that sense. For instance, the patient may be a young child, or someone who is physiologically mature but mentally severely handicapped. In these sorts of cases, someone has to make the decision for the incompetent person. But who?

Traditionally, it was assumed that the family or next-of-kin played that role. With the rise of modern medicine, as the decision-making function was gradually assumed by the physician even in ordinary contexts, it became the practice to let the physician assume the role of decision-maker for incompetent persons. In the last twenty years, the pendulum has swung the other way. The family has again become the primary decision-maker for incompetent persons. The article by Bernard Dickens explores the role of the family from a legal perspective.

However, the family may not always function appropriately in this regard. The case of *re S.D.*, excerpts from which are reproduced below, illustrates the court's concerns in this regard. Among other things, it is noteworthy for its attempt to introduce the notion of substituted judgement into the Canadian legal setting.

The Supreme Court of Canada, in the case of *Eve*, rejected substituted judgement for the Canadian setting. It characterized substituted judgement as legal sleight-of-hand. The court went further. It outlined what it considered to be its primary concern when safeguarding the interests of incompetent persons. The case itself deals specifically only with the involuntary sterilization of a mentally handicapped person. However, the reasoning of the court has wider application. In his commentary on the *Eve* case, Kluge points out some of the ethical shortcomings of the Supreme Court's decision, and gives a sketch of how an alternative approach to proxy decision-making might be developed.

RE S.D.

The subject of these proceedings is a severely retarded boy approaching 7 years, who shortly after birth suffered profound brain damage through meningitis which inflamed the lining of his brain and left him with no control over his faculties, limbs or bodily functions. At the age of 5 months life-support surgery was performed by implanting a shunt which is a plastic tube which drains excess cerebro-spinal fluid from head to another body cavity from which it is expelled or absorbed.

As perceived by his parents the boy is legally blind, with atrophied optic nerves, partly deaf, incontinent, cannot hold a spoon to feed himself, cannot stand, walk, talk or hold objects. They say that he has no method of communicating with his environment and think he is in pain. The sounds he makes are too soft to be heard from any distance. He is subject to seizures despite anti-convulsant medication. He is restrained by splints which are bandages on his arms to keep his elbows straight so that he cannot chew on his hands and roughly handle his face. Staff carry him from bed to wheelchair, which has a molded "insert" to ensure he is held securely and he is belted in with a hip belt.

This description applies to his condition as it existed when he was a patient in Sunnyhill Hospital before the shunt stopped operating. About 6 weeks ago a blockage in the shunt was detected and the parents gave their consent to remedial surgery but, after a day's reflection, withdrew their consent on the ground that the boy should be allowed to die with dignity rather than continue to endure a life of suffering. They continue to maintain that position.

Because of the parent's refusal the Superintendent of Family and Child Service, acting under the Act which creates his office (S.B.C. 1980 C.11) and mindful of the provision (s.2) which makes the safety and well-being of a child the paramount consideration in administering and interpreting the Act, considered this child "in need of protection" and acted under s.9 to apprehend him. The quoted words, as defined in s.1, have several meanings, in relation to a child, including that he is "deprived of necessary medical attention".

Following apprehension, the Superintendent, conforming with s.11, presented a written report to the Provincial Court of British Columbia and asked for an order that the custody of the child be retained by him pending a hearing to determine whether the child was in need of protection. Following 5 days of hearing and a weekend's contemplation and writing, the Provincial Court Judge read in open court a 29-page oral judgment on 14 March 1983 which ordered the Superintendent to return the child to his parent's custody. The Judge identified the issue as:

> ... who may exercise an incompetent's right to refuse life sustaining treat-

Re S.D. (1983)3 W.W.R. 618 (B.C.S.C.).

ment if no directive exists and the incompetent is unable to do so?

The Judge appears to have held that this right belongs in the family, in consultation with their medical advisors. Where treatment would serve "only to prolong a life inflicted with an incurable condition" rather than cure or improve the patient's condition, the interest of the state in the preservation of life is overridden by the wishes of the people whose duty it is to make the decision.

Adopting the distinction between treatment that "cures" and treatment that simply "prolongs life where there is no hope of recovery" the Judge found that the shunt revision fell into the latter category.

The Judge found that the shunt revision in S.'s case constituted an "extraordinary surgical intervention", and not "necessary medical attention". Since S. was therefore not deprived of "necessary medical attention" there was no basis for the belief that S. was not a "well-cared-for and loved child", and she concluded that she should order that he be returned to his parents under s.11(2)(b) of the Family and Child Service Act. S.11 sets out the procedure for review of the Superintendent's decision to apprehend a child pending a hearing on the question of whether the child is in need of protection. The Judge also held that the shunt revision would constitute a violation of S.'s right not to be subjected to cruel and unusual treatment under s.12 of the Canadian Charter of Rights and Freedoms ...

I think that the Superintendent's petition is accurate in contending that the learned Judge:

1) Held that a life saving operation does not amount to necessary medical attention as defined in s.1.

2) Did not consider as paramount the safety and well-being of the child as required in s.2.

3) Held that the shunt revision constituted cruel and unusual punishment under s.12 of the Canadian Charter of Rights and Freedoms.

4) Did not consider s. 7 of the Charter.

By referring to the proceedings in Provincial Court and to the disposition of those proceedings I have done so for narrative reasons only because, as I conceive it, the *parens patriae* jurisdiction of the Supreme Court in this matter takes precedence over the proceedings in Provincial Court and allows this court to act as if the matter came before it in the first instance. Confirmation of this view is contained in s.21 of the Act.

> Nothing in this Act limits the inherent jurisdiction of the Crown, through the Supreme Court, over infants, as parens patriae, and the Supreme Court may rescind a permanent order where it is satisfied that to do so is conducive to a child's best interest and welfare.

Time does not permit me to expand on this aspect or on other important aspects of this case, such as the standing of Philip J. Russell, President of the British Columbia Association for the Mentally Retarded or of the Public Trustee for the Province of British Columbia, who come before the court as petitioners in a petition separate from that instituted by the Superintendent. Because of the urgency of the situation I will act on the assumption, which I believe to be sound, that the Superintendent unquestionably has standing and that the other petitioners are duplicating his arguments, or, at least, are duplicating his argument that this court should exercise its inherent jurisdiction as *parens patriae* and authorize medical and surgical treatment as required by the boy. Indeed, the parents seek the invocation of the same jurisdiction but ask that it be applied to support their position.

> I propose to examine the matter from the *parens patriae* point of view as expressed by Lord Eldon, L.C. in *Wellesley v. Duke of Beaufort* (1827) 2 Russ. 1 at 18, 38 E.R., affirmed 2 Bligh N.S. 124, 4 E.R. 1078 ... by the House of Lords...

...

In considering the application of the *parens patriae* jurisdiction I recognize that the central concern is to discover what is in S.'s best interest. This is not a "right to die" situation where the courts are concerned with people who are terminally ill from incurable conditions. Rather it is a question of whether S. has the right to receive appropriate medical and surgical care of a relatively simple kind which will assure to him the continuation of his life, such as it is.

I am satisfied that the laws of our society are structured to preserve, protect and maintain human life and that in the exercise of its inherent jurisdiction this court could not sanction the termination of a life except for the most coercive reasons. The presumption must be in favour of life. Neither could this court sanction the wilful withholding of surgical therapy where such withholding could result not necessarily in death but in a prolongation of life for an indeterminate time but in a more impoverished and more agonizing form.

I do not think that it lies within the prerogative of any parent or of this court to look down upon a disadvantaged person and judge the quality of that person's life to be so low as not to be deserving of continuance.

The matter was well put in an American decision — *re Weberlist* (1974), 360 N.Y.S. (2d) 783, 79 Misc. 2d 753 (N.Y. Co, Ct.),where Justice Asch said at p. 787:

> There is a strident cry in America to terminate the lives of *other* people — deemed physically or mentally defective.... Assuredly, one test of civilization is its concern with the survival of the unfittest, a reversal of Darwin's formulation.... In this case, the court must decide what its ward would choose, if he were in a position to make a sound judgment ...

This last sentence puts it right. It is not appropriate for an external decision maker to apply his standards of what constitutes a livable life and exercise the right to impose death if that standard is not met in his estimation. The decision can only be made in the context of the disabled person viewing the worthwhileness or otherwise of his life in its own context as a disabled person — and in that context he would not compare his life with that of a person enjoying normal advantages. He would know nothing of a normal person's life having never experienced it ...

...

I respect and have given anxious consideration to the views of the parents. In so doing I must give some weight to the fact that they were divorced in mid-1980 after extended matrimonial discord. Also I must give weight to my conclusion based on the evidence that they thought S. better dead long before the need for the critical decision arose about replacement of the shunt. Despite the evidence of highly qualified professionals, in whom I place great reliance, they are satisfied S. will promptly die if treatment is denied. My finding is that it is by no means a certainty that death will soon follow and a real possibility exists that his life will go on indefinitely but in pain and progressive deterioration. I must reject their assertion that they would consent to the operation if they could be assured that he would thereafter be comfortable and free of pain when at the same time they reject the opinions of competent professionals that such will probably be the case. I believe that their minds are firmly made up and closed shut.

I regret having to make such findings.

Further, I find that the professionals who have been treating and observing S.

since late 1982 are better qualified than they are to assess his condition and capacities because they, the parents, have hardly seen him. I do not criticize them for this but simply observe it as a fact.

I cannot accept their view that S. would be better off dead. If it is to be decided that "it is in the best interests of S. that his existence cease", then it must be decided that, for him, non-existence is the better alternative. This would mean regarding the life of a handicapped child as not only less valuable than the life of a normal child, but so much less valuable that it is not worth preserving. I tremble at contemplating the consequences if the lives of disabled persons are dependent upon such judgments.

To refer back to the words of Templeman, L.J., I cannot in conscience find that this is a case of severe proved damage "where the future is so certain and where the life of the child is so bound to be full of pain and suffering that the court might be driven to a different conclusion". I am not satisfied that "the life of this child is demonstrably going to be so awful that in effect the child must be condemned to die". Rather I believe that "the life of this child is still so imponderable that it would be wrong for her to be condemned to die".

There is not a simple choice here of allowing the child to live or die according to whether the shunt is implanted or not. There looms the awful possibility that without the shunt the child will endure in a state of progressing disability and pain. It is too simplistic to say that the child should be allowed to die in peace.

In conclusion I order that interim custody be granted to the Superintendent pending a hearing pursuant to s.13 of the Family and Child Service Act and while in that interim custody the surgical procedure be carried out pursuant to the authority of this court. The matter is remitted to the Provincial Court for the s.13 hearing.

Eve v. Mrs. E

Supreme Court of Canada

La Forest J. — These proceedings began with an application by a mother for permission to consent to the sterilization of her mentally retarded daughter who also suffered from a condition that makes it extremely difficult for her to communicate with others. The application was heard by McQuaid J. of the Supreme Court of Prince Edward Island — Family Division. In the interests of privacy, he called the daughter "Eve", and her mother "Mrs. E".

BACKGROUND

... [Mr. Justice McQuaid, the trial judge, on the basis of the evidence before him, found that the following description summed up Eve's situation:]

> The evidence established that Eve is 24 years of age, and suffers what is described as extreme expressive aphasia. She is unquestionably at least mildly to moderately retarded.

Re Eve (1987), 3 D.L.R.(4th) 1 (S.C.C.).,[1987] 2 S.C.R. 388 (S.C.C.).

She has some learning skills, but only to a limited level. She is described as being a pleasant and affectionate person who, physically, is an adult person, quite capable of being attracted to, as well as attractive to, the opposite sex. While she might be able to carry out the mechanical duties of a mother, under supervision, she is incapable of being a mother in any other sense. Apart from being able to recognize the fact of a family unit, as consisting of a father, a mother, and children residing in the same home, she would have no concept of the idea of marriage, or indeed, the consequential relationship between, intercourse, pregnancy and birth. Expressive aphasia was described as a condition in which the patient is unable to communicate outwardly thoughts or concepts which she might have perceived. Particularly in the case of a person suffering from any degree of retardation, the result is that even an expert such as a psychiatrist is unable to determine with any degree of certainty if, in fact, those thoughts or concepts have actually been perceived, or whether understanding of them exists. Little appears to be known of the cause of this condition, and even less of its remedy. In the case of Eve, this condition has been diagnosed as extreme

From the evidence, he [Mr. Justice McQuaid] further concluded:

> [t]hat Eve is not capable of informed consent, that her moderate retardation is generally stable, that her condition is probably non-inheritable, that she is incapable of effective alternative means of contraception, that the psychological or emotional effect of the proposed operation would probably be minimal, and that the probable incidence of pregnancy is impossible to predict.

Mrs. E. wanted to be sure she had a right to consent to the sterilization of Eve, so she applied ... for the following remedies:

(a) that Eve be declared a mentally incompetent pursuant to the provisions of the Mental Health Act;

(b) that Mrs. E. be appointed the committee of the person of Eve;

(c) that Mrs. E. be authorized to consent to a tubal ligation operation being performed on Eve.

... Having reviewed the Canadian and English case law and found no governing authorities, McQuaid J. considered whether the court should, in the exercise of its parens patriae jurisdiction, intervene on behalf of Eve. He had no doubt that the court could authorize a surgical procedure necessary to health even though a side-effect might be sterilization, and he postulated that it could also do so where the public interest clearly required it, though he found it difficult to come up with an example. However, McQuaid J. was of the view that Eve, like other individuals, was entitled to the inviolability of her person, a right that superseded her right to be protected from pregnancy. That this might result in inconvenience and even hardship to others was irrelevant. The law must protect those who are unable to protect themselves; it must ensure the protection of the higher right. He, therefore, concluded that the court had no authority or jurisdiction to authorize a surgical procedure on a mentally retarded person, the intent and purpose of which was solely contraceptive. It followed that, except for clinically therapeutic reasons, parents or others similarly situated could not give a valid consent to such a surgical procedure either, at least in the absence of clear and unequivocal statutory authority. He, therefore, denied the application.

An appeal to the Supreme Court of Prince Edward Island, *in banco*, was launched, and an order was then made appointing the Official Trustee as Guardian ad litem for Eve. The appeal was allowed. The general view of the court is set forth in an addendum to its notes of judgment as follows:

> In rendering judgment in this matter, we are unanimously of the opinion that the Court has, in proper circumstances, the authority and jurisdiction to authorize the sterilization of a mentally incompetent person for non-therapeutic reasons. The jurisdiction of the Court originates from its parens patriae powers towards individuals who are unable to look after themselves and gives the Court authority to make the individual a ward of the Court.

The court, however, differed on the evidence. A majority (Large and Campbell JJ.) was of the view, MacDonald J. dissenting, that there was sufficient evidence to warrant the sterilization of Eve. The court therefore ordered that:

(a) "Eve" be appointed a ward of the Court pursuant to the *parens patriae* jurisdiction for the sole purpose of facilitating and authorizing her sterilization;

(b) the Court authorizes the sterilization of "Eve" by a competent medical practitioner;

(c) the Court reserves its approval of the method of sterilization to be followed pending further submissions of counsel as to the medically preferred surgical procedure.

... Leave to appeal to this Court was then granted to Eve's Guardian *ad litem* by the Prince Edward Island Supreme Court, Appeal Division. The major issues raised in this appeal are substantially as follows:

1. Is there relevant provincial legislation that gives a court jurisdiction to appoint a committee vested with the power to consent to or authorize surgical procedures for contraceptive purposes on an adult who is mentally incompetent?
2. In the absence of statutory authority, does the court's *parens patriae* jurisdiction allow the court to consent to the sterilization of an adult who is mentally incompetent?
3. What is the appropriate standard of proof to be applied in a case where an application is made to the court for its substituted consent to a non-therapeutic procedure on behalf of a mentally incompetent adult? Upon whom is the onus of proof?
4. If the court has jurisdiction to provide substituted consent for a non-therapeutic procedure on behalf of a mentally incompetent adult, did the Supreme Court of Prince Edward Island, *in banco*, properly exercise its jurisdiction in granting an order authorizing the sterilization of Eve?
5. Does the Canadian Charter of Rights and Freedoms protect an individual against sterilization without that individual's consent?
6. If the Charter provides such protection, when will it permit the non-therapeutic sterilization of a mentally incompetent who is incapable of giving consent?
7. Does the Charter give an individual the right to choose not to procreate, and if so does the court have jurisdiction to make that choice on behalf of an individual who is unable to do so?

GENERAL CONSIDERATIONS

Before entering into a consideration of the specific issues before this Court, it may be useful to restate the general issue briefly. The Court is asked to consent, on behalf of

Eve, to sterilization since she, though an adult, is unable to do so herself. Sterilization by means of a tubal ligation is usually irreversible. And hysterectomy, the operation authorized by the Appeal Division, is not only irreversible; it is major surgery. Eve's sterilization is not being sought to treat any medical condition. Its purposes are admittedly non-therapeutic. One such purpose is to deprive Eve of the capacity to become pregnant so as to save her from the possible trauma of giving birth and from the resultant obligations of a parent, a task the evidence indicates she is not capable of fulfilling. As to this, it should be noted that there is no evidence that giving birth would be more difficult for Eve than for any other woman.

A second purpose of the sterilization is to relieve Mrs. E. of anxiety about the possibility of Eve's becoming pregnant and of having to care for any child Eve might bear.

... [Mr. Justice LaForest then discusses the history and rationale of proxy decision-making in the UK and the roles of the courts. He then turns to the US and discusses two approaches to proxy decision-making that have been used there.]

... While many state courts have, in recent cases, been prepared to recognize an inherent power in courts of general jurisdiction to authorize sterilization of mentally incompetent persons, they differ on the standard of review. Two distinct approaches have emerged: the "best interests" approach and the "substituted judgment" approach. In five of the nine states in which equitable jurisdiction to authorize the non-consensual sterilization of a mentally incompetent person is recognized, that jurisdiction is based on the inherent equitable power of the courts to act in the best interests of the mentally incompetent person; ... The test necessarily leads to uncertainties ... and in an effort to minimize abuses, American courts have developed guidelines to assist in determining whether the best interests of the affected person would be furthered through sterilization....

.... As noted these facts indicate that the courts of the United States in acting under the best interests test have a very wide discretion.

The second approach, the substituted judgment test, raises Charter implications.

... The primary purpose of the substituted judgment test is to attempt to determine what decision the mental incompetent would make, if she were reviewing her situation as a competent person, but taking account of her mental incapacity as one factor in her decision. It allows the court to consider a number of factors bearing directly upon the condition of the mental incompetent. Thus the court may consider such issues as the values of the incompetent, any religious beliefs held by her, and her societal views as expressed by her family. In essence, an attempt is made to determine the actual interests and preferences of the mental incompetent. This, it is thought, recognizes her moral dignity and right to free choice. Since the incompetent cannot exercise that choice herself, the court does so on her behalf. The fact that a mental incompetent is, either because of age or mental disability, unable to provide any aid to the court in its decision does not preclude the use of the substituted judgment test.

The respondent submitted that this test should be adopted in this country. As in the case of the best interests test, various guidelines have been developed by the courts in the United States to ensure the proper use of this test.

... [I]t is easy to understand the natural feelings of a parent's heart. ...[However] a court ... must exercise great caution to avoid being misled by this all too human mixture of emotions and motives. So we are left to consider whether the purposes underlying the operation are necessarily for Eve's benefit and protection.

The justifications advanced are the ones commonly proposed in support of non-therapeutic sterilization ... Many are demonstrably weak. The [Law Reform] Commission dismisses the argument about the trauma of birth by observing at p. 60 [Working paper 24, *Sterilization: Implications for Mentally Retarded and Mentally Ill Persons.* Ottawa: Minister of Supply and Services, 1978]:

> For this argument to be held valid would require that it could be demonstrated that the stress of delivery was greater in the case of mentally handicapped persons than it is for others. Considering the generally known wide range of post-partum response would likely render this a difficult case to prove.

The argument relating to fitness as a parent involves many value-loaded questions. Studies conclude that mentally incompetent parents show as much fondness and concern for their children as other people; see *Sterilization, supra,* p. 33 et seq., 63-64. Many, it is true, may have difficulty in coping, particularly with the financial burdens involved. But this issue does not relate to the benefit of the incompetent; it is a social problem, and one, moreover, that is not limited to incompetents. Above all it is not an issue that comes within the limited powers of the courts, under the *parens patriae* jurisdiction, to do what is necessary for the benefit of persons who are unable to care for themselves. Indeed, there are human rights considerations that should make a court extremely hesitant about attempting to solve a social problem like this by this means. It is worth noting that in dealing with such issues, provincial sterilization boards have revealed serious differences in their attitudes as between men and women, the poor and the rich, and people of different ethnic backgrounds.

As far as the hygienic problems are concerned, the following view of the Law Reform Commission (*[Sterilization]* at p. 34) is obviously sound:

> ... if a person requires a great deal of assistance in managing their own menstruation, they are also likely to require assistance with urinary and fecal control, problems which are much more troublesome in terms of personal hygiene.

Apart from this, the drastic measure of subjecting a person to a hysterectomy for this purpose is clearly excessive.

The grave intrusion on a person's rights and the certain physical damage that ensues from non-therapeutic sterilization without consent, when compared to the highly questionable advantages that can result from it, have persuaded me that it can never safely be determined that such a procedure is for the benefit of that person. Accordingly, the procedure should never be authorized for non-therapeutic purposes under the parens patriae jurisdiction.

To begin with, it is difficult to imagine a case in which non-therapeutic sterilization could possibly be of benefit to the person on behalf of whom a court purports to act, let alone one in which that procedure is necessary in his or her best interest. And how are we to weigh the best interests of a person in this troublesome area, keeping in mind that an error is irreversible? Unlike other cases involving the use of the parens patriae jurisdiction, an error cannot be corrected by the subsequent exercise of judicial discretion. That being so, one need only recall Lord Eldon's remark, ... that "it has always been the principle of this Court, not to risk damage to children which it cannot repair" to conclude that non-therapeutic sterilization may not be authorized in the exercise of the parens patriae jurisdiction. McQuaid J. was, therefore, right in concluding that he had no authority or jurisdiction to grant the application.

Nature or the advances of science may, at least in a measure, free Eve of the incapacity from which she suffers. Such a possibility should give the courts pause in extending their power to care for individuals to such irreversible action as we are called upon to take here. The irreversible and serious intrusion on the basic rights of the individual is simply too great to allow a court to act on the basis of possible advantages which, from the standpoint of the individual, are highly debatable. Judges are generally ill-informed about many of the factors relevant to a wise decision in this difficult area. They generally know little of mental illness, of techniques of contraception or their efficacy. And, however well presented a case may be, it can only partially inform. If sterilization of the mentally incompetent is to be adopted as desirable for general social purposes, the legislature is the appropriate body to do so. It is in a position to inform itself and it is attuned to the feelings of the public in making policy in this sensitive area. The actions of the legislature will then, of course, be subject to the scrutiny of the courts under the Canadian Charter of Rights and Freedoms and otherwise.

... The foregoing, of course, leaves out of consideration therapeutic sterilization and where the line is to be drawn between therapeutic and non-therapeutic sterilization. On this issue, I simply repeat that the utmost caution must be exercised commensurate with the seriousness of the procedure. Marginal justifications must be weighed against what is in every case a grave intrusion on the physical and mental integrity of the person.

... I cannot agree that a court can deprive a woman of that privilege for purely social or other non-therapeutic purposes without her consent. The fact that others may suffer inconvenience or hardship from failure to do so cannot be taken into account. The Crown's *parens patriae* jurisdiction exists for the benefit of those who cannot help themselves, not to relieve those who may have the burden of caring for them.

I should perhaps add ... that sterilization may, on occasion, be necessary as an adjunct to treatment of a serious malady, but I would underline that this, of course, does not allow for subterfuge or for treatment of some marginal medical problem.

The foregoing remarks dispose of the arguments based on the traditional view of the *parens patriae* jurisdiction as exercised in this country. Counsel for the respondent strongly contended, however, that the Court should adopt the substituted judgment test recently developed by a number of state courts in the United States. That test, he submitted, is to be preferred to the best interests test because it places a higher value on the individuality of the mentally incompetent person. It affords that person the same right, he contended, as a competent person to choose whether to procreate or not.

There is an obvious logical lapse in this argument. I do not doubt that a person has a right to decide to be sterilized. That is his or her free choice. But choice presupposes that a person has the mental competence to make it. It may be a matter of debate whether a court should have the power to make the decision if that person lacks the mental capacity to do so. But it is obviously fiction to suggest that a decision so made is that of the mental incompetent, however much the court may try to put itself in her place. What the incompetent would do if she or he could make the choice is simply a matter of speculation. The sophistry embodied in the argument favouring substituted judgment has been fully revealed in *Eberhardy* ... where ... the court stated:

> The fault we find in the New Jersey case is the *ratio decidendi* of first concluding, correctly we believe, that the right to sterilization is a personal choice, but then equating a decision made by others with the choice of the person to be sterilized. It clearly is not a personal choice, and no amount of legal legerdemain can make it so.
>
> ...
>
> We conclude that the question is not choice because it is sophistry to refer to it as such, but rather the question is whether there is a method by which others, acting in behalf of the person's best interests and in the interests, such as they may be, of the state, can exercise the decision. Any governmentally sanctioned (or ordered) procedure to sterilize a person who is incapable of giving consent must be denominated for what it is, that is, the state's intrusion into the determination of whether or not a person who makes no choice shall be allowed to procreate.

Counsel for the respondent ... argued that there is what he called a fundamental right to free procreative choice. Not only, he asserted, is there a fundamental right to bear children; there is as well a fundamental right to choose not to have children and to implement that choice by means of contraception. ... [H]e appears to base this argument on s. 7 of the Charter. But assuming for the moment that liberty as used in s. 7 protects rights of this kind (a matter I refrain from entering into), counsel's contention seems to me to go beyond the kind of protection s. 7 was intended to afford. All s. 7 does is to give a remedy to protect individuals against laws or other state action that deprive them of liberty. It has no application here.

Another Charter related argument must be considered. In response to the appellant's argument that a court-ordered sterilization of a mentally incompetent person, by depriving that person of the right to procreate, would constitute an infringement of that person's rights to liberty and security of the person under s. 7 of the Canadian Charter of Rights and Freedoms, counsel for the respondent countered by relying on that person's right to equality under s. 15(1) of the Charter, saying "that the most appropriate method of ensuring the mentally incompetent their right to equal protection under s. 15(1) is to provide the mentally incompetent with a means to obtain non-therapeutic sterilizations, which adequately protects their interests through appropriate judicial safeguards." A somewhat more explicit argument along the same lines was made by counsel for the Public Trustee of Manitoba. His position was stated as follows:

> It is submitted that in the case of a mentally incompetent adult, denial of the right to have his or her case presented by a guardian *ad litem* to a Court possessing jurisdiction to give or refuse substituted consent to a non-therapeutic procedure such as sterilization, would be tantamount to a denial to that person of equal protection and equal benefit of the law. Such a denial would constitute discrimination on the basis of mental disability, which discrimination is prohibited by Section 15 of The Canadian Charter of Rights and Freedoms.

Section 15 of the Charter was not in force when these proceedings commenced but, this aside, these arguments appear flawed. They raise in different form an issue already dealt with, i.e. that the decision made by a court on an application to consent to the sterilization of an incompetent is somehow that of the incompetent. More troubling is that the issue is, of course, not raised by the incompetent, but by a third party. The court undoubtedly has the right and duty to protect those who are unable to take care of themselves, and in doing so it has a wide discretion to do what it considers to be in their best interests. But this function must not, in my view, be transformed so as to create a duty obliging the court, at the behest of a third party, to make a choice between the two alleged constitutional rights — the right to procreate or not to procreate — simply because the individual is unable to make that choice. All the more so since, in the case of non-therapeutic sterilization as we saw, the choice is one the courts cannot safely exercise.

... Since, barring emergency situations, a surgical procedure without consent ordinarily constitutes battery, it will be obvious that the onus of proving the need for the procedure is on those who seek to have it performed. And that burden, though a civil one, must be commensurate with the seriousness of the measure proposed. In conducting these procedures, it is obvious that a court must proceed with extreme caution; otherwise ... it would open the way for abuse of the mentally incompetent.... I would allow the appeal and restore the decision of the judge who heard the application.

After "Eve": Whither Proxy Decision-Making?

Eike-Henner W. Kluge

One of the most difficult problems facing physicians is how to approach proxy decisions made on behalf of congenitally incompetent patients. The author considers two recent court cases that attempt to provide guidelines: *Re Stephen Dawson,* which opts for a substituted-judgement approach, and *Eve v. Mrs. E.,* which enjoins best-interests considerations. The author explores the impact of *Eve v. Mrs. E.* as superseding *Re Stephen Dawson,* considers its ethical implications and attempts to clarify the best-interests criterion by sketching some guidelines for its interpretation. In so doing, he tries to reconcile the two decisions by laying bare their common underlying ethical rationale. The author concludes by pointing out some ethically questionable implications of *Eve v. Mrs. E.* in the allocation of health care resources.

One of the most difficult situations that physicians may face is one involving an incompetent patient. Normally, following what could be called a fiduciary model of the physician-patient relationship, physicians may feel that they have fulfilled their professional obligation when they have advised the patient of the various pertinent modalities of treatment, expressed an opinion and made a recommendation, and have done all this in language that the patient can and does understand. Whatever decision the patient then makes will be legally

Eike-Henner W. Kluge, "After 'Eve': Whither Proxy Decision-Making?" *Canadian Medical Association Journal* , 137 (October 15, 1987) 715-720.

and ethically acceptable. If it should not accord with the physician's own better judgement, he or she may of course attempt to reason and persuade but not coerce; and all other things being equal, the physician may not overrule the patient's determination. *Reibl v. Hughes*[1] is very clear on that point. If all else fails and the physician cannot in good conscience accept the patient's decision, there is always the option of referring the patient to another physician and withdrawing from the case.[2] At no point, however, with the exceptions of emergency and therapeutic privilege, is the physician called on to assume the role of proxy decision-maker or to examine the ethical acceptability of the decision itself.

The case of the incompetent patient, however, is different. Here the physician must assume an evaluative role. As front-line workers, so to speak, physicians have to examine the way in which the proxy decision-makers — usually the next-of-kin — make the decision in order to assure themselves that it is the product of reflective consideration and not the offhand result of a hasty reaction. Furthermore, they must consider the criteria used by the proxy decision-makers in reaching the decision in order to make sure that they do not simply reflect the proxies' own standards, feelings or expectations but rather are ethically appropriate. When there is any doubt, the physician must engage the appropriate administrative or legal channels to prevent what may be an unacceptable exercise of proxy authority.[3]

To some degree, of course, this is a matter of subjective assessment on the part of the physician, but not entirely so. In cases in which the patient was once competent but is competent no longer, the physician will balance the quality of life expected from the various treatment options against the wishes and expectations expressed by the patient when competent in order to assess the reasonableness or acceptability of the particular proxy decision. The testimony of next-of-kin as well as formal and informal data to which the physician may have access will provide invaluable assistance. As to situations in which there is no evidence that the patient expressed preferences when competent, the physician will proceed on the basis of the quality-of-life standards that are currently accepted by the ordinary person, standards that are based not on the concept of social utility (whether defined within the ambit of the immediate family or social grouping or drawn more widely to include society as a whole) but rather on criteria that flow from the concept of the patient as a person. The physician will take into account the distinction between the continuation or sustaining of merely biologic life and support of the patient as a person who has (or retains the capacity for) sapient cognitive awareness and the possibility of meaningful social interaction.[4] Again, while this will involve a certain amount of subjectivity on the part of the physician, it need not and does not occur in complete isolation. Physicians can draw on the more or less standard perception of quality of life that prevails in society and are aided by their sensitivity to the cost of the various treatment options to the patient in purely human terms. Their professional knowledge of the nature and likelihood of the outcomes expected from the various modalities of treatment is invaluable, as is their awareness of what other, competent patients under similar circumstances have decided. Together, all this gives the physician a fairly good idea of what the ordinary reasonable person would decide under similar circumstances and provides a basis against which to measure the proxy decision. And although this sort of approach may present difficulties on occasion, it generally is workable and presents no serious ethical problems.

As to the case of the currently incompetent patient who never has been competent but in all likelihood will become competent in the future — i.e., an otherwise normal child — it, too, does not present the physician with fundamentally new issues. The physician will proceed on the assumption that, all other things being equal, the child's sensible experience and qualitative perception of the world is essentially like that of an adult and that the factor of incompetence involves the cognitive and judgemental plane. It is therefore entirely appropriate for the physician to take into account the child's subjective expressions (in so far as they are present or available) and balance them against the objective standard of what a reasonable person would decide when considering the proxy decision. The function of the proxy is to supply the cognitive and judgemental want of the child. Consequently, if the physician finds that the proxy decision-maker has introduced his or her own, nonstandard values in making the decision, the physician must challenge the decision. The situation becomes a little more complicated when the child has given assent in a particular direction, but even here it is not a matter of purely subjective evaluation. The assent must be seen as guiding, although not necessarily determining, depending on the facts of the cases.[5,6] Finally, in all cases of doubt, the courts must be the ultimate forum of appeal.

THE RADICALLY CONGENITALLY INCOMPETENT PATIENT

The case of the congenitally incompetent patient who, so far as medical science can tell, not only is barely at the limits of sapient cognitive awareness but also in all probability will never become competent is radically different. The sort of balancing of subjective expression against an objective standard that can at least be attempted in other cases seems inappropriate here. This is so not because the patient is not reasonable — no incompetent patient is — but because the presumption on which such balancing is based may be false in such cases. The quality of life of the radically congenitally incompetent patient may be so fundamentally different from the norm that both the use of the objective standard of what a reasonable person would decide as a balance and the attempt to use the patient's own subjective expression would be untoward. The very significance of the latter may be fundamentally misconstrued because it would be based on the world experience of the physician, someone who fits the norm of the reasonable person. Consequently, there exists a danger that the use of the objective standard would violate the individuality of the patient and that the attempt to circumvent this by using subjective indicators from the patient would be so out of line with his or her actual experience that any treatment decision based on these criteria would be experienced as cruel and unusual treatment.[7,8]

If this is true, the physician who monitors proxy decisions made for radically congenitally incompetent patients is faced with a serious problem: What criteria — indeed, what evaluative approach — ought he or she to apply?

THE STEPHEN DAWSON DECISION

It was at least in part for this reason that the 1983 British Columbia Supreme Court decision *Re Stephen Dawson*[9] was welcomed by some members of the medical community. The case concerned a 7-year-old boy who had contracted meningitis shortly after birth, suffered severe brain damage and become hydrocephalic and as a consequence was exceedingly retarded, with no control over his faculties or limbs. At 5 months of age a shunt had been inserted and had been revised over the years, and at the time of application to the courts revision was again required. The reason for the court intervention was that the parents, as proxy decision-maker, had initially agreed to the revision, but after taking into account what they considered to be appropriate quality-of-life considerations from the perspective of the ordinary person — considerations involving the capacity for sapient cognitive awareness, the possibility of relatively pain-free and physically comfortable existence, and the potential for meaningful social interaction — and after consultation with a pediatric neurosurgeon they had withdrawn their permission. The superintendent of child welfare for the province intervened, and the matter came to trial in provincial court. The test used by the court to evaluate the parents' decision was whether, under the circumstances, the proposed revision constituted extraordinary treatment. The court decided in the affirmative and held in favour of the parents. On appeal to the British Columbia Supreme Court, the decision was reversed and an order for treatment was made. Stephen subsequently received treatment and continues to live.

It was the reasoning stated by the British Columbia Supreme Court that made the decision so important for the medical community. For the first time in Canadian medicolegal history the courts issued a ruling that explicitly addressed the question of what criteria and approach a proxy decision-maker and a physician should use when dealing with a congenitally incompetent person. Mr. Justice L. McKenzie, who decided the issue, ruled 1) that a congenitally incompetent person does not lose the rights to health care normally enjoyed by other persons simply in virtue of his or her incompetence, 2) that the duty of exercising this right normally rests in the parents as appropriate proxy decision-makers, 3) that their decision-making authority is appropriately challenged when it is not exercised in the best interests of the incompetent person, and 4) that what counts as being in the best interests of the incompetent person must not be determined from the point of view of the objective reasonable person. Rather, 5) it must be determined from the perspective of the incompetent person. As Judge McKenzie put it, "I do not think that it lies within the prerogative of any parent or of this court to look down upon a disadvantaged person and judge the quality of that person's life to be so low as not to be deserving of continuance." Quoting with approval Judge Asch in the US case *In the Matter of Eugene Weberlist* ("In this case, the court must decide what its ward would choose, if he were in a position to make a sound judgment.") he went on to say:

> This last sentence puts it right. It is not appropriate for an external decision-maker to apply his standards of what constitutes a livable life and exercise the right to impose death if that standard is not met in his estimation. The decision can only be made in the context of the disabled person viewing the worthwhileness or otherwise of his life in its own context as a disabled person — and in that context he would not compare his life with that of a person enjoying normal advantages. He would know nothing of a normal person's life having never experienced it.

In adopting this position, Judge McKenzie was enunciating what had become known as a substituted-judgement approach to proxy decision-making for congenitally incompetent persons. As one US commentator put it, proxy decision-makers should try to put themselves as much as possible into the situation of the incompetent person and then decide in the way and from the perspective from which the latter would decide, were he or she able.[10]

The Stephen Dawson case injected an element of clarity into the Canadian context. The Canadian physician faced with the question of how to proceed in these sorts of cases now had definite guidelines on how to interpret "best interests" considerations and evaluate the appropriateness of a particular proxy decision. However, while definitive and clarifying, Judge McKenzie's decision was not without problems, some of which I pointed out at the time.[11] In the context of proxy decision-making the most important problem was the concept of a substituted-judgement approach itself. As I said then, the demand that the perspective of the congenitally incompetent person should constitute the basis of quality-of-life considerations by the proxy decision-maker and that any acceptance or rejection of medical treatment should be grounded on this basis is not only unworkable in practical terms but also and, indeed above all, logically incoherent. If the incompetent person lacks sapient cognitive awareness — or, less severely, if he or she lacks any standards or criteria — then, trivially, neither standards nor criteria can be ascribed to the person. That fact is definitive of the situation in which such people find themselves and characterizes their very nature. It is therefore logically impossible to determine what their wishes are or would be if they could make them known. To proceed otherwise is to do one of two things: to assume that despite this lack they have standards or criteria after all — a flat contradiction — or to project some other standards or criteria into the situation by substitution and thereby treat incompetent people as though they were not incompetent. In either case, however, the very concept of substituted judgement, of viewing the situation from the perspective of the incompetent person, "in its own context", is a fiction.

If this analysis was correct, the position of the physician faced with a congenitally incompetent patient was not improved but rather was worsened by the Stephen Dawson case: uncertainty over how to proceed had indeed been replaced by certainty, but at the price of logical impossibility.

THE CASE OF "EVE"

Then came *Eve v. Mrs. E.,*[12] which altered the whole picture. On the facts, the case was entirely different from that of Stephen Dawson. "Eve" was a 24-year-old moderately retarded woman suffering from extreme expressive aphasia. She was described to the courts as an extremely pleasant and affectionate person who, being physically adult, was capable of being attractive to and attracted by men. Her mother, of advancing years, feared that Eve might become pregnant, and since Eve was unable to take care of a child, the mother saw herself faced with the prospect of having to care for Eve's progeny. She found this unmanageable. She also felt that both pregnancy and childbirth would be incomprehensible to Eve. Consequently, acting as proxy decision-maker, she requested that Eve be sterilized.

The court of first instance rejected the request. It ruled that except for clinically therapeutic reasons, parents or other appropriate proxy decision-makers could not give valid proxy consent to such a procedure. On appeal to the Supreme Court of Prince Edward Island, the judgement was reversed and sterilization by hysterectomy was ordered. However, leave was granted to appeal the decision to the Supreme Court of Canada. On Oct. 23, 1986, that court handed down its ruling. It reinstated the trial court's order and rejected sterilization. Mr. Justice La Forest, writing the unanimous decision of the court, gave two reasons. One dealt with the historical nature of the *parens patriae* powers of the court. Here the thrust of Mr. Justice La Forest's deliberations was that these powers could be exercised only in the best interests of the incompetent person, no matter what the position of society or next-of-kin. The second reason was an attempt to clarify the way in which such best interests could be determined. He here focused on the position advanced by the attorneys for Mrs. E. They had argued that as proxy decision-maker Mrs. E. had the duty to exercise Eve's rights for her and had argued further that, indeed, these rights ought to be exercised on the basis of what would be in Eve's best interests. However, they insisted that Eve's best interests could be determined only in a subjective fashion: by approximating as closely as possible the kind of situation in which Eve found herself and then making the kind of decision that she herself would make. In other words, they reasoned that a "substituted-judgement" approach to the determination of "best interests" would be appropriate "because it places a higher value on the individuality of the incompetent person".[12] Using such an approach, they argued, would result in a decision for sterilization.

For the purposes of this essay, it is irrelevant whether the logic of Mrs. E.'s position is valid. What is important is the court's reaction to the line of reasoning. While accepting the concept of best interests as appropriate, the court roundly rejected the contention that best interests could be appropriately determined with the substituted-judgement approach. In fact, the court brusquely rejected the concept of substituted judgement itself. Substituted judgement, it reasoned, is an attempt to determine what choice the incompetent person would make were he or she able. However, the court stated,[12]

> Choice presupposes that a person has the mental competence to make it. It may be a matter of debate whether a court should have the power to make the decision if that person lacks the mental capacities to do so. But it is obviously a fiction to suggest that a decision so made is that of the incompetent, however much the court may try to put itself in her place. What the incompetent would do if she or he could make a choice is simply a matter of speculation.

Mr. Justice La Forest went on to speak of "the sophistry embodied in the argument favouring substituted judgment" and quoted with approval from *Matter of Eberhardy* (a US case), in which the court had stated:[13]

> We conclude that the question is not choice because it is sophistry to refer to it as such, but rather the question is whether there is a method by which others, acting on behalf of the person's best interests and in the interests, such as they may be, of the state, can exercise the decision.

Neither the US court nor the Supreme Court of Canada went on to detail such a method. They agreed in their focus on best interests considerations. One thing, however, was clear: by characterizing the substituted-judgement approach as legal "legerdemain", the Supreme Court effectively ruled out the very test enjoined by the Stephen Dawson case.

Of course, it could be argued that all this holds only for sterilization, that it leaves all other cases unaffected. That, however, is unlikely for three reasons. First, it would contradict the very *raison d'être* of Supreme Court decisions. They are, and are supposed to be, models for general types of cases. While *Eve v. Mrs. E.* is representative of sterilization cases, it is also and, indeed, above all representative of a type of case that deals with the problem of proxy decision-making for incompetent people. All cases of proxy decision for such people are thereby affected. The fact that the court itself saw it in this light is evidenced by the fact that the precedential cases it considered and cited in reaching its decision were drawn from a whole spectrum of cases proposing medical procedures for incompetent people, not only those advocating sterilization. Second, the fact that the Supreme Court intended its decision to have wider ambit is indicated by the fact that its rejection of substituted judgement is not explicitly directed to sterilization cases. It is couched independently of that issue in response to the argument that a substituted-judgement approach as such "is to be preferred to the best interests test because it places a higher value on the individuality of the mentally incompetent person".[12] In other words, it was a reply to the argument that because the substituted-judgement approach is the appropriate test for incompetent people in general, it should also be used in this case. It is to this general claim that the court replied in the negative. Its rejection, therefore, has general implications. Finally, there is this to consider. Undoubtedly there are many strands intertwined in this case. However, to construe the rejection of substituted judgement in a limited fashion is to ascribe to the Supreme Court the position that different principles of law and of ethics hold for the very same problem — proxy decision-making — in different material cases. Not only would that undermine the very notion of the uniformity of legal and ethical principles, but also it lacks basis in any of the court's dicta.

I suggest, therefore, that *Eve v. Mrs. E.* ought to be seen as having general import. But if that is the case, it presents the Canadian physician with a problem: How to interpret best interests? The fact that the court recalled with approval Lord Eldon's remarks in *Wellesley v. Wellesley* ("It has always been the principle of this court, not to risk damage to children ... which it cannot repair"[12]) may be considered guiding. However, that merely pushes the interpretational uncertainty onto the word "damage". Did the court intend this to apply to physiologic damage only, or did it intend to encompass psychologic, mental and emotional deficit as well as other repercussions? There are indications that it intended the wider construal; for example, it inveighed against a "grave intrusion on the physical and mental integrity of the person"[12] and included "health problems, religious upbringing and protection against harmful association".[12] But we do lack a really explicit statement. The physician is thus once again left in a domain of uncertainty. Only three — negative — guidelines are clear: physicians may not use a substituted-judgement approach to evaluate the appropriateness of proxy decisions, they may not accept a decision based on the proxy decision-maker's own idiosyncratic standards, and they may not use their own values, standards and expectations.

ATTEMPT AT A RESOLUTION

However, both the reasoning advanced in *Re Stephen Dawson* and that given in *Eve v. Mrs. E.* do point in the direction in which more positive criteria may be sought.[14] These stem not from the assumption of equality of life experience, which is the contentious concept, but from the assumption that whatever his or her handicap, the radically and congenitally incompetent patient is still a person. If this assumption is true — and here only incontrovertible evidence of the permanent lack of capability for sapient cognitive awareness can count as an indication to the contrary — that patient has the same panoply of rights as all other persons. More important, it follows that he or she must be treated as a person in all respects. This in turn means that the quality of life that the patient faces in the future as well as the quality at the present time, while it may be admitted to differ in degree of sophistication from that of the competent person, nevertheless cannot be held to differ in kind: no matter what the difference in degree, the quality itself, in its very nature, must be that of a person. This, however, immediately entails that the evaluative criteria that are appropriate in the case of all other persons must be applied here as well. Not, of course, in a straightforward fashion. That would be to ignore the difference in degree between the respective qualities of life. Rather, what it means is that the physician must use the quality of life of an otherwise healthy person with similar type and degree of incompetence as an evaluative baseline and consider the relative changes that would result in that quality under the various treatment options being considered. In this it is appropriate for the physician to take into account the incompetent person's subjective expressions of satisfaction with physical life, the psychologic affect and other attendant factors and balance these against the likelihood of retention of or improvement in sapient cognitive awareness, the possibility of meaningful social interaction at that level and the cost of the various options to the patient in purely human terms. Let us call this a comparative quality-of-life coefficient. The physician must then do a similar evaluation, with due alteration of detail, for an ordinary competent patient with a similar medical problem to determine what the comparative quality-of-life coefficient would be in his or her case. The physician must then compare the two coefficients. If, on balance, the comparative quality-of-life coefficient for the incompetent patient is the same as or higher than that for the competent patient, and if in the case of the latter the decision would normally be in favour of treatment (or of some specific form of treatment), the decision must be in favour of treatment for the incompetent patient as well. If the proxy decision-maker's decision is against treatment, the physician must oppose it, if necessary through administrative and judicial channels. In all other cases, he or she need not.

This way of approaching the problem provides a procedure that can be implemented in practice. At the same time, however — or perhaps precisely because of this — it allows us to reconcile *Eve v. Mrs. E.* with *Re Stephen Dawson*. For, in this way, Judge McKenzie's injunction to consider the situation of the radically congenitally incompetent person in the "context of the disabled person" can be given an interpretation that avoids the sophistry of substituted judgement while satisfying Mr. Justice La Forest's conclusion that the "best interests" of the person should be guiding.

A FINAL PROBLEM

At the same time, however, the case of Eve leaves the health care professional with a problem. The considerations that I have sketched are appropriate from the perspective of the incompetent person and under the *parens patriae* powers of the court. Ethically, however, they are insufficient. Medical decisions, after all, are not made in a vacuum, nor can health care decisions be reached in isolation from the overall context in which they must be implemented. The resources that will be involved in health care decisions and their distribution have ineluctable social implications. It is here that *Eve v. Mrs. E.* fails. By being focused narrowly within the *parens patriae* doctrine as traditionally understood, the decision paints an unrealistic picture. The rights of the incompetent person must never be less than those of the competent person solely by virtue of their incompetence, to be sure. However, justice and equality demand that they not be more either. It is ethically unacceptable to engage in reverse discrimination that accords a favoured ethical status to the incompetent person solely by virtue of his or her incompetence. That, however, would in fact occur if the powers of Eve's rights, as captured in the best-interests clause as expressed in the judgement, were to be given automatic precedence over the rights of others; if, in the words of Mr. Justice La Forest, we were to "sympathize with Mrs. E." but insist, as he did, that in cases such as these only the rights of the incompetent person are decisive.[12] The point of *Eve v. Mrs. E.* and analogous court actions surely is to insist that the rights of the incompetent person must be given due weight because incompetent people are persons. That, however, also means that with due alteration of detail their rights must be treated as subject to the same balancing process to which the rights of all other persons are subject under similar conditions. By rejecting the weight of the competing rights of Mrs. E. and the rest of society, Mr. Justice La Forest has created a special class of persons who are immune from the restrictive and balancing considerations that apply to everyone else. This seems to suggest that the physician who monitors proxy decisions for such people must refrain from taking into account the considerations of equity and justice that guide the allocation of resources in all other cases. Not only are the ethics of this highly questionable, but also it may lead to a distributive nightmare.

NOTES

1. *Reibl v. Hughes,* 14 CCLT 1 (SCC 1980)
2. *Code of Ethics,* Can Med Assoc, Ottawa, 1978: 15
3. Dickens, B.: The role of the family in surrogate medical consent. *Health Law Can* 1980; 1 (3): 49-52
4. Keyserlingk, E.W.: Sanctity of life or quality of life. In *The Context of Ethics, Medicine and Law,* Law Reform Commission of Canada, Ottawa, 1979: 49-72
5. McCormick, R.A.: Proxy consent in the experimentation situation. *Perspect Biol Med* 1974; 18: 2-20
6. Ramsey, P.: *The Patient as Person,* Yale U Pr, New Haven, Conn, 1970: 1-58
7. *Superintendent of Belchertown State School v. Saikewicz,* 370 NE (2d) 417 (Mass 1977)
8. Annas, G.: Reconciling Quinlan and Saikewicz: decision making for the terminally ill incompetent. *Am J Law Med* 1979; 4: 367-396
9. *Re Stephen Dawson,* 3 WWR 618 (BC SC 1983) reversing 3 WWR 597 (BC Prov Ct 1983)

10. Annas, G.: The incompetent's right to die: the case of Joseph Saikewicz. *Hastings Cent Rep* 1978; 8 (1): 21-23
11. Kluge, E.-H.W.: In the matter of Stephen Dawson: right v. duty of health care. *Can Med Assoc J* 1983; 129: 815-818
12. *Eve v. Mrs. E.,* SCC, judgement handed down Oct 23, 1986, SCR 16654
13. *Matter of Eberhardy,* 307 NW (2d) 881 (Wis 1981)
14. Magnet, J.E., Kluge, E.-H.W.: *Withholding Treatment From Defective Newborn Children,* Brown Legal Pubns, Cowansville, PQ, 1985: 3-306

FURTHER READINGS

American College of Physicians, in "Cognitively Impaired Subjects," *Annals of Internal Medicine* 111: 10 (Nov. 15, 1989), 843–848.

Buchanan, Allen E. and Dan W. Brock
Deciding for Others: The Ethics of Surrogate Decision Making. (Cambridge and New York: Cambridge University Press, 1989).

Gaylin, W. and R. Macklin, eds.
Who Speaks for the Child? The Problems of Proxy Consent. (New York and London: Plenum Press, 1982).

Keyserlingk, Edward W.
The Unborn Child's Right to Prenatal Care: A Comparative Law Perspective. (Montreal: McGill Legal Studies No. 5, 1984) .

Savage, H. and Carla McKague
"Competency and Proxy Decision-Making," from H.Savage and Carla McKague, *Mental Health Law in Canada.* (Toronto and Vancouver: Butterworths, 1987)114-124.

Wikler, D.
"Paternalism and the Mildly Retarded," *Philosophy and Public Affairs* 8 (1979) 337–392.

CHAPTER 9 PROXY DECISION-MAKING AND EXPERIMENTATION

INTRODUCTION

It is difficult to act as proxy decision-maker in the ordinary therapeutic setting. The problems are compounded when the treatment that is suggested is experimental or innovative in nature. Nevertheless, sometimes there is no choice but to involve such incompetent subjects in experimental protocols. The factors that make them incompetent may be the very reasons why the protocol is developed in the first place.

For instance, children differ from adults not simply because they are younger, smaller and know less. In many cases, their organs function differently from the way they function in adults. This is important when it comes to trying to determine how drugs function in children. We cannot simply scale down the dosage proportionally on the basis of size and body-weight. The pharmacokinetic function of the drug, the metabolization process, etc. may be quire different. Therefore, children really are the only subjects on whom we can find out how a drug works on children.

Similar remarks apply to people who suffer from organic psychiatric diseases, as well as the elderly. There are conditions that strike mainly elderly persons. Alzheimer's disease is a good example. The disease typically leaves the stricken individual incompetent. Therefore such a person cannot meet the ordinary standards of informed consent. Yet to exclude this population group from research and experimentation is to exclude precisely the group about whom we need data if we are going to be able to develop appropriate methods of treatment.

The Law Reform Commission of Canada suggest that experimenting on and doing research with human subjects is both ethical and legal. In its working paper *Biomedical Experimentation Involving Human Subjects*, the Commission addresses the issue — but at the same time maintains that special safeguards should be in place. The selection from *Biomedical Experimentation* outlines some of the safeguards envisioned by the Commission. It presents the Commission's perspective on experimenting with prisoners, children, the mentally disabled, and embryos and foetuses. Since the function of the Law Reform Commission is to suggest legislation to the Minister of Justice, the considerations it raises are of considerable importance.

Brown considers the topic from the point of view of elderly populations. Since most of us will fall into this category of elderly, this selection may be of special interest.

Biomedical Experimentation Involving Human Subjects

Law Reform Commission of Canada

SPECIAL CASES

I. PRISONERS

In the last few years a great deal has been written about experimentation on prisoners, and in the United States the topic has been the subject of lively legal and ethical debate. The major relevant international documents, the Nuremberg Code and the Helsinki Declaration, do not expressly prohibit the use of prison populations in scientific and medical research.[85] Furthermore, a comparison between the first draft and the version finally adopted at Helsinki in 1964 shows that the total ban on the use of prisoners found in the initial draft was deliberately omitted from the final version. On the other hand, the resolution passed by the United Nations General Assembly on December 18, 1982[86] clearly appears to prohibit it, as does a resolution of the Council of Europe.[87]

A number of studies, including those conducted by the Belmont Commission of which we spoke above, have shown that experimentation on prisoners is a phenomenon almost exclusively confined to the United States.[88] European countries, including France[89] and the Federal Republic of Germany,[90] expressly prohibit this practice. England and most other countries, although they do not prohibit it, do not engage in it. In Canada, it appears to be prohibited in federal and provincial institutions. For instance, section 21 of the *Regulation respecting Houses of Detention*[91] made under the *Act respecting Probation and Houses of Detention*[92] reads as follows:

> 21. An imprisoned person may not be subjected to medical and scientific experiments that may be detrimental to his mental or physical integrity.[93]

Law Reform Commission of Canada, Working Paper 61 *Biomedical Experimentation Involving Human Subjects*. (Ottawa: Minister of Supply and Services, 1989).

Experimentation on prisoners in the United States really began during World War II with the pharmacological testing of treatments for infectious diseases that might be contracted by members of the armed forces. Various abuses came to light during the 1950s and 1960s and were strongly denounced. In some states the practice was completely banned. In its recommendations the Belmont Commission took a position somewhere between permissiveness and total prohibition. It considered that an unconditional ban on experimentation involving prisoners was inappropriate, but that certain precautions should be taken to ensure that consent would be freely given. Based on these recommendations, DHEW issued regulations which are even more restrictive than those proposed by the Belmont Commission.[94]

In the course of its investigations, the Belmont Commission made a number of interesting observations. First, contrary to what might be expected, almost all of the-more recent experiments on prisoners involved the testing of medications or new cosmetic products that involved little risk. Next, payments to prisoners for their participation were always very small, making it doubtful whether economic incentives played much of a role in obtaining their consent. Finally, the Commission noted that in most cases the same experiments could have been conducted as rigorously and successfully using subjects from the general population.

Why are prisoners so attractive to researchers? The answer is simple. Prisoners are a captive population leading a routine existence. Their lifestyle greatly facilitates the administration of research protocols and the collection of data, especially where the research is related to new medications and pharmaceutical products.

Both advocates and adversaries of the legalization of research using prisoners advance substantial arguments in support of their positions. The main argument of those who oppose legalization is as follows: in experimentation (where the subject derives no personal benefit), it is absolutely essential that consent be freely given. The fact that the prisoner is in a prison environment means that there are several reasons why he is unable to give free consent. He is more susceptible to undue influence; his motive for participating is often not disinterested, but rather related to his hopes for improving his lot (breaking the monotony, earning money or privileges, making a good impression on authorities, obtaining early release, having his sentence reduced or being granted parole). His being deprived of freedom makes his consent suspect and, given the possibilities for abuse, justifies an outright ban.

Proponents of the opposite view argue that an outright ban on the use of prisoners is discriminatory and unfair. They note that, in general, prisoners are highly motivated and that performing a socially useful, altruistic act that gives them a sense of self-worth is often an expression of their desire to make amends. They also argue that, while participation in an experiment should never be linked to a reduced sentence or parole, the desire to break the monotony of prison life or to improve one's lot is perfectly legitimate. Finally, one can only speak of coercion where there really is a threat. To offer a prisoner a tempting reward for his participation is not to threaten but merely to encourage, and does not in any way undermine his freedom to choose.

Nevertheless, no one would seriously dispute that the voluntary nature of a prisoner's consent must be considered more critically than in the case of a person having the exercise of his freedom. It must also be admitted that, except for research on the condition of prisoners themselves, prison populations tend to be used more out of convenience than out of scientific necessity. The same type of research can be conducted in the same manner on subjects who are not imprisoned, even though with more difficulty.

The mere existence of additional difficulties is not, in our opinion, a sufficient reason for legalizing experimentation on prisoners. We believe that the danger of abuse is too great. The fact that prisoners, unlike children or the mentally ill, do not constitute a distinct biomedical group, and that there will always be uncertainty about how free their consent is, whatever precautions may be taken, in our opinion also justifies a formal ban on the use of prisoners as experimental subjects and thus the maintenance of the status quo. Faced with this dilemma, the Commission believes it is necessary to consider the issue further before taking a position either in favour of a total ban or of acceptance under some conditions of experimentation on prisoners in Canadian prisons. We are also very interested in hearing from concerned parties and the public.

II. CHILDREN

...

Experiments involving children continue to be highly controversial. The legal profession is sharply divided on the issue.[95] There is agreement on only one point: experimentation of a therapeutic nature, that is to say which offers a reasonable hope of benefiting the child (such as the testing of a new medication in the treatment of leukemia) is legitimate and legal under ordinary conditions because its ultimate aim is to provide an individual benefit. Where the controversy arises is with respect to non-therapeutic experimentation.

Before we consider the arguments in support of each position, a few remarks are in order. First, everyone agrees that experimentation on children should be prohibited where adults capable of giving consent could be used just as well. Second, it is clear that from a scientific standpoint some experiments can be performed only on children. This is true for most research on childhood diseases (such as infantile leukemia, cystic fibrosis, chorea) and on certain congenital deformities. The issue must be faced squarely: an outright ban on any research involving children would limit the growth of scientific knowledge concerning these diseases and disorders and thereby adversely affect the development of cures and remedies, so the stakes are considerable.

Everyone agrees that a child is more vulnerable than an adult because it is impossible for him to weigh all the factors that should guide him in making a decision. The same holds true for an adult whose mental faculties are impaired. Whatever solution is chosen, in a society such as ours the law must, because of the possibilities for abuse, provide enhanced protection for its most vulnerable members.

This issue was the subject of a controversy between two American theologians, Ramsey[96] and McCormick.[97] Ramsey opposed any type of non-therapeutic experimentation involving children. He considered children incapable of adhering to the objectives pursued by the researcher. He felt it would be immoral to allow consent by a representative (parent or guardian), since non-therapeutic experimentation could not be of direct benefit to the child. The preservation of the health and enhancement of the well-being of a child were the only objectives to which a third party could consent on that child's behalf. Since non-therapeutic experimentation serves neither of these purposes, it should be totally prohibited.

McCormick and others[98] replied to this reasoning with two arguments. First, they advanced the notion of social utility. To ban all research involving children would be to condemn other children, since advances in the treatment of childhood diseases would no longer be possible. Second, although consent remains an important and even vital element, it should not necessarily be the one and only factor. Essentially, consent is given to indicate acceptance of the risks inherent in an experiment; the risk factor should thus be the major focus in any debate on the subject. In the name of what principle, it could then be asked, should there be a ban on an experiment of major scientific value and which involves no risk for the child? For those who support the second position, the legality of experimentation on children must therefore be determined primarily in terms of the risk involved in the experiment. Consent in the form of parental permission should continue to be required. However, if the risks involved in an experiment are humanly acceptable, the impossibility of obtaining the subject's own consent should not to be used to justify an absolute ban.

Most of the national and international documents dealing with ethical issues favour the second position. For instance, the Venice amendments to the Helsinki Declaration allow experimentation involving children. Where a child is able to consent, his consent must be obtained, in addition to that of his parents of course. In the United States, the Belmont Commission found non-therapeutic experimentation on children to be legitimate provided that certain conditions were fully met: the experiment cannot be properly performed on any other groups; consent of children over seven has to be obtained; the risk has to be minimal and assessed by an independent ethics committee; and the research has to be of major scientific importance.[99]

Article 20 of the Quebec *Civil Code* expresses an uncommon position. It distinguishes between a minor "capable of discernment" and one who is not. It forbids any experimentation on a child in the second category. However, it does allow experimentation involving children in the first category, on two conditions: first, there must be consent from a person having parental authority, and there must be authorization by a Superior Court judge; and, second, the experiment must not constitute a "serious risk" to the child's health. According to article 20, in the case of a person of legal age the risk must not be "disproportionate to the benefit anticipated." In the case of a minor, there can be no question of an acceptable ratio. Any experiment presenting a *serious* risk is prohibited, even if the risk/benefit ratio is otherwise acceptable.

This position is considerably relaxed under article 18 of Bill 20, which allows, in principle, experiments on minors under fourteen years of age with the permission of the court and the consent of the person having parental authority. However, the new provisions stipulate that the risk may not be disproportionate to the anticipated benefit and that the refusal of a minor who has reached fourteen years of age precludes experimentation.

In 1978, the first report of the Medical Research Council of Canada included both a majority and a minority position. A majority of the working group was of the opinion that research on children was legitimate, provided that substituted consent was obtained and that the risk/benefit ratio was acceptable. The minority, on the other hand, advocated a total ban on non-therapeutic experimentation on the grounds that when the parent or guardian consents on a child's behalf they are acting as "fiduciaries" and must therefore act in the child's exclusive interest. They should therefore have no authority to consent to an act that is not in his interest. In its second report, the Council reaffirmed the majority position and recognized the legitimacy of experimentation involving children, adding however that the child has to be properly consulted and his opinion taken into account.

In Canada, as elsewhere, there is a tendency to reject a total ban on non-therapeutic experimentation involving children. We believe that this is a reasonable position and that a complete ban is not called for. We also believe that the ethical and legal guarantees proposed in some of the above-mentioned models are highly desirable.

Recommendation

4. The Commission recommends that the legality of non-therapeutic biomedical experimentation involving children should be recognized in a general federal statute on experimentation, provided that all the following conditions are met:

   (a) the research is of major scientific importance and it is not possible to properly conduct it using adult subjects capable of giving consent;

   (b) the research is in close, direct relation to infantile diseases or pathologies;

   (c) the experiment does not involve any serious risks for the child;

   (d) the consent of a person having parental authority and of an independent third party (a judge, an ombudsman or the child's lawyer) is obtained; and

   (e) where possible, the consent of the child should be obtained. Moreover, whatever the child's age, his refusal should always be respected.

III. THOSE WITH MENTAL DISORDERS

Experimentation on persons with a mental disorder or illness raises problems similar in some respects to those raised by experimentation on prisoners and in other respects to those raised by experimentation on children. In effect, such persons are often not free, and the observations we made in connection with prisoners therefore apply to them. But regardless of whether or not they are confined, their situation resembles that of children in that they are in theory incapable of giving valid consent.

It is therefore not surprising that issues affecting those with mental disorders and children are frequently discussed together, since the principles that apply to the one generally apply to the other.

First, for the same reasons that experimentation on prisoners has been banned, experimentation on confined, mentally disordered people should be banned where the choice of subjects is based solely on grounds of ease of observation and analysis of results.

It should also be pointed out that the mentally disordered do not form as well-defined a group as, for instance, children. It is a very heterogeneous group and includes people who are institutionalized as well as those who are not. If the term mental disorder is taken in a broad sense, the category also includes those in a state of irreversible coma. Finally, mental disorder and mental illness may be temporary or permanent, and can vary greatly in severity, to the extent that one affected person may be absolutely incapable of understanding an experiment and giving his consent, whereas another may have this capability.

Article 11 of the Helsinki Declaration permits experimentation on a mentally disordered person, but requires that person's representative to give consent in accordance with national legislation. The 1977 Hawaii Declaration[103] of the World Psychiatric Association states that only those experiments that contribute to the growth of psychiatric knowledge are permissible. On the other hand, the Council of Europe's Committee of Ministers has taken the opposite position: it wants to see non-therapeutic experimentation on persons with mental disorders banned.[104]

The Belmont Commission in the United States has published a number of recommendations on the subject.[105] They reveal the difficulty the Commission had arriving at a firm position. There were two reasons for this. First, there are no solid, detailed guiding principles in positive law. Second, this kind of experimentation gives rise to conflicts and ethical difficulties. The Commission finally decided in favour of legalizing experimental research on the mentally disordered, mainly because a complete ban would very probably amount to hindering progress in the fight against mental illnesses and disorders and would destroy the prospects for improving the lot of this segment of the population. The Commission nevertheless rightly observed that historically the most flagrant abuses have been of the mentally disordered and that strong protective mechanisms were in order. In this regard, experimentation should be subject to two basic conditions. First, only minimal risk is acceptable. Second, the subject's approval should be obtained if at all possible, while that of his legal representative should be necessary in all cases. To all intents and purposes, the rules would in fact be the same as those governing research on children.[106]

In France, on the contrary, it appears that all experimentation on mental incompetents of legal age is prohibited on grounds of public policy. A recent case, in which a doctor experimented on persons in a state of brain death, gave rise to a major controversy. The National Ethics Committee, condemned the practice outright on the following grounds.[107] First, it is unethical to subject a sick person to tests not connected with the treatment of his illness. Second, it is impossible to obtain valid consent and, in the Committee's opinion, it would even be illegal to accept the consent of next of kin to legitimize an experiment. In its report mentioned above, the Conseil d'État was in favour of a total ban on non-therapeutic experimentation on the mentally incompetent.

The Medical Research Council of Canada has never taken a clear position on the issue. It points out the need to distinguish legal incapacity from incapacity to consent to a medical act. Just because a person is under guardianship should not mean he should automatically be deprived of the right to express his opinion regarding a medical act, if at the time he possesses the necessary capacity and understanding. Like the French National Ethics Committee, the Council, in view of the *Canadian Charter of Rights and Freedoms*, questions the legality of consent by another in these cases. Can the right to integrity be, in effect, subject to waiver by a third party? The Council seems prepared to acknowledge only research involving no risks, but its position remains unclear.

It is possible to interpret article 20 of the Quebec *Civil Code* as completely excluding the mentally disabled from the class of persons on whom experiments may be performed. In fact, by analogy with minors, it could be argued that experimentation should be prohibited where a mentally disabled person lacks sufficient discernment, but should be permitted where this is not the case.

In this regard, the provisions of Bill 20 give rise to a problem of interpretation. Article 18 allows experimentation with the permission of the court and the tutor or curator, provided that the risk assumed is not disproportionate to the anticipated benefit. However, article 20 stipulates that the court ruling on the application for permission shall satisfy itself that the experiment is "in the interest of the person concerned," which would limit the scope of article 18 in the case of non-therapeutic experimentation.

With respect to ethical principles, the legal problem is therefore complex. An absolute ban on experimentation involving the mentally deficient can be objected to on the same grounds that we discussed in connection with children: it precludes certain kinds of desirable progress in the treatment of mental illnesses. On the other hand, and again as in the case of children, permitting experimentation with no restrictions requires disregarding the basic condition that consent be obtained, at least where the handicap is such as to deprive the subject of all discernment. As the Cameron affair at McGill University's Allan Memorial Institute clearly shows, abuses are possible and, because the mentally deficient form a more heterogeneous group, they are probably even more vulnerable than children. If law and ethics are to allow experimentation on the mentally deficient, strict requirements must therefore be laid down.

In the Commission's opinion, non-therapeutic biomedical experimentation should be allowed on persons with a mental deficiency, but it should be surrounded with ethical and legal guarantees.

Recommendation

5. The legality of non-therapeutic biomedical experimentation on mentally deficient persons should be recognized, in a general federal statute on experimentation provided that the following conditions are met:

   (a) the research is of major scientific importance and it is not possible to properly conduct it using adult subjects capable of giving consent;

   (b) the research is in close, direct relation to the subject's mental illness or deficiency;

   (c) the research does not involve any serious risks for the subject;

   (d) the consent of the incompetent person's representative and of an independent third party (a judge, an ombudsman or the incompetent person's lawyer) is obtained; and

   (e) where possible, the incompetent person's consent is to be obtained, and his refusal is always to be respected.

IV. EMBRYOS AND FOETUSES

The ethical and legal issues raised by research on embryos and foetuses are extremely complex, and as likely as not to provoke highly emotional responses because they are linked to the controversy surrounding abortion and each person's own position on the subject. Moreover, experimentation on embryos and foetuses touches on a very difficult philosophical, theological and ethical problem: the beginning of human life.[111] At what moment in the development of the product of conception are we dealing with a human being or a human person? What value should society place on embryonic and foetal life?

The Law Reform Commission, in Working Paper 58, *Crimes Against the Foetus*, defined the term foetus as "the product of a union in the womb of human sperm cells and egg cells at all stages of its life prior to becoming a person" : the term does not therefore include embryos fertilized *ex utero*. This is the meaning the word will have here.

Historically, experimentation began on the foetus. According to a special report of the Belmont Commission, it has taken four main directions.[114] First, research on the physiology and development of foetal tissue, hence on the growth of the foetus. Second, research relating to the diagnosis and detection of foetal diseases and congenital deformities. Third, some research has been done on foetal therapy and pharmacology, in particular on the possible effects of certain medications. This type of research, it should be said, is mainly retrospective and based on observation of aborted foetuses. It is this type of research that led to the discovery that the German measles vaccine could penetrate the placental barrier in women and have a teratological effect on the foetus, which was not the case with monkeys. Finally, there is research on foetuses that are not viable outside the womb, to determine whether they can be saved by somehow reproducing the uterine environment. This research has sometimes been described in layman's terms as the creation of an "artificial womb." As well, recent developments in France and the United States include experiments using the thymus glands of dead foetuses to produce a growth hormone, and those using foetal tissue to research the etiology of cancer.

Directly connected with the problem of experimentation on foetuses is the use of tissues from dead foetuses for the treatment of some diseases. Some current research offers hope that the implantation in the brain of certain foetal tissues or substances could have curative properties in the case of, for instance, Alzheimer's disease and Parkinson's disease. It should be noted in this connection that in principle these bodily substances are taken only from dead foetuses and that in strictly legal terms the taking of tissue from corpses is already regulated. From an ethical standpoint, however, there are those who object to the practice for a number of reasons. First, there is the connection with abortion, around which, as we know, there is nothing resembling a social consensus. Second, some fear that society will come to close its eyes to the production of foetuses solely for tissues and substances. The problem is complex and will not be dealt with here since it is, strictly speaking, outside the bounds of biomedical experimentation.

In addition to the above, research is also being done on *in vitro* fertilization techniques using embryos a few days old. Not every embryo formed as a result of *in vitro* fertilization is necessarily reimplanted. The ethical and legal problems posed by surplus embryos are complex. May they be frozen? Destroyed? Experimented on? The situation of the embryo is in fact different from that of the foetus. It should be remembered that at a few days old the embryo consists of just a few undifferentiated cells. Although it possesses life, it is not viable and, because of the total absence of even a primitive nervous system, it cannot feel any pain. Embryo research is also of real interest, making possible a better understanding of the very process of the creation and development of human life. It has important consequences for embryo conservation and freezing techniques as well as for the development of artificial reproductive technologies. Finally, with regard to genetic research, it makes possible the hope that one day ways will be found to repair the errors of nature and to correct genetic deficiencies in as yet unborn infants. This set of problems has given rise to a number of studies.[115]

B. General Principles Governing Experimentation on Embryos and Foetuses

The Commission is of the opinion that any policy in the area of non-therapeutic biomedical experimentation should have to comply with certain fundamental principles. The first is respect for all forms of human life, whatever its stage of development. The rules governing experimentation should therefore also reflect respect for the sanctity of human life from its beginnings.

Second, the law should never treat embryos and foetuses as mere objects. Accordingly, their commercialization or the commercialization of research on them should be strictly prohibited, although this prohibition should clearly not extend to the use of embryonic or foetal tissue for therapeutic purposes.

Third, it seems clearly unethical to allow the creation of embryos solely for experimental purposes. In other words, only surplus embryos conceived in connection with an *in vitro* fertilization program and not reimplanted should be used in experiments rather than simply be destroyed. We will return to this question below.

Fourth, the Commission is of the opinion that, with respect to experimentation on foetuses, research policy should be clearly dissociated from abortion policy. A woman's right to have an abortion and her decision to do so does not necessarily mean that science may freely dispose of the aborted foetus. Consequently, the prospect of abortion should not affect the criteria determining the admissibility and legitimacy of research. However, if an experiment has been found to be ethically acceptable for foetuses in general, it seems legitimate to prefer to conduct it on a foetus to be aborted rather than on one intended to be brought to term, since this would decrease the risks even further.

Fifth, the Commission considers it important that permissible types of research be strictly defined. Like many others, the Commission is of the opinion that some experiments should by their very nature be considered unethical and contrary to public policy.

It is important to establish controls for monitoring embryo and foetal research. Within the broad framework established by legislation, there should be provision for ensuring that research is ethical before it is undertaken. It is also necessary to ensure that it remains ethical during the period of experimentation and, once the experimentation has been completed, to ascertain the ethical value of the lessons to be learned for the future. The Commission is of the opinion that peer review is absolutely indispensable, as being the only way of properly evaluating the scientific aspects of a protocol and ensuring that it is ethical. It is also of the opinion that the ethics committees that presently approve research would do well both to include members from other disciplines (ethicists and jurists) and to play a wider role. In effect, in most cases these committees now do nothing more than accept or reject protocols. Once they approve an experiment because they consider it ethical, they have no authority to monitor it.

Finally, there is the question of the consent of parents to do research on their embryos or foetuses. The issue is even more sensitive when the foetus is in the womb, but the problem remains the same.

With respect to the question of consent, one thing is clear from the outset: no experiments should be allowed on a foetus *in utero* without the mother's free and informed consent. But is it useful, necessary or even desirable to obtain the father's consent as well? Three positions are possible. According to the first, the mother's consent should be sufficient, since she is in the best possible position to make an informed decision, and requiring the father's consent could be perceived as an undue restriction on the woman's rights over her own body.

The second position is to the opposite effect: non-therapeutic experimentation is purely elective and the child to be born is also the father's child. Requiring his consent is considered as providing additional protection.

Finally, there are some who, arguing that it is sometimes difficult if not impossible to identify the father, consider that where he is known, the mother's consent should still suffice unless he objects to the experiment.

Upon consideration, the Commission is of the opinion that the consent of both parents should be necessary. It seems important, on the one hand, to underline the fact that a child has two parents and hence to grant the father the right of refusal and, on the other hand, to respect his moral, religious or personal reasons for withholding consent. We would also extend this rule to experimentation on embryos since the underlying reasoning applies in that case as well.

Recommendation

6. Non-therapeutic biomedical experimentation on embryos and foetuses should be recognized, in a general federal statute on experimentation, provided that all the following conditions are met:
   (a) the experimentation has received the prior approval of a multidisciplinary ethics committee responsible for ensuring that the research is ethical and scientifically genuine and having direct authority to monitor and control it;
   (b) the embryo or foetal research is carried out in centres or hospitals recognized by the appropriate public authorities; and
   (c) the consent of both parents of the embryo or foetus has been obtained.

C. The Differences Between the Embryo and the Foetus

From a biological standpoint, there are differences between an embryo and a foetus. It is known that, in the current state of science, the embryo cannot continue to develop outside the womb beyond a certain period of time. On the other hand, the development of the foetus is a slow process ending in the birth of a person: at a certain point, the foetus is endowed with nervous perception; at another, the foetus is viable even if expelled from its mother's body. For this reason, it seems to us essential to distinguish between these two stages in the development of the product of conception, each of which gives rise to different scientific, ethical and legal questions despite their undeniable common denominator: the existence of a potential human being.

1. Experimentation on Embryos

As we mentioned above, embryo research (we are speaking here of embryos fertilized *ex utero*: see the definition of the foetus given above) is currently being carried out on embryos produced by *in vitro* fertilization as a solution to the problem of sterility and which end up not being reimplanted. What might come to mind here is, of course, the deliberate creation of embryos solely for purposes of scientific research, something that will be that much easier when science discovers how to freeze oocytes. Researchers with frozen sperm and oocyte banks at their disposal will in theory no longer have to rely on the therapeutic process of *in vitro* fertilization for a supply of embryos. However, for the time being most jurists and ethicists look askance at the production of embryos for purely experimental purposes. They consider it to be in conflict with the respect due to human life even in a primitive state. The situation is not the same with respect to surplus embryos. There are three possibilities for embryos that are not reimplanted in the woman who provided the oocyte required for their creation: they could be destroyed, donated to another sterile couple or, before being destroyed, be used for research. The Commission is of the view that, if circumstances do not permit donation, experimentation to advance knowledge seems to be preferable to outright destruction.

Recommendation

7. (1) The creation of embryos solely for purposes of scientific research should be prohibited and punished as a criminal offence.

The fate of the embryo that has been used for experimental purposes poses another problem. As we will see further on, the current international consensus is that the period during which research may be carried out should be limited (to fourteen days, generally speaking). Furthermore, the Commission agrees with the unanimous opinion of medical and legal authorities that embryos that have already been used for experimental purposes should not be reimplanted in a woman. The risk that such experimentation would leave traces is indeed too great.

Recommendation

7. (2) The re-implantation of embryos that have been used for experimental purposes should be prohibited and subject to criminal penalty.

Let us now return to the main problems raised by embryo research. The first question is to determine how standards relating to embryo experimentation should be defined by law. The view of the Commission is that not all types of research on embryos should be permitted. Moreover, the scientific community itself disapproves of certain types of research, and in this it has the support of ethicists and of all the governmental and quasi-governmental reports on the subject. Among these types of research are cloning, ectogenesis, parthenogenesis, and the crossing of human and animal gametes. The Commission shares this point of view and considers that certain types of research on embryos should be prohibited and criminally punished. A description and a complete list of them should be drawn up in consultation with the scientific community.

Recommendation

7. (3) Certain types of experimentation on embryos, in particular cloning, ectogenesis, parthenogenesis, and the crossing of human and animal gametes, should be prohibited by criminal law; a complete list of types of experiment should be drawn up after consultation with scientific authorities.

The second question involves determining until what point *in vitro* research on embryos is ethically acceptable. Currently there is some international consensus that a limit of fourteen (sometimes seventeen) days should be imposed. In scientific terms the figure is, of course, arbitrary, but a number of reasons can be put forward to justify it. To begin with, after fourteen days of cellular development the embryo *ex utero* cannot be reimplanted. Furthermore, it is at this point that it becomes known if the embryo is going to twin. Finally, it is towards the fourteenth or even the seventeenth day that the neural tube, that is to say the central nervous system, begins to develop.

While we are aware that this fourteen-day limit is arbitrary the Commission nevertheless considers that, given the current state of knowledge, it is appropriate to agree to a standard that enjoys broad international support, if only to ensure that research done in Canada will be as respected as that done in the rest of the world.

Recommendation

8. (1) Experimentation on embryos should be prohibited after the fourteenth day of embryonic development.

Like sperm, the human embryo may be frozen. Medical science has already produced living children from embryos that had been frozen. However, freezing raises certain problems. First, science does not yet really know what the effects of prolonged freezing are. Second, if freezing extends over a long period of time, the very principle of generations may be disrupted: think of the prospect — science fiction for the time being, but already theoretically possible — of the reimplantation some fifty years hence of an embryo created in 1989. Such difficulties have prompted most countries to impose time limits on freezing. Given the current state of knowledge, these limits are of course completely arbitrary. However, a figure of five years seems to meet with more or less general approval. The Commission agrees with this position.

Recommendation

8. (2) The freezing of embryos should be allowed, but it should not be prolonged for more than five years.

2. Experimentation on Foetuses

Non-therapeutic biomedical experimentation on foetuses also raises sensitive questions. Some criteria are the same as for experimentation on embryos (authorization by an ethics committee, prior approval of the team or centre, the impossibility of obtaining the same results by experimentation on animals or adults, consent of both parents). But the foetus also poses a special problem that should be dealt with in somewhat more detail.

Experimentation on the foetus may take place either inside or outside the mother's womb. In *ex utero* experimentation, a new factor comes into play: either the foetus is dead or doomed because nonviable, or else it is viable. In the case of an already dead foetus, experiments are presently limited to the taking of foetal tissue. As we have seen, the law requires various kinds of authorization. If on the other hand the foetus is viable, from both a legal and ethical standpoint it must be treated as a human being with all the rights of a person.

In effect, a foetus that has proceeded completely and permanently from its mother's body becomes a "person" as defined in the Law Reform Commission's proposed new Criminal Code. In this connection, the reader is referred to Working Paper 58, *Crimes Against the Foetus*. Therefore the conditions set out above in the case of experimentation involving children apply.

Unlike the embryo, which is to be destroyed in any event, a foetus inside the womb raises the question of whether the risks are proportionate to the expected benefits. As we have seen, in the case of competent adults the law requires that there be no serious risk to life or health. Naturally, this requirement should continue to apply to the mother whose body is subjected, even indirectly, to an experiment that primarily concerns the foetus. That said, the Commission considers that when it is impossible for experimental subjects themselves to give consent, they should be provided with additional protection. For children and the incompetent, the Commission recommended that experimentation be allowed where it did not involve serious risk. Since the whole life, integrity and health of the unborn child can be compromised by experimentation on the foetus, the Commission considers acceptable only those experiments involving no risk or only minimal risk, this being defined as a risk normally associated with pregnancy.

Recommendation

9. The only experiments on the foetus that should be considered acceptable are those involving no risk or only minimal risk, this being defined as a risk normally associated with pregnancy.

NOTES

86. Resolution 37-194 (111th plenary session), December 18, 1982. "The Principles of Medical Ethics relevant to the role of health personnel, particularly physicians, in the protection of prisoners against torture and other cruel, inhuman, or degrading treatment" appear in (1983) 37:3 *WHO CHRONICLE* at 91-92.
87. Resolution 73-5, February 12, 1987.
88. See National Commission for the Protection of Human Subjects of Biomedical and Behavioral Research, *Research Involving Prisoners* (Washington, D.C.: Department of Health, Education & Welfare, 1976).
89. *Code de procédure pénale*, art. D380(3) and Law of 20 December 1988, art. 209.3.
90. Medicines Act, August 24, 1976. Bundesgesetzblatt 1, 2445.
91. R.R.Q. 1981, c. P-26, r.1 art. 21.
92. R.S.Q. 1977, c. P-26.
93. For federal regulations, see: *Penitentiary Service Regulations*, C.R.C., c. 1251.
94. See National Commission for the Protection of Human Subjects of Biomedical and Behavioral Research, *supra*, note 88.
95. See the first report of the Medical Research Council of Canada, *supra*, note 9.
96. P. Ramsey, *The Patient as Person: Explorations in Medical Ethics*, (New Haven: Yale University Press, 1970); "The Enforcement of Morals: Non Therapeutic Research on Children" (1976) 6:4 *Hast. Cent. Rep.* 21; "Children as Research Subjects: A Reply" (1977) 7:2 *Hast. Cent. Rep.* 40.
97. R.A. McCormick, "Proxy Consent in the Experimentation Situation" (1974) 18 *Perspectives in Biology and Medicine* 2; "Experimentation in Children: Sharing in Sociality" (1976) 6:6 *Hast. Cent. Rep.* 41.

98. See B. Freedman, "A Moral Theory of Consent" (1975) 5:4 *Hast. Cent. Rep.* 32; H.K. Beecher, *Research and the Individual: Human Studies* (Boston: Little, Brown, 1970) at 63.
99. National Commission for the Protection of Human Subjects of Biomedical and Behavioral Research, *Research Involving Children: Report and Recommendations* (Bethesda, Md.: The Commission, 1977).
103. The full text of the Declaration appears in D. Clarence and D. Blomquist "From the Oath of Hippocrates to the Declaration of Hawaï" (1977) 4 *Ethics in Science and Medicine* 139.
104. Rec. No. R-83 (1983).
105. National Commission for the Protection of Human Subjects of Biomedical and Behavioral Research, *Research Involving Those Institutionalized as Mentally Infirm: Report and Recommendations* (Bethesda, Md.: The Commission, 1978).
106. See G. Schaefer, "Limited Guardianship: Additional Protection for Mentally Disabled Research Subjects Used in Biomedical and Behavioral Research" (1980-81) 16 *The Forum* 796; B. Barber, *Informed Consent in Medical Therapy and Research* (New Jersey: Rutgers University Press, 1980) at 177 ff.
107. Comité national d'éthique, *Avis sur les expérimentations sur des malades en état végétatif chronique*, February 24, 1986.
111. M. Rivet, "Le droit à la vie ou l'hominisation du XXI^{c} siècle: l'éthique et le droit répondant à la science," in D. Turp and G.A. Beaudoin, eds., *Perspectives canadiennes et européennes des droits de la personne* (Cowansville, Que.: Yvon Blais, 1986) at 445.
114. National Commission for the Protection of Human Subjects of Biomedical and Behavioral Research, *Research on the Fetus: Report and Recommendations* (Bethesda, Md.: The Commission, 1975).
115. For Britain, see *inter alia, Report of the Committee of Inquiry into Human Fertilization and Embryology, supra*, note 57.

     For the Federal Republic of Germany, see the report of the Benda Commission, *supra*, note 53.

     For Australia, see the *Report on the Disposition of Embryos Produced by In Vitro Fertilization, supra*, note 58; *Report of the Special Committee Appointed by the Queensland Government Inquiry into the Laws Relating to Artificial Insemination, In Vitro Fertilization and Other Matters*, 1984; *South Australia Report on Artificial Insemination and Related Matters*, 1984.

     For France, see *Sciences de la vie: de l'éthique au droit, supra*, note 52.

     For Canada, Ontario Law Reform Commission, *Report on Human Artificial Reproduction and Related Matters, supra*, note 59, vol. II, Recommendation 31 at 281; Medical Research Council of Canada, *supra*, note 9 at 32-35; Barreau du Québec, *Les enjeux éthiques et juridiques des nouvelles technologies de reproduction* (Montréal, 1988).

Proxy Consent for Research on the Incompetent Elderly

Barry F. Brown

In the past decade, the ethical issues of research with the elderly have become of increasing interest in gerontology, medicine, law, and biomedical ethics. In particular, the issue has been raised whether the elderly deserve special protection as a dependent group (Ratzan 1980). One of the most profound difficulties in this area of reflection is that of the justification of proxy consent for research on borderline or definitely incompetent patients.

Some diseases of the elderly, such as Alzheimer's disease, cause senile dementia: devastating for the patient and family and, in future, a considerable burden for society. This condition, in turn, renders a patient incapable of giving informed, voluntary consent to research procedures designed to learn about the natural history of the disease, to control it, and to find a cure. The research must be done on human subjects, since there is not as yet a suitable animal model; indeed some feel that there never can be such a model. A protection of the patient, rooted in concern for his best interests, from procedures to which he cannot give consent gives rise to a paradox: "If we can only perform senile dementia research using demented patients, but should not allow them to participate because they are incompetent, then we are left in a quandary. We cannot ethically conduct senile dementia research using demented patients because they are incompetent; but we cannot technically perform it using competent subjects because they are not demented" (Ratzan 1980: 36). Such a position seems to protect demented patients at the expense of their exposure, as a class, to prolonged misery or death.

If the patient cannot give consent, is the proxy consent of relatives ethically valid? That is, do the relatives have the moral right or capacity to give consent for procedures that may not offer much hope for the patient in that they may not offer a direct benefit to him?

Such procedures have by recent convention been called non-therapeutic. They might offer a possible benefit for other sufferers in the future, but little hope of benefit for *this* patient, here and now.

At present, an impasse has developed regarding such research. It appears that such procedures might be illegal under criminal laws on assault. If the research is strictly non-therapeutic, then no benefit is to be found for the patient-subject. If the requirement of therapeutic experimentation is that a direct, or fairly immediate, improvement in the patient's condition is the sole benefit that could count, then it is difficult to see how this could be discovered. For unlike the case of a curable disease or research on preventive measures for childhood diseases, such as polio, the Alzheimer's patients suffer from a presently terminal illness. Studies of the causation of this condition may hold little or no hope of alleviating the condition in them.

Barry F. Brown, "Proxy Consent for Research on Incompetent Elderly," from James E. Thornton and Earl R. Winkler, eds., *Ethics and Aging: The Right to Live, The Right to Die*. (Vancouver: The University of British Columbia Press, 1988) 183-193.

There appears to be no present or future benefit directly accruing to them. Others may benefit, but they likely will not. Thus, it seems, there is no benefit in view.

If, in fact, such procedures, even relatively innocuous ones, are illegal, then such research cannot go ahead. If so, such persons will remain "therapeutic orphans" just as surely as infants and children unless proxy consent is valid. If proxy consent is also legally invalid, then the legal challenge to this impasse may be either legislative or judicial. In either case, ethical arguments must be offered as justification for the case that proxy consent is or ought to be legally valid. The following explorations are a contribution to that debate.

Can some kind of benefit for the demented be found in research that offers no immediate hope of improvement? I believe that it can, but the nature of that benefit will be unfamiliar or unacceptable to those who are sure that there are only two mutually exclusive alternatives: a utilitarian conception of the social good pitted against a deontological notion of the individual's rights.

Contemporary biomedical ethics routinely employs three principles in its effort to resolve such dilemmas (Reich 1970; Beauchamp & Childress 1983). These are the principle of beneficence, which demands that we do good and prevent harm; the principle of respect for persons (or the principle of autonomy), from which flows the requirement of informed consent; and the principle of justice, which demands the equitable distribution of the benefits and burdens of research. But the first two obviously conflict with each other in human experimentation: the principle of beneficence, which mandates research to save life and restore health, especially if this is seen as directed to the good of society, is in tension with the principle of respect for persons, which requires us to protect the autonomy of subjects. Moreover, the principle of beneficence requires us not only to benefit persons as patients through research, but also to avoid harming them as research subjects in the process. So there is an internal tension between moral demands created by the same principle. Finally, demented patients are no longer fully or sufficiently autonomous. Standard objections to paternalism do not apply. Consequently paternalism of the parental sort is not inappropriate, but rather necessary in order to protect the interest of the patient.

Simple application of these principles, therefore, will not provide a solution. Underlying the manner in which they are applied are radically different conceptions of the relationship of the individual good to the societal or common good.

In the present framework of philosophical opinion, there appear to be two major positions. On the one hand, some consequentialist arguments for non-therapeutic research justify non-consensual research procedures on the grounds that individual needs are subordinate to the general good conceived as an aggregate of individual goods. This good, that of the society as a whole, can easily be seen to take precedence over that of individuals. This is especially so if the disease being researched is conceptualized as an "enemy" of society. On the other hand, a deontological position argues that the rights of the individual take precedence over any such abstract general good as the advancement of science, the progress of medicine, or the societal good. In this view, to submit an individual incapable of giving or withholding consent to research procedures not for his own direct benefit is to treat him solely as a means, not as an end in himself. In this debate, one side characterizes the general good proposed by the other as much too broad and inimical to human liberty; the other sees the emphasis on individual rights as excessively individualistic or atomistic.

There are strengths and weaknesses in both approaches. The consequentialist rightly insists on a communal good, but justifies too much; the deontologist rightly protects individual interests, but justifies too little. I contend that if we are to resolve the dilemma concerning the incompetent "therapeutic orphan," it is necessary to go between these poles. In order to do so, I wish to draw upon and develop some recent explorations concerning non-therapeutic research with young children. In at least one important respect, that of incompetence, children and the demented are similar. We ought to treat similar cases similarly. I wish also to argue that research ethics requires: (1) a conception of the *common good* that is at once narrower than that of society as a whole and yet transcends immediate benefit to a single individual; and (2) a conception of the common good that sees it not in opposition to the individual good but including it, so that the good is seen as distributed to individuals.

THE LESSON OF RESEARCH WITH CHILDREN

As to the first, we may learn much from the discussions concerning research with children, particularly as they bear upon the distinction between therapeutic and non-therapeutic experimentation. In the 1970s a spirited debate took place between the noted ethicists Paul Ramsey and Richard McCormick on the morality of experimentation with children (Ramsey 1970, 1976, 1977; McCormick 1974, 1976). Ramsey presented a powerful deontological argument against non-therapeutic experimentation with children. Since infants and young children cannot give consent, an essential requirement of the canon of loyalty between researcher and subject, they cannot be subjected ethically to procedures not intended for their own benefit. To do so, he contended, is to treat children solely as means to an end (medical progress), not as ends in themselves (Ramsey 1970).

McCormick, arguing from a natural law position similar to that developed in the next section, argued that since life and health are fundamental natural goods, even children have an obligation to seek to preserve them. Medical research is a necessary condition of ensuring health, and this is a desirable social goal. Consequently children, as members of society, have a duty in social justice to wish to accept their share of the burdens of participating in research that promise benefit to society and is of minimal or no risk. Thus the parents' proxy consent is a reasonable presumption of the child's wishes if he were able to consent (McCormick 1974).

There are two major puzzles generated by this debate over non-therapeutic research in children. First, Ramsey stressed that the condition to which a child may be at risk need not reside within his skin, but could be an epidemic dread disease. Thus, testing of preventive measures such as polio vaccine on children is justified; indeed it counts for Ramsey as therapeutic. This is interesting for several reasons. First, the therapeutic benefit may be indirect or remote, not necessarily immediate. Second, it embodies the concept of a group or population at risk smaller than society as a whole. Third, it apparently allows for considerable risk. There was a risk of contracting polio from the vaccine. Although the risk might have been slight statistically, the potential damage was grave. By Ramsey's own account, a slight risk of grave damage is a grave risk. Thus, he was prepared to go beyond the limit of minimal or no risk on the grounds that the polio vaccine was *therapeutic,* while McCormick attempted to justify *non-therapeutic* research on children, but confined the risk to minimal or none. It is odd that in the subsequent protracted debate, this difference was not contested.

The second major puzzle arises from McCormick's view that fetuses, infants, and children ought to participate in low- or no-risk non-therapeutic research in order to share in the burden of social and medical progress in order that all may prosper. Note that only *burdens* are to be shared, not benefits. This is because the topic by definition was non-therapeutic experimentation. By putting it this way he seemed to many to be subordinating the interests of such subjects to a very broadly construed societal good. But let us remember that the argument for such research in the first place was that without it, infants and children would be "therapeutic orphans." That is, without pediatric research, there could be fewer and slower advances in pediatric therapy.

Although not of direct benefit, such research is intended for the long-term benefit of children, and is thus indirectly or remotely therapeutic. It is not conducted for "the benefit of society" or for "the advancement of medical science"; it is for children in the future. Otherwise, it could be carried out on adults. Thus, such research should be construed as done not in view of broad social benefit but for the benefit of children as a group or a sub-set of society. Of course, if advances are made in medicine for the sake of children, society benefits as well, but this is incidental and unnecessary. The sole justification is provided by the benefits now and to come for *children.* At the same time, such benefits set one of the limits for such research: it should be confined to children's conditions, and should not be directed at conditions for which the research may be done on competent persons.

THE COMMON GOOD OF A DISEASE COMMUNITY

Some of the hints arising from the foregoing debate can now be developed. It is indeed wrong to experiment on an incompetent person for "the benefit of society" if the research is unrelated to that person's disease and he is made a subject simply because he is accessible and unresistant. But is it necessarily unethical to conduct experiments on an incompetent person which attempt to discover the cause of the condition which causes the incompetence, and which may cure it or prevent it in others, even if he will not himself be cured?

In a "third way" of conceptualizing the relation between the individual and the group, the good in view is neither that of society as a whole nor that of a single individual. It involves the group of persons with a condition, such as Alzheimer's disease. Here I turn to a conception of the common good articulated by John Finnis of Oxford. Finnis defines the common good not as the "greatest good for the greatest number" but as "a set of conditions which enables the members of a community to attain for themselves reasonable objectives, or to realize reasonably for themselves the value[s] for the sake of which they have reason to collaborate with each other [positively and/or negatively] in a community" (Finnis 1980: 155).

The community may be either the complete community or the political one, or it may be specialized, such as the medical community, the research community, or the community of children with leukemia, and so on. The common good is thus not the sum total of individual interests, but an ensemble of conditions which enable individuals to pursue their objectives or purposes, which enable them to flourish. The purposes are fundamental human goods: life, health, play, esthetic experience, knowledge, and others. Relevant to this discussion are life, health, especially mental integrity, and the consequent capacity for knowledge, all of which are threatened by diseases which cause dementia.

For my purposes, the community should be considered to be, at a minimum, those suffering from Alzheimer's disease. They have, even if they have never explicitly associated with each other, common values and disvalues: their lost health and the remaining health and vitality they possess. It could be said with McCormick that if they could do so, they would reasonably wish the good of preventing the condition in their relatives and friends.

But the community may be rightly construed more broadly than this. It naturally includes families with whom the patients most closely interact and which interact in voluntary agencies devoted to the condition, the physicians who treat them, the nurses, social workers, and occupational therapists who care for them, and the clinical and basic researchers who are working to understand, arrest, cure, and prevent the disease.

The participation of the patient, especially the demented patient, may be somewhat passive. He is a member of the specialized community by accident, not by choice, unless he has indicated his wish to become a research subject while still competent. Efforts to determine what a demented or retarded person would have wished for himself had he been competent have been made in American court decisions involving an incompetent patient's medical care. These "substituted judgment" approaches may have some worth, especially if the patient had expressed and recorded his wishes while still competent.

An individual might execute a document analogous to a human tissue gift — a sort of pre-dementia gift, in which he would officially and legally offer his person to medical research if and when he became demented. This might alleviate the problem of access to some extent, but it has its own difficulties. A pre-dementia volunteer cannot know in advance what types of research procedures will be developed in future, and so cannot give a truly informed consent except to either very specific procedures now known or to virtually anything. Such a pre-commitment may give some support to the decision to allow him to be a subject. But that decision, I contend, is justified by the claim, if valid, that it is for the common good of the dementia-care-research community, of which he is a member and to which, it is presumed, he would commit himself if he were capable of doing so at the time.

It is true, of course, that one might not ever have wished to participate in research procedures. In this case, the individual should be advised to register his or her objection in advance, along the lines that have been suggested for objection to organ donation in those countries that have a system of presumed consent for such donation. This can be achieved by carrying a card on which such an opt-out is recorded, or by placing one's name on a registry which might be maintained by support organizations. I suggest that unless one opt out in this manner, in the early stages of the disease, he or she be considered to have opted-in. That is, there should be a policy of presumed consent. In any event, as experience with organ retrieval has shown, in the final analysis it is the permission of relatives that is decisive in both those cases in which an individual has consented and those in which he or she has not made his or her wishes known.

The other members of the community may not all know each other. They do, however, have common values and, to a considerable degree, common objectives. There can be a high level of deliberate and active interaction, especially if there is close communication between the researchers, family, and volunteers in the voluntary health agencies.

What, then, is the ensemble of conditions which constitute the common good of the Alzheimer's community? Insofar as the purposes of collaboration include the effort to cure or to alleviate the disease, the common good would embrace, in addition to caring health professionals, a policy of promoting research, its ethical review, a sufficient number of committed clinical and scientific researchers, the requisite physical facilities and funding (some or all of which may be within other communities such as hospitals and medical schools), availability of volunteers for research, an atmosphere of mutual trust between research and subject, and finally ongoing research itself. This list is not exhaustive.

If access to the already demented is not allowed, and if this is essential for research on the disease to continue, it may well be impossible to find the answers to key questions about the disease. The common good of the Alzheimer's community would be damaged or insufficiently promoted. Since the goods of life and mental health are fundamental goods, this insufficiency would be profound.

One essential aspect of this common good is distributive justice. Each patient-subject shares not only in the burdens of research in order that all may prosper, but also the benefits. The benefits are not necessarily improved care or cure for the subject, but generally improved conditions for all such patient-subjects: a more aggressive approach to research, improved knowledge of the disease, increased probabilities for a cure, and others. Since the individual participates wholly in that good, he will be deprived of it in its entirety if it is not pursued. The common good is not so much a quantity of benefits as a quality of existence. It can therefore be distributed in its fullness to each member of the community. So, too, each can suffer its diminution.

Richard McCormick (1974) left his description of the common good unnecessarily broad and sweeping. According to some natural law theorists (Maritain 1947) the common good is always a distributed good, not simply the sum of parts. It is construed as flowing back upon the individual members of the community, who are not simply parts of a whole but persons, to whom the common good is distributed in its entirety. Thus, not only can the common good of which McCormick speaks be narrowed to that of children as a group (equivalent to Ramsey's population at risk) but the benefits of such research can be seen as redistributed to the individuals of the group. The benefits are not to be taken in the sense of an immediately available therapy, but in the sense of improved general conditions under which a cure, amelioration, or prevention for all is more likely.

CONCLUSION

Some of these observations can now be applied to the case of the elderly demented. First, the debate showed the inadequacy of the simple distinction between therapeutic and non-therapeutic experimentation, which has been challenged on several grounds in past years. For example, May (1976: 83) includes diagnostic and preventive types of research under therapeutic experimentation, whereas Reich (1978: 327) observes that the terms "therapeutic" and "non-therapeutic" are inadequate because they do not seem to include research on diagnostic and preventive techniques. In the area of the development of experimental preventive measures such as vaccines for epidemic diseases, and in the area of diseases in which research is carried out on terminal patients with little or no expectation of immediate benefit for these patients, the distinction is somewhat blurred. In each case, there is a defined population at risk: one without the disease but at great risk of contracting it, the other with a disease but with little hope of benefiting from the research.

Such types of research seem to constitute an intermediate category: the "indirectly therapeutic," involving the hope of either prevention or alleviation or cure. This category as applied to dementia shows some characteristics of therapeutic experimentation in the accepted sense, since it is carried out on persons who are ill and it is directed to their own illness. But it also shares some properties of non-therapeutic research, since it is not for their immediate treatment and, therefore, benefit. The good to be achieved is more remote, both in time and in application, since it is less sharply located in the individual than is therapy as such.

It must be admitted that there is a difference between the testing of a vaccine for prevention of disease in young, healthy children and research on elderly, seriously ill patients. In the former, the child-subjects will benefit if the vaccine is successful, or at least be protected from harm. In the latter, the subjects will not benefit by way of prevention or cure of their disease, but rather simply by being part of a community in which those goals are being actively pursued. The identification of the demented patient's good with that common good is doubtless less concrete than the identification of the child's good with that of his peers. But it seems to me that underlying both these cases is a notion of the common good required to justify all cases of research that do not promise a hope of direct benefit to a person who is, here and now, ill.

Years ago, Hans Jonas (1969) noted that a physician-researcher might put the following question to a dying patient: "There is nothing more I can do for you. But there is something you can do for me. Speaking no longer as your physician but on behalf of medical science, we could learn a great deal about future cases of this kind if you would permit me to perform certain experiments on you. It is understood that you yourself would not benefit from any knowledge we might gain; but future patients would." Although greatly vulnerable and deserving of maximum protection, such a patient might be ethically approached to be a research subject, because the benefits to future patients are in a way a value to him: "At least that residue of identification is left him that it is his own affliction by which he can contribute to the conquest of that affliction, his own kind of suffering which he helps alleviate in others; and so *in a sense it is his own cause*" (Jonas 1969: 532, emphasis mine).

In this case, the individual apprehends a good greater than his personal good, less than that of society: that of his disease class, which is *his* good. Of course, the identification of which Jonas speaks is psychological: he would likely not agree with the approach herein outlined and might require that such participation be through a conscious, free choice of the patient. Nevertheless, it is a real, objective good which justifies his choice and prevents us from asking him to participate in research unrelated to his disease. Can a relative, a son or daughter perhaps, ethically make that decision for an incompetent, demented Alzheimer's patient? If so, it is because, in a sense, it is the patient's cause, the patient's good as a member of a community which justifies that choice. It is not a matter of enforcing a social duty or minimal social obligation here, but seeking a good that lies in the relationship one has to others with the same disease. That same good, as noted above, limits the participation of the subject to research related precisely to his disease, not to anything else.

What is the implication of this for risk and the limits of risk? As has been seen, some wish to allow for exposure of subjects to greater than minimal risk provided only that it is classified as "therapeutic" (though the subjects are not ill). Others, in spite of the fact that the research is intended for the benefit of a group at risk, classify it as non-therapeutic and limit the acceptable risk to minimal levels. Are these the only alternatives? One advisory group has allowed, in the case of the mentally incompetent, for a "minor increase over minimal risk" in such circumstances (National Commission for the Protection of Human Subjects 1978: 16). This is presumably permitted because the research is "of vital importance for the understanding or amelioration of the type of disorder or condition of the subjects" or "may reasonably be expected to benefit the subjects in future" (17). But what counts as minor increase in risk? Proposed research into Alzheimer's might involve invasive procedures such as brain biopsies, implantation of electrodes, spinal taps, and injections of experimental drugs. Are these of greater risk than that specified by the National Commission simply because they are invasive of the human brain? Or is there clear statistical risk of serious added damage to the brain? These are matters for empirical study. The invasiveness per se should not rule out a procedure. The major limitations should be whether the procedure is painful, causes anxiety, or adds to the already serious damage to the brain. If research involving procedures of greater risk than "minor increase over minimal" is ever to be justified, it must be so by the intent to avert the proportional evils of death or mental incapacity. If these are insufficient, then I fail to see what grounds might be available upon which to base a case for legislative change.

It is clear, then, that should such research be acceptable, it also demands that stringent protective procedures be established in order to ensure that the demented are not drafted into research unrelated to their disease class. This is because the standard, being broader than that of "direct or fairly immediate benefit," is open to an accordionlike expansion, and therefore to abuse. Such safeguards could include: rigorous assurance that the proxy's consent (in reality, simply a permission) is informed and voluntary, the provision of a consent auditor, and various layers of administrative review and monitoring, from a local institutional review board up to a judicial review with a guardian appointed to represent the patient-subject's rights. These procedures may prove to be onerous. But we are on dangerous ground, and as we try to avoid overprotection, which may come at the expense of improved therapy for all, we must also avoid opening up a huge door to exploitation.

REFERENCES

Beauchamp, T.L., & Childress, J.F. (1983). *Principles of Biomedical Ethics.* 2nd ed. New York: Oxford University Press

Finnis, J. (1980). *Natural Law and Natural Rights.* Oxford: Clarendon Press

Jonas, H. (1969). Philosophical reflections on experimenting with human subjects. In T. Beauchamp and L. Walters (Eds.), *Contemporary Issues in Bioethics.* 2nd ed. Belmont, CA: Wadsworth

Maritain, J. (1947). *The Person and the Common Good.* New York: Charles Scribner's Sons

May, W. (1976). Proxy consent to human experimentation. *Linacre Quarterly, 43,* 73-84

McCormick, R. (1974). Proxy consent in the experimentation situation. *Perspectives in Biology and Medicine, 18,* 2-20

McCormick, R. (1976). Experimentation in children: sharing in sociality. *Hastings Center Report, 6,* 41-46

National Commission for the Protection of Human Subjects (1978). *Report and Recommendations: Research Involving Those Institutionalized as Mentally Infirm.* Washington, DC

Ramsey, P. (1970). *The Patient as Person.* New Haven: Yale University Press

Ramsey, P. (1976). The enforcement of morals: Non-Therapeutic research on children *Hastings Center Report, 4,* 21-30

Ramsey, P. (1977). Children as research subjects: a reply. *Hastings Center Report, 2,* 40-41

Ratzan, R. (1980). "Being old makes you different": The ethics of research with elderly subjects. *Hastings Center Report, 5,* 32-42

Reich, W. (1978). Ethical issues related to research involving elderly subjects *Gerontologist, 18,* 326-37

FURTHER READINGS

In the Matter of Kristie Lee F, P.C.C. (F.D.) Ontario (1072/88).

Coughlan, M.J. and E. Anscombe

"Using People," *Bioethics* 4:1 (1990) 55-65.

Levine, Robert J.

Ethics and Regulations of Clinical Research. (New Haven and London: Yale University Press, 1988) Chapters 10-13.

Mason, J.K.

Medico-Legal Aspects of Reproduction and Parenthood. (Brookfield, VT.:Gopwer, 1990) 280-296, "Consent to Treatment and Research in Children".

Medical Research Council of Canada

Guidelines on Research Involving Human Subjects 1987. (Ottawa: Minister of Supply and Services, 1987).

National Commission for the Protection of Human Subjects of Biomedical and Behavioral Research

The Belmont Report: Ethical Principles for the Protection of Human Subjects of Research, (Washington, DC: US Government Printing Office, 1978) pub. no. 78–0012.

McCormick, R.

"Proxy Consent in Experimentation Situations," *Perspectives in Biology and Medicine* 18:1(1974).

Nicholson, Richard H., ed.

Medical Research With Children: Ethics, Law, and Practice. (New York and Tokyo: Oxford University Press, 1986).

Picard, E.I.

Legal Liability of Doctors and Hospitals in Canada (Toronto: Carswell, 1984) Chapter 3, "Consent".

Ramsey, P.

The Ethics of Fetal Research. (New Haven: Yale University Press, 1975).

Superintendent of Belchertown State School v. Saikewicz, 370 N.E. (2d) C 417 (Mass. S.C. 1977).

Wasserstrom, R.

"Ethical Issues Involved in Experimentation on the Non-Viable Human Foetus," National Commission for the Protection of Human Subjects of Biomedical and Behavioral Research, *Appendix: Research on the Foetus.* (1975) DHEW No. (05) 76–128.

PART 3 DELIBERATE DEATH

CHAPTER 10 PERSONHOOD

INTRODUCTION

Until fairly recently, the distinction between being a person and being a member of the species *homo sapiens* was of interest only to philosophers and theologians. It was generally assumed that any living human being was a person, and *vice versa*. Not only our tradition, but also our laws reflect that fact.[1]

Three recent developments in health care have challenged this assumption. First, medical technology such as respirators, kidney machines, etc. were developed to the point that people could be kept alive considerably beyond the time when otherwise they would have died. However, in many cases the people who were thus saved were left in a permanent vegetative coma, because their higher brain centres had been destroyed. These individuals were therefore biologically alive but without any possibility of a return to sentient cognitive awareness. In fact, in some cases, not only were their higher brain centres destroyed, but their whole brain—and yet the bodies could be kept alive for a time. The question therefore arose, are these individuals still persons?

The thrust of the question was sharpened by the scarcity of medical resources. It therefore came to be asked whether it was ethically appropriate to spend scarce resources to sustain someone who was only biologically living, when that would deprive others of appropriate and possibly beneficial health care?

A second development that influenced the debate and expanded it considerably was the advent of transplantation. It soon became evident that organs from living donors had a much better chance of not being rejected than organs from cadavers. This increased the pressure for examining the validity of the distinction between being biologically alive only, and being alive as a person.

Finally, the distinction between humanity and personhood was pressed when abortion became a public issue, and when the federal government attempted to draft abortion laws that satisfied the multicultural and multi-religious makeup of Canadian society. This pushed the debate about personhood to the beginning of human life. It forced an examination of the question of whether a human being is a person from the moment of conception, or acquires personhood at some later stage.

In the course of the debate, it became evident to many that the question of when someone is dead is really the question of when someone is *no longer* a person, and that this question could not ethically be divorced from the question of when someone is *already* a person. Whatever notion of personhood was ultimately to be developed, and however it was to be related to the concept of a human being, it would have to be applicable in a consistent fashion in both cases.

The selections below give an indication of some of the range of considerations that have been covered in the course of the debate. On the issue of developing personhood, one extreme is presented by Rosenberg's editorial from the Federation of Medical Women's *Newsletter*. The position paper of the Committee on Ethics of the Canadian Medical Association reflects an attempt by the senior advisory committee of organized Canadian medicine to steer a somewhat less radical course.

On the issue of when someone is no longer a person, the cases of *R. v. Kitching and Adams* and *R. v. Green* represent two different approaches that the law has taken.

Finally, the discussion by Roland Pucetti, who is a philosopher, deals with the question of those who are in permanent vegetative state. These individuals do not meet the whole-brain criterion, yet there is no question that they no longer have the capacity for sentient cognitive awareness. Are they dead as persons? The issue is especially important in light of the chronic shortage of health care resources and the cost involved in keeping these individuals alive. The issues of resource allocation, right to health care, etc., dealt with by selections in preceding chapters, here become relevant.

NOTE

1. The political and legal position on personhood is another matter. It involves judicial recognition of individuals as having the rights that are normally associated with other individuals who are recognized as persons in a judicial sense. Women were not recognized as legal persons in Canada until 1929, when the Privy Council of Great Britain extended that recognition by stating that the word "person" contained in the British North America Act extended to women as well as men. It is interesting to note that in this sense, children are still not recognized as persons.

Say "No" to Fetal Personhood

Frances Rosenberg

A woman is her fetus. Until the fetus is born, there is only one person, the mother.

Why has it become so easy for society to propose that a pregnant woman can be treated as more than one person? Perhaps the partial answer lies with the progressive fragmentation of the family and the individual that has followed industrialization. Increasingly, we live in two worlds. The private world (largely a world of women) is concerned with the "natural" areas of our lives; sex, reproduction and the emotional aspects of relationships. The public world, on the other hand, is primarily the domain of man, and is concerned, first and foremost, with production and efficiency. This is the world of work and business, where productivity takes precedence over feelings.[1] Concurrent with this division in family life, the individual has felt increasingly alienated from the community. For men, the performance of work that has no apparent relationship to a larger whole has eroded their image of themselves as valuable members of society. For women, the displacement of family tradition on childbearing and rearing by societal authorities has reduced their perceived social stature.

When we move from the person as a whole to their parts we see increasing fragmentation. Women have long been compelled to disown their intelligence, given the widely held beliefs that brains and beauty do not mix and that beauty is the quality desired in women. More recently, parts of our bodies, including sperm, ova, and embryos can be moved from person to person, and out of and back into the same person.[1]

These processes for artificial reproduction have tended to obscure the integrity of mother and fetus that is intrinsic to natural reproduction.

Coupled with the fragmentation evident within society, there has been the production orientation of medicine toward childbearing; in which the health care deliverers could be likened to factory management with women being the laborers and the infant the product. Contemporary efforts at returning childbirth to a more natural state fail to address the erosion of women's integrity that has resulted from the practice of "commodity oriented" obstetrics. One has but to read much that is written about artificial reproduction and fetal rights to realize that there has been little change in the attitude toward women's childbearing role.

Now here is the insidious thing ... we are all so shaped by the thinking that has given rise to the question of fetal rights and the implied fetal personhood that we find it very difficult to explore the issue. Yet we must if society is to be informed by the insight of women. We must transcend those beliefs and attitudes instilled by the forces that created this dilemma and express our feelings on this issue. We must examine for ourselves how it would feel if bureaucrats, doctors, lawyers, were determining how we should behave when we were pregnant and there were "pregnancy police" (a term now in use in the US) to monitor our behaviour. If that would not be comfortable, then say "no" to fetal personhood.

---

* Revised from "Editorial," *Newsletter of the Association of Medical Women of Canada*: "Say 'No' to Fetal Personhood." 1990.

Trust your instinct and assert your womanhood. Let us reestablish organic unity between the fetus and the mother through the recognition of only one person prior to childbirth, the mother.

Frances Rosenberg MD PhD FRCP(C), Department of Laboratories, St. Paul's Hospital.

NOTE

1. See E. Martin, *The Woman in the Body*. Boston: Beacon Press (1987).

The Status of the Human Foetus

Canadian Medical Association, Commitee on Ethics

Fertilization marks the beginning of human embryonic development. From its very beginning, therefore, a human foetus is a member of the species *Homo sapiens*. Physicians, scientists and ordinary members of the community agree on this point. Thereafter, however, opinions diverge. Some see no difference between being a human being in a biological sense (i.e., being a member of the species *Homo sapiens*) and being a human being or person in an ethical sense. Indeed, they characterize any attempt to draw such a distinction as untenable and pernicious. Others maintain that there is a difference. They believe that membership in the species *Homo sapiens* has only biological importance. They believe that what conveys ethical status is not membership in a biological species but the fulfillment of certain criteria. They maintain that these criteria involve such characteristics as the capacity for sapient cognitive awareness, the capacity for self-awareness, and the like.

The opposition between these two approaches has usually been cast as the opposition between a biologically and a functionally oriented notion of personhood. The biologically oriented position contends that human beings are persons in an ethical sense from the very moment of conception. The functionally oriented position maintains that only those living organisms who satisfy certain functional criteria — some of which have been mentioned — can be considered persons.

Recent developments have cast doubt on the acceptability of the biologically oriented position.[1] They have done so from a medical as well as from a legal perspective. Developments in medicine have reached a point where a biologically human being may be kept alive long after any semblance of sapient capacity has been irremediably destroyed. Medically, therefore, it has become appropriate to distinguish between a human being who is biologically alive but no longer a person, and someone who is biologically alive as well as a person. The acceptance of the Harvard criteria for the determination of brain death was but the professional recognition of this development. The concept has since been refined in various ways and has found legal acceptance in most jurisdictions.

Canadian Medical Association, "The Status of the Human Foetus," from *Proceedings of the 123rd General Council, 1991,* pp.4-14.

In Canada, legal acceptance of brain-centred criteria for the determination of death occurred in the case of *Regina v. Kitching and Adams.*[2] The courts here recognized that while some human beings may be biologically alive, the fact that their brains are irreparably dysfunctional allows us to consider them legally dead and therefore persons no longer. At this time, only Manitoba has enacted a statute which fixes this distinction. However the distinction is generally accepted for most purposes in Canada as well as elsewhere.[3] Indeed, the practice of harvesting organs from biologically alive but brain-dead human beings would otherwise not be defensible: It would amount to murder.

These developments did not take place in isolation. They went hand-in-hand with a fundamental reorientation in ethical perspective. It became widely accepted as matter of general principle that what is ethically central to the issue of personhood is not whether a given individual is alive or even belongs to the species *Homo sapiens.* Instead, the possession of certain capacities became widely recognized as ethically central: specifically, the capacity for some level of self-awareness and sapient cognitive awareness.

By drawing on these historical developments, the Committee does not mean to equate a developing foetus with a brain-dead human being; nor does the Committee intend to suggest that the process of dying is an exact analogue as the process of gestation. The Committee recognizes that there are fundamental differences. They include the fact that a foetus is developing and has a potential for increased functioning, whereas this is precisely what is absent in the case of a brain-dead human being.

Nevertheless, the Committee feels that the analogy has a point. Abstracting from philosophical niceties that centre around the notion of potentiality itself, the analogy lies in the functional aspects of the case. Death is not an instantaneous event. It is a process of increasing dissolution and dysfunction. Brain cells die, and their death contributes to the dysfunction of the brain as a whole. At some point in this process, this dysfunction is so cumulative that a threshold is crossed. At that point the individual is said to be dead, the fact of continued cellular and even organic life notwithstanding.

The development of the human foetus also involves a functional gradation. The difference is that it occurs in reverse fashion. There is a gradual increase in neurological complexity from the first identifiable neural cells which do not as yet function in an integrated fashion, to the integrated brain structure of the foetus at term. The capacity for sapient cognitive awareness is absent at the beginning of that development. There is not even capacity for somatic sensation. These capacities are acquired as the neurological structure of the foetus grows and increases. They constitute as it were an inverse of the process of death. Consistency and equality require that if the integrated functioning presence of such structures, and the presence of such capacities, are deemed necessary for human beings to be considered persons, they must be applied to the human foetus as well as to human beings that have already been born.

The fact that the foetus has the potential for development may be thought to make a difference. However, the Committee on Ethics believes that is not the case. In the *first* place, a potential does not give whoever has that potential the same status as someone who actually exhibits the relevant characteristic. A fertilized and incubating egg is a foetal bird. For all that, however, the incubating egg does not have the same status, and in an intuitively clear sense is not materially the same, as the hatched bird which it will become. In order to attain that status, the foetal bird has to develop under appropriate conditions of incubation. To equate a fertilized and developing egg with a bird who has been hatched, and to treat them the same, is to ignore the very fundamental difference between the two: A difference that involves their present material natures.[4] Of course this does not prevent society from bestowing the same *legal* status on both, or from protecting the two by the same (or at least essentially similar) sanctions. However, that would be the result of a deliberate decision by society on societal or other grounds. Logically it would neither be necessary nor would it follow from the material nature of the case.

In the *second* place, to say that something has a potential by that very fact is to distinguish it from something in which the potential is actualized. Otherwise the distinction would be pointless. Therefore to say that the two have the same status — the same ethical status — requires a premise which says that something which has a mere potential and something in which this potential is actualized *should* be treated the same way. But that is the very point at issue. Simply to assert that their status is the same is to settle the matter by definition. It is to beg the question. An example may serve to illustrate the point: If someone who is a potential sufferer from Huntington disease (someone who carries the genetic determinant for it) has the same status as someone who is an actual sufferer from Huntington disease in virtue of that potentiality, then the potential sufferer should be treated the same way as the actual sufferer. However to treat the two in the same way would be entirely inappropriate: psychologically, socially and above all medically.[5]

The Committee therefore proposes the following:

Recommendation 1:

A human foetus becomes a person when it meets the criteria for personhood that must be met by all other human beings.

Recommendation 2:

These criteria are met when the foetal nervous system has developed to the point where it has the basic capacity for sapient cognitive awareness irrespective of level of sophistication.

These considerations suggests that while ethical considerations are always relevant with respect to the human foetus, they increase in gravity and change in nature as the gestation progresses. As the pregnancy progresses, the foetus increasingly becomes an object of ethical concern.[6,7] This means that in actions that impact on a human foetus, respect for the life of the foetus increasingly has to be balanced against the right to self-determination of the pregnant woman and to the integrity of her person. However, once the foetus has become a person, the ethical deliberations that are now appropriate no longer consist in a weighing of the value of respect for life of the foetus against the principle of autonomy of the pregnant woman. They now involve a balancing of the right to life against the right to integrity and self-determination. At this point the existence of competing right-claims is no longer at issue. What is at issue is their relative strengths.

In other words, although a human foetus is an object of serious ethical concern prior to approximately twenty weeks, it is not the ethical equal of the mother before that time. The reason lies in the development of its functional capacity. If one were to depict this capacity on a linear scale, it could be represented as a line with variable but increasing slope. The line begins at a minimal level when fertilization occurs and rises steadily until around the twentieth week. According to current understanding, the line appears to cross a critical point of quantum-like proportions around that time. The reason is that according to current understanding it is around that time that the capacities of the foetus meet the minimal requirements that are otherwise considered necessary for someone to be considered a person.

What this means in practical terms may be illustrated by considering the case of a pregnant woman who requires medical treatment. Ethical considerations require that the attending physician take the life and welfare of the foetus into account when evaluating the treatment options for the woman no matter what the stage of development of the foetus.[8] The physician must balance the competing claims of the woman against considerations concerning the foetus. However, the strength of that balancing will not be uniform at all stages of foetal development. Instead, the weight given to foetal concerns in this balancing process will be functionally determined by the level of development of the foetus and the threat to the health of the pregnant woman.

Care must be taken not to understand this notion of balancing in too liberal a fashion. It does not mean that only passing and token consideration should be given to the foetus. Instead, it means is that the reasoning process that leads to a medical decision must attempt a genuine balancing, with serious consideration being given to the foetus as well as to the pregnant woman. This is in keeping with resolution of the 1989 General Council of the CMA which directed the Committee on Ethics to consider the proposition that "in the decision concerning a abortion, both parties must consider the existence of the unborn child and respect its rights." In any abortion counselling, therefore, or in any situation involving the human foetus, the status of that foetus must be taken into account.[9]

Furthermore, it should be kept in mind that history is replete with examples where individuals have been denied appropriate treatment because they have been denied the status of persons. The fate of women prior to their enfranchisement, of slaves, of ethnic and religious minorities in general are all-too familiar examples. The Committee is solicitous that not recognizing the foetus as an object of ethical concern from its very beginning may be seen in this light. It therefore wants to go on record as rejecting completely, emphatically and utterly the suggestion that any and all actions towards a foetus are licit simply because the foetus has not as yet been born. Society has certain standards and values which, while not ethical principles, nevertheless function as fundamental principles of acceptable conduct. One of these was referred to above. It is the principle of respect for human life. No human being, whatever its stage of development, may be deprived without good reason of the protection that this principle affords. Therefore it is the position of the Committee that all other things being equal the human foetus, whatever its stage of development, is also entitled to appropriate and respectful treatment.[10]

Among other things, this means that so far as the Committee is concerned, the standard of conduct to be observed towards a human foetus who has not as yet attained to the stage where it becomes a person must, as a minimal benchmark, satisfy the requirements embodied in humane legislation: The fact that a foetus does not have the same status as an ordinary member of society does not mean that it should be accorded even less respect than non-human living beings. Furthermore, the Committee believes that a human foetus which has not as yet attained to being an object of fullfledged ethical concern may be involved in undertakings that are of no benefit to itself only on the condition that there are overwhelming ethical reason (rooted in the rights of extant and fullfledged members of society) that outweigh the considerations which stem from the principle of respect for human life. In other words, the Committee believes that the human foetus should not be involved in non-therapeutic endeavours or undertakings that are not mandated by overwhelming social or individual ethical considerations.

The Committee on Ethics therefore suggests the following as a further fundamental guideline for all actions involving the human foetus:

Recommendation 3:

The principle of respect for human life is of fundamental importance in medical practice. Therefore any action involving a human foetus must always be evaluated in light of this principle, and departures from it must always be justified in terms of the principles of medical ethics.

VIABILITY

So far, no reference has been made to the concept of viability. The reason lies in the dubious ethical validity that attaches to the notion of viability itself.

In the foetal context, "viability" usually refers to the capacity of the foetus to stay alive when removed from or independent of the body of its mother. In a state of nature and in the absence of medical intervention, that capacity depends solely on the state of the individual foetus: on its development, its present capacities and the like. This is no longer true in the contemporary setting. Viability is no longer an independent variable which, all other things being equal, finds its basis in the state of the foetus itself. Given the advances of modern medicine and technology, it has largely become a function of the sophistication of the external supports that are available, on the readiness to use them — as well as on the willingness of society to use all available scientific means to push back still further the current practical limits on sustaining life.

What this means in ethical terms is that to consider viability as determinative of the ethical status of anyone is to make the ethical status of that individual dependent on the willingness of society to develop and use means to use life support systems. More specific to the foetal context, to attach ethical significance to the notion of foetal viability is to ignore the criteria for personhood that are considered relevant in all other contexts. It is to replace considerations that depend on the state and development of the foetus with considerations that depend on the sophistication of available medical technology and on society's willingness to use it.

It is worth mentioning in this regard that such an approach would constitute an ethical anomaly: The fact that someone is dependent on a respirator, a kidney machine or other external support system is generally not considered sufficient reason for not treating that individual as an object of fullfledged ethical concern. Consistency demands that the human foetus should not be treated differently.

Implications for the Physician

(a) With Respect to Everyday Practice

These considerations have important consequences for physicians in actual practice. The first consequence, and in many ways perhaps the most important, is that such physicians ought to consider the foetus an object of ethical concern almost from the beginning, and that the foetus should be considered a genuine patient at the latest at twenty weeks gestation. This would hold true irrespective of whether the foetus was in utero or in an artificial environment.

Furthermore, current developments in reproductive technology and reproductive care, as well as advances in perinatal medicine and associated disciplines, have made it clear that the fetal environment during gestation has a profound effect on the development of the foetus itself. What is done to the foetus — or, for that matter, to the mother — may shape its later life profoundly. In anticipation of considerations to be dealt with later, the Committee therefore suggests the following as a guiding principle:

Recommendation 4:

A physician should always act on the assumption that the foetus is likely to become a person unless there are clear indications to the contrary.

(b) Indications to the Contrary

(i) However, there are cases where the exceptive clause of Consideration 5 will in fact be met. *For instance,* the foetus may suffer from such severe and irreparable congenital or other deficits that it will never fulfil the material requirements for becoming a person. In such cases, while the physician's actions should still be guided by respect for life, the physician's primary concern should be the pregnant woman.

Recommendation 5:

When it is medically certain that the foetus will never become a person, the physician's obligations towards the foetus are those agreed to by the pregnant woman and otherwise owed living beings of a comparable level of development. The primary concern of the physician, however, should be the pregnant woman.

ii) A *second* indication to the contrary obtains when, according to the best medical knowledge available under the circumstances, the foetus suffers from such deficits that if it were to be born, its life would be tantamount to a continuous state of injury, or the life that the foetus could reasonably be expected to live would be describable only in terms of inhumanity, indignity and suffering.[11] In such cases, the aim of the physician should be to try to prevent the actualization of continuous and irremediable harm. The sorts of situations that would warrant such considerations may include Trisomy 13, Tay-Sachs, anencephaly and similar conditions that are usually grouped under the term "medical indications for abortion."

Recommendation 6:

When, in the best understanding of the physician, the foetus can only attain an existence that is significantly lacking in human quality or one that is fraught with irremediable pain and suffering, then the physician may ethically terminate the pregnancy. The treatment of the mother should be from a humanitarian perspective, recognizing her loss. Under certain circumstances, termination of the foetus' existence even after 20 weeks gestation may be appropriate.

The last statement should be seen as a partial clarification of the CMA's current position on abortion, which states that "Elective termination of pregnancy after fetal viability may be indicated under exceptional circumstances."[12]

(iii) A *third* exceptive condition obtains when the pregnant woman's life is in danger and it is medically certain that her life can be saved — but only through a procedure that will kill the foetus.

In a case like this, the physician's primary obligation is towards the pregnant woman. However, the Principle of Autonomy entails that the woman has the right to decide whether she wishes her life to be saved or, alternatively, wants the life and welfare of the foetus to receive priority. The physician therefore has an obligation to try and determine the woman's wishes. Once these wishes have been determined, the physician must follow them. If it is not possible to ascertain what the woman's wishes are, Recommendation 5 takes over and the woman's life and welfare become the physician's primary concern.

Recommendation 7:

When the physician is faced with a choice between the life of the pregnant woman and the life of the foetus and if the pregnant woman has indicated in a competent and informed fashion that the life of the foetus should be given priority, then the physician must follow those wishes.

Recommendation 8:

When the physician is faced with a choice between the life of the pregnant woman and the life of the foetus and if there is no way of reasonably determining the wishes of the pregnant woman, the physician should attempt to save both. If that should prove to be unfeasible, the life of the mother should be the physician's first priority.

However, there may be cases where the course selected by the pregnant woman may conflict with the private values of the physician. In such cases, if the physician were to follow the wishes of the woman, the physician would be forced to go against his or her own conscience. However, the Code of Ethics of the Canadian Medical Association makes it clear, and indeed it is generally accepted, that all other things being equal, a physician has the right to follow his or her conscience in the conduct of his or her practice. Therefore if the values of the physician differ or likely to differ from those of the pregnant woman, and if that difference is likely to impact on the willingness or ability of the physician to respect the woman's wishes or to follow standard medical practice, then the physician has an obligation so to inform the woman at the inception of the physician-patient relationship.

This may present problems in individual cases. The process of communicating such personal values is always a delicate matter. However, it is a general and fundamental requirement of informed consent that a patient be informed of any relevant and important differences between the physician's standards and those of the general medical community, and that the patient must be told of any factors that are likely to affect the physician's ability to acquiesce in the patient's informed and competent directives based on the patient's values. These fundamental duties do not lapse in the case of pregnancy.

Recommendation 9:

If the physician's private morality differs or is likely to differ from the generally accepted standards of society, or if the physician's private morality places the physician into conflict with the competent and informed value-directives of the pregnant woman (or if it is likely to do so) then the physician should inform the pregnant woman of that fact at the earliest appropriate opportunity. At that time, the physician should also inform the woman that she has the option to consult another physician.

Other Contexts

There remains a whole domain of actions that involve the foetus prior to twenty weeks gestation. Experimental protocols from the side of the physician, lifestyle and behaviour patterns from the side of the pregnant woman, etc. are here implicated.[13] In these cases a distinction should be drawn between situations where the foetus is intended (or expected) to complete the gestational period and ultimately be born, and situations where the intention (or expectation) is that this will not occur.

If the intention (or expectation) is that the foetus will develop to the point where it becomes a person, then any action or inaction that impacts negatively on the developmental chances of the foetus, whatever its stage of development, will be *prima facie* indefensible.

The reason lies in the ethics of causality. In general terms, the argument may be stated as follows: To initiate a train of events that predictably and foreseeably will have an injurious outcome, or to allow such a train of events to occur when it lies within the powers of the individual actor to prevent it without undue harm to the actor him- or herself, confers responsibility for that outcome on the actor.[14]

In the case of foetal development, knowingly to initiate a train of events that predictably and foreseeably will have this sort of outcome, or to allow such a train of events to occur when it lies within the powers of the individual to prevent it, is to initiate a train of events that predictably and foreseeable would result in harm to the foetus once it becomes a person. Anyone who finds her- or himself in such a position acquires a degree of responsibility for the outcome. The degree of responsibility that attaches to the person will be commensurate with the extent the individual's involvement (or deliberate failure to become involved) contributed to the outcome itself.

These considerations apply not only to the pregnant woman or the physician; they also are valid for all other persons whose actions or inactions have a measurable causal impact on the development of the foetus. Therefore they also apply to the medical staff, the nursing staff and anyone else who may be involved in an appropriate capacity. Still, in the medical setting it applies primarily to the physician. It is the physician who has ultimate responsibility for the medical environment. Therefore there lies a special ethical obligation on the attending physician not to ignore these considerations.[15]

Recommendation 10:

When the foetus has become a person, or when there is the intention or reasonable expectation that the foetus will become a person, the physician has an obligation to try and prevent harm to the foetus insofar as that is compatible with other obligations the physician may have.

SPECIAL CONSIDERATIONS

(a) When it is not intended/expected that the foetus will survive beyond twenty weeks gestation

Not all pregnancies are intended to go to term or are expected to do so. A pregnancy where the woman intends to have an abortion is an example of the former; a pregnancy where the constitution of the foetus is incompatible with survival beyond twenty weeks is an example of the latter. In cases such as these, non-therapeutic and research activities, when conducted prior to 20 weeks gestation and in accordance with otherwise applicable standards, are ethically permissible if certain conditions are met. These include the following:

(1) the pregnant woman and/or other appropriate alternate decision-maker has given informed consent; and

(2) the research protocol or procedure has been duly approved by an appropriate Ethics Review Board according to national and uniform guidelines set out by the Medical Research Council of Canada, the National Council on Bioethics in Human Research, and any other relevant and applicable body; and

(3) the foetus will not survive beyond twenty weeks gestation.

Recommendation 11:

Non-therapeutic, experimental, innovative or otherwise unusual procedures are permissible on a foetus with maternal and/or other appropriate consent if it is intended and certain that the foetus will never become a person and will never develop beyond twenty weeks gestation. Such procedures or undertakings, however, must meet all otherwise applicable standards of treatment and/or experimentation and must have been approved by an appropriate ethics review board. They should also be in keeping with Recommendation 3 above.

(b) Situations where the bodily integrity of the pregnant woman is the central issue.

The right to integrity of the person is a logical consequence of the Principle of Autonomy and Respect for Persons. It therefore follows that every person, irrespective of gender, age or other qualitative distinctions, has the right to insist on such integrity against all others. Nevertheless, no right is absolute. All are conditioned by the circumstances under which they arise and the circumstances in which they are claimed. Consequently there are situations where the right to the integrity of the person may be rendered ineffective and may be overruled by the competing and weightier rights of others.

Women who become pregnant are almost always willing to undergo a considerable measure of self-sacrifice in order to benefit their foetuses. The voluntary inception of a pregnancy itself, with all that this entails, bears vivid testimony to this fact. Therefore the best way to assure that a conflict between maternal and foetal considerations does not arise in the first instance is to make every effort to ensure that pregnancies are wanted, and that mothers themselves are the beneficiaries of appropriate social, economic and psychological conditions. The benefits that would redound to the foetus from such a perspective will of course be quite patent.

Nevertheless, even under the best of circumstances, it may sometimes happen that a conflict between maternal and foetal interests arises. For instance, the pregnant woman may refuse to cooperate in the medical care designed to benefit the foetus, she may create a potentially hazardous environment for the foetus, or she may refuse to accept the need for a Caesarian delivery because of the implications that such undertakings have for the woman herself. In such cases, great care should be taken that the limitations of medical knowledge are taken into account, that due weight is given to the fallibility inherent in medical predictions of this nature, and that the limitations on the reliability of diagnostic procedures are factored into the equation.

Still, even when all of these factors are given due weight, the physician may be of the opinion that an intervention would be necessary for the sake of the foetus. In almost all cases, such a conflict will be resolvable through judicious and appropriate education and counselling of the pregnant woman, and through a conscientious and co-operative examination of the relevant options.[16] However, there may be cases where such a process will not lead to a resolution. This will be especially troublesome in the later stages of pregnancy when the foetus has become a person and a surgical or medical intervention is considered necessary to save the life of the foetus yet the woman claims the right of inviolability of her body. In such cases, it may be appropriate for the physician to request a judicial ruling to determine whether such a breach of personal integrity or interference with her autonomy should take place.

In emergency cases, where such a judicial review is not possible, the physician has the duty to do what is medically appropriate and possible under the circumstances, in keeping with the reasoning indicated above.[17] In defense of this, the physician may point to the doctrine of emergency, the principle of beneficence, and the fact that the foetus has become a person. Furthermore, failure to engage in the appropriate and medically indicated action may well constitute an abandonment of the foetal patient.

Recommendation 12:

The physician's duty towards the foetus during the third trimester may require that the physician resort to the judicial process in order to try to ensure the survival and wellbeing of the foetus. Such a step should be taken only after due consideration of the gravity of such a step and after all alternatives that are reasonably available have been exhausted. In emergency contexts, the physician's duty is governed by the doctrine of emergency.18

CONCLUSIONS

The practice of medicine goes to the heart of human life. More than any other professional activity, therefore, medicine requires an exquisite adherence to ethical standards and a respect for the fundamental values that shape our social outlook. Recommendations 1- 12 are an attempt to provide such standards and to implement such values. Doubtless, these Recommendations will strike some as restricting the interests of certain parties too severely; equally as predictably, they will strike others as not going far enough. The task of the Committee on Ethics is to combine ethical sensitivity with practicality. The preceding Recommendations are an attempt to do just that.

Approved by the Committe on Ethics, Canadian Medical Association; principal author, E. -H.W. Kluge, Director, Department of Ethics and Legal Affairs, Canadian Medical Association

NOTES

1. The most noteworthy recent example is *R. v. Morgentaler* [1988] 1 S.C.R. 30.
2. *R. v Kitching and Adams* (1976), 32 C.C.C. (2d) 159, [1976] 6 W.W.R. 697.
3. The recent case of *R. v. Green,* [1988] B.C.J. No. 1807, Vernon Registry No. 18024, June 27, 1988, does not contradict the reasoning in *Kitching and Adams.* As the presiding judge in *Green* made very clear, he rejected the position of *Kitching and Adams* specifically for legal reasons of practicality: reasons that do not obtain in the medical setting:

   > The suggestion that brain death or the irreversible cessation of brain function be the legal standard for determining when death occurs may be suitable in the medical context and even in the civil law context, but in my view it is a completely impractical standard to apply in the criminal law. ... If the onus is on the Crown to satisfy this jury beyond a reasonable doubt that Mr. Frie was still alive — that is to say that his brain function had not yet irreversibly ceased — when the Accused Green "pumped" two bullets into him, it can be seen that such an onus would be impossible to discharge — unless someone had happened along with an EEG monitor and applied same to Mr. Frie either before or immediately after the two shots allegedly fired by Green.
   >
   > As I have said both the medical profession and the Law Reform Commission are principally concerned with the moral and legal issues arising out of artificially sustained life and human transplant procedures. The legal issues raised are approached from what is primarily a civil law point of view — in other words the administration of the criminal law does not appear to have been of paramount concern in the approach taken by either group.
   >
   > On the face of it I see no reason why the same legal definition of death must be applied in both a civil and criminal context. Indeed there are good reasons why the same criteria should not apply. The criminal law seeks to deter the incidence of, inter alia, violent crime by holding accountable those whose conduct endangers the lives and safety of others. The civil law, in the context under discussion, seeks to ensure that societies' moral and personal values are not compromised in the pursuit of bona fide efforts to prolong or save meaningful life.

4. This difference was traditionally recognized by the Judaeo-Christian Islamic religions, who characterized the conceptus as a "clot of blood" and accepted it as having a human ethical status only after a series of developments had occurred. The distinction between a potential person and an actual person was clearly recognized in canon law. See *Corpus Juris Canonici Emendatum et Notis Illustratum cum Glossae: Decretalium Gregori Papae Noni Compilatio* (Rome, 1585), *Glossa ordinaria,* Bk. 5, t. 12, c. 20, p. 1713. For a good historical discussion, see J. Donceel, "Abortion: Medicate v. Immediate Animation," *Continuum* 5(Spring 1967) pp. 167-171, and "Immediate Animation and

Delayed Hominization," *Theological Studies* 13 (March 1970), pp. 76-105; E.-H.W. Kluge, "St. Thomas, Abortion and Euthanasia," *Philosophical Research Archives* (September, 1981).

5. For a fuller discussion of the notion of potentiality and its ethical implications, see E.-H.W. Kluge, *The Ethics of Deliberate Death* (Yale University Press: New Haven and London, 1975), Chap. 1; H.T. Engelhardt, Jr., *The Foundations of Bioethics* (Oxford University Press: New York and Oxford, 1986) 110-113.
6. See Law Reform Commission Working Paper 58, pp. 40 ff. *et pass.* for considerations along similar lines.
7. See H.T. Engelhardt, Jr., *The Foundation of Bioethics* (Oxford: Oxford University Press, 1986) Chap. 6; Paul Ramsey, *The Patient As Person* (New Haven and London: Yale University Press, 1977) Chap. 2; Helmut Thielicke, "The Doctor as Judge of Who Shall Live and Who Shall Die," in Kenneth Vaux, ed., *Who Shall Live? Medicine, Technology, Ethics,* (Philadelphia, 1970); Karl Rahner, "Gedanken Ueber das Sterben," *Arzt und Christ* 15, 1969; etc.
8. Resolutions of the 122nd General Council of the Canadian Medical Association, Quebec City, 1989.
9. Resolutions of the 122nd General Council of the Canadian Medical Association, Quebec City, 1989.
10. For a recent discussion indicating agreement with according the fetus some status, see George J. Annas, "A French Homonculus in a Tennessee Court," *Hastings Center Report* 19:6 (Nov. Dec. 1989) 20-22, at 20 "Every national commission worldwide that has examined the status of the human embryo to date has placed it in this third category: neither people no products, but nonetheless entities of unique symbolic value that deserves society's respect and protection."
11. For various discussions of this concept, see Margin Kohl, ed., *Infanticide and the Value of Life* (Buffalo: Prometheus, 1978); Ruth Macklin, *Mortal Choices: Bioethics in Today's World* (New York: Pantheon, 1987) chapter 8, "The `Best Interest' of the Child; Richard A. McCormick, "To Save or Let Die: The Dilemma of Modern Medicine," *Journal of the American Medical Association* 229 (July 8, 1974); President's Commission for the Study of Ethical Problems in Medicine and Biomedical and Behavioral Research, *Deciding to Forego Life-Sustaining Treatment* (U.S. Govt. Printing Office: Washington, 1983); Magnet and Kluge, *Withholding Treatment from Defective Newborn Children* (Cowansville: Brown Legal Publications, 1985) Chapter Three; etc.
12. CMA Policy Summary, "Induced Abortion".
13. For an extended discussion, see Edward E. Keyserlingk, "The Unborn Child's Right to Prenatal Care," *Health Law in Canada* 3:1 (1987) 10-21. See also Law Reform Commission, Working Paper 58, *Crimes Against the Foetus* (Law Reform Commission of Canada: Ottawa, 1989), pp. 50 ff., "A New Foetus Title" 1. Foetal Destruction or Harm:

    (1) Everyone commits a crime who

(a) purposely, recklessly or negligently causes destruction or serious harm to a foetus; or

(b) being a pregnant woman, purposely causes destruction or serious harm to her foetus by any act or by failing to make reasonable provision for assistance in respect of delivery.

The Committee differs from the Commission in that it believes that provision against causing harm should take into account the difference between a foetus that is intended or expected to go to term and a foetus where the opposite is expected or intended.

14. Cf. Law Reform Commission of Canada, Working Paper 46 *Omission, Negligence and Endangering* (Law Reform Commission of Canada: Ottawa, 1985). See also Working Paper 45, *Secondary Liability — Participation in Crime and Inchoate Offenses* (Law Reform Commission of Canada: Ottawa, 1985). See also E.-H.W. Kluge, *The Ethics of Deliberate Death* (Port Washington N.Y. & London: National University Publications, 1981) pp. 12-13.

15. See Law Reform Commission, Working Paper 58, "A New Foetus Title."

16. See The American College of Obstetricians and Gynecologists, Committee on Ethics, "Patient Choice: Maternal-Fetal Conflict," *WHI* 1:1 (Fall, 1990) 13-15.

17. There has been an increase in court cases dealing with emergency requests for non-consensual Caesarean sections. The various jurisdictions have split on whether such sections are legally allowable. However, the Committee sees a danger in equating what is ethical with what is legal. It does not believe that the law is necessarily an appropriate guide to what is or should be ethical behaviour. As an example, the Committee would point to the sterilization laws that were lately repealed by the various provinces, or the laws that declared women and children nonpersons. For a contrary view to the one expressed above, see George J. Annas, "Pregnant Women as Fetal Containers," *Hastings Center Report* 16:6 (December, 1986) 13-14.

18. It should be noted that Recommendation 12 does not constitute a novelty in the Canadian context. There are several Canadian court decisions that deal with the issue consideration. [e.g., *Re Children's Aid Society of City of Belleville, Hastings Country and T et al.*]

R. v. Green

. . .

In this case the issue of when death, as an event, occurs is raised in the evidence by the statements of the Accused Green who told police that Roche Charles Frie, the person named in the indictment, was already dead when he "pumped two bullets into him".

The evidence establishes that three bullets were fired into the head of Mr. Frie. All three individually were fatal wounds in the sense that no amount of treatment could have saved Mr. Frie's life if any one — and only one — had been inflicted alone. As I understand the evidence all three bullets severely damaged the base of the brain and/or the brain stem from which the respiratory function is controlled. As a consequence with the first shot fired, whichever one it was, Mr. Frie likely ceased breathing. The evidence however is also capable of supporting the conclusion that his heart would have continued to beat for anywhere from three to five minutes after the first shot. The opinion of Dr. Currie to this effect is supported by his finding that all three bullet tracks showed evidence of arterial bleeding, a phenomena which can only occur as long as the heart beats.

On the evidence as a whole it is open to the jury to conclude that Harrison fired the first shot to the top of Mr. Frie's head and that Green then, sometime thereafter, fired two more shots to the left side of Mr. Frie's head — one through and the other behind his ear. If Mr. Frie was already dead when the first of these two shots was fired then Green cannot be convicted of murder except by virtue of the application of Section 21(1), which the Crown relies upon in its theory that Green aided and abetted Harrison in the killing. Thus it becomes crucial for the jury to know, as a matter of law, when death can be said to occur.

Mr. Brunear urges me to accept the wisdom of both the medical profession and the Law Reform Commission on this subject and to instruct the jury that death takes place when a person becomes brain dead in the medical sense of that term. Mr. Van Alstine argues that the traditional approach to the question should prevail, namely that life continues until all vital functions of the human body have ceased to operate.

In recent years the medical profession has been concerned with this question for obvious reasons. As the miracle of human transplants has become almost routine the need for live donors of organs has grown. The moral or ethical implications not to mention the legal consequences of removing vital organs from one not yet dead in order to save the life of another, who but for such help must die, have troubled doctors, lawyers, philosophers and theologians alike.

The Law Reform Commission, in its report on the criteria for the determination of death, has sought to address this specific problem and has proposed a legislative definition of when death occurs, based on the best advice and assistance it has been able to receive from all interested groups. That proposal — and it is nothing more than that — emphasizes brain function as the criterion by which death

---

R. v. Green. Vernon Registry No. 18024 [1988] B.C.J. No. 1807

is determined. Thus the common expression "brain dead" which was bandied about during the cross-examination of Dr. Currie. From the evidence it would appear that the medical profession considers a person to be brain dead when 24 hours of continuous EEG monitoring produces no sign of any brain activity whereas the Law Reform Commission proposes that the "irreversible cessation of brain function be determined by the prolonged absence of spontaneous circulatory and respiratory function."

As I have said both the medical profession and the Law Reform Commission are principally concerned with the moral and legal issues arising out of artificially sustained life and human transplant procedures. The legal issues raised are approached from what is primarily a civil law point of view — in other words the administration of the criminal law does not appear to have been of paramount concern in the approach taken by either group.

The suggestion that brain death or the irreversible cessation of brain function be the legal standard for determining when death occurs may be suitable in the medical context and even in the civil law context, but in my view it is a completely impractical standard to apply in the criminal law. The present case is a good example of why it is not feasible to apply such a concept to the criminal law. If the onus is on the Crown to satisfy this jury beyond a reasonable doubt that Mr. Frie was still alive — that is to say that his brain function had not yet irreversibly ceased — when the Accused Green "pumped" two bullets into him, it can be seen that such an onus would be impossible to discharge — unless someone had happened along with an EEG monitor and applied same to Mr. Frie either before or immediately after the two shots allegedly fired by Green.

On the face of it I see no reason why the same legal definition of death must be applied in both a civil and a criminal context. Indeed there are good reasons why the same criteria should not apply. The criminal law seeks to deter the incidence of, inter alia, violent crime by holding accountable those whose conduct endangers the lives and safety of others. The civil law, in the context under discussion, seeks to ensure that societies' moral and personal values are not compromised in the pursuit of bona fide efforts to prolong or save meaningful life.

In *Regina versus Kitching and Adams* (1976) ... the Manitoba Court of Appeal considered the issue from the opposite perspective. There the accused, who were convicted of manslaughter, caused serious injury to the deceased who thereafter was kept alive artificially until his kidneys were removed for transplant purposes at which point the life support system was disconnected and he died. The issue in that case was the cause of death — not when death occurred. The Court of Appeal, therefore, did not have to deal with the issue before me. ...

In my view the criminal law should, whenever possible, strive for certainty and simplicity in its approach to such definitional problems. The traditional criterion described by Mister Justice O'Sullivan has both virtues:

> Traditionally, both law and medicine have been unanimous in saying that it is not safe to pronounce a man dead until after his vital functions have ceased to operate. The heart has always been regarded as a vital organ.

I adopt that traditional approach in this case. I propose to tell this jury that as a matter of law Mr. Frie was alive so long as any of his vital organs — which would include his heart — continued to operate. It will, of course, be for them to decide, on the evidence, whether any of Rocky Frie's vital organs continued to function after the first shot was fired into his head. If they conclude that no vital organs continued to function after the first shot, or if they are left with a reasonable doubt on that issue then they must give the Accused Green the benefit of that doubt and conclude that Mr. Frie was dead before the second and third shots were fired.

R. v. Kitching and Adams

Matas J.A. (dissenting in part) (Monnin J.A. concurring): — The appellants, Adams and Kitching, were charged with causing the death of D. G. Junor by means of an unlawful act, thereby committing manslaughter. They were convicted on the charge after a trial before Hunt J. and a jury, and were sentenced to penitentiary for five years and four years respectively. This is an appeal from conviction and sentence.

Around midnight, 23rd July 1975, Junor was seen at the Vibrations Discotheque, a bar attached to the St. Charles Hotel in Winnipeg. Junor ordered a drink, and shortly after was seen sitting in a chair with his feet up on another chair, his head slouched forward and his chin resting on his chest. (It became known later that Junor had a blood alcohol reading of 267 milligrams per 100 millilitres of blood.) One of the waiters employed at the Vibrations tried to rouse him but was unsuccessful.

Within a few minutes Junor was taken outside by two men and dropped onto the concrete sidewalk. A cab driver stationed near the hotel saw the manoeuvre and said that when Junor was dropped, his face hit the sidewalk, making a sound which was described as: "A. Just a squishy sound, like, say a tomato hitting against concrete."

...

An ambulance was called. On arrival, the ambulance attendant examined Junor, did not detect any sign of life and tried resuscitative procedures. Junor was taken to the Health Sciences Centre, with the procedures being continued. On arrival at the hospital, shortly after 1:00 a.m. on 24th July, Junor was examined by Dr. Donan, the resident in charge of the intensive care unit. Dr. Donan noted that the patient had no respiration, pulse, or activity of the heart. Seven minutes after continued resuscitative procedures, a pulse was obtained and respiration was restored. Junor was admitted to the intensive care unit. During the early morning he was attached to a respirator and to several monitoring devices.

At 7:00 a.m. on 24th July Dr. Tweed, an anaesthetist, examined Junor and found he was deeply unconscious, totally unresponsive to voice or deep painful stimulation and with no significant neurological signs. When removed from the respirator he breathed spontaneously but his breath-

R. v. Kitching and Adams (1976) 6 W.W.R. 697 (Manitoba Court of Appeal).

ing was shallow and inadequate. Dr. Tweed diagnosed a brain injury. At 11:30 p.m., the same day, Dr. Tweed found, in summary, that Junor had a complete absence of function at any level of his brain and that his outlook for recovery was hopeless.

Dr. A. J. Gomori, a neurologist, was called in as a consultant and he examined Junior in the early afternoon of 24th July and at 11:00 a.m. on 25th July. On the second examination, Dr. Gomori found that Junor was unable to breathe on his own, there was no evidence of response to external painful stimuli and there were no reflexes; Dr. Gomori could not detect any brain stem function; all of this indicated "brain death" and no chance of any recovery.

In the early afternoon of 25th July Junor suffered a cardiac arrest, which normally would have ended his life. However, Junor's bodily functions were maintained until his kidneys could be removed for transplant purposes. The purpose of maintaining the bodily functions, latterly, was to preserve Junor's organs, not his life. After removal of the kidneys the artificial respirator was turned off; the E.K.G., monitoring the heart, continued to show electrical activity for 13 minutes.

The formal death certificate was completed upon removal of the kidneys.

Dr. J. R. Taylor, a pathologist, conducted an autopsy on the morning of 26th July 1975. He said there were two major findings: two hairline fractures of the base of the skull and extensive degenerative changes within the brain itself. The injuries to the skull and brain were consistent with a fall. According to Dr. Taylor, the principal injury was "the brain lesion, the total and absolute death of the brain". Dr. Taylor summarized his findings as follows:

> Well, as I have said at the time of autopsy I found several things. He had an absence of kidneys for one thing. Incidently he had evidence of highly bronchial pneumonia. Thirdly, he had, and most significantly to my mind he had evidence of severe and irreversible brain injury at the time of death. How that injury came about can be interpreted in one of two ways. At least, but primarily it was I think due to a blow which was sufficient to crack his skull. It was sufficient to produce subarachnoid hemorrhage, and it might, but I can't prove this, it might have been sufficient at the time to have damaged this man's brain. It could have damaged the hypothalamus, or some other part of the brain. At the time of autopsy all I can suggest is one of two pathways of this finding of the final condition of the brain. Either it was caused at the time of the initial injury or the death of the brain was a result of a sequence of events starting with the injury and the brain swelling, compression of blood vessels, and from the compression of the blood vessels to the death of the brain, with the same final end result. At the time of autopsy it is not possible to say when or which pathway this man took. I think it would require other evidence of the state of his nervous system, the function especially of his hypothalamus at the time that he was admitted, to be able to elucidate and at this point I cannot expand on that factor.

The jury heard detailed evidence from all the doctors who were called by the Crown on the several tests given Junor and his progressive medical condition; as well, there was an exhaustive exploration of the difficult criteria for determining death and the basis for use of those criteria.

Adams' notice of appeal listed 28 grounds of alleged error and Kitching's notice of appeal set out 22 grounds. I will deal only with those points which, in my view, warrant comment; since there is an element of duplication, the grounds will be considered in groups.

...

5. There were a series of objections made to the summing up with respect to ss. 207 to 209 of the Criminal Code, R.S.C. 1970, c. C-34, dealing with questions of death which might have been prevented, death from treatment of injury and acceleration of death. It was part of appellants' case that it was something which the doctors had done, or omitted to do, arising from the kidney transplant, which brought about the death of Junor. In my view, the argument is without merit.

The question of the cause of death was left to the jury for their decision. They obviously decided, after weighing all the evidence, including the extensive medical testimony, and the judge's charge, that Junor had died as a result of acts of appellants. In my view, the learned trial judge, if anything, gave more credence than was warranted to the defence that death was caused by the doctors, in respect of the transplant.

O'Sullivan J.A.: — Counsel for the accused argued that their clients should not be convicted of manslaughter because there was a possibility on the evidence that the deceased, Mr. Junor, was killed not as a result of the acts of the accused, but as a result of the acts of doctors at Health Sciences Centre in Winnipeg, who removed the deceased's kidneys and shut off a life-supporting ventilator.

The actions of the accused took place on 24th July 1975 about 1:00 a.m., when Mr. Junor was dropped on the sidewalk while being taken out of the Vibrations.

On 25th July 1975, at about 1:00 p.m., the deceased's heart was beating spontaneously and his lungs were breathing with the help of a ventilator.

At that time the deceased's body was taken to an operating room and both kidneys were removed for potential transplantation.

About 2:10 p.m., following removal of the kidneys, the ventilator was shut off. The heart continued to beat on its own for 13 minutes. Then the heart stopped beating.

It was only after the kidneys were removed that Dr. W. A. Tweed certified the death of Mr. Junor. No one at Health Sciences Centre had pronounced him dead before the removal of the kidneys.

The contentions of counsel raise far-reaching questions of law relating to death, its definition, and the time of death.

By traditional criteria, there is no question that Mr. Junor was alive when his kidneys were removed. Traditionally, both law and medicine have been unanimous in saying that it is not safe to pronounce a man dead until after his vital functions have ceased to operate. The heart has always been regarded as a vital organ.

Since the introduction of organ transplantation, however, many physicians and moralists have sought to establish new and different criteria for determining the time and the fact of death.

It is apparent that the fresher the kidneys, the better chance the recipient will have. It is apparent that in the case of a heart transplant there is no use transplanting a dead heart. The heart must be alive if the recipient of it is to have any chance of life. The problem facing medicine and society in recent years is: How do you get a living heart out of a dead body? If a person is not dead until after his heart ceases to function, it is practically impossible to imagine a successful heart transplant except by taking a living heart out of a still living person. But this is abhorrent to the conscience of many people.

So a substantial body of medical opinion has come forward with the suggestion that the concept of death itself should be redefined.

Some have said, if a man is "as good as dead", we will call him "dead" and then there will be no ethical problem about taking out his vital organs.

Some doctors have said that a person is as good as dead, and is therefore dead, if he is in such a condition that it can be predicted with confidence that he will never again be able to be restored to meaningful life.

Others have advanced the proposition that death is not an event but a process and when the process of death reaches a stage where a doctor is of the opinion that the process is irreversible the person should be declared dead.

Dr. Tweed advanced this view in this case before the jury and the learned trial judge appears to have adopted it for he said to the jury, "It appears that death is a process, not an event, as I stated earlier."

This is a most controversial statement, at variance with centuries of religious tradition. It is a statement vigorously disputed in many medico-legal books, for example, in Grey's *Attorney's Textbook of Medicine*, (3d) 1975 (Supp.), vol. 1B, para. 29.11. Religion has taught us that death is an event. Dying may be process, but death is an event. Except for some small sects, such as those in Rumania, who believe that death is a process during which the soul is in a state of suspended animation (hence, perhaps residing in vampire bats), the overwhelming weight of religious teaching all over the world is that the moment of death occurs when the soul leaves the body. This is true not only of Christians, who believe in the personal immortality of the individual soul and the immediacy of judgment after death, but also of eastern religions which believe in the transmigration of souls at the moment of death.

Furthermore, by common consent, it has been held by all civilized people that no one, for however laudable a purpose, has the right to dispatch a dying man so as to hasten his death. Most moralists agree that it is not wrong to withhold extraordinary treatment to prolong the life of a dying man. It is not wrong to let him die. But directly to dispatch him by cutting out his heart or his lungs or his kidneys is contrary to every principle of civilized morality, as held by large numbers of citizens.

Another large body of medical opinion, I think the most substantial body, accepts the fact that death is an event and not a process. They say that the criteria for "defining" death are really criteria for determining the manifestations of death. It is true that the fact of death is manifested where all the vital signs, including heartbeat, have ceased. But, they say, it is equally true that the fact of death is manifested if all activity of the brain has ceased for a sufficient period of time. If the brain of a man is dead, then it is safe to say that the whole man is dead. It is the activities operated through the brain which differentiate man from an animal. If the brain is dead, he is dead.

This approach has gained widespread support not only among doctors but among moralists as well and has received legislative recognition in some states and in the Province of Manitoba.

This opinion does not proceed on the principle that if a man will surely die, then it is safe to call him already dead. It operates on the principle that, if a man's brain is dead, he is dead.

The trouble is that it is not always obvious when brain death occurs. There are well documented cases where a man's brain has shown absolutely no sign of activity for two days or more and yet he has recovered and survived. This is particularly so where a man has ingested large quantities of central nervous system depressants such as barbiturates.

There has been a great deal of debate about this subject and the debate is likely to go on for some time.

Many eminent physicians, including an ad hoc committee of doctors of Harvard University, have established certain criteria for determining brain death. Among the requirements are flat E.E.G.s taken 24 hours apart. The possibility of barbiturate consumption being excluded, they say that if there is no sign of brain activity during a 24-hour period, it is then safe to say that the brain is dead and hence that the man is dead.

In the case of the deceased, Mr. Junor, the Harvard criteria were not followed. Twenty-four hours before the kidney transplant there was evidence of brain stem activity. Neither were the criteria proposed by Cornell University doctors followed.

Faced with the difficulties inherent in establishing universally acceptable criteria for determining brain death, many doctors have said that the safe course is to have at least two doctors certify death before allowing removal of vital organs.

Thus, a world assembly on medicine held in Australia in 1968 said, "If transplantation of an organ is involved, the decision that death exists should be made by two or more physicians, and the physician determining the moment of death should in no way be immediately concerned with the performance of the transplantation."

Many hospitals have regulations requiring such certificates of death prior to removal of vital organs. According to the evidence, the Health Sciences Centre has no such protection for potential donors.

These questions are important and they may have to be considered by the courts some day. In my opinion, however, they were not properly before the court in the case before us.

The legal and ethical implications of the conduct of doctors are no doubt under constant and careful review by peer review committees, by the Colleges of Physicians and Surgeons, and by others.

I think it is regrettable that the doctors at Health Sciences Centre were subjected to the lengthy questioning in this case. I do not think that the trial in this case, or in cases similar to it, affords a suitable forum for discussing these important questions.

I think that counsel for the accused proceeded on a fundamental misconception of the law. They assumed that, if it could be shown that death resulted in this case from the removal of the kidneys, then the accused should be acquitted because there would be a reasonable doubt that they had been the cause of death.

The assumption underlying counsel's conduct in this case is that there can be only one cause of death. I think the law is that the conduct of a defendant in a criminal trial need not be shown to be the sole or "the effective" cause of a crime. It is sufficient if it is a cause.

Sections 207 to 209 of the Criminal Code, R.S.C. 1970, c. C-34, extend liability in certain cases; they do not affect the principle that it is not necessary to prove that a criminal is the sole cause of his crime.

The law is discussed on this subject in 11 Hals. (4th) at paras. 8 and 1156. The statements in the latter paragraph must be read with the qualifications raised by Lord Widgery C.J. in *Regina v. Cato,* [1976] 1 All E.R. 260.

I think the authorities are clear that there may be two or more independent operative causes of death.

Without in this case criticizing the doctors of Health Sciences Centre or suggesting that they were guilty of any improper conduct, I am of the opinion that their conduct was irrelevant to the questions before the jury. Even if it could be shown that the actions of the doctors constituted an operative cause of Mr. Junor's death — and I emphasize that I do not suggest that the evidence would support such a conclusion — still that would not exonerate the accused unless the evidence left a reasonable doubt that the accused's actions also constituted an operative cause of the deceased's death.

On that question, the evidence was overwhelming. Whether or not the kidneys had been removed, the deceased could not have lasted more than a short period of time even with artificial assistance.

The jury had to decide not whether the doctors were ethical or not but simply, did the accused cause the death of the deceased by unlawful means? The question of causation was put to the jury plainly; they decided that the accused did cause the death. The evidence was overwhelmingly in favour of their verdict.

On the matters raised by defence counsel on the subject of conviction, I am in substantial agreement with the reasons of my brother Matas.

I would not say, however, that the learned trial judge answered the jury's question satisfactorily. Although he said that criminal negligence was not the jury's major problem, it is obvious, I think, that the jury had directed its mind toward the possibility of finding the accused liable on the basis of their criminal negligence. I think the trial judge left the jury with the impression that they could convict the accused of manslaughter if they concluded that the accused caused death not by unlawful act but by criminal negligence.

The accused were acting in the course of a duty. Their actions amounted to the unlawful act of assault only if they used more force than was reasonably necessary.

A wanton and reckless disregard for the deceased's safety might have made the accused guilty of manslaughter by criminal negligence but they were not charged with that.

Had the charge been worded suitably, this distinction would not have been material. But the Crown chose to charge only manslaughter by unlawful act. Why the Crown did so we do not know. But the Crown is bound by the charge it brings. Otherwise the accused might be convicted of that of which they have had no proper notice.

Nevertheless, I am prepared to apply the provisions of s. 613(1)(*b*)(iii) because I am satisfied that the jury could not, as reasonable men, have done otherwise than find the accused guilty of manslaughter by unlawful act.

...

Does Anyone Survive Neocortical Death?

Roland Puccetti

A person is dead when an irreversible cessation of all that person's brain functions has occurred. The cessation of brain functions can be determined by the prolonged absence of spontaneous cardiac and respiratory functions.

Law Reform Commission of Canada Working Paper 23 (1979, pp. 58-59)

An individual with irreversible cessation of all functions of the entire brain, including the brain stem, is dead.

Defining Death, President's Commission ([15], p. 162)

One day on a very cold morning, I started the engine of my car without opening the garage door, then retreated to the kitchen to let it warm up. At that moment there was a long distance phone call from my publisher, and I spent a half hour haggling over the terms of a contract. Upon returning to the garage I found there, alongside the car, my dog Fido. Of course I immediately opened the automatic door and carried him outside into the fresh air. When I saw he wasn't breathing I pressed rhythmically on his chest cavity, and sure enough his heart and lungs started to respond. But still he did not wake up, so I took him to the vet's on the way to the university. The vet said Fido appeared to be comatose as a result of carbon monoxide poisoning, and advised that I prepare myself for the worst. He said it seemed the dog would not recover consciousness because the top of the brain was destroyed, although the brain stem must be intact, since Fido could breathe unaided. What should I do?

Now suppose I told you that I did the following. I took Fido home, made a special bed for him, shaved his body and fitted him with diapers, learned to feed him intravenously and nasogastrically, and arranged to have him turned in his bed often so he would not develop pressure sores. Evenings I would watch TV alongside Fido, stroking his warm body and listening to his breathing, though never again did he go for a walk with me, fetch the newspaper, bark, or do anything dogs normally do.[1] Would you think I am a rational person? Or worse, suppose I asked the vet to put Fido down for me and he replied that he couldn't do that to a comatose canine capable of spontaneous breathing, *because the law forbade it.* Would you think this a rational society?

If your answers to those questions are, as I think they would be, resoundingly negative, then presumably the main reason for your negative response is simply that my ministrations would do *no good* for Fido, who has permanently lost consciousness even if he is nonapneic; for the same reason, *no harm* can be done to him by stopping his breathing. In other words, a permanently unconscious dog is, for all practical purposes, a dead dog anyway.

Now change the above apocryphal story in just one detail. Instead of it being Fido on the garage floor, it is my neighbor's infant son, little Bobby. I rush him to a children's hospital, but with the same result. Now could what was agreed to be irrational

Roland Pucetti, "Does Anyone Survive Neocortical Death?" in Richard M. Zaner, ed., *Death: Beyond Whole-Brain Criteria.* Dordrecht: Kluwer Academic Publishers, 1988 pp. 75-90.

behavior in Fido's case become rational in Bobby's case? That a human life is much more valuable and worth preserving at all costs is completely irrelevant, since we agreed before that the main consideration was simply that one can do neither good nor harm to an irreversibly comatose being, and that should hold true independently of his species identity.

Yet, and this is what I find amazing, a great number of otherwise very able people in the legal and health professions think just the opposite. But before we examine their arguments, let us get one point absolutely straight. No matter what your calling, any position you adopt on this issue is going to be a *philosophical* stand. For the question we are addressing here is quintessentially philosophical: namely, *what constitutes* (in this world anyway, to avoid begging religious questions) *personal death?* This does not mean a poll of professional philosophers will settle the matter, for by that standard the Earth must have been flat in the Middle Ages, before it became spherical again in the Renaissance. Nevertheless, you cannot offer argument as to when a person may be safely considered dead without doing philosophy. The question, of course, is whether you are doing philosophy well or badly. I begin with an example of what I consider bad philosophizing on this subject.

I. WALTON ON CEREBRAL VS. ENCEPHALIC DEATH

In his recent book [17], Douglas N. Walton asks why proponents of the cerebral or neocortical criterion of brain death are not even more selective.

> The reply (that it is the cerebrum which mediates cognitive activity in the brain) is still not entirely satisfactory. However, it seems equally plausible to say that mental activity of the higher cognitive sort takes place essentially in the cerebral cortex, the thin membraneous *(sic)* substance that forms a mantle over the cerebrum. Why include the lobes of the cerebrum under the cortex if lower parts of the midbrain or the cerebellum and brain stem are excluded? ... [The cerebral death advocate] might argue that it is safer to include the whole cerebrum, because there is a possibility of indeterminacy or error. But then, if tutiorism (chancing error to be on the safe side) is brought in, why not be even safer and take into account the whole-brain ([18], p. 50)?

To which one can counter: if it is better to err on the side of safety, why not wait until complete somatic death (including, e.g., cartilage cells in the knee) occurs, thereby foregoing organ transplantation? The reason cerebral death includes the lobes of the cerebrum beneath the cortical surface is that these are composed of association fibers (white matter) that interconnect neocortical motor and sensory areas (grey matter); if these are selectively destroyed (e.g., in asphyxiation), the result is a shattered self with isolated conscious functions [5]. If, on the other hand, the neocortical surface is itself selectively destroyed, which as we shall see is the case with apallic syndrome, that is sufficient to obliterate all conscious functions.

The case for excluding other subcortical structures mentioned by Walton in passing has nothing at all to do with tutiorism anyway. The midbrain is of course just the top of the brain stem, where the superior and inferior colliculi trigger orientating reflexes related, respectively, to sources of visual and auditory stimuli: such reflexive responses do not require conscious mediation, as we all know from finding ourselves turned towards an abrupt movement in the peripheral visual field, or in the direction of a sudden sound, before such stimuli register in consciousness. If a brain structure does its job unconsciously, then there is no reason to think its integrity in a comatose patient is evidence of residual conscious functions. Similarly with the cerebellum, which preorchestrates complex bodily movements, and under therapeutic electrode stimulation does not yield clear sensations [3]. The cerebellum probably also stores learned subroutines of behavior, like swimming or typing: precisely the kinds of things you do better when not concentrating on them. Why then is it necessary for the cerebellum to be dead in order to have a dead person on your hands?

Yet Walton seems to think that everything above the level of C^1 directly contributes to a conscious mental life. His attitude seems to be that if something moves, it must or at least might have a life of its own, with its own kind of feeling. For example, of the pupillary reflex mediated by the lower brain stem he says:

> The pupillary reflex could, for all we know, indicate some presence of feeling or sensation even if the higher cognitive faculties are absent. Even if we cannot resolve the issue with the precision we would like and, indeed, just because of that, we should be on the safe side ... Following my tutiorist line of argument, it is clear that we cannot rule out the possibility that brain stem reflexes could indicate some form of sensation or feeling, even if higher mental activity is not present ([18], p. 69).

The statement fairly reeks of superstition. As we all know, when the doctor flashes his penlight on the eye, we do not feel the pupil contract, then expand again when he turns the light off. If not, then why in the world does Walton suppose that a deeply comatose patient feels anything in the same testing situation? The whole point of evolving reflexes like this, especially in large brained animals that do little peripheral but lots of central information processing, is to shunt quick-response mechanisms away from the cerebrum so that the animal can make appropriate initial responses to stimuli *before* registering them consciously. If one could keep an excised human eye alive *in vitro* and provoke the pupillary reflex, the way slices of rat hippocampus have been stimulated to threshold for neuronal excitation, would Walton argue that the isolated *eye* might feel something as its pupil contracts?[2]

Apparently he would, since in his view the entire encephalon must be safely dead to justify a finding of personal death. The spinal cord, he agrees, presents no obstacle to a determination of death, because of the relative sparsity of its neurons and its accessibility to tactile stimuli exclusively. I quote:

> The upshot is that brain death should include the whole-brain but nothing more. I would add that specially if we emphasize the element of reflective selfconsciousness or awareness ... the tactile stimuli accessible from the spinal cord need not be thought significant if, in the absence of a brain, there is no possibility of awareness of these stimuli. The presence of a tactile reflex by itself need not indicate mental activity or consciousness ([18], p. 75).

But what is sauce for the goose is sauce for the gander. Why does a pinprick in the foot or hand, provoking a withdrawal reflex in that limb because of residual electrical activity in the spinal arc nerve pathways, count as a tactile sensation in the case of a cerebrally dead patient, but not in the case of an encephalically dead one? For consider: there is no such thing as a non-localized tactile sensation; to the question, "Where did the accused touch you on your person?" there always is and must be a fairly specific answer. Even a statement like "I felt the spring sun warm my body all over, like a gentle kiss," is in a sense localized: it refers to all the skin surface on one side of the body, that facing the sun. Now what brain mechanism localizes sensations of touch? Surely it is the somatosensory strip posterior to the Rolandic fissure in both cerebral hemispheres (Brodmann's area 3), which is clearly gone in the cerebrally dead patient. No localization, no tactile sensation: thus Walton's unconcern for spinal cord-mediated nerve impulses from the skin surface is logically extendable to the entire subcortical architecture of the brain.

Walton nevertheless expresses deep puzzlement over this matter, and in fact at times comes perilously close to committing the Fallacy of Ad Ignorantium. For example, wondering whether perception or awareness might not occur in the absence of higher cognitive functions, he writes:

> It is hard to know how to define exactly what is meant by "higher cognitive faculties," so it is hard to be sure that we mean by this phrase something that definitely excludes all types of perception that might persist in deeper parts of the brain ([18], pp. 75-76).

But surely ignorance of whether a statement is true does not imply that we know it is false; the admitted complexity of the human brain does not carry with it the imputation that we cannot say *some* things about it with confidence. One thing I feel reasonably confident in stating is that sensations are not experienced without recruitment of populations of neurons in the grey matter on the cerebral cortical surface. And it is easy to see why this is so: the phylogenetic novelty of *neo*cortex is due to brain expansion in primates beginning about 50 million years ago to accommodate increasing intelligence, for where else could new cell layers appear but on the outer surface of the brain [9]? That being the case, sensation migrated there as well, and although deeper structures certainly contribute complexly to the sentient input, this is not transduced as sensation until, at a minimum, some 10^4 neurons are provoked to discharge on the surface of at least one cerebral hemisphere at the same time [16]. It is also plain why the contribution of subcortical mechanisms to this input does not itself implicate conscious perception. If it did, we would have sensations in *seriatum:* a baseball leaving the pitcher's hand would be seen as arriving by the hitter several times in succession as neural impulses course from retina to optic chiasm to geniculate body through the optic radiation to primary visual cortex in the occipital lobe. From an evolutionary viewpoint, that would be a recipe for disaster.

Walton makes the claim that, to be on the safe side, "we should presume that the whole-brain is required to produce mental activity" ([18], p. 74). Normally, of course, that is true, but from this it would hardly follow that, when the ultimate neuronal destination of neural input is no longer there, or is dead, sensations still occur. We can liken this proposal to having an express elevator that whisks passengers from the ground floor to executive offices on the top floor. If a nuclear strike blows off the top floor, it would be unreasonable to suppose that you could nevertheless conduct your business at still-standing intermediate floors. What Walton is doing is confusing the normally necessary contribution of subcortical mechanisms to sensation with the sufficient condition of neocortical functions. In the case of the primary visual system in man this is indisputable: destruction of Brodmann's area 17 alone, say by shrapnel wounds, brings permanent total blindness [7]; whereas a peripherally blind person with intact visual cortex can be induced to experience visual sensations by direct electrode stimulation of that grey matter [2].

Probably the sensation we worry most about in irreversibly comatose patients is *pain*. Now Walton may know that depth electrode stimulation intended to relieve intractable "central" or "thalamic" pain (where the pain is not localized at all), indicates that there are discrete "pain centers" in the thalami [14, 17], and these are certainly subcortical structures that could survive neocortical death. Would this fact not tend to show that such patients might nevertheless experience pain, in line with Walton's tutioristic cautions?

Such a suggestion would be, I think, doubly wrong. It is wrong, first, because it incorporates an excessively *homuncular* view of the relation between brain structures and conscious experience. The "little men in the thalami getting pain messages" picture is absurd: it is *we* who get the pains, not those structures. And it is wrong, secondly, because if the firing of thalamic pain centers by itself gave rise to pain experience, then it surely follows that if we could excise this tissue, keep it alive *in vitro,* stimulate it electrically to threshold for discharge and record the neurons' discharging, we would have to say that there is pain going on *in the vat!* Anyone who would believe this is beyond reason.

II. PEOPLE AS BRAIN STEMS

I want now to consider a specific case of neocortical death without brain stem death, in order to show the utter futility of acting on the stand Walton defends. There are many cases like this one, and in some somatic survival subsequent to cerebral destruction far surpasses the present case.[3] Nevertheless, the case history here is remarkably complete. I give it *in extenso* so that I cannot be accused of glossing over some crucial fact [8].

> *Case 8.* The patient (Th. Sv.) was a female who had been born in 1936. In July 1960, at the age of 24, she suffered severe eclampsia during pregnancy with serial epileptic attacks, followed by deep coma and transient respiratory and circulatory failure. In the acute phase, Babinski signs were present bilaterally and there was a transitory absence of pupillary, corneal and spinal reflexes. A left-sided carotid angiogram showed a slow passage of contrast medium and signs of brain edema. An EEG taken during the acute phase did not reveal any electrical activity. The EEG remained isoelectric for the rest of the survival time (seventeen years). After the first three to four months the patient's state became stable with complete absence of all higher functions.
>
> Examination ten years after the initial anoxic episode showed the patient lying supine, motionless, and with closed eyes. Respiration was spontaneous, regular and slow with a tracheal cannula. The pulse was regular. The systolic blood pressure was 75-100 mm. Hg. Severe flexion contractures had developed in all extremities. Stimulation with acoustic signals, touch or pain gave rise to primitive arousal reactions including eye-opening, rhythmic movement of the extremities, chewing and swallowing, and withdrawal reflexes. The corneal reflex was present on the left side. When testing was done on the right side, transient

horizontal nystagmus movements were elicited. Pupillary reflexes were present and normal on both sides. On passive movements of the head, typical vestibulo-ocular reflexes were elicited. The spinal reflexes were symmetrical and hyperactive. Patellar clonus was present bilaterally. Divergent strabismus was found when the eyes were opened (by the examiner). Measurement of the regional cerebral blood flow on the left side (ten years after the initial anoxic episode) showed a very low mean hemisphere flow of 9 ml/100g/min. The distribution of the flow was also abnormal, high values being found over the brain stem. The patient's condition remained essentially unchanged for seven more years and she died seventeen years after the anoxic episode after repeated periods of pulmonary edema.

Autopsy showed a highly atrophic brain weighing only 315 grams. The hemispheres were especially atrophied and they were in general transformed into thin-walled yellow-brown bags. The brain stem and cerebellum were sclerotic and shrunken. On the basal aspect some smaller parts of preserved cortex could be seen, mainly in the region of the unci. Microscopically the cerebral cortex was almost totally destroyed with some remnants of a thin gliotic layer and underneath a microcystic spongy tissue with microphages containing iron pigment. The basal ganglia were severely destroyed, whereas less advanced destruction was found in the subfrontal basal cortex, the subcallosal gyrus, the unci, the thalamus and hypothalamus, and in the subicular and entorhinal areas. In the cerebellum the Purkinji cells had almost completely disappeared and were replaced by glial cells. The granular layer was partly destroyed. The cerebellar white matter was partly demyelinated. In the brain stem some neurons had disappeared and a diffuse gliosis was found. Several cranial nuclei remained spared. The long sensory and motor tracts were completely demyelinated and gliotic, whereas transverse pontine tracts remained well myelinated ([8], pp. 196-198).

This clinical picture, confirmed by the autopsy findings, is known in the literature as "neocortical death without brain stem death," or more recently and appropriately, as "the apallic syndrome," for its characteristic feature is precisely destruction of the paleum, that cortical mantle of grey matter covering the surface of the cerebrum or telencephalon. As it happens, neurons composing the paleum are the most vulnerable to oxygen deprivation during transient cardiac arrest or, as in the above case, asphyxiation. Whereas in encephalic or whole-brain death, therefore including the brain stem that monitors respiration (which in turn provokes cardiac activity), the patient can be sustained on a ventilator for only up to a week in adults and two weeks in children before cardiac standstill, the apallic patient breathes spontaneously and demonstrates cephalic reflexes (also brain stem mediated), so that if fed nasogastrically or intravenously and kept free from infection, he or she can sustain somatic life for years or even decades after losing the top of the brain.

I said "somatic life," for without a paleum the basis for a conscious and hence a personal life in this world is gone forever. But then what are we doing supplying intensive care to apallic syndrome patients? For surely the quality of life in a patient like Th.Sv. during all those seventeen years differed not one jot from the quality of life of someone buried underground for seventeen years. It was zero. Permanent unconsciousness is permanent unconsciousness whether the condition is associated with a body that lives by virtue of being able to breathe spontaneously or not. To deny this is to elevate spontaneous breathing to a principle of human life, something I find incredible. Yet this is actually the emerging consensus of the medico-legal community in North America, as indicated by my earlier quotations from the Reform Commission's Report in Canada for 1979, and the U.S. President's Commission's Report of 1981. Are there any good arguments to support this astonishing attitude?

The President's Commission goes out of its way to justify regarding a whole-brain dead person sustained on a respirator as a dead person whose organs are therefore freely transplantable, whereas cerebrally dead persons are still to be considered alive and requiring heroic maintenance procedures. Listen to this passage:

> While the respirator and its associated medical techniques do substitute for the functions of the intercostal muscles and the diaphragm, which without neuronal stimulation from the brain cannot function spontaneously, they cannot replace the myriad functions of the brain stem or of the rest of the brain. The startling contrast between bodies lacking *all* brain functions and patients with intact brain stems (despite severe neocortical damage) manifests this. The former lie with fixed pupils, motionless except for the chest movements produced by their respirators. The latter can not only breathe, metabolize, maintain temperature and blood pressure, and so forth, *on their own* but also sigh, yawn, track light with the eyes, and react to pain or reflex stimulation ([15], p. 35).

One is tempted to cry out: *So what?* I can not only breathe, metabolize, maintain temperature and blood pressure, *on my own,* but also sigh, yawn, and react to reflex stimulation (such as the patellar reflex) when in a deep, dreamless sleep. Admittedly I cannot track light with my eyes, or react to pinprick in the foot, without awakening, but that is because, with an intact reticular formation and intact primary visual system, the light I am tracking causes visual sensations, and with an intact somatosensory strip pinprick in the foot wakes me up because I feel it as such. The apallic syndrome patient *can* do both these things without awakening, of course, because those neocortical structures are permanently missing. In fact, he or she cannot do *anything* consciously anymore, because there is no one home in that head to wake up.[4]

This consideration seems to make no difference to members of the President's Commission, who then go on to say:

> It is not easy to discern precisely what it is about patients in this latter group that makes them alive while those in the other category are not. It is in part that in the case of the first category (i.e., absence of all brain functions) when the mask created by the artificial medical support is stripped away what remains is not an integrated organism but "merely a group of artificially maintained subsystems." Sometimes, of course, an artificial substitute can forge the link that restores the organism as a whole to unified functioning. Heart or kidney transplants, kidney dialysis, or an iron lung used to replace physically-impaired breathing ability in a polio victim, for example, restore the integrated functioning of the organism as they replace the failed function of a part. Contrast such

> situations, however, with the hypothetical of a decapitated body treated so as to prevent the outpouring of blood and to generate respiration: continuation of bodily functions in that case would not have restored the requisites of human life ([15], pp. 35-36).

But what *are* the requisites of human life according to the President's Commission? Evidently they are the ability to breathe spontaneously, demonstrate cephalic reflexes, regulate body temperature, metabolism, and blood pressure, etc.: in other words, *to perform unaided the janitorial functions of the Central Nervous System, which requires no conscious direction or reflection whatsoever.* Thus by the standards of the Commission, a hypothetical decapitated human body treated so as to prevent the outpouring of blood, but with brain stem left intact so that these janitorial functions are performed unaided, qualifies as a live person with all the requisites of human life, whereas if someone lops off the stem and substitutes a mechanical respirator in its place, the patient becomes a dead person thereby. Again, what is the difference in quality of life, or even prospects for the quality of life, in the two cases? And again the answer seems undeniable: none whatever.

To sum up: either human life is rooted in brain stem function or it is rooted in the capacity for personal experience. If the former, then all vertebrate species are on an equal footing and what counts in medical ethics is just long-term organic functioning independently of our capacity to intervene. If the latter, then there is no ethically relevant difference in the status of encephalically and cerebrally dead people: they have both lost the neocortical basis of an ongoing personal life. The only surprising fact to come out of the apallic syndrome is, or should be, that corpses are really of two kinds: the vast majority that cannot breathe unaided, and a small minority that nevertheless can do this. Apneic or nonapneic, a corpse is still a corpse.

III. THE DIAGNOSTIC PROBLEM

In a still more recent writing Walton [19] returns to defense of the whole-brain criterion of death. He begins by restating his earlier scepticism about our ability to avoid negative error in diagnosis of the apallic syndrome. He says:

> However, physicians have not yet developed or tested proven, certainly safe criteria for the apallic syndrome or other so-called "vegetative states" more highly localized in dysfunction than whole-brain death. For the present, tutioristic reasoning dictates cleaving to criteria for whole-brain death ([19], p. 270).

I do not know what Walton understands by "certainly safe" criteria for diagnosis of apallic syndrome; since the practice of medicine is an empirical science, there is always room for error. However, an accumulation of diagnostic results like those given in the case of Th. Sv. seems strongly conclusive. If one can safely exclude the possibility of hypothermia or intoxication with a C.N.S. depressive, which drastically lowers oxygen requirements of the neocortex, a repeated finding of diminished cerebral blood flow, to less than 20% of normal, is itself powerful evidence of pallial destruction. In fact Lassen *et al.* [10] reported firm correlations between increases in blood flow to specific regions of the cortex of patients in the waking, conscious state when problem solving, and also a significant overall increase in blood flow to the cerebrum as a whole of about 10 per cent during such activity. It therefore seems exceedingly unlikely that any kind of conscious experience is going on in a brain with use for less than a fifth of normal blood flow.[5]

However, with the advent of Positron Emission Tomography, all reasonable grounds for doubt can be removed. In PET scanning, the uptake of oxygen and particularly glucose in selective subregions of cerebral cortex can be measured and displayed in color on a video screen: yellow or green for normal metabolic activity, blue or purple for low or no uptake. Although as of a couple years ago the PET scan had apparently not been used to confirm a diagnosis of apallic syndrome [4], nothing could be safer, easier or more certain: the entire surface of the brain would be displayed in blue or purple. While such deep subcortical structures as the brain stem itself are not visualizable using the PET scan [11], the absence of apnea is by itself evidence of the integrity of the stem. So much for Walton's concerns about negative error in diagnosing apallic syndrome.

IV. SEEDS OF DOUBT

Before leaving Walton's contrary stand on this issue, I want to reply to two further points he makes in that more recent defense of the whole-brain criterion. Neither is really very important, but they illustrate the tendency in philosophical debate to sow confusion among your opponents by almost any means at hand.

First, Walton says that even in the face of a repeated isoelectric EEG, where there is not death of the whole-brain there can be *restoration* of cortical activity through reactivation of the brain stem arousal system. The imputation, of course, is that cortical destruction may itself be reversible. Where there is breath there is always hope.[6]

But Walton refers to only one case [6]. And he does not go on to say that the patient, victim of a motorcycle fall, was treated with electrode stimulation for only 19 days following five months' akinetic mutism, gave only partial signs of arousal, and at no time recovered spontaneous motor activity, leading to abandonment of the treatment. If this patient *had* recovered consciousness, then he could not have been correctly diagnosed as a case of post-traumatic apallic syndrome, for the fact is that no one, after age 16 or so, sprouts new central neurons. The failure in this case to secure sustained arousal is indeed confirmation of post-traumatic pallial destruction, and remains, sadly, incurable.

Walton's second fresh point in the debate alludes to findings by Lober (reported in [12]), that some people recovered from infantile hydrocephaly, thus growing up with severely reduced cerebral hemispheres, can nevertheless function well: an example being that of a university student, IQ 126, who gained first class honors in mathematics. This Walton takes to be evidence that the neocortex is neither the sole seat of consciousness nor, perhaps, crucial to the return of conscious functions.

One wants to scream aloud a commonplace of clinical psychopathology: When neural plasticity enters the picture, all bets are off! The neural plasticity of the infant brain allows a lot less than the normal quantity of grey matter to take over a wide range of functions that are usually diffused in greater brain space. This is strikingly and uncontroversially demonstrated in complete hemispherectomy for infantile hemiplegia, where control of the whole body (except for distal finger movements in the arm contralateral to the missing half brain) is found in adulthood [1]. Furthermore, as Epstein has said (quoted in [12]), hydrocephalus is principally a disease of the *white* matter of the brain (the cerebral ventricles, swelled by overproduction of cerebrospinal fluid, disrupt the axons of association fibers around them). It is precisely the *sparing* of nerve cells in the grey matter, even in severe cases of hydrocephalus, that explains the retention of conscious functions and high-performance IQs.

To summarize against Walton on both these points, *for those who have a normal history of neocortical development,* the integrity of the neocortex is essential to the continuance of a mental, and hence a personal, life. It follows from this that pallial destruction is equivalent to personal demise, and this has nothing to do with a residual capacity for spontaneous respiration. Thus both the wholly brain dead and the cerebrally dead patient are dead people, and it is only superstition to make a vital dichotomy between them.

V. ETHICAL CONSIDERATIONS

Many who have followed me so far would nevertheless balk at the problem of disposing of human remains capable of breathing spontaneously. They would say that active intervention to stop the breathing prior to preparation for burial is not only presently illegal (laws can be changed, and already have, to facilitate organ harvesting), but morally murder; and it is often argued that passive (by the non-continuance of treatment) as opposed to active euthanasia is the more humane course.

Both these replies miss the point. You can stab a corpse, but you cannot *kill* it, for it is already dead whether breathing or not. If neocortical death is agreed to constitute personal death, then a firmly diagnosed apallic syndrome patient is in no better or worse situation than the encephalically dead patient sustained on a respirator, whom we all agree is dead though still breathing artificially. Similarly, "euthanasia" means "mercy killing," but one cannot be merciful to a cadaver, for cadavers are beyond pain and indeed all further experience of this world. Indeed, if it were *my* nonapneic remains causing the problem, I want to insist in advance that the breathing be stopped, for by treating my body as if *I* were still alive, hospital personnel would be stripping me of human dignity: it is enough to have others change your diapers in the first years of life.[7]

Someone might suggest that the difference between defenders of the whole-brain criterion and defenders of the neocortical standard is that they envisage different logical subjects: the former taking that to be a still living, spontaneously breathing human *body,* the latter a *mind* now gone from this world. But if this were just a verbal dispute, it ought not to matter much to the disposal problem in a more enlightened age. But in fact it does matter. Those taking the first view would have to say to enquiring relatives and friends, "He's still alive but permanently unconscious, so we're going to let him die of dehydration, starvation, or infection, whichever comes first." Whereas those taking the second view, which is my own, would logically respond in words like these: "She's dead but her body is still breathing, so we're going to stop the breathing and prepare her body for burial."

Needless to say, the latter formulation seems to me less cruel.

NOTES

1. He might, however, occasionally wag his tail. Apparently this is spinal cord mediated, as dogs coming out of anesthesia often wag their tails. I owe this suggestion to John Fentress.
2. Of course no such contraction would occur, since the pupillary reflex is brain stem mediated; the point is strictly hypothetical.
3. McWhirter gives the following case: "The longest recorded coma was that undergone by Elaine Esposito (b. Dec. 3, 1934) of Tarpon Springs, Florida. She never stirred after an appendectomy on Aug. 6, 1941, when she was 6, in Chicago, Illinois, and she died Nov. 24, 1978 aged 43 years 357 days, having been in a coma for 37 years 111 days" ([13], p. 37).
4. Conversely, selective damage to the brain stem alone can produce a similar result, for without input from the brain stem's reticular activating system, untouched neocortical cells cannot be alerted to incoming stimuli and the patient never wakes up. In the apallic syndrome the lines, so to speak, are still up but no one is home; whereas with brain stem lesions sparing cells that monitor respiration, there is someone home but permanently slumbering because the lines are down. In either case a personal life in this world has ended, so the same remarks made in the section of this paper entitled "Ethical Considerations" will apply. It is perhaps confusion of the necessary contribution of the brain stem reticular formation to achieving conscious awareness with conscious awareness itself that motivates superstitious attitudes towards the apallic syndrome.
5. D. H. Ingvar has recently reported that cerebral blood flow in apallic patients has been measured using Xenon 133 gas inhalation and 254 scintillators that monitor oxygen and glucose uptake in as many square centimeters of superficial cerebral cortex on each side of the head. The video display is uniform: dark blue or purple on the entire screen, indicating little or no uptake of blood, because "these patients have no neocortex to supply with blood" (Ingvar, in a Symposium organized by the Faculty of Medicine, University of Montreal, entitled "Two Hemispheres: One Brain," on May 18, 1984).
6. An anatomist once suggested to me that there is hope for eventual restoration of cortical activity in experiments where embryonic fetal tissue has been successfully transplanted into homologous lesioned areas of the adult rat brain. While this may be encouraging with regard to treatment of, say, expressive aphasia, I do not see how one could hope to replace an entire neocortex that way; surely the survivor of such an operation would not be the original person.
7. This point was originally supplied by a former student of mine who has nursed apallic syndrome patients (name withheld).

BIBLIOGRAPHY

1. Basser, L. S.: 1962, 'Hemiplegia of Early Onset and the Faculty of Speech with Special Reference to the Effects of Hemispherectomy', *Brain* 85, 427-460.
2. Brindley, G. A. and Lewin, W. S.: 1968, 'The Sensations Produced by Electrical Stimulation of the Visual Cortex', *Journal of Physiology 196,* 479-493.
3. Cooper, I. S. et al.: 1974, 'The Effect of Chronic Stimulation of Cerebellar Cortex on Epilepsy in Man', in I. S. Cooper, M. Riklan and R. S. Snider (eds.), *The Cerebellum, Epilepsy, and Behavior,* Plenum Press, New York and London, pp. 119-171.
4. Feindel, W.: 1982, Personal Communication.
5. Geschwind, N. et al.: 1968, 'Isolation of the Speech Area', *Neuropsychologia* 6, 327-340.
6. Hassler, R. et al.: 1969, 'Behavioural and EEG Arousal Induced by Stimulation of Unspecific Projection Systems in a Patient with Post-traumatic Apallic Syndrome', *Electroencephalography and Clinical Neurophysiology* 27, 306-310.
7. Holmes, G.: 1945, 'The Organization of the Visual Cortex in Man', *Proceedings of the Royal Society* (Biology) 132, 348-361.
8. Ingvar, D. H. et al.: 1978, 'Survival After Severe Cerebral Anoxia, with Destruction of the Cerebral Cortex: The Apallic Syndrome', *Annals of the New York Academy of Sciences* 315, 184-214.
9. Jerison, H. J.: 1973, *Evolution of the Brain and Intelligence,* Academic Press, New York and London.
10. Lassen, N. A. et al.: 1978, 'Brain Function and Blood Flow', *Scientific American* 239, 62-71.
11. LeBlanc, M.: 1983, Personal Communication.
12. Lewin, R.: 1980, 'Is Your Brain Really Necessary?', *Science* 210, 1232-1234.
13. McWhirter, N. D.: 1984, *Guinness Book of World Records,* Bantam, New York.
14. Melzack, R.: 1973, *The Puzzle of Pain,* Penguin, London.
15. President's Commission for the Study of Ethical Problems in Medicine and Biomedical and Behavioral Research: 1981, *Defining Death: Medical, Legal, and Ethical Issues in the Determination of Death,* U.S. Government Printing Office, Washington, D.C.
16. Puccetti, R.: 1981, 'The Case of Mental Duality: Evidence from Split-brain Data and Other Considerations', *The Behavioral and Brain Sciences* 4, 92-123.
17. Sem-Jacobsen, C.: 1968, *Depth-Electrographic Stimulation of the Human Brain and Behavior,* Thomas, Springfield, Illinois.
18. Walton, D. N.: 1980, *Brain Death: Ethical Considerations,* Purdue University Press, West Lafayette, Indiana.
19. Walton, D. N.: 1981, 'Epistemology of Brain Death Determination', *Metamedicine* 2, 259-274.

FURTHER READINGS

"A Definition of Irreversible Coma: Report of the Ad Hoc Committee of the Harvard Medical School to Examine the Definition of Death," *Journal of the American Medical Association* 205 (1968) 337.

Adamkiewicz, V.W.

"What are the bonds between the fetus and the uterus?" *Canadian Nurse*. 1976 Feb; 72 (2): 26-8.

Curran, W.J.

"An historical perspective on the law of personality and status with special regard to the human fetus and the rights of women." *Milbank Memorial Fund Quarterly* 1983 Winter; 61 (1): 58-75.

Gillon, R.

"Pregnancy, obstetrics and the moral status of the fetus," *Journal of Medical Ethics* 1988 Mar; 14 (1): 3-4.

Goldenring, J.M.

"The brain-life theory: towards a consistent biological definition of humanness." *Journal of Medical Ethics* 1985 Dec; 11 (4): 198-204.

Jonas, Hans

"Against the Stream: Comments on the Definition and Redefinition of Death," in T.L. Beauchamp and S. Perlin, eds., *Ethical Issues in Death and Dying* (Englewood Cliffs, N.J.: Prentice Hall, 1978) 51-59.

Justin, R.G. and Rosner, F.

"Maternal/fetal rights: two views." *Journal of the American Medical Women's Association* 1989 May-June; 44 (3): 90-5.

Kluge, E.H.

"When caesarean section operations imposed by a court are justified." *Journal of Medical Ethics* 1988 Dec; 14 (4): 206-11.

Sharpe, Gilbert S.

"Determination of Death," from G.S. Sharpe, *The Law and Medicine in Canada* (Toronto and Vancouver: Butterworths, 1987).

Strong, C. and Anderson, G.

"The moral status of the near-term fetus." *Journal of Medical Ethics* 1989 Mar; 15 (1): 25-7.

The Canadian Medical Association

"Guidelines for the Diagnosis of Brain Death. *CMAJ* 136 (January 15, 1987) 220A-B.

Theoretical Medicine 5(1984). The whole issue devoted to the definition of Death. Issue editor, D.A. Walton. 16

Tomlinson, Tom

"The Conservative Use of the Brain-Death Criterion: A Critique," *The Journal of Medicine and Philosophy* 9:4 (1984) 377-393.

Zaner, Richard M., ed.

Death: Beyond Whole-Brain (Dordsrecht and Boston: Kluwer Academic Publishers, 1988).

CHAPTER 11 EUTHANASIA

INTRODUCTION

Historically, people used to die by accident, through a disease, or simply as a result of gradual physical deterioration and old age. Most of the time, the way the death occurred had nothing formalized about it. It just happened — expectedly or otherwise — and there was not much anyone could do. Most of the time, too (accidents excepted), it occurred at home.

Modern scientific medicine and modern health care have changed all that. Death and dying have moved into the institutionalized setting of the hospital or health care facility. Consequently, death and dying have become increasingly medicalized not only in terms of the criteria that are used to determine death, but also in the sense that dying itself has become imbued with the nimbus of medical practice, and the ethos of the medical profession has tended to determine the shape a particular dying will take.

This has raised several problems. One is that the traditional ethos of the health care professions in general, and of the medical profession in particular, is to save and/or sustain life. That makes it psychologically very difficult for these professionals to allow death to occur. Health care professionals tend to see death as a failure.

However, not everyone sees death as a failure. Sometimes death is seen as a release. Sometimes, when death seems inevitable anyway and continued living means only a meaningless prolongation of indignity and suffering, patients may want to hasten that dying — or at least not oppose or delay it. Patients who see it that way therefore do not approach death as something that the health care professionals should try to prevent at all cost. With this, there arises the issue of deliberate death.

According to the latest available public opinion poll, the majority of Canadians feel that deliberately bringing about death is quite acceptable. A July 24, 1989, Gallup poll indicated that the proportion of Canadians who believe that a physician should be allowed to end an incurably ill patient's life has gone up from 66% in 1984, to 77%.[1] This appears to put the ethos of the health care professions squarely into conflict with the preferences of Canadian society.

To provide a patient only with comfort measures and allow death to occur is usually called passive euthanasia; to bring about the death of a patient deliberately by active means is referred to as active euthanasia. The health care professions have usually maintained that the two are different. For instance, while the Hippocratic Oath requires physicians to refrain from deliberately bringing about death, it does not prohibit physicians from letting nature take its course if death is inevitable and the prolongation of life would only be a prolongation of suffering.[2]

On the other hand, Canadian statute law has taken a firmer stance. It maintains that taking active steps to bring about the death of a patient is murder;[3] and goes on to say that once medical treatment has been started, the professional is under a duty to continue it if failure to do so is likely to imperil the life or health of the patient.[4]

On this issue, therefore, the strength of Canadian public opinion is fundamentally at odds with the position of the health care professions and the law. This raises several important questions: Are the tradition and the law really in touch with current ethical perceptions, or do they merely reflect a privately held morality? Are active and passive euthanasia really different, as the medical profession claims? Is the law correct in condemning both? Is public opinion correct in accepting both? And if public opinion should be respected, how should this respect be translated into medical practice and law?

Some of these questions are addressed in the selections from the Law Reform Commission and by James Rachels. The two present opposing views on the tenability of the distinction.

Most countries and most medical associations tend to agree with the Law Reform Commission that there is a difference between active and passive euthanasia. However, there is one medical association which does not: the Royal Dutch Medical Society. It maintains that the distinction is bogus, and together with the Dutch Crown it has worked out a carefully controlled protocol under which it is permissible for a physician deliberately to bring about the death of a patient. Despite the almost universal public rejection of the Dutch stance, at least some North American physicians make no bones about the fact that they also reject the distinction, and that on occasion they also engage in so-called active euthanasia.[5] The selections by Doerflinger (a Dutch physician opposed to the Dutch practice) and by Wanzer *et al.* (US physicians who appear to condone euthanasia) reflect this international diversity of opinion.

NOTES

1. L. Bozinoff and P. MacIntosh, *Gallup*, Gallup Canada Inc., July 24, 1989. The regional distribution is as follows: 81% in Québec, 77% in Ontario and BC, 72% in Atlantic Canada, and 71% in the Prairie provinces. The results are considered accurate within four percentage points, nineteen times out of twenty. A recent Gallup poll from the Fall of 1991 shows only a 2% variation in these figures.
2. Similar prohibitions were traditional for other health care professionals.
3. See the various provisions in the Revised Statutes of Canada 1985, c.C-46; especially Part VIII, "Offenses Against the Person."
4. See above, s. 216, 217, 219, 220 *et pass.*
5. Jude Carlson, "Bioethics Comes to Life," *Calgary Alumni* (Spring, 1992), p.4. reports that, in a recent study by D. Kinsella, 51% of Alberta physicians would accept active euthanasia.

The Need for Reform

Law Reform Commission of Canada

The onus is on those suggesting a change, it is said, to show that the change is desirable and represents an improvement over the existing situation. The consultations held between the publication of Working Paper 28 and the drafting of this Report provide clear evidence that the legal profession, the public and those working in the health professions are in favour of legal reforms or at least clarifications in the area of euthanasia, aiding suicide and cessation of treatment.

Without necessarily espousing the views expressed in the Working Paper, lawyers, university professors and scholars who were consulted agreed that the present *Criminal Code* provisions are ambiguous and vague, and much in need of revision. The Bar of one province has even made a formal recommendation to that effect.

Certain provisions, including sections 14, 45, 198, 199 and 229 of the *Criminal Code,* were drafted at a time when the specific problems confronted in this paper had not then arisen. For example, modern medical technology was not yet available to the medical profession. Sophisticated and scientific palliative care was either unknown or at best in its infancy. Indeed, the very practice of medicine and hospital management was radically different from what it is now.

Those provisions, drafted in general language, were adequate to meet the problems of the era for which they were conceived. However, they were never supplemented, as they perhaps should have

Law Reform Commission of Canada, "The Need for Reform," from Law Reform Commission of Canada, Report 20, *Euthanasia, Aiding Suicide and Cessation of Treatment.* (Ottawa: Minster of Supply and Services, 1983) pp. 7-13, 17-20, 22-28.

been, by amendments adapting them to changed realities. The Commission believes that these *Criminal Code* sections now need to be re-examined and revised in the light of current conditions and problems. Consultations carried out by the Commission have served to confirm this view. A legal scholar commenting on Working Paper 28 aptly observed that the legislator must now provide judges and courts with a clearer indication of legal policy in this area rather than forcing them to guess at it on the basis of outdated laws.

Moreover, the *Criminal Code* provisions which are the object of the Commission's reform proposals have never really been subjected to a sophisticated and clear judicial interpretation in the context of these life-and-death issues. It is possible to undertake a lengthy theoretical discussion to determine the interpretation which the courts might apply to a given word or section of the *Criminal Code.* It may indeed constitute an interesting and stimulating exercise. However, in real life and perhaps to an even greater extent in criminal law, rules should have a certain degree of predictability, especially in matters as crucial as the life or death of an individual. The great majority of those consulted felt strongly that clarification of existing law was overdue. Moreover, many of those who were not convinced of the need for amendments nevertheless had to admit that they could not predict with any certainty what interpretation the courts might give to particular provisions if applied in the current medical context regarding a decision to cease life-supporting treatment.

The view that reform is needed and even urgent is shared by medical and hospital personnel and others working in the health professions.

Health care professionals, perhaps because they are less accustomed than lawyers to reading and interpreting legal provisions, have frequently indicated how ambiguous, imprecise and vague they find the existing provisions of the *Criminal Code.* They have also told us that a number of sections, namely sections 45 and 199, seem to cast real doubt on the legality of various medical and hospital practices. We believe that these concerns are genuine and serious and sometimes have a very negative impact on medical practice. The ambiguities and doubts encourage some physicians to be excessively conservative in the practice of medicine. As one of those consulted told us, referring to section 199 of the *Criminal Code,* there are two alternatives. One is to hope that the present law does not actually mean what is seems to say and to practice medicine as it should be practiced, that is, in the patient's best interests. The other is to believe that the law intends to say what it does and therefore to practice a defensive type of medicine, one which is not always in the best interests of the patient.

Even if in practice there are hardly any criminal prosecutions in the medical context, this legislative imprecision nevertheless encourages uncertainty and tension which is to everyone's benefit to eliminate.

In effect we were told by many of those consulted that on such important issues the law should not speak in riddles, but rather should set out clearly and precisely, in language accessible to the general public, the exact parameters of permitted behaviour. The Commission agrees with that view.

The Commission believes that these reform proposals are useful and meet a genuine need. As will become apparent, these proposals do not represent a complete overhaul of the traditional legal rules, but rather a clarification and necessary supplement to them. The proposed reform will undoubtedly not completely eliminate the possibility of conflict and uncertainty. It would be naive to think so. The Commission believes, however, that the reform will have achieved its main objective if the proposed amendments allow everyone to better understand the limits governing conduct in these matters, and enable courts to identify more clearly the basic principles underlying the revised legislative policy.

These basic principles were discussed at length in Working Paper 28 and in other documents published by the Law Reform Commission in the *Protection of Life* series. They may be briefly summarized here. The first is that in the medical context the presumption in favour of life should always be recognized. Our law regards the protection of human life as a fundamental value. Any law reform must be based on that value. The proposed system of rules should never depart from the principle that in the absence of reasons to the contrary the patient should always be presumed to want to live, and that the patient would prefer life to death even when unable to express that preference. In practical terms, this principle may be expressed by the rule that if a treatment is reasonable and useful for the purpose of preserving the health or life of a human being, it should be assumed that a patient unable to express a choice would choose to receive the treatment and not to refuse it. Accordingly, a physician should normally have a duty to treat an unconscious patient admitted to hospital. This principle and presumption does not however oblige extraordinary measures. First of all, the presumption is not absolute and, secondly, it applies only if the proposed treatment is reasonable and useful. But according to this first principle the onus is on those who stop or do not initiate life-supporting treatment to provide justification for that decision.

The second principle is that of the patient's autonomy and right to self-determination. The Commission, which has repeatedly upheld this principle, continues to be of the view that it should be explicitly affirmed in law. Within the bounds of public order, morality and the rights of others, human beings must remain masters of their fate. They should therefore have the right, based on the notion of free and informed consent, to make decisions concerning themselves. No one should have the right to impose such decisions on patients against their will. The law should clearly acknowledge this right to autonomy and self-determination, and penalize any interference with it.

It is interesting to note that only one person among those consulted argued in favour of compelling a competent patient to undergo treatment.

A third principle which any reform proposals should acknowledge is that human life should be considered not only from the "quantitative" perspective, but also from the "qualitative" perspective. When patients freely choose to refuse treatment, their choice is often based upon quality-of-life considerations. In the Commission's view such considerations should be respected. We believe that the law should now clearly recognize the right of patients, exercising their free and informed choice, not to undertake treatment if they feel it would deprive them of, or not provide, an adequate quality of life for the time remaining. Inasmuch as such a decision is based on a value-judgment, there is room for argument when patients are unable to express wishes because they are too young or too old, or are unconscious or mentally handicapped. As the Commission emphasized in its Working Paper, the law should provide special measures to protect the incompetent. It should also be noted that all provinces currently have specific provisions for the exercise of what is called in law substituted consent. It is not the Commission's task to scrutinize these laws and regulations or to substitute its judgment for that of the provincial legislators. The Commission can only lay down a rule or general standard of conduct for criminal law purposes. Incompetent patients in every province of Canada have various means to enforce their rights when they are infringed upon. Moreover, the very definition of what constitutes legal incapacity varies from province to province.

The Commission wishes to prevent the possibility that a patient's inability to give or refuse consent would seem to impose on the physician a legal duty to provide aggressive treatment. If the quality of life is a value which the law should always respect, then it should also be respected and weighed when the patient is incompetent.

These are in brief the main principles underlying the proposed reform recommended by the Commission in Working Paper 28. Months of consultation have demonstrated that in Canada there currently exists a broad consensus regarding these principles. The dissenting views, which will be examined below, tend to apply especially to the question of enforcement. Some feel, for instance, that the principle of personal autonomy is so important that it would justify an individual's demand for assistance in committing suicide and that, therefore, such assistance should be completely decriminalized.

In concluding Part One of this Report, we should again recall the precise role played by legislative reform. One should not expect the lawmaker to provide a detailed and definitive guideline or manual to enable physicians to decide in a mechanical fashion whether he can or cannot discontinue treatment. All that the lawyer, or the health care professional, or the patient or the general public is entitled to expect from the legislator are general guidelines indicating the path to take and the path to avoid. Should a case involving these issues be brought before a court, it would be left to the court to determine whether or not the conduct of the accused conformed to the law by evaluating the special nature and circumstances of that case.

In its Working Paper, the Commission asked three basic questions:

(1) Should active euthanasia be legalized, or at least decriminalized?

(2) Should aiding suicide be decriminalized by the repeal of section 224 of the *Criminal Code?*

(3) Should sections 14, 45, 198, 199 and 229 of the *Criminal Code* be revised to define the legal parameters of the refusal and cessation of medical treatment?

Generally speaking the vast majority of those consulted believed that these questions were well formulated and to the point. In these final recommendations to Parliament, it is appropriate therefore to consider each of them again, partly in the light of the proposals and criticisms responding to the earlier Working Paper on these issues.

I. EUTHANASIA

The word "euthanasia" is somewhat ambiguous and has several possible meanings. Hence it is appropriate to explain what we mean by the term whenever it is used. For the purposes of this Report, euthanasia will mean the act of ending the life of a person, from compassionate motives, when he is already terminally ill or when his suffering has become unbearable.

A. The Voluntary Aspect

The Commission's final position remains that even if such a patient requests that he be killed, such an act should not be legalized. With few exceptions, the comments received have all supported the Commission's position in this matter. A country like Canada could not, without violating its social traditions and history, tolerate and give a legal veneer to a policy of active euthanasia, not even voluntary euthanasia.

The argument will undoubtedly be raised that if persons are the masters of their own bodies, they ought to have the right to demand that society allow someone else to end their life if it has become unbearable. We cannot and need not repeat and review here the pro and con arguments explored in detail in the Working Paper. As maintained in that Working Paper, the legalization of euthanasia is unacceptable to the Commission because it would indirectly condone murder, because it would be open to serious abuses, and because it appears to be morally unacceptable to the majority of the Canadian people. The Commission believes that there are better answers to the problems posed by the sufferings of the terminally ill. The development of palliative care and the search for effective pain control methods constitute a far more positive response to the problem than euthanasia on demand. To allow euthanasia to be legalized, directly or indirectly, would be to open the door to abuses, and hence indirectly weaken respect for human life.

The Commission therefore recommends against legalizing or decriminalizing voluntary active euthanasia in any form and is in favour of continuing to treat it as culpable homicide.

B. The Mercy Aspect

As the Commission stated in Working Paper 28, when the actor's chief motive for killing is compassion for that suffering person, there are three possible options by way of legal response: to preserve the status quo; to create a special category of homicide; or to add a specific provision aimed at mitigating the sentence.

The Commission received many comments on this subject. None were in favour of complete decriminalization. Responses favouring one or another of the three options were roughly equal in number, although the supporting arguments were quite varied.

Those in favour of the first and third options were agreed on one thing: a specific offence should definitely not be created. The reasons given were several. Some argued that a door to a number of problems and abuses would thereby be opened. Some maintained that the inclusion of motive as one of the elements of an offence would result in an extremely complex evidentiary problem — that of reaching a precise determination of the "purity" of the motives of the accused. In the opinion of some this would be quite impossible. The Commission does not necessarily agree. It believes, and current criminal law in fact bears this out, that it is indeed legally possible, though difficult, to prove the motive behind an accused's act.

The creation of a specific offence for mercy killing is technically compatible with the present law. But is it compatible with our traditions? As one of our correspondents noted, adding another type of homicide to the *Criminal Code* is not really a solution, since the enforcement of such a provision is bound to create difficulties in practice. How could the offences of ordinary murder and mercy killing be effectively distinguished if the only real difference between the two is to be found not in the intent to kill but in the proof of motive? One group of scholars has suggested that mercy killing be made a lesser offence included in that of culpable homicide.

Many of our correspondents, however, especially those not belonging to the legal profession, were adamantly opposed to any change. A change either in the definition of the offence or in sentencing would, in their view, amount to accepting a devaluation of human life. The most prevalent fears were the dangers posed by any weakening of legislative policy. Proponents of the first option felt that any change would open the door to abuses of all sorts.

As previously stated in the Working Paper, the Commission feels that formulating a fair and just solution of this issue is far from easy. Each of the options has its defenders and arguments in its favour, and in the final analysis the choice is a matter of personal conviction, at least on an individual level. However, the choice of policy must be made in harmony with general legislative policy on the criminal law.

All things considered, the Commission agrees with those who feel that the law on this point should not be altered, and that mercy killing should not be treated as a separate or included offence, nor entail as of right a reduction of sentence. It should be recalled that our legal system has internal regulating mechanisms which offset the apparent harshness of the law. It is possible that in some circumstances the accused would be allowed to plead guilty to a lesser charge. We also feel that our trial system, and the conclusions and verdicts reached by our juries, should be trusted. Finally, in truly exceptional cases, the authorities already have it within their discretion to decide not to prosecute.

The Commission therefore recommends that mercy killing not be made an offence separate from homicide and that there be no formal provision for special modes of sentencing for this type of homicide other than what is already provided for homicide.

II. AIDING SUICIDE

One of our correspondents brought to our attention an incident involving a charge laid under section 224 of the *Criminal Code* ("Counselling or Aiding Suicide"). Twenty years ago in Northern Canada charges were laid under that section against a certain Inuit. The accused had helped one of his elderly parents load the rifle with which the latter finally killed himself. The accused was found guilty and given a suspended sentence.

The Commission's tentative recommendation was that the offence of aiding suicide should be retained, even if in practice it is rarely invoked. To reinforce the present approach of restraint in appealing to this section of the *Code,* and to accentuate the exceptional nature of such a charge, the Commission recommended that prosecution on the basis of this section should be permitted only on written authorization from the Attorney General.

This recommendation touched off a lively debate among those we consulted or who sent us their reactions and observations. With two exceptions, all our correspondents were in agreement that the offence of aiding suicide should remain in the *Code.* A number of correspondents wrote in effect that although one may sympathize with a person who assists a terminally ill family member or friend to end his life, such sympathy should not necessarily be translated into an explicit approval of the legality of that assistance. Moreover, there can be other cases in which aiding suicide is done for far less altruistic motives, and which do warrant a legal penalty.

The Commission agrees with that view and does not recommend that aiding suicide be decriminalized.

What, however, of the recommendation requiring the written authorization of the Attorney General in order to prosecute? Contrary to the Commission's expectation when drafting the Working Paper, this suggestion encountered fairly strong opposition. These objections led the Commission to review its position and to withdraw this particular recommendation.

The first objection, cogently expressed by one of our legal correspondents, was that in this case it is preferable to let the law take its normal course. Decisions made by the Attorney General about whether or not to prosecute may be perceived, no doubt erroneously, as having political overtones. In life-and-death matters, it may not be advisable to make such a sensitive legal matter depend upon a decision which could be interpreted as politically motivated. Another correspondent suggested that the decision about whether or not to prosecute should not be left in the hands of the Attorney General himself, but rather with his regional representative. Although we agree that this suggestion could go a long way towards dispelling the above objection, we feel that it does not wholly remove the possibility of misunderstanding.

The second objection, which appears equally serious to the Commission, is that if prosecution of the offence were to depend on the Attorney General's authorization, significant differences in the manner in which the law is enforced in the various provinces could be expected. Here again, our correspondents felt that such differences involving fundamental issues and principles, might give the impression that life does not have the same value everywhere in Canada.

Finally, on a practical level, the Commission considers that since this offence is almost never prosecuted, requiring an additional procedure would amount to its *de facto* abolition. In conclusion, for the reasons given above and in the Working Paper, the Commission's view is that the offence should not be removed from the *Code* or revised.

The Commission therefore recommends retaining section 224 of the *Criminal Code* in its present form.

III. CESSATION AND REFUSAL OF TREATMENT

The Commission found near unanimous approval for the proposal originally made in Working Paper 26 and repeated in Working Paper 28. Any competent person should have the right to refuse treatment of any kind and to insist that treatment already begun be discontinued either temporarily or permanently. In other words, treatment should never be imposed against a patient's will. The physician's duty in such a case is to inform the patient of the options open to him and of their consequences, and consent to treatment or to its discontinuance must adhere to the guidelines established by court decisions to date, that is, it should be informed and freely given. If these requirements are satisfied, then whatever personal reasons motivate a person to accept or refuse a given course of treatment should not be questioned by physicians or courts and the individual's freedom of choice should be universally respected.

Provision for the formal and explicit recognition of this principle in the *Criminal Code* was widely supported. The first subsection of the *Code* amendment proposed below, subsection 199.1(*a*), contains our recommended addition to do just that. However, it was not considered advisable to add a provision specifying that physicians who treat patients against their wishes commit a specific criminal offence. Treatment by force or the continuation of treatment already undertaken against the wishes of the patient constitutes an assault, an offence already provided for and penalized under the appropriate provisions of the *Criminal Code.* Furthermore, this act is also a tort, or a delict in civil law, giving rise to civil remedies.

Our recommendation concerning palliative care also received unanimous approval. Some felt that it was the most important recommendation in the Working Paper. It was brought to our attention however that palliative care may sometimes be very aggressive and that, here too, it is important to be assured of the patient's consent or the consent of those who are responsible for making decisions concerning that patient. Palliative care is subject, in fact, to all the rules governing medical treatment, including the requirements that it be reasonable and that consent must be sought and provided.

Some of our correspondents drew to our attention an infelicitous expression on page 71 in Working Paper 28 regarding palliative care. The Commission agrees with its correspondents that the current provisions of the *Criminal Code* should not prevent a physician from undertaking or continuing palliative care when necessary, only because it might have an effect on the patient's life expectancy. Our proposed section 199.2 now clearly accommodates the proposition just stated.

The Commission therefore recommends that it be specified in the *Criminal Code* that a physician cannot be held criminally liable merely for undertaking or continuing the administration of appropriate palliative care in order to eliminate or reduce the suffering of an individual, only because of the effect that this action might have on the latter's life expectancy.

If, as we believe, the opinion of our correspondents is representative of the Canadian people as a whole, it is clear that there is a desire to eliminate the ambiguity unintentionally created by the present wording of section 199. Interpreted literally, it appears to place an unqualified duty on the physician to continue treatment once he has begun it, even if the treatment in question has become useless or unreasonable. On this question, too, the Commission's proposals received the support and approval of our consultants, subject to certain objections pertaining to matters of form.

The Commission therefore recommends an amendment to the *Criminal Code* to remove the ambiguity created by some of the current provisions, in particular by section 199.

The longest and most complex discussions revolved around the problems posed by the non-initiation or the discontinuance of treatment with people who, because of their age, their state of unconsciousness or mental handicap are unable to give a valid consent. The recent *Dawson* case in British Columbia has fueled debate and has undoubtedly increased public awareness of the issues involved. Accordingly, a systematic review of the general principles which should govern any attempts to resolve these complex problems is in order.

On the basis of submissions from various organizations representing those suffering from mental handicaps, the Commission remains convinced about the soundness of the tentative proposal in the Working Paper. The law must avoid and guard against any involuntary discrimination against handicapped people. A person's inability to give consent should not be invoked to deny to that person the rights granted to competent individuals. In the context of this discussion, a person's incompetence alone should not oblige or empower a physician to begin or continue a therapeutically useless treatment when its only result will be to prolong unnecessarily the patient's agony. Incompetent persons, like all others, have the right to die with dignity, assisted by whatever palliative care is needed. Accordingly, the law should attempt to eliminate any difference in that regard between a competent and an incompetent person. In either case, the continuance or initiation of useless or inappropriate medical treatment should not be promoted or condoned by criminal law. Heroic or aggressive therapeutic measures which would not be used in the case of a competent person, should also not be used in the case of an incompetent person.

The Commission also reaffirms the position it expressed on the subject of newborns in its Working Paper. The decision to treat or not to treat should be made on the basis of the medical facts of each case and in the best interests of that newborn patient, not for eugenic reasons. For example, the Commission feels that it is a physician's duty to perform corrective surgery for atresia of the digestive tract in the case of a trisomic newborn if the risks of the operation are acceptable and if, apart from the trisomy 21, there are no other serious and incurable defects. The decision ought to be made according to whether the problem can be corrected or not, and by considering the newborn's quality of life, just as would be the case for an adult patient. If, according to the present state of medical science, the seriously handicapped newborn is already dying, he or she should be treated in the same way one would treat a conscious or unconscious terminally ill adult. However, if the infant could benefit from a form of treatment which offers reasonable hope for an acceptable quality of life, then that treatment should be provided. The Commission is well aware of the ambiguity in the expression, "acceptable quality of life". In medical practice the resolution of this dilemma seems to present fewer difficulties for the adult patient. It also acknowledges that it is essentially a question of fact, the differences in each case making generalization impossible. It is as well a question of sound medical judgment based not only on medical experience, but also on consultation with the appropriate party or parties, such as the parents, the spouse, the family and the next of kin. The purpose of criminal law is not to tell the physician how to act in each and every case. It exists only to draw general lines and punish abuses. In each particular case it is up to the courts to determine whether or not a particular decision was reasonable and acceptable under the circumstances. A decision that would only prolong the dying patient's agony would not be reasonable in the Commission's opinion; nor would a decision be reasonable which would force a newborn or adult to undergo an exceptional series of operations or treatments, resulting in great suffering, only to end up with a medically unacceptable quality of life. On the other hand, the mere existence of a physical or mental handicap in a newborn, even if serious, should not be a pretext to refuse treatment on the basis of what are essentially eugenic considerations.

A third question meriting discussion here is that of substituted consent for those incapable of expressing their wishes. It is a difficult problem and the Commission is particularly grateful to those correspondents who helped to shed light on the principles involved or who submitted a variety of typical cases for our consideration.

The Commission stated in its Working Paper that there are essentially three systems or mechanisms for ensuring consent to treatment or to discontinuance of treatment for persons themselves incapable of making or expressing that decision. We stated that we would take a definitive position on the question in the report to Parliament. The first mechanism could be called the "judicial model". The decision would be made either by a judge or by a quasi-judicial body, such as a hospital committee. A large majority of our correspondents were against resorting to institutionalizing such a system on the grounds that it can be unwieldy, complex and, above all, inappropriate for dealing with the type of decision which has to be made. The ideal decision-making model for such cases is in fact one which seeks a consensus among the various people involved (the physician, other involved health care professionals, the family and the next of kin). A confrontational model of the adversary sort is clearly not ideal under normal circumstances. Rejection of this first model as the normal decision-making mechanism does not mean, however, the elimination of any recourse to the courts. Should any of the parties be opposed to or in disagreement with a decision to treat or not to treat an incompetent patient, it should always be possible to ask a court to resolve the conflict in order to provide the best available protection to the patient. But what we wish to emphasize is that, solely from the point of view of criminal law, there appears to be no point in requiring that every decision concerning the treatment of an incompetent person be automatically subject to a formal and initial order by a court or quasi-judicial body. We have no intention of excluding the involvement of courts in this type of decision when the exceptional need arises.

A second possible decision-making mechanism is to allow those who represent the incompetent person (e.g. next of kin, parents, curator, guardian and so forth) to make the decision by themselves alone for the incompetent person. This solution is favoured by a number of individuals and organizations in Canada at the present time. The Commission sees two possible dangers if this approach were to prevail. The first is the unfairness involved in placing an extremely heavy psychological burden on those who are perhaps not really in a position to bear it. The second is the possibility that conscious or unconscious conflicts of interest might arise, risking an injustice being done to the incompetent person.

This explains why the Commission recommended that the decision be primarily medical in nature, believing that there is no ideal solution and that, all things considered, this option remains the least unsatisfactory. It must be noted, however, that a rejection of the second solution as the basic legislative policy naturally does not mean the exclusion of those persons from the decision-making process. On the contrary, even if the physician must remain ultimately responsible for the decision in the eyes of the law, the decision must necessarily be made after discussion, explanation and consultation with those close to the patient. This option, which the Commission maintains in its final recommendations, merits further explanation.

In the first place, we do not intend and indeed we are not empowered to express an opinion on the matter as a whole. Many aspects of medical treatment for the incompetent come wholly or in part under provincial jurisdiction. Each province has particular laws and regulations relating to the rights and protection of infants, and which regulate the powers of parents, tutors and guardians. The Law Reform Commission therefore cannot and does not wish to express an opinion on the content of such provincial legislation. The sole question which the Commission may ask itself is the following: When may a person be held criminally liable for discontinuing or failing to initiate medical treatment for an incompetent person? The Commission's answer is the following: Such liability should not exist when the discontinuance or non-initiation is based on a valid medical decision, that is, one which is reasonable in the circumstances, is in the best interests of the incompetent person and in conformity with other standards set by criminal law.

The requirement proposed by the Commission is therefore necessarily a minimum requirement, only what is necessary for an acceptable standard of criminal liability. As a minimum standard for purposes of criminal liability, it in no way precludes the adoption of more detailed and sophisticated formulas which could offer the incompetent patient more protection. Quite the contrary. The following are some examples. A formal decision regarding treatment must be made by the physician on the basis of medical facts and expertise, but it can and should be made after consultation with the family, the spouse, the next of kin or tutor, or guardian. Such a decision can also be made and normally is, after an independent second medical consultation. It may be made or contributed to by an interdisciplinary hospital committee. All that the criminal law seeks to ensure is that the physician has made a reasonable decision in terms of his expertise, the medical data and the particular circumstances. It is not within the scope of criminal law, which can only dictate a general standard of conduct, to say exactly how that decision should be reached, what advice may be sought and who may participate in the decision-making process.

Nothing of course should preclude anticipatory recourse to a court, as in the *Dawson* case, in order that the appropriateness and legality of a contemplated medical decision may be determined, especially when there is an obvious conflict of opinion among the interested parties about what should be done.

On the other hand, since it is physicians who normally bear the onerous burden of possible criminal liability, it is only fair to clarify for their sake the rather ambiguous provisions of the *Criminal Code.* We hope the proposed amendments do just that.

The Commission therefore recommends that a physician should not incur any criminal liability if he decides to discontinue or not initiate treatment for an incompetent person, when that treatment is no longer therapeutically useful and is not in the person's best interest.

Active and Passive Euthanasia

James Rachels

ABSTRACT

The traditional distinction between active and passive euthanasia requires critical analysis. The conventional doctrine is that there is such an important moral difference between the two that, although the latter is sometimes permissible, the former is always forbidden. This doctrine may be challenged for several reasons. First of all, active euthanasia is in many cases more humane than passive euthanasia. Secondly, the conventional doctrine leads to decisions concerning life and death on irrelevant grounds. Thirdly, the doctrine rests on a distinction between killing and letting die that itself has no moral importance. Fourthly, the most common arguments in favor of the doctrine are invalid. I therefore suggest that the

James Rachels, "Active and Passive Euthanasia," *New England Journal of Medicine* 292:2 (Jan 9, 1975) 78-80.

> American Medical Association policy statement that endorses this doctrine is unsound.

The distinction between active and passive euthanasia is thought to be crucial for medical ethics. The idea is that it is permissible, at least in some cases, to withhold treatment and allow a patient to die, but it is never permissible to take any direct action designed to kill the patient. This doctrine seems to be accepted by most doctors, and it is endorsed in a statement adopted by the House of Delegates of the American Medical Association on December 4, 1973:

> The intentional termination of the life of one human being by another — mercy killing — is contrary to that for which the medical profession stands and is contrary to the policy of the American Medical Association.
>
> The cessation of the employment of extraordinary means to prolong the life of the body when there is irrefutable evidence that biological death is imminent is the decision of the patient and/or his immediate family. The advice and judgment of the physician should be freely available to the patient and/or his immediate family.

However, a strong case can be made against this doctrine. In what follows I will set out some of the relevant arguments, and urge doctors to reconsider their views on this matter.

To begin with a familiar type of situation, a patient who is dying of incurable cancer of the throat is in terrible pain, which can no longer be satisfactorily alleviated. He is certain to die within a few days, even if present treatment is continued, but he does not want to go on living for those days since the pain is unbearable. So he asks the doctor for an end to it, and his family joins in the request.

Suppose the doctor agrees to withhold treatment, as the conventional doctrine says he may. The justification for his doing so is that the patient is in terrible agony, and since he is going to die anyway, it would be wrong to prolong his suffering needlessly. But now notice this. If one simply withholds treatment, it may take the patient longer to die, and so he may suffer more than he would if more direct action were taken and a lethal injection given. This fact provides strong reason for thinking that, once the initial decision not to prolong his agony has been made, active euthanasia is actually preferable to passive euthanasia, rather than the reverse. To say otherwise is to endorse the option that leads to more suffering rather than less, and is contrary to the humanitarian impulse that prompts the decision not to prolong his life in the first place.

Part of my point is that the process of being "allowed to die" can be relatively slow and painful, whereas being given a lethal injection is relatively quick and painless. Let me give a different sort of example. In the United States about one in 600 babies is born with Down's syndrome. Most of these babies are otherwise healthy — that is, with only the usual pediatric care, they will proceed to an otherwise normal infancy. Some, however, are born with congenital defects such as intestinal obstructions that require operations if they are to live. Sometimes, the parents and the doctor will decide not to operate, and let the infant die. Anthony Shaw describes what happens then:

> ... When surgery is denied [the doctor] must try to keep the infant from suffering while natural forces sap the baby's life away. As a surgeon whose natural inclination is to use the scalpel to fight off death, standing by and watching a salvageable baby die is the most emotionally exhausting

experience I know. It is easy at a conference, in a theoretical discussion, to decide that such infants should be allowed to die. It is altogether different to stand by in the nursery and watch as dehydration and infection wither a tiny being over hours and days. This is a terrible ordeal for me and the hospital staff — much more so than for the parents who never set foot in the nursery.

I can understand why some people are opposed to all euthanasia, and insist that such infants must be allowed to live. I think I can also understand why other people favor destroying these babies quickly and painlessly. But why should anyone favor letting "dehydration and infection wither a tiny being over hours and days?" The doctrine that says that a baby may be allowed to dehydrate and wither, but may not be given an injection that would end its life without suffering, seems so patently cruel as to require no further refutation. The strong language is not intended to offend, but only to put the point in the clearest possible way.

My second argument is that the conventional doctrine leads to decisions concerning life and death made on irrelevant grounds.

Consider again the case of the infants with Down's syndrome who need operations for congenital defects unrelated to the syndrome to live. Sometimes, there is no operation and the baby dies, but when there is no such defect, the baby lives on. Now, an operation such as that to remove an intestinal obstruction is not prohibitively difficult. The reason why such operations are not performed in these cases is, clearly, that the child has Down's syndrome and the parents and doctor judge that because of that fact it is better for the child to die.

But notice that this situation is absurd, no matter what view one takes of the lives and potentials of such babies. If the life of such an infant is worth preserving, what does it matter if it needs a simple operation? Or, if one thinks it better that such a baby should not live on, what difference does it make that it happens to have an unobstructed intestinal tract? In either case, the matter of life and death is being decided on irrelevant grounds. It is the Down's syndrome, and not the intestines, that is the issue. The matter should be decided, if at all, on that basis, and not be allowed to depend on the essentially irrelevant question of whether the intestinal tract is blocked.

What makes this situation possible, of course, is the idea that when there is an intestinal blockage, one can "let the baby die," but when there is no such defect there is nothing that can be done, for one must not "kill" it. The fact that this idea leads to such results as deciding life or death on irrelevant grounds is another good reason why the doctrine should be rejected.

One reason why so many people think that there is an important moral difference between active and passive euthanasia is that they think killing someone is morally worse than letting someone die. But is it? Is killing, in itself, worse than letting die? To investigate this issue, two cases may be considered that are exactly alike except that one involves killing whereas the other involves letting someone die. Then, it can be asked whether this difference makes any difference to the moral assessments. It is important that the cases be exactly alike, except for this one difference, since otherwise one cannot be confident that it is this difference and not some other that accounts for any variation in the assessments of the two cases. So, let us consider this pair of cases:

In the first, Smith stands to gain a large inheritance if anything should happen to his six-year-old cousin. One evening while the child is taking his bath, Smith sneaks into the bathroom and drowns the child, and then arranges things so that it will look like an accident.

In the second, Jones also stands to gain if anything should happen to his six-year-old cousin. Like Smith, Jones sneaks in planning to drown the child in his bath. However, just as he enters the bathroom Jones sees the child slip and hit his head, and fall face down in the water. Jones is delighted; he stands by, ready to push the child's head back under if it is necessary, but it is not necessary. With only a little thrashing about, the child drowns all by himself, "accidentally," as Jones watches and does nothing.

Now Smith killed the child, whereas Jones "merely" let the child die. That is the only difference between them. Did either man behave better, from a moral point of view? If the difference between killing and letting die were in itself a morally important matter, one should say that Jones's behavior was less reprehensible than Smith's. But does one really want to say that? I think not. In the first place, both men acted from the same motive, personal gain, and both had exactly the same end in view when they acted. It may be inferred from Smith's conduct that he is a bad man, although that judgment may be withdrawn or modified if certain further facts are learned about him — for example, that he is mentally deranged. But would not the very same thing be inferred about Jones from his conduct? And would not the same further considerations also be relevant to any modification of this judgment? Moreover, suppose Jones pleaded, in his own defense, "After all, I didn't do anything except just stand there and watch the child drown. I didn't kill him; I only let him die." Again, if letting die were in itself less bad than killing, this defense should have at least some weight. But it does not. Such a "defense" can only be regarded as a grotesque perversion of moral reasoning. Morally speaking, it is no defense at all.

Now, it may be pointed out, quite properly, that the cases of euthanasia with which doctors are concerned are not like this at all. They do not involve personal gain or the destruction of normal healthy children. Doctors are concerned only with cases in which the patient's life is of no further use to him, or in which the patient's life has become or will soon become a terrible burden. However, the point is the same in these cases: the bare difference between killing and letting die does not, in itself, make a moral difference. If a doctor lets a patient die, for humane reasons, he is in the same moral position as if he had given the patient a lethal injection for humane reasons. If his decision was wrong — if, for example, the patient's illness was in fact curable — the decision would be equally regrettable no matter which method was used to carry it out. And if the doctor's decision was the right one, the method used is not in itself important.

The AMA policy statement isolates the crucial issue very well; the crucial issue is "the intentional termination of the life of one human being by another." But after identifying this issue, and forbidding "mercy killing," the statement goes on to deny that the cessation of treatment is the intentional termination of a life. This is where the mistake comes in, for what is the cessation of treatment, in these circumstances, if it is not "the intentional termination of the life of one human being by another?" Of course it is exactly that, and if it were not, there would be no point to it.

Many people will find this judgment hard to accept. One reason, I think, is that it is very easy to conflate the question of whether killing is, in itself, worse than letting die, with the very different question of whether most actual cases of killing are more reprehensible than most actual cases of letting die. Most actual cases of killing are clearly terrible (think, for example, of all the murders reported in the newspapers), and one hears of such cases every day. On the other hand, one hardly ever hears of a case of letting die, except for the actions of doctors who are motivated by humanitarian reasons. So one learns to think of killing in a much worse light than of letting die. But this does not mean that there is something about killing that makes it in itself worse than letting die, for it is not the bare difference between killing and letting die that makes the difference in these cases. Rather, the other factors — the murderer's motive of personal gain, for example, contrasted with the doctor's humanitarian motivation — account for different reactions to the different cases.

I have argued that killing is not in itself any worse than letting die; if my contention is right, it follows that active euthanasia is not any worse than passive euthanasia. What arguments can be given on the other side? The most common, I believe, is the following:

> The important difference between active and passive euthanasia is that, in passive euthanasia, the doctor does not do anything to bring about the patient's death. The doctor does nothing, and the patient dies of whatever ills already afflict him. In active euthanasia, however, the doctor does something to bring about the patient's death: he kills him. The doctor who gives the patient with cancer a lethal injection has himself caused his patient's death; whereas if he merely ceases treatment, the cancer is the cause of the death.

A number of points need to be made here. The first is that it is not exactly correct to say that in passive euthanasia the doctor does nothing, for he does do one thing that is very important: he lets the patient die. "Letting someone die" is certainly different, in some respects, from other types of action — mainly in that it is a kind of action that one may perform by way of not performing certain other actions. For example, one may let a patient die by way of not giving medication, just as one may insult someone by way of not shaking his hand. But for any purpose of moral assessment, it is a type of action nonetheless. The decision to let a patient die is subject to moral appraisal in the same way that a decision to kill him would be subject to moral appraisal: it may be assessed as wise or unwise, compassionate or sadistic, right or wrong. If a doctor deliberately let a patient die who was suffering from routinely curable illness, the doctor would certainly be blame for what he had done, just as he would be to blame he had needlessly killed the patient. Charges against him would then be appropriate. If so, it would be no defense all for him to insist that he didn't "do anything." He would have done something very serious indeed, for he let his patient die.

Fixing the cause of death may be very important from legal point of view, for it may determine whether criminal charges are brought against the doctor. But I do not think that this notion can be used to show a moral difference between active and passive euthanasia. The reason why it is considered bad to be the cause of someone's death is that death is regarded as a great evil — and so it is. However if it has been decided that euthanasia — even passive euthanasia — is desirable in a given case, it has also been decided that in this instance death is no greater an evil than the patient's continued existence. And if this is true the usual reason for not wanting to be the cause of someone's death simply does not apply.

Finally, doctors may think that all of this is only of academic interest — the sort of thing that philosophers may worry about but that has no practical bearing on their own work. After all, doctors must be concerned about the legal consequences of what they do, and active euthanasia is clearly forbidden by the law. But even so, doctors should also be concerned with the fact that the law is forcing upon them a moral doctrine that may well be indefensible, and has a considerable effect on their practices. Of course, most doctors are not now in the position of being coerced in this matter, for they do not regard themselves as merely going along with what the law requires. Rather, in statements such as the AMA policy statement that I have quoted, they are endorsing this doctrine as a central point of medical ethics. In that statement, active euthanasia is condemned not merely as illegal but as "contrary to that for which the medical profession stands," whereas passive euthanasia is approved. However, the preceding considerations suggest that there is really no moral difference between the two, considered in themselves (there may be important moral differences in some cases in their *consequences,* but, as I pointed out, these differences may make active euthanasia, and not passive euthanasia, the morally preferable option). So, whereas doctors may have to discriminate between active and passive euthanasia to satisfy the law, they should not do any more than that. In particular, they should not give the distinction any added authority and weight by writing it into official statements of medical ethics.

Assisted Suicide: Pro-Choice or Anti-Life?

Richard Doerflinger

The intrinsic wrongness of directly killing the innocent, even with the victim's consent, is all but axiomatic in the Jewish and Christian worldviews that have shaped the laws and mores of Western civilization and the self-concept of its medical practitioners. This norm grew out of the conviction that human life is sacred because it is created in the image and likeness of God, and called to fulfillment in love of God and neighbor.

With the pervasive secularization of Western culture, norms against euthanasia and suicide have to a great extent been cut loose from their religious roots to fend for themselves. Because these norms seem abstract and unconvincing to many, debate tends to dwell not on the wrongness of the act as such but on what may follow from its acceptance. Such arguments are often described as claims about a "slippery slope," and debate shifts to the validity of slippery slope arguments in general.

Since it is sometimes argued that acceptance of assisted suicide is an outgrowth of respect for personal autonomy, and not lack of respect for the inherent worth of human life, I will outline how autonomy-based arguments in favor of assisting suicide do entail a statement about the value of life. I will also distinguish two kinds of slippery slope argument often confused with each other, and argue that those who favor social and legal acceptance of assisted suicide have not adequately responded to the slippery slope claims of their opponents.

Richard Doerflinger, "Assisted Suicide: Pro-Choice or Anti-Life?" *Hastings Center Report* 19:1(Jan/Feb. 1989) suppl. 16-19.

ASSISTED SUICIDE VERSUS RESPECT FOR LIFE

Some advocates of socially sanctioned assisted suicide admit (and a few boast) that their proposal is incompatible with the conviction that human life is of intrinsic worth. Attorney Robert Risley has said that he and his allies in the Hemlock Society are "so bold" as to seek to "overturn the sanctity of life principle" in American society. A life of suffering, "racked with pain," is "not the kind of life we cherish."[1]

Others eschew Risley's approach, perhaps recognizing that it creates a slippery slope toward practices almost universally condemned. If society is to help terminally ill patients to commit suicide because it agrees that death is objectively preferable to a life of hardship, it will be difficult to draw the line at the seriously ill or even at circumstances where the victim requests death.

Some advocates of assisted suicide therefore take a different course, arguing that it is precisely respect for the dignity of the human person that demands respect for individual freedom as the noblest feature of that person. On this rationale a decision as to when and how to die deserves the respect and even the assistance of others because it is the ultimate exercise of self-determination — "ultimate" both in the sense that it is the last decision one will ever make and in the sense that through it one takes control of one's entire self. What makes such decisions worthy of respect is not the fact that death is chosen over life but that it is the individual's own free decision about his or her future.

Thus Derek Humphry, director of the Hemlock Society, describes his organization as "pro-choice" on this issue. Such groups favor establishment of a constitutional "right to die" modeled on the right to abortion delineated by the U.S. Supreme Court in 1973. This would be a right to choose *whether or not* to end one's own life, free of outside government interference. In theory, recognition of such a right would betray no bias toward choosing death.

LIFE VERSUS FREEDOM

This autonomy-based approach is more appealing than the straightforward claim that some lives are not worth living, especially to Americans accustomed to valuing individual liberty above virtually all else. But the argument departs from American traditions on liberty in one fundamental respect.

When the Declaration of Independence proclaimed the inalienable human rights to be "life, liberty, and the pursuit of happiness," this ordering reflected a long-standing judgment about their relative priorities. Life, a human being's very earthly existence, is the most fundamental right because it is the necessary condition for all other worldly goods including freedom; freedom in turn makes it possible to pursue (without guaranteeing that one will attain) happiness. Safeguards against the deliberate destruction of life are thus seen as necessary to protect freedom and all other human goods. This line of thought is not explicitly religious but is endorsed by some modern religious groups:

> The first right of the human person is his life. He has other goods and some are more precious, but this one is fundamental — the condition of all the others. Hence it must be protected above all others.[2]

On this view suicide is not the ultimate exercise of freedom but its ultimate self-contradiction: A free act that by destroying life, destroys all the individual's future earthly freedom. If life is more basic than freedom, society best serves freedom by discouraging rather than assisting self-destruction. Sometimes one must limit particular choices to safeguard freedom itself, as when American society chose over a century ago to prevent people from selling themselves into slavery even of their own volition.

It may be argued in objection that the person who ends his life has not truly suffered loss of freedom, because unlike the slave he need not continue to exist under the constraints of a loss of freedom. But the slave does have some freedom, including the freedom to seek various means of liberation or at least the freedom to choose what attitude to take regarding his plight. To claim that a slave is worse off than a corpse is to value a situation of limited freedom less than one of no freedom whatsoever, which seems inconsistent with the premise of the "pro-choice" position. Such a claim also seems tantamount to saying that some lives (such as those with less than absolute freedom) are objectively not worth living, a position that "pro-choice" advocates claim not to hold.

It may further be argued in objection that assistance in suicide is only being offered to those who can no longer meaningfully exercise other freedoms due to increased suffering and reduced capabilities and lifespan. To be sure, the suffering of terminally ill patients who can no longer pursue the simplest everyday tasks should call for sympathy and support from everyone in contact with them. But even these hardships do not constitute total loss of freedom of choice. If they did, one could hardly claim that the patient is in a position to make the ultimate free choice about suicide. A dying person capable of making a choice of that kind is also capable of making less monumental free choices about coping with his or her condition. This person generally faces a bewildering array of choices regarding the assessment of his or her past life and the resolution of relationships with family and friends. He or she must finally choose at this time what stance to take regarding the eternal questions about God, personal responsibility, and the prospects of a destiny after death.

In short, those who seek to maximize free choice may with consistency reject the idea of assisted suicide, instead facilitating all choices *except* that one which cuts short all choices.

In fact proponents of assisted suicide do *not* consistently place freedom of choice as their highest priority. They often defend the moderate nature of their project by stating, with Derek Humphry, that "we do not encourage suicide for any reason except to relieve unremitting suffering." It seems their highest priority is the "pursuit of happiness" (or avoidance of suffering) and not "liberty" as such. Liberty or freedom of choice loses its value if one's choices cannot relieve suffering and lead to happiness; life is of instrumental value insofar as it makes possible choices that can bring happiness.

In this value system, choice as such does not warrant unqualified respect. In difficult circumstances, as when care of a suffering and dying patient is a great burden on family and society, the individual who chooses life despite suffering will not easily be seen as rational, thus will not easily receive understanding and assistance for this choice.

In short, an unqualified "pro-choice" defense of assisted suicide lacks coherence because corpses have no choices. A particular choice, that of death, is given priority over all the other choices it makes impossible, so the value of choice as such is not central to the argument.

A restriction of this rationale to cases of terminal illness also lacks logical force. For if ending a brief life of suffering can be good, it would seem that ending a long life of suffering may be better. Surely the approach of the California "Humane and Dignified Death Act" — where consensual killing of a patient expected to die in six months is presumably good medical practice, but killing the same patient a month or two earlier is still punishable as homicide — is completely arbitrary.

SLIPPERY SLOPES, LOOSE CANNONS

Many arguments against sanctioning assisted suicide concern a different kind of "slippery slope": Contingent factors in the contemporary situation may make it virtually inevitable in practice, if not compelling at the level of abstract theory, that removal of the taboo against assisted suicide will lead to destructive expansions of the right to kill the innocent. Such factors may not be part of euthanasia advocates' own agenda; but if they exist and are beyond the control of these advocates, they must be taken into account in judging the moral and social wisdom of opening what may be a Pandora's box of social evils.

To distinguish this sociological argument from our dissection of the conceptual *logic* of the rationale for assisted suicide, we might call it a "loose cannon" argument. The basic claim is that socially accepted killing of innocent persons will interact with other social factors to threaten lives that advocates of assisted suicide would agree should be protected. These factors at present include the following:

The psychological vulnerability of elderly and dying patients. Theorists may present voluntary and involuntary euthanasia as polar opposites; in practice there are many steps on the road from dispassionate, autonomous choice to subtle coercion. Elderly and disabled patients are often invited by our achievement-oriented society to see themselves as useless burdens on younger, more vital generations. In this climate, simply offering the *option* of "self-deliverance" shifts a burden of proof, so that helpless patients must ask themselves why they are *not* availing themselves of it. Society's offer of death communicates the message to certain patients that they *may* continue to live if they wish but the rest of us have no strong interest in their survival. Indeed, once the choice of a quick and painless death is officially accepted as rational, resistance to this choice may be seen as eccentric or even selfish.[3]

The crisis in health care costs. The growing incentives for physicians, hospitals, families, and insurance companies to control the cost of health care will bring additional pressures to bear on patients. Curt Garbesi, the Hemlock Society's legal consultant, argues that autonomy-based groups like Hemlock must "control the public debate" so assisted suicide will not be seized upon by public officials as a cost-cutting device. But simply basing one's own defense of assisted suicide on individual autonomy does not solve the problem. For in the economic sphere also, offering the option of suicide would subtly shift burdens of proof.

Adequate health care is now seen by at least some policymakers as a human right, as something a society owes to all its members. Acceptance of assisted suicide as an option for those requiring expensive care would not only offer health care providers an incentive to make that option seem attractive — it would also demote all other options to the status of strictly private choices by the individual. As such they may lose their moral and legal claim to public support — in much the same way that the U.S. Supreme Court, having protected abortion under a constitutional "right of privacy," has quite logically denied any government obligation to provide public funds for this strictly private choice. As life-extending care of the terminally ill is increasingly seen as strictly elective, society may become less willing to appropriate funds for such care, and economic pressures to choose death will grow accordingly.

Legal doctrines on "substituted judgment." American courts recognizing a fundamental right to refuse life-sustaining treatment have concluded that it is unjust to deny this right to the mentally incompetent. In such cases the right is exercised on the patient's behalf by others, who seek either to interpret what the patient's own wishes might have been or to serve his or her best interests. Once assisted suicide is established as a fundamental right, courts will almost certainly find that it is unjust not to extend this right to those unable to express their wishes. Hemlock's political arm, Americans Against Human Suffering, has underscored continuity between "passive" and "active" euthanasia by offering the Humane and Dignified Death Act as an amendment to California's "living will" law, and by including a provision for appointment of a proxy to choose the time and manner of the patient's death. By such extensions our legal system would accommodate nonvoluntary, if not involuntary, active euthanasia.

Expanded definitions of terminal illness. The Hemlock Society wishes to offer assisted suicide only to those suffering from terminal illnesses. But some Hemlock officials have in mind a rather broad definition of "terminal illness." Derek Humphry says "two and a half million people alone are dying of Alzheimer's disease."[4] At Hemlock's 1986 convention, Dutch physician Pieter Admiraal boasted that he had recently broadened the meaning of terminal illness in his country by giving a lethal injection to a young quadriplegic woman — a Dutch court found that he acted within judicial guidelines allowing euthanasia for the terminally ill, because paralyzed patients have difficulty swallowing and could die from aspirating their food at any time.

The medical and legal meaning of terminal illness has already been expanded in the United States by professional societies, legislatures, and courts in the context of so-called passive euthanasia. A Uniform Rights of the Terminally Ill Act proposed by the National Conference of Commissioners on Uniform State Laws in 1986 defines a terminal illness as one that would cause the patient's death in a relatively short time if life-preserving treatment is *not* provided — prompting critics to ask if all diabetics, for example, are "terminal" by definition. Some courts already see comatose and vegetative states as "terminal" because they involve an inability to swallow that will lead to death unless artificial feeding is instituted. In the *Hilda Peter* case, the New Jersey Supreme Court declared that the traditional state interest in "preserving life" referred only to "cognitive and sapient life" and not to mere "biological" existence, implying that unconscious patients are terminal, or perhaps as good as dead, so far as state interests are concerned. Is there any reason to think that American law would suddenly resurrect the older, narrower meaning of "terminal illness" in the context of *active* euthanasia?

Prejudice against citizens with disabilities. If definitions of terminal illness expand to encompass states of severe physical or mental disability, another social reality will increase the pressure on patients to choose death: long-standing prejudice, sometimes bordering on revulsion, against people with disabilities. While it is seldom baldly claimed that disabled people have "lives not worth living," able-bodied people often say they could not live in a severely disabled state or would prefer death. In granting Elizabeth Bouvia a right to refuse a feeding tube that preserved her life, the California Appeals Court bluntly stated that her physical handicaps led her to "consider her existence meaningless" and that "she cannot be faulted for so concluding." According to disability rights expert Paul Longmore, in a society with such attitudes toward the disabled, "talk of their 'rational' or 'voluntary' suicide is simply Orwellian newspeak."[5]

Character of the medical profession. Advocates of assisted suicide realize that most physicians will resist giving lethal injections because they are trained, in Garbesi's words, to be "enemies of death." The California Medical Association firmly opposed the Humane and Dignified Death Act, seeing it as an attack on the ethical foundation of the medical profession.

Yet California appeals judge Lynn Compton was surely correct in his concurring opinion in the *Bouvia* case, when he said that a sufficient number of willing physicians can be found once legal sanctions against assisted suicide are dropped. Judge Compton said this had clearly been the case with abortion, despite the fact that the Hippocratic Oath condemns abortion as strongly as it condemns euthanasia. Opinion polls of physicians bear out the judgment that a significant number would perform lethal injections if they were legal.

Some might think this division or ambivalence about assisted suicide in the medical profession will restrain broad expansions of the practice. But if anything, Judge Compton's analogy to our experience with abortion suggests the opposite. Most physicians still have qualms about abortion, and those who perform abortions on a full-time basis are not readily accepted by their colleagues as paragons of the healing art. Consequently they tend to form their own professional societies, bolstering each other's positive self-image and developing euphemisms to blunt the moral edge of their work.

Once physicians abandon the traditional medical self-image, which rejects direct killing of patients in all circumstances, their new substitute self-image may require ever more aggressive efforts to make this killing more widely practiced and favorably received. To allow killing by physicians in certain circumstances may create a new lobby of physicians in favor of expanding medical killing.

The human will to power. The most deeply buried yet most powerful driving force toward widespread medical killing is a fact of human nature: Human beings are tempted to enjoy exercising power over others; ending another person's life is the ultimate exercise of that power. Once the taboo against killing has been set aside, it becomes progressively easier to channel one's aggressive instincts into the destruction of life in other contexts. Or as James Burtchaell has said: "There is a sort of virginity about murder; once one has violated it, it is awkward to refuse other invitations by saying, 'But that would be murder!'"[6]

Some will say assisted suicide for the terminally ill is morally distinguishable from murder and does not logically require termination of life in other circumstances. But my point is that the skill and the instinct to kill are more easily turned to other lethal tasks once they have an opportunity to exercise themselves. Thus Robert Jay Lifton has perceived differences between the German "mercy killings" of the 1930s and the later campaign to annihilate the Jews of Europe, yet still says that "at the heart of the Nazi enterprise ... is the destruction of the boundary between healing and killing."[7] No other boundary separating these two situations was as fundamental as this one, and thus none was effective once it was crossed. As a matter of historical fact, personnel who had conducted the "mercy killing" program were quickly and readily recruited to operate the killing chambers of the death camps.[8] While the contemporary United States fortunately lacks the anti-Semitic and totalitarian attitudes that made the Holocaust possible, it has its own trends and pressures that may combine with acceptance of medical killing to produce a distinctively American catastrophe in the name of individual freedom.

These "loose cannon" arguments are not conclusive. All such arguments by their nature rest upon a reading and extrapolation of certain contingent factors in society. But their combined force provides a serious case against taking the irreversible step of sanctioning assisted suicide for any class of persons, so long as those who advocate this step fail to demonstrate why these predictions are wrong. If the strict philosophical case on behalf of "rational suicide" lacks coherence, the pragmatic claim that its acceptance would be a social benefit lacks grounding in history or common sense.

NOTES

1. Presentation at the Hemlock Society's Third National Voluntary Euthanasia Conference, "A Humane and Dignified Death," September 25-27, 1986, Washington, DC. All quotations from Hemlock Society officials are from the proceedings of this conference unless otherwise noted.
2. Vatican Congregation for the Doctrine of the Faith, *Declaration on Procured Abortion* (1974), para. 11.
3. I am indebted for this line of argument to Dr. Eric Chevlen.
4. Denis Herbstein, "Campaigning for the Right to Die," *International Herald Tribune,* 11 September 1986.
5. Paul K. Longmore, "Elizabeth Bouvia, Assisted Suicide, and Social Prejudice," *Issues in Law & Medicine* 3:2 (1987), 168.
6. James T. Burtchaell, *Rachel Weeping and Other Essays on Abortion* (Kansas City: Andrews & McMeel, 1982), 188.
7. Robert Jay Lifton, *The Nazi Doctors: Medical Killing and the Psychology of Genocide* (New York: Basic Books, 1986), 14.
8. Yitzhak Rad, *Belzec, Sobibor, Treblinka* (Bloomington, IN: Indiana University Press, 1987), 11, 16-17.

The Physician's Responsibility Toward Hopelessly Ill Patients

A Second Look

*Sidney H. Wanzer, Daniel D. Federman, S. James Adelstein, M.D., Christine K. Cassel, M.D., Edwin H. Cassem, Ronald E. Cranford, Edward W. Hook, Bernard Lo, Charles G. Moertel, M.D., Peter Safar, Alan Stone, and Jan van Eys.**

ABSTRACT

Physicians have a specific responsibility toward patients who are hopelessly ill, dying, or in the end stages of an incurable disease. In a summary of current practices affecting the care of dying patients, we give particular emphasis to changes that have become commonplace since the early 1980s. Implementation of accepted policies has been deficient in certain areas, including the initiation of timely discussions with patients about dying, the solicitation and execution in advance of their directives for terminal care, the education of medical students and residents, and the formulation of institutional guidelines.

The appropriate and, if necessary, aggressive use of pain-relieving substances is recommended, even when such use may result in shortened life. We emphasize the value of a sensitive approach to care — one that is adjusted continually to suit the changing needs of the patient as death approaches. Possible settings for death are reviewed, including the home, the hospital, the intensive care unit, and the nursing home. Finally, we consider the physician's response to the dying patient who is rational and desires suicide or euthanasia.

S.H. Wanzer, D.D. Federman, S.J. Adelstein ,et al.,"Letter," *New England Journal of Medicine* (1989) 320:844-849.

* From Emerson Hospital, Concord, Mass. (S.H.W.); Harvard Medical School, Boston (D.D.F., S.J.A.); the Pritzker School of Medicine, Chicago (C.K.C.); Masssachusetts General Hospital, Boston (E.H.C.); Hennepin County Medical Center, Minneapolis (R.E.C.); University of Virginia Medical Center, Charlottesville (E.W.H.); University of California School of Medicine, San Francisco (B.L.); Mayo Clinic and Medical School, Rochester, Minn. (C.G.M.); the International Resuscitation Research Center, University of Pittsburgh Medical School, Pittsburgh (P.S.); Harvard Law School, Cambridge, Mass. (A.S.); and the University of Texas System Cancer Center and School of Medicine, Houston (J.v.E.). Address reprint requests to Dr. Wanzer at Harvard Law School Health Services, 1563 Massachusetts Ave., Cambridge, MA 02138.

Formulated at a meeting at the Countway Library of Medicine, Boston, October 29 to 31, 1987, held under the auspices of the Society for the Right to Die, New York. Dr. Federman was chairman of the meeting.

Supported by a grant in memory of Joseph S. Kornfeld.

Some of the practices that were controversial five years ago[1] in the care of the dying patient have become accepted and routine. Do-not-resuscitate (DNR) orders, nonexistent only a few years ago, are now commonplace. Many physicians and ethicists now agree that there is little difference between nasogastric or intravenous hydration and other life-sustaining measures. They have concluded, therefore, that it is ethical to withdraw nutrition and hydration from certain dying, hopelessly ill, or permanently unconscious patients. The public and the courts have tended to accept this principle. Most important, there has been an increase in sensitivity to the desires of dying patients on the part of doctors, other health professionals, and the public. The entire subject is now discussed openly. Various studies and reports from governmental bodies, private foundations, the American Medical Association, and state medical societies reflect these advances in thinking.[2-9]

The increased awareness of the rights of dying patients has also been translated into new laws. Thirty-eight states now have legislation covering advance directives ("living wills"), and 15 states specifically provide that a patient's health care spokesperson, or proxy, can authorize the withholding or withdrawal of life support.[10,11]

The courts have continued to support patients' rights and have expanded the legal concept of the right to refuse medical treatment, upholding this right in more than 80 court decisions.[12] As a general rule, the cases in the early 1980s involved terminally ill patients whose death was expected whether or not treatment was continued, and the treatment at issue — for instance, prolonged endotracheal intubation, mechanical ventilation, dialysis, or chemotherapy — was often intrusive or burdensome. The courts recognized the patient's common-law right to autonomy (to be left alone to make one's own choices) as well as the constitutional right to privacy (to be protected from unwanted invasive medical treatment).

Currently, the courts are moving closer to the view that patients are entitled to be allowed to die, whether or not they are terminally ill or suffering. Many recent cases have permitted treatment to be terminated in patients who are permanently unconscious, indicating that the right to refuse treatment can be used to put an end to unacceptable conditions even if the patients are not perceptibly suffering or close to death. In such court opinions, many of which have dealt with artificial feeding, the cause of the patient's death continues to be attributed to the underlying disease, rather than to the withholding or withdrawal of treatment.[13]

Popular attitudes about the rights of dying patients have also changed, often in advance of the attitudes of health care providers, legislators, and the courts. The results of one public-opinion poll indicated that 68 percent of the respondents believed that "people dying of an incurable painful disease should be allowed to end their lives before the disease runs its course."[14]

Health professionals have also become much more aware of patients' rights. In states with laws legitimizing living wills, hospitals have become responsive to patients' wishes as expressed in their advance directives, and hospital accreditation by the Joint Commission on Accreditation of Health Care Organizations now requires the establishment of formal DNR policies. The frequency with which DNR orders are used in nursing homes has also increased. In 1987 the California Department of Health Services became the first state agency to develop clear guidelines for the removal of life support, including tube feeding, in the state's 1500 nursing homes and convalescent hospitals.[15]

GAPS BETWEEN ACCEPTED POLICIES AND THEIR IMPLEMENTATION

Many patients are aware of their right to make decisions about their health care, including the refusal of life-sustaining measures, yet few actually execute living wills or appoint surrogates through a health care proxy. Although such documents can be very helpful in clarifying the patient's wishes, they are all too infrequently discussed in standard medical practice. Furthermore, at present, advance directives do not exert enough influence on either the patient's ability to control medical decision making at the end of life or the physician's behavior with respect to such issues in hospitals, emergency rooms, and nursing homes. There remains a considerable gap between the acceptance of the directive and its implementation. There is also a large gap between what the courts now allow with respect to withdrawal of treatment and what physicians actually do. All too frequently, physicians are reluctant to withdraw aggressive treatment from hopelessly ill patients, despite clear legal precedent.

Physicians have a responsibility to consider timely discussions with patients about life-sustaining treatment and terminal care. Only a minority of physicians now do so consistently.[16] The best time to begin such discussions is during the course of routine, nonemergency care, remembering that not all patients are emotionally prepared, by virtue of their stage in life, their psychological makeup, or the stage of their illness. Nevertheless, as a matter of routine, physicians should become acquainted with their patients' personal values and wishes and should document them just as they document information about medical history, family history, and sociocultural background. Such discussions and the resultant documentation should be considered a part of the minimal standard of acceptable care. The physician should take the initiative in obtaining the documentation and should enter it in the medical record.

These issues are not sufficiently addressed in medical schools and residency programs. Medical educators need to recognize that practitioners may not sufficiently understand or value the patient's role in medical decision-making or may be unwilling to relinquish control of the decision-making process. The interests of patients and physicians alike are best served when decisions are made jointly, and medical students and residents should learn to pursue this goal. These topics ought to be specifically included as curriculums are revised.

In general, health care institutions must recognize their obligation to inform patients of their right to participate in decisions about their medical care, including the right to refuse treatment, and should formulate institutional policies about the use of advance directives and the appointment of surrogate decision-makers. Hospitals, health maintenance organizations, and nursing homes should ask patients on admission to indicate whether they have prepared a living will or designated a surrogate. It seems especially important that nursing homes require a regular review of patient preferences, with each patient's physician taking responsibility for ensuring that such information is obtained and documented. In the case of patients who lack decision-making capacity, surrogate decision-makers should be identified and consulted appropriately. (We prefer the term "decision-making capacity" to "competency" because in the medical context, the patient either has or does not have the capacity to make decisions, whereas competency is a legal determination that can be made only by the courts.)

Although we advocate these approaches, we recognize that the mechanisms of appointing a surrogate and executing a living will do present certain problems. Obviously, it may happen that a surrogate appointed previously is unavailable for consultation when problems arise in the treatment of a patient who lacks decision-making capacity. In addition, there is the problem of determining what constitutes an outdated living will or surrogate appointment and how often they need to be reaffirmed. Laws in most states provide that a living will is valid until it is revoked, but patients need to be encouraged to update and reconfirm such directives from time to time.

SETTINGS FOR DYING

Home

Dying at home can provide the opportunity for quiet and privacy, dignity, and family closeness that may make death easier for the patient and provide consolation for the bereaved. Assuming that a stable and caring home environment exists, emotional and physical comfort is most often greatest at home, with family and friends nearby.

Patients and their families need reassurance that dying at home will not entail medical deprivation. They should be carefully instructed in the means of coping with possible problems, and appropriate community resources should be mobilized to assist them. The provision of care should be guided by the physician and implemented with the help of well-trained, highly motivated personnel from the hospice units that now serve many communities in this country, since home care often becomes too difficult for the family to handle alone. Hospice, a form of care in which an interdisciplinary team provides palliative and support services to both patient and family, is a concept whose time has come.

Recent cost-containment measures for expensive hospital care have given the home hospice movement considerable impetus, resulting in an emphasis on alternatives such as home care.[17] On the other hand, hospice care at home, which should be adequately financed by insurance as a cost-effective way to care for the patient, is often poorly reimbursed, and many hospice programs struggle to stay solvent. There is too much emphasis on reimbursement for high-technology care in the home, as opposed to hands-on nursing care. More adequate financing is clearly indicated for hospice and other home care providers, since it is clear that, overall, care at home usually costs much less than in other settings.

Nursing Home

When an admission to a nursing home is planned for a terminally ill patient, it is important to specify the treatment plans and goals at the outset. The nursing home should inquire about the patient's wishes with regard to life-sustaining procedures, including DNR orders and artificial nutrition and hydration. The patient should be encouraged to execute an advance directive, appoint a surrogate, or both. The possibility that it may be necessary to transfer the patient to a general hospital should be discussed in advance (transfer may become indicated, but usually it is not). All parties should anticipate that the final phases of the dying process will occur in the nursing home without a transfer to the hospital, unless the patient cannot be kept reasonably comfortable in the nursing home.

Even though care can clearly be given more cost-effectively in the nursing home setting than in the general hospital, a major drawback to using the nursing home as a place for dying is that often insurance does not cover the cost of the nursing home care (just as it often does not cover the cost of care at home). Currently, there is almost no private insurance for nursing home care, and Medicare now covers only about 3 percent of nursing home days. The rest must be covered by a combination of Medicaid, to be eligible for which a patient must be pauperized, and private pay. It is essential that federal and private health care plans be modified to make nursing home care more accessible to patients of limited means.

Hospital

As much as one third of the patients cared for at home and expected to die there actually die in the hospital, even when hospice techniques of home care are used. The symptoms or anxiety generated by an impending death may overwhelm the family, and recourse to the hospital is appropriate whenever any treatment program, including a psychosocial one, cannot palliate the distress felt by the patient, the family, or both.

To accommodate such families and patients, hospitals should consider the development of specialized units, with rooms appointed so as to provide pleasant surroundings that will facilitate comfortable interchange among patient, family, and friends. The presence of life-sustaining equipment would be inappropriate in such an environment.

The intensive care unit should generally be discouraged as a treatment setting for the hospitalized patient who is dying, unless intensive palliative measures are required that cannot be done elsewhere. Too often, life-sustaining measures are instituted in the intensive care unit without sufficient thought to the proper goals of treatment. Although the courts have held that in the treatment of the hopelessly ill there is no legal distinction between stopping treatment and not starting it in the first place, there is a bias in the intensive care unit toward continuing aggressive measures that may be inappropriate. Though difficult, it is possible for a patient to die in the intensive care unit with dignity and comfort, since medical hardware itself has no capacity to dehumanize anyone. The important point is that the physician set a tone of caring and support, no matter what the setting.

Although the physicians and nurses in intensive care units may be less prepared than other professionals to switch from aggressive curative care to palliation and the provision of comfort only, they have all seen many situations in which clear decisions to limit treatment have brought welcome relief. Since these care givers often have considerable emotional energy invested in patients who have previously been receiving aggressive curative treatment, they may need consultation with colleagues from outside the intensive care unit to decide when to change the treatment goals.

TREATING THE DYING PATIENT — THE IMPORTANCE OF FLEXIBLE CARE

The care of the dying is an art that should have its fullest expression in helping patients cope with the technologically complicated medical environment that often surrounds them at the end of life. The concept of a good death does not mean simply the withholding of technological treatments that serve only to prolong the act of dying. It also requires the art of deliberately creating a medical environment that allows a peaceful death. Somewhere between the unacceptable extremes of failure to treat the dying patient and intolerable use of aggressive life-sustaining measures, the physician must seek a level of care that optimizes comfort and dignity.

In evaluating the burdens and benefits of treatment for the dying patient — whether in the hospital, in a nursing home, or at home — the physician needs to formulate a flexible and adjustable care plan, tailoring treatment to the patient's changing needs as the disease progresses. Such plans contrast sharply with the practice, frequent in medicine, in which the physician makes rounds and prescribes, leaving orders for nurses and technicians, but not giving continual feedback and adjustment. The physician's actions on behalf of the patient should be appropriate, with respect to both the types of treatments and the location in which they are given. Such actions need to be adjusted continually to the individual patient's needs, with the physician keeping primarily in mind that the benefits of treatment must outweigh the burdens imposed.

When the patient lacks decision-making capacity, discussing the limitation of treatment with the family becomes a major part of the treatment plan. The principle of continually adjusted care should guide all these decisions.

Pain and Suffering

The principle of continually adjusted care is nowhere more important than in the control of pain, fear, and suffering. The hopelessly ill patient must have whatever is necessary to control pain. One of the most pervasive causes of anxiety among patients, their families, and the public is the perception that physicians' efforts toward the relief of pain are sadly deficient. Because of this perceived professional deficiency, people fear that needless suffering will be allowed to occur as patients are dying.[18] To a large extent, we believe such fears are justified.

In the patient whose dying process is irreversible, the balance between minimizing pain and suffering and potentially hastening death should be struck clearly in favor of pain relief. Narcotics or other pain medications should be given in whatever dose and by whatever route is necessary for relief. It is morally correct to increase the dose of narcotics to whatever dose is needed, even though the medication may contribute to the depression of respiration or blood pressure, the dulling of consciousness, or even death, provided the primary goal of the physician is to relieve suffering. The proper dose of pain medication is the dose that is sufficient to relieve pain and suffering, even to the point of unconsciousness.

Dying patients often feel isolated and doubt seriously that their physician will be there to relieve their pain when the terminal phase is near. Early in the course of fatal disease, patients should be offered strong reassurance that pain will be controlled and that their physician will be available when the need is greatest. Both the patient and the family should be told that addiction need not be a source of concern and that the relief of pain will have nothing but a salutary effect from both the physical and the emotional standpoint. When possible, pain medication should be given orally to maximize patient autonomy, but usually a continuous parenteral route is needed for the adequate medication of patients in the near-terminal or terminal state. Under no circumstances should medication be "rationed." For episodic pain, patients should be encouraged to take medication as soon as they are conscious of pain, instead of waiting until it becomes intense and far more difficult to control. For continuous or frequently recurring pain, the patient should be placed on a regular schedule of administration. Some patients will choose to endure a degree of pain rather than experience any loss of alertness or control from taking narcotics — a choice that is consistent with patient autonomy and the concept of continually adjusted care.

If pain cannot be controlled with the commonly used analgesic regimens of mild or moderate strength, the patient should be switched quickly to more potent narcotics. It is important that doses be adequate; the textbook doses recommended for short-term pain are often grossly inadequate for long-term pain in the patient dying of cancer. The physician should be familiar with two or three narcotics and their side effects and appropriate starting dosages. Doses should be brought promptly to levels that provide a reliable pain-free state. Since adequate narcotic management seems to be an unfamiliar area to many physicians, we urge that educational material be distributed to them from a noncommercial source.[19] To allow a patient to experience unbearable pain or suffering is unethical medical practice.

Legal Concerns

The principles of medical ethics are formulated independently of legal decisions, but physicians may fear that decisions about the care of the hopelessly ill will bring special risks of criminal charges and prosecution. Although no medical decision can be immune from legal scrutiny, courts in the United States have generally supported the approaches advocated here.[20-23] The physician should follow these principles without exaggerated concern for legal consequences, doing whatever is necessary to relieve pain and bring comfort, and adhering to the patient's wishes as much as possible. To withhold any necessary measure of pain relief in a hopelessly ill person out of fear of depressing respiration or of possible legal repercussions is unjustifiable. Good medical practice is the best protection against legal liability.

Preparing for Death

As sickness progresses toward death, measures to minimize suffering should be intensified. Dying patients may require palliative care of an intensity that rivals even that of curative efforts. Keeping the patient clean, caring for the skin, preventing the formation of bed sores, treating neuropsychiatric symptoms, controlling peripheral and pulmonary edema, aggressively reducing nausea and vomiting, using intravenous medications, fighting the psychosocial forces that can lead to family fragmentation — all can tax the ingenuity and equanimity of the most skilled health professionals. Even though aggressive curative techniques are no longer indicated, professionals and families are still called on to use intensive measures — extreme responsibility, extraordinary sensitivity, and heroic compassion.

In training programs for physicians, more attention needs to be paid to these aspects of care. Progress has been made in persuading house staff and attending physicians to discuss DNR orders and to include clear orders and notes in the chart about limits on life-sustaining therapies, but patients are too rarely cared for directly by the physician at or near the time of death. Usually it is nurses who care for patients at this time. In a few innovative training programs, most notably at the University of Oregon, the hands-on aspects of care of the dying are addressed,[24] and such techniques should be presented at all training institutions.

ASSISTED SUICIDE

If care is administered properly at the end of life, only the rare patient should be so distressed that he or she desires to commit suicide. Occasionally, however, all fails. The doctor, the nurse, the family, and the patient may have done everything possible to relieve the distress occasioned by a terminal illness, and yet the patient perceives his or her situation as intolerable and seeks assistance in bringing about death. Is it ever justifiable for the physician to assist suicide in such a case?

Some physicians, believing it to be the last act in a continuum of care provided for the hopelessly ill patient, do assist patients who request it, either by prescribing sleeping pills with knowledge of their intended use or by discussing the required doses and methods of administration with the patient. The frequency with which such actions are undertaken is unknown, but they are certainly not rare. Suicide differs from euthanasia in that the act of bringing on death is performed by the patient, not the physician.

The physician who considers helping a patient who requests assistance with suicide must determine first that the patient is indeed beyond all help and not merely suffering from a treatable depression of the sort common in people with terminal illnesses. Such a depression requires therapeutic intervention. If there is no treatable component to the depression and the patient's pain or suffering is refractory to treatment, then the wish for suicide may be rational. If such a patient acts on the wish for death and actually commits suicide, it is ethical for a physician who knows the patient well to refrain from an attempt at resuscitation.

Even though suicide itself is not illegal, helping a person commit suicide is a crime in many states, either by statute or under common law. Even so, we know of no physician who has ever been prosecuted in the United States for prescribing pills in order to help a patient commit suicide.[25] However, the potential illegality of this act is a deterrent, and apart from that, some physicians simply cannot bring themselves to assist in suicide or to condone such action.

Whether it is bad medical practice or immoral to help a hopelessly ill patient commit a rational suicide is a complex issue, provoking a number of considerations. First, as their disease advances, patients may lose their decision-making capacity because of the effects of the disease or the drug treatment. Assisting such patients with suicide comes close to performing an act of euthanasia. Second, patients who want a doctor's assistance with suicide may be unwilling to endure their terminal illness because they lack information about what is ahead. Even when the physician explains in careful detail the availability of the kind of flexible, continually adjusted care described here, the patient may still opt out of that treatment plan and reject the physician's efforts to ease the dying process. Also, what are the physician's obligations if a patient who retains decision-making capacity insists that family members not be told of a suicide plan? Should the physician insist on obtaining the family's consent? Finally, should physicians acknowledge their role in a suicide in some way — by obtaining consultation, or in writing? Physicians who act in secret become isolated and cannot consult colleagues or ethics committees for confirmation that the patient has made a rational decision. If contacted, such colleagues may well object and even consider themselves obligated to report the physician to the Board of Medical Licensure or to the prosecutor. The impulse to maintain secrecy gives the lie to the moral intuition that assistance with suicide is ethical.

It is difficult to answer such questions, but all but two of us (J.v.E. and E.H.C.) believe that it is not immoral for a physician to assist in the rational suicide of a terminally ill person. However, we recognize that such an act represents a departure from the principle of continually adjusted care that we have presented. As such, it should be considered a separate alternative and not an extension of the flexible approach to care that we have recommended. Clearly, the subject of assisted suicide deserves wide and open discussion.

EUTHANASIA

Some patients who cannot carry out suicide plans themselves, with or without assistance, may ask their physicians to take a more active part in ending their lives. In the case of suicide, the final act is performed by the patient, even when the physician provides indirect assistance in the form of information and means. By contrast, euthanasia requires the physician to perform a medical procedure that causes death directly. It is therefore even more controversial than assisted rational suicide, and various arguments have been mustered through the years for and against its use.[26,27]

In the Netherlands, the practice of euthanasia has gained a degree of social acceptance. As a result of a 1984 decision by the Dutch Supreme Court, euthanasia is no longer prosecuted in certain approved circumstances. The Dutch government authorized the State Commission on Euthanasia to study the issue, and the commission's report favored permitting doctors to perform euthanasia with certain safeguards, but the Dutch parliament, the States-General, has not yet acted to change the law.

Many Dutch physicians believe, however, that the medical treatments and actions needed to keep dying patients comfortable may at times be extended to include the act of euthanasia. Some of them hold that a continuum of measures can be brought into play to help the patient, and occasionally the injection of a lethal dose of a drug (usually a short-acting barbiturate, followed by a paralyzing agent) becomes necessary, representing the extreme end of that continuum. This occurs between 5000 and 10 000 times a year in the Netherlands, according to van der Werf[28] (and Admiraal P: personal communication).

The medical community in the Netherlands has developed criteria that must be met for an act of euthanasia to be considered medically and ethically acceptable.[29] The patient's medical situation must be intolerable, with no prospect of improvement. The patient must be rational and must voluntarily and repeatedly request euthanasia of the physician. The patient must be fully informed. There must be no other means of relieving the suffering, and two physicians must concur with the request.

In recent years, euthanasia has been discussed more openly in the United States, and the public response has been increasingly favorable. When a Roper poll asked in 1988 whether a physician should be lawfully able to end the life of a terminally ill patient at the patient's request, 58 percent said yes, 27 percent said no, and 10 percent were undecided. (This poll, taken for the National Hemlock Society by the Roper Organization of New York City, surveyed 1982 adult Americans in March 1988.)

Presumably, the majority of physicians in the United States do not favor the Dutch position. Many physicians oppose euthanasia on moral or religious grounds, and indeed it raises profound theological questions. All religions address the matter of whether it is proper to decide the time of one's death. Whatever attitudes society may develop toward assisted suicide or euthanasia, individual physicians should not feel morally coerced to participate in such approaches. Many physicians oppose euthanasia because they believe it to be outside the physician's role, and some fear that it may be subject to abuse. (Some physicians and laypersons fear that active voluntary euthanasia, as practiced in the Netherlands, could lead to involuntary euthanasia and to murder, as practiced by the Nazis. Ethically, however, the difference is obvious.) In addition, the social climate in this country is very litigious, and the likelihood of prosecution if a case of euthanasia were discovered is fairly high

— much higher than the likelihood of prosecution after a suicide in which the physician has assisted. Thus, the prospect of criminal prosecution deters even the hardiest advocates of euthanasia among physicians.

Nevertheless, the medical profession and the public will continue to debate the role that euthanasia may have in the treatment of the terminally or hopelessly ill patient.

We are indebted to Marjorie B. Zuckerman, Ph.D., and Peg Cameron for assistance in the preparation of the manuscript.

REFERENCES

1. Wanzer SH, Adelstein SJ, Cranford RE, et al. The physician's responsibility toward hopelessly ill patients. *N Engl J Med* 1984; 310:955-9.
2. President's Commission for the Study of Ethical Problems in Medicine and Biomedical and Behavioral Research. *Deciding to forego life-sustaining treatment: a report on the ethical, medical and legal issues in treatment decisions.* Washington, D.C.: Government Printing Office, 1983.
3. Office of Technology Assessment. *Life-sustaining technologies and the elderly.* Washington, D.C.: Government Printing Office, 1987.
4. Senate Special Committee on Aging. *A matter of choice: planning ahead for health care decisions.* Washington, D.C.: Government Printing Office, 1987.
5. *Guidelines on the termination of life-sustaining treatment and the care of the dying: a report by the Hastings Center.* Briarcliff Manor, N.Y.: Hastings Center, 1987.
6. Current Opinions of the Council on Ethical and Judicial Affairs of the American Medical Association — 1986. *Withholding or withdrawing life-prolonging treatment.* Chicago: American Medical Association, 1986.
7. Executive Board of the American Academy of Neurology. *Position of the American Academy of Neurology on certain aspects of the care and management of the persistent vegetative state patient.* Minneapolis: American Academy of Neurology, 1988.
8. Ruark JE, Raffin TA, Stanford University Medical Center Committee on Ethics. Initiating and withdrawing life support. *N Engl J Med* 1988; 318:25-30.
9. Safar P, Bircher N. *Cardiopulmonary cerebral resuscitation: an introduction to resuscitation medicine*. 3rd ed. Philadelphia: W.B. Saunders, 1988.
10. Society for the Right to Die. *Handbook of living will laws.* New York: Society for the Right to Die, 1987.
11. *Appointing a proxy for health care decisions.* New York: Society for the Right to Die, 1988.
12. *Adult right to die case citations.* New York: Society for the Right to Die, 1988.
13. *Right to die court decisions: artificial feeding.* New York: Society for the Right to Die, 1988.
14. Associated Press/Media General. Poll no. 4. Richmond, Va.: Media General, February 1985.
15. California Department of Health Services. *Guidelines regarding withdrawal or withholding of life-sustaining procedure(s) in longterm care facilities,* August 7, 1987.

16. Bedell SE, Pelle D, Maher PL, Cleary PD. Do-not-resuscitate orders for critically ill patients in the hospital: how are they used and what is their impact? *JAMA* 1986; 256:233-7.
17. Bulkin W, Lukashok H. Rx for dying: the case for hospice. *N Engl J Med* 1988; 318:376-8.
18. Angell M. The quality of mercy. *N Engl J Med* 1982; 306:98-9.
19. Payne R, Foley KM, eds. Cancer pain. *Med Clin North Am* 1987; 71:153-352.
20. *Bartling v. Superior Court* (Glendale Adventist Medical Center), 163 Cal. App. 3d 186, 209 Cal. Rptr. 220 (Ct. App. 1984).
21. *Bouvia v. Superior Court* (Glenchur), 179 Cal. App. 3d 1127, 225 Cal. Rptr. 297 (Ct. App. 1986), review denied (Cal. June 5, 1986).
22. *Brophy v. New England Sinai Hosp., Inc.,* 398 Mass. 417, 497, N.E. 2d 626 (1986).
23. *In re Culham,* No. 87-340537-AC (Mich. Cir. Ct., Oakland County, Dec. 15, 1987) (Breck J).
24. Tolle SW, Hickham DH, Larson EB, Benson JA. Patient death and house-staff stress. *Clin Res* 1987; 35:762A. abstract.
25. Glantz LH. Withholding and withdrawing treatment: the role of the criminal law. Law *Med Health Care* 1987-88; 15:231-41.
26. Van Bommel H. *Choices for people who have a terminal illness, their families and their caregivers.* Toronto: NC Press, 1986.
27. Angell M. Euthanasia. *N Engl J Med* 1988; 319:1348-50.
28. van der Werf GT. Huisarts en euthanasie. *Medisch Contact* 1986; 43:1389.
29. The Central Committee of the Royal Dutch Medical Association. *Vision on euthanasia.* Utrecht, the Netherlands, 1986.

FURTHER READINGS

Ashley, B.A. and K.D. O'Rourke
Health Care Ethics: A Theological Analysis. (The Catholic Health Association of the United States: St. Louis, 1982).
Beauchamp, T.L.
"A Reply to Rachels on Active and Passive Euthanasia," in Beauchamp and Perlin, *Ethical Issues in Death and Dying.* (Englewood Cliffs, N.J.: Prentice Hall, 1978).
Engelhardt, Jr., H.T.
"Euthanasia and Children: The Injury of Continued Existence," *Journal of Paediatrics* 83:170 (1073).
Foot, P.
"Euthanasia," *Philosophy and Public Affairs* 6: 2 (Winter 1977).
Gould, J. and L. Craigmyle
Your Death Warrant: The Implications of Euthanasia. (London: Chapman, 1971).
Kamisar, Yale
"Some Non-Religious Objections Against Proposed Mercy-Killing Legislation," *Minnesota Law Review* 42 (May 1958) 969–1042.
Kluge, E.-H.W.
The Practice of Death. (New Haven: Yale University Press, 1975).

Law Reform Commission of Canada
Report 20, *Euthanasia, Aiding Suicide and Cessation of Treatment.* (Ottawa: Minister of Supply and Services, 1983).
Law Reform Commission of Canada
Working Paper 46, *Omission, Negligence and Endangering.* (Ottawa: Law Reform Commission, 1985).
Macklin, R.
Mortal Choices. (N.Y.: Pantheon Books, 1987).
Magnet, J.E. and E.-H.W. Kluge
Withholding Treatment from Defective Newborn Children. (Cowansville: Brown Legal Publications, 1985).
Pope Pius XII
"Prolongation of Life: Allocution to an International Congress of Anesthesiologists," Nov. 24, 1957, *Osservatore Romano* 4 (1957).
Rachels, James
The End of Life: Euthanasia and Morality. (Oxford: Oxford University Press, 1986).
Ramsey, P.
"On (Only) Caring for the Dying," in *The Patient as Person.* (New Haven and London: Yale University Press, 1970), 120–123.
Rosner, F.
Modern Medicine and Jewish Law. (New York: Yeshiva University, 1972).
Sade, R.M. and A.B. Redfern
"Euthanasia," *New England Journal of Medicine* 292: 16 (April 17, 1975). 96ff.
Society for the Right to Die
Handbook of Living Will Laws. (New York: Society for the Right to Die, 1987).
Vaux, K., ed.
Who Shall Live? Medicine, Technology, Ethics. (Philadelphia: Fortress Press, 1970).
Veatch, R.
Death, Dying, and the Biological Revolution: Our Last Quest for Responsibility. (New Haven and London: Yale University Press, 1970).

CHAPTER 12 ADVANCE DIRECTIVE AND LIVING WILLS

INTRODUCTION

The push for autonomy that has characterized so many recent developments in the ethics of health care delivery has begun to assert itself in the sphere of dying. Sometimes people who are dying wish to die faster; sometimes people who are not dying want to die, and yet the institutionalized circumstances in which they find themselves have taken what little control they previously had over the dying process out of their hands and placed it into the hands of the health care professionals. This development has prompted a movement to put control of the dying process — insofar as such control is ever possible — into the hands of the individual.

The selections that follow reflect this patient- and autonomy-oriented movement. The case of *Malette v. Shulman* shows the conflict between the traditional ethos of the medical profession, which feels that its obligation is to save life whenever medically possible and appropriate, against the patient's claim to autonomy.

Malette v. Shulman says that if a patient has explicitly given an advance directive about not using a specific procedure, then health care professionals are duty-bound to respect that wish. The judgment therefore accepts that a patient has the right to exercise her or his autonomy, even if that means that the patient will die. However, the judgment in *Malette v. Shulman* states explicitly that it is not intended to legalize so-called living wills: documents in which patients state under what circumstances they do not wish to be kept alive.

The discussion by Fisher and Meslin (a physician and an ethicist respectively) provides a series of perspectives on the pros and cons on the issue.

The position of the Canadian Medical Association, which was formally adopted by the Association at its 124th general Council in August of 1991, shows how organized Canadian medicine has tried to look behind the mere legalism of *Malette* to the underlying ethical justification of the decision, and how it has attempted to develop a policy that accepts the principle of the autonomy of the patient.

Malette v. Shulman et al.

I

In the early afternoon of June 30, 1979, Mrs. Georgette Malette, then age 57, was rushed, unconscious, by ambulance to the Kirkland and District Hospital in Kirkland Lake, Ontario. She had been in an accident. The car in which she was a passenger, driven by her husband, had collided head-on with a truck. Her husband had been killed. She suffered serious injuries.

On arrival at the hospital, she was attended by Dr. David L. Shulman, a family physician practising in Kirkland Lake who served two or three shifts a week in the emergency department of the hospital and who was on duty at the time. Dr. Shulman's initial examination of Mrs. Malette showed, among other things, that she had severe head and face injuries and was bleeding profusely. The doctor concluded that she was suffering from incipient shock by reason of blood loss, and ordered that she be given intravenous glucose followed immediately by Ringer's Lactate. The administration of a volume expander, such as Ringer's Lactate, is standard medical procedure in cases of this nature. If the patient does not respond with significantly increased blood pressure, transfusions of blood are then administered to carry essential oxygen to tissues and to remove waste products and prevent damage to vital organs.

At about this time, a nurse discovered a card in Mrs. Malette's purse which identified her as a Jehovah's Witness and in which she requested, on the basis of her religious convictions, that she be given no blood transfusions under any circumstances. The card, which was not dated or witnessed, was printed in French and signed by Mrs. Malette. Translated into English, it read:

NO BLOOD TRANSFUSION!

> As one of Jehovah's Witnesses with firm religious convictions, I request that no blood or blood products be administered to me under any circumstances. I fully realize the implications of this position, but I have resolutely decided to obey the Bible command: "Keep abstaining ... from blood." (Acts 15:28, 29). However, I have no religious objection to use the nonblood alternatives, such as Dextran, Haemaccel, PVP, Ringer's Lactate or saline solution.

Dr. Shulman was promptly advised of the existence of this card and its contents.

Mrs. Malette was next examined by a surgeon on duty in the hospital. He concluded, as had Dr. Shulman, that, to avoid irreversible shock, it was vital to maintain her blood volume. He had Mrs. Malette transferred to the X-ray department for X-rays of her skull, pelvis and chest. However, before the X-rays could be satisfactorily completed, Mrs. Malette's condi-

Malette v. Shulman, (1990) 72 O.R. (2d) 417 (C.A.).pp. 17-42. The decision has since been affirmed by the Supreme Court of Canada.

tion deteriorated. Her blood pressure dropped markedly, her respiration became increasingly distressed, and her level of consciousness dropped. She continued to bleed profusely and could be said to be critically ill.

At this stage, Dr. Shulman decided that Mrs. Malette's condition had deteriorated to the point that transfusions were necessary to replace her lost blood and to preserve her life and health. Having made that decision, he personally administered transfusions to her, in spite of the Jehovah's Witness card, while she was in the X-ray department and after she was transferred to the intensive care unit. Dr. Shulman was clearly aware of the religious objection to blood manifested in the card carried by Mrs. Malette and the instruction that "NO BLOOD TRANSFUSION!" be given under any circumstances. He accepted full responsibility then, as he does now, for the decision to administer the transfusions.

Some three hours after the transfusions were commenced, Mrs. Malette's daughter, Celine Bisson, who had driven to Kirkland Lake from Timmins, arrived at the hospital accompanied by her husband and a local church elder. She strongly objected to her mother being given blood. She informed Dr. Shulman and some of the other defendants that both she and her mother were Jehovah's Witnesses, that a tenet of their faith forbids blood transfusions, and that she knew her mother would not want blood transfusions. Notwithstanding Dr. Shulman's opinion as to the medical necessity of the transfusions, Mrs. Bisson remained adamantly opposed to them. She signed a document specifically prohibiting blood transfusions and a release of liability. Dr. Shulman refused to follow her instructions. Since the blood transfusions were, in his judgment, medically necessary in this potentially life-threatening situation, he believed it his professional responsibility as the doctor in charge to ensure that his patient received the transfusions. Furthermore, he was not satisfied that the card signed by Mrs. Malette expressed her current instructions because, on the information he then had, he did not know whether she might have changed her religious beliefs before the accident; whether the card may have been signed because of family or peer pressure; whether at the time she signed the card she was fully informed of the risks of refusal of blood transfusions; or whether, if conscious, she might have changed her mind in the face of medical advice as to her perhaps imminent but avoidable death.

As matters developed, by about midnight Mrs. Malette's condition had stabilized sufficiently to permit her to be transferred early the next morning by air ambulance to Toronto General Hospital where she received no further blood transfusions. She was discharged on August 11, 1979. Happily, she made a very good recovery from her injuries.

II

In June, 1980, Mrs. Malette brought this action against Dr. Shulman, the hospital, its executive director and four nurses, alleging, in the main, that the administration of blood transfusions in the circumstances of her case constituted negligence and assault and battery and subjected her to religious discrimination. The trial came on before Donnelly J. who, in reasons now reported at 63 O.R. (2d) 243, 47 D.L.R. (4th) 18, 43 C.C.L.T. 62, dismissed the action against all defendants save Dr. Shulman. With respect to Dr. Shulman, the learned judge concluded that the Jehovah's Witness card validly restricted his right to treat the patient, and there was no rationally founded basis upon which the doctor could ignore that restriction. Hence, his administration of blood transfusions constituted a battery on the plaintiff. The judge awarded her damages of $20,000 but declined to make any award of costs.

Dr. Shulman now appeals to this court from that judgment. Mrs. Malette cross-appeals the judge's dismissal of the action against the hospital and his order with respect to costs.

In his reasons for judgment, Donnelly J. fully and carefully set out the facts of this case as he found them. I see no need to restate those facts in any greater detail than I already have. Nor do I see any need to repeat the arguments that were advanced in both the appeal and the cross-appeal by which the parties seek to impugn the judge's findings in certain particulars. I think it sufficient to say that I am of the opinion that the judge's factual conclusions are unassailable. His findings were properly made within his province as the trier of fact and are supported by the evidence. It is not this court's function to weigh conflicting evidence or to determine the relative effect of contradictory medical opinions with respect either to bloodless medicine or to the benefits and risks of blood transfusions. The legal issues to be determined in this appeal must be dealt with on the basis of the findings made at trial.

I should perhaps underscore the fact that Dr. Shulman was not found liable for any negligence in his treatment of Mrs. Malette. The judge held that he had acted "promptly, professionally and was well-motivated throughout" and that his management of the case had been "carried out in a competent, careful and conscientious manner" in accordance with the requisite standard of care. His decision to administer blood in the circumstances confronting him was found to be an honest exercise of his professional judgment which did not delay Mrs. Malette's recovery, endanger her life or cause her any bodily harm. Indeed, the judge concluded that the doctor's treatment of Mrs. Malette "may well have been responsible for saving her life".

Liability was imposed in this case on the basis that the doctor tortiously violated his patient's rights over her own body by acting contrary to the Jehovah's Witness card and administering blood transfusions that were not authorized. His honest and even justifiable belief that the treatment was medically essential did not serve to relieve him from liability for the battery resulting from his intentional and unpermitted conduct...

III

What then is the legal effect, if any, of the Jehovah's Witness card carried by Mrs. Malette? Was the doctor bound to honour the instructions of his unconscious patient or, given the emergency and his inability to obtain conscious instructions from his patient, was he entitled to disregard the card and act according to his best medical judgment?

To answer these questions and determine the effect to be given to the Jehovah's Witness card, it is first necessary to ascertain what rights a competent patient has to accept or reject medical treatment and to appreciate the nature and extent of those rights.

The right of a person to control his or her own body is a concept that has long been recognized at common law. The tort of battery has traditionally protected the interest in bodily security from unwanted physical interference. Basically, any intentional nonconsensual touching which is harmful or offensive to a person's reasonable sense of dignity is actionable. Of course, a person may choose to waive this protection and consent to the intentional invasion of this interest, in which case an action for battery will not be maintainable. No special exceptions are made for medical care, other than in emergency situations, and the general rules governing actions for battery are applicable to the doctor-patient relationship. Thus, as a matter of common law, a medical intervention in which a doctor touches the body of a patient would constitute a battery if the patient did not consent to the intervention. Patients have the decisive role in the medical decision-making process. Their right of self-determination is recognized and protected by the law. As Justice Cardozo proclaimed in his classic statement: "Every human being of adult years and sound mind has a right to determine what shall be done with his own body; and a surgeon who performs an operation without his patient's consent commits an assault, for which he is liable in damages": *Schloendoff v. Society of New York Hospital,* 211 N.Y. 125 (1914). See also, *Videto v. Kennedy* (1981), 33 O.R. (2d) 497, 125 D.L.R. (3d) 127, 17 C.C.L.T. 307 (C.A.); Linden, *Canadian Tort Law,* 4th ed. (1988), at pp. 40-3 and p. 59 *et seq.;* Prosser & Keeton, *The Law of Torts,* 5th ed. (1984), at pp. 39-42; and Fleming, *The Law of Torts,* 7th ed. (1987), at pp. 23-4.

The doctrine of informed consent has developed in the law as the primary means of protecting a patient's right to control his or her medical treatment. Under the doctrine, no medical procedure may be undertaken without the patient's consent obtained after the patient has been provided with sufficient information to evaluate the risks and benefits of the proposed treatment and other available options. The doctrine presupposes the patient's capacity to make a subjective treatment decision based on her understanding of the necessary medical facts provided by the doctor and on her assessment of her own personal circumstances. A doctor who performs a medical procedure without having first furnished the patient with the information needed to obtain an informed consent will have infringed the patient's right to control the course of her medical care, and will be liable in battery even though the procedure was performed with a high degree of skill and actually benefitted the patient.

The right of self-determination which underlies the doctrine of informed consent also obviously encompasses the right to refuse medical treatment. A competent adult is generally entitled to reject a specific treatment or all treatment, or to select an alternate form of treatment, even if the decision may entail risks as serious as death and may appear mistaken in the eyes of the medical profession or of the community. Regardless of the doctor's opinion, it is the patient who has the final say on whether to undergo the treatment. The patient is free to decide, for instance, not to be operated on or not to undergo therapy or, by the same token, not to have a blood transfusion. If a doctor were to proceed in the face of a decision to reject the treatment, he would be civilly liable for his unauthorized conduct notwithstanding his justifiable belief that what he did was necessary to preserve the patient's life or health. The doctrine of informed consent is plainly intended to ensure the freedom of individuals to make choices concerning their medical care. For this freedom to be meaningful, people must have the right to make choices that accord with their own values regardless of how unwise or foolish those choices may appear to others...

IV

The emergency situation is an exception to the general rule requiring a patient's prior consent. When immediate medical treatment is necessary to save the life or preserve the health of a person who, by reason of unconsciousness or extreme illness, is incapable of either giving or withholding consent, the doctor may proceed without the patient's consent. The delivery of medical services is rendered lawful in such circumstances either on the rationale that the doctor has implied consent from the patient to give emergency aid or, more accurately in my view, on the rationale that the doctor is privileged by reason of necessity in giving the aid and is not to be held liable for so doing. On either basis, in an emergency the law sets aside the requirement of consent on the assumption that the patient, as a reasonable person, would want emergency aid to be rendered if she were capable of giving instructions.

On the facts of the present case, Dr. Shulman was clearly faced with an emergency. He had an unconscious, critically ill patient on his hands who, in his opinion, needed blood transfusions to save her life or preserve her health. If there were no Jehovah's Witness card he undoubtedly would have been entitled to administer blood transfusions as part of the emergency treatment and could not have been held liable for so doing. In those circumstances he would have had no indication that the transfusions would have been refused had the patient then been able to make her wishes known and, accordingly, no reason to expect that, as a reasonable person, she would not consent to the transfusions.

However, to change the facts, if Mrs. Malette, before passing into unconsciousness, had expressly instructed Dr. Shulman, in terms comparable to those set forth on the card, that her religious convictions as a Jehovah's Witness were such that she was not to be given a blood transfusion under any circumstances and that she fully realized the implications of this position, the doctor would have been confronted with an obviously different situation. Here, the patient, anticipating an emergency in which she might be unable to make decisions about her health care contemporaneous with the emergency, has given explicit instructions that blood transfusions constitute an unacceptable medical intervention and are not to be administered to her. Once the emergency arises, is the doctor none the less entitled to administer transfusions on the basis of his honest belief that they are needed to save his patient's life?

The answer, in my opinion, is clearly no. A doctor is not free to disregard a patient's advance instructions any more than he would be free to disregard instructions given at the time of the emergency. The law does not prohibit a patient from withholding consent to emergency medical treatment, nor does the law prohibit a doctor from following his patient's instructions. While the law may disregard the absence of consent in limited emergency circumstances, it otherwise supports the right of competent adults to make decisions concerning their own health care by imposing civil liability on those who perform medical treatment without consent.

The patient's decision to refuse blood in the situation I have posed was made prior to and in anticipation of the emergency. While the doctor would have had the opportunity to dissuade her on the basis of his medical advice, her refusal to accept his advice or her unwillingness to discuss or consider the subject would not relieve him of his obligation to follow her instructions. The principles of self-determination and individual autonomy compel the conclusion that the patient may reject blood transfusions even if harmful consequences may result and even if the decision is generally regarded as foolhardy. Her decision in this instance would be operative after she lapsed into unconsciousness, and the doctor's conduct would be unauthorized. To transfuse a Jehovah's Witness in the face of her explicit instructions to the contrary would, in my opinion, violate her right to control her own body and show disrespect for the religious values by which she has chosen to live her life...

V

The distinguishing feature of the present case — and the one that makes this a case of first impression — is, of course, the Jehovah's Witness card on the person of the unconscious patient. What then is the effect of the Jehovah's Witness card?

In the appellant's submission, the card is of no effect and, as a consequence, can play no role in determining the doctor's duty toward his patient in the emergency situation existing in this case. The trial judge, the appellant argues, erred in holding both that the Jehovah's Witness card validly restricted the doctor's right to administer the blood transfusions, and that there was no rationally founded basis for ignoring the card. The argument proceeds on the basis, first, that, as a matter of principle, a card of this nature could not operate in these circumstances to prohibit the doctor from providing emergency health care and, second, that in any event, as a matter of evidence, there was good reason to doubt the card's validity.

The appellant acknowledges that a conscious rational patient is entitled to refuse any medical treatment and that a doctor must comply with that refusal no matter how ill-advised he may believe it to be. He contends, however, to quote from his factum, that "a patient refusing treatment regarded by a doctor as being medically necessary has a right to be advised by the doctor, and the doctor has a concomitant duty to advise the patient of the risks associated with that refusal". Here, because of the patient's unconsciousness, the doctor had no opportunity to advise her of the specific risks involved in refusing the blood transfusions that he regarded as medically necessary. In those circumstances, the appellant argues, it was not possible for the doctor to obtain, or for the patient to give, an "informed refusal". In the absence of such a refusal, the argument proceeds, Dr. Shulman was under a legal and ethical duty to treat this patient as he would any other emergency case and provide the treatment that, in his medical judgment, was needed to preserve her health and life. In short, the argument concludes, Mrs. Malette's religiously motivated instructions, prepared in contemplation of an emergency, directing that she not be given blood transfusions in any circumstances, were of no force or effect and could be ignored with impunity.

In challenging the trial judge's finding that there was no rationally founded evidentiary basis for doubting the validity of the card and ignoring the restriction contained in it, the appellant puts forth a number of questions which he claims compel the conclusion that he was under no duty to comply with these instructions. He argues that it could properly be doubted whether the card constituted a valid statement of Mrs. Malette's wishes in this emergency because it was unknown, for instance, whether she knew the card was still in her purse; whether she was still a Jehovah's Witness or how devout a Jehovah's Witness she was; what information she had about the risks associated with the refusal of blood transfusion when she signed the card; or whether, if she were conscious, she would refuse blood transfusions after the doctor had an opportunity to advise her of the risks associated with the refusal.

With deference to Mr. Royce's exceedingly able argument on behalf of the appellant, I am unable to accept the conclusions advocated by him. I do not agree, as his argument would have it, that the Jehovah's Witness card can be no more than a meaningless piece of paper. I share the trial judge's view that, in the circumstances of this case, the instructions in the Jehovah's Witness card imposed a valid restriction on the emergency treatment that could be provided to Mrs. Malette and precluded blood transfusions.

I should emphasize that in deciding this case the court is not called upon to consider the law that may be applicable to the many situations in which objection may be taken to the use or continued use of medical treatment to save or prolong a patient's life. The court's role, especially in a matter as sensitive as this, is limited to resolving the issues raised by the facts presented in this particular case. On these facts, we are not concerned with a patient who has been diagnosed as terminally or incurably ill who seeks by way of advance directive or "living will" to reject medical treatment so that she may die with dignity; neither are we concerned with a patient in an irreversible vegetative state whose family seeks to withdraw medical treatment in order to end her life; nor is this a case in which an otherwise healthy patient wishes for some reason or other to terminate her life. There is no element of suicide or euthanasia in this case.

Our concern here is with a patient who has chosen in the only way possible to notify doctors and other providers of health care, should she be unconscious or otherwise unable to convey her wishes, that she does not consent to blood transfusions. Her written statement is plainly intended to express her wishes when she is unable to speak for herself. There is no suggestion that she wished to die. Her rejection of blood transfusions is based on the firm belief held by Jehovah's Witnesses, founded on their interpretation of the Scriptures, that the acceptance of blood will result in a forfeiture of their opportunity for resurrection and eternal salvation. The card evidences that "as one of Jehovah's Witnesses with firm religious convictions" Mrs. Malette is not to be administered blood transfusions "under any circumstances"; that, while she "fully realize[s] the implications of this position", she has "resolutely decided to obey the Bible command"; and that she has no religious objection to "nonblood alternatives". In signing and carrying this card Mrs. Malette has made manifest her determination to abide by this fundamental tenet of her faith and refuse blood regardless of the consequences. If her refusal involves a risk of death, then, according to her belief, her death would be necessary to ensure her spiritual life.

Accepting for the moment that there is no reason to doubt that the card validly expressed Mrs. Malette's desire to withhold consent to blood transfusions, why should her wishes not be respected? Why should she be transfused against her will? The appellant's answer, in essence, is that the card cannot be effective when the doctor is unable to provide the patient with the information she would need before making a decision to withhold consent in this specific emergency situation. In the absence of an informed refusal, the appellant submits that Mrs. Malette's right to protection against unwanted infringements of her bodily integrity must give way to countervailing societal interests which limit a person's right to refuse medical treatment. The appellant identifies two such interests as applicable to the unconscious patient in the present situation: first, the interest of the state in preserving life and, second, the interest of the state in safeguarding the integrity of the medical profession.

VI

The state undoubtedly has a strong interest in protecting and preserving the lives and health of its citizens. There clearly are circumstances where this interest may override the individual's right to self-determination. For example, the state may in certain cases require that citizens submit to medical procedures in order to eliminate a health threat to the community or it may prohibit citizens from engaging in activities which are inherently dangerous to their lives. But this interest does not prevent a competent adult from refusing life-preserving medical treatment in general or blood transfusions in particular.

The state's interest in preserving the life or health of a competent patient must generally give way to the patient's stronger interest in directing the course of her own life. As indicated earlier, there is no law prohibiting a patient from declining necessary treatment or prohibiting a doctor from honouring the patient's decision. To the extent that the law reflects the state's interest, it supports the right of individuals to make their own decisions. By imposing civil liability on those who perform medical treatment without consent even though the treatment may be beneficial, the law serves to maximize individual freedom of choice. Recognition of the right to reject medical treatment cannot, in my opinion, be said to depreciate the interest of the state in life or in the sanctity of life. Individual free choice and self-determination are themselves fundamental constituents of life. To deny individuals freedom of choice with respect to their health care can only lessen, and not enhance, the value of life. This state interest, in my opinion, cannot properly be invoked to prohibit Mrs. Malette from choosing for herself whether or not to undergo blood transfusions.

Safeguarding the integrity of the medical profession is patently a legitimate state interest worthy of protection. However, I do not agree that this interest can serve to limit a patient's right to refuse blood transfusions. I recognize, of course, that the choice between violating a patient's private convictions and accepting her decision is hardly an easy one for members of a profession dedicated to aiding the injured and preserving life. The patient's right to determine her own medical treatment is, however, paramount to what might otherwise be the doctor's obligation to provide needed medical care. The doctor is bound in law by the patient's choice even though that choice may be contrary to the mandates of his own conscience and professional judgment. If patient choice were subservient to conscientious medical judgment, the right of the patient to determine her own treatment, and the doctrine of informed consent, would be rendered meaningless. Recognition of a Jehovah's Witness' right to refuse blood transfusions cannot, in my opinion, be seen as threatening the integrity of the medical profession or the state's interest in protecting the same.

In sum, it is my view that the principal interest asserted by Mrs. Malette in this case — the interest in the freedom to reject, or refuse to consent to, intrusions of her bodily integrity — outweighs the interest of the state in the preservation of life and health and the protection of the integrity of the medical profession. While the right to decline medical treatment is not absolute or unqualified, those state interests are not in themselves sufficiently compelling to justify forcing a patient to submit to nonconsensual invasions of her person. The interest of the state in protecting innocent third parties and preventing suicide are, I might note, not applicable to the present circumstances.

VII

The unique considerations in this case arise by virtue of Mrs. Malette's aim to articulate through her Jehovah's Witness card her wish not to be given blood transfusions in any circumstances. In considering the effect to be given the card, it must, of course, be borne in mind that no previous doctor-patient relationship existed between Dr. Shulman and Mrs. Malette. The doctor was acting here in an emergency in which he clearly did not have, nor could he obtain, her consent to his intervention. His intervention can be supported only by resort to the emergency doctrine which I outlined in Part IV of these reasons.

Under that doctrine, the doctor could administer blood transfusions without incurring liability, even though the patient had not consented, if he had no reason to believe that the patient, if she had the opportunity to consent, would decline. In those circumstances, it could be assumed that the patient, as a reasonable person, would consent to aid being rendered if she were able to give instructions. The doctor's authority to make decisions for his patient is necessarily a limited authority. If he knows that the patient has refused to consent to the proposed procedure, he is not empowered to overrule the patient's decision by substituting his decision for hers even though he, and most others, may think hers a foolish or unreasonable decision. In these circumstances the assumption upon which consent is set aside in an emergency could no longer be made. The doctor has no authority to intervene in the face of a patient's declared wishes to the contrary. Should he none the less proceed, he would be liable in battery for tortiously invading the patient's bodily integrity notwithstanding that what he did may be considered beneficial to the patient.

In this case, the patient, in effect, issued standing orders that she was to be given "NO BLOOD TRANSFUSION!" in any circumstances. She gave notice to the doctor and the hospital, in the only practical way open to her, of her firm religious convictions as a Jehovah's Witness and her resolve to abstain from blood. Her instructions plainly contemplated the situation in which she found herself as a result of her unfortunate accident. In light of those instructions, assuming their validity, she cannot be said to have consented to blood transfusions in this emergency. Nor can the doctor be said to have proceeded on the reasonable belief that the patient would have consented had she been in a condition to do so. Given his awareness of her instructions and his understanding that blood transfusions were anathema to her on religious grounds, by what authority could he administer the transfusions? Put another way, if the card evidences the patient's intent to withhold consent, can the doctor none the less ignore the card and subject the patient to a procedure that is manifestly contrary to her express wishes and unacceptable to her religious beliefs?

At issue here is the freedom of the patient as an individual to exercise her right to refuse treatment and accept the consequences of her own decision. Competent adults, as I have sought to demonstrate, are generally at liberty to refuse medical treatment even at the risk of death. The right to determine what shall be done with one's own body is a fundamental right in our society. The concepts inherent in this right are the bedrock upon which the principles of self-determination and individual autonomy are based. Free individual choice in matters affecting this right should, in my opinion, be accorded very high priority. I view the issues in this case from that perspective.

VIII

The appellant's basic position, reduced to its essentials, is that unless the doctor can obtain the patient's informed refusal of blood transfusions he need not follow the instructions provided in the Jehovah's Witness card. Nothing short of a conscious, contemporaneous decision by the patient to refuse blood transfusions — a decision made after the patient has been fully informed by the doctor of the risks of refusing blood in the specific circumstances facing her — will suffice, the appellant contends, to eliminate the doctor's authority to administer emergency treatment or, by the same token, to relieve the doctor of his obligation to treat this emergency patient as he would any other.

In my opinion, it is unnecessary to determine in this case whether there is doctrine of informed refusal as distinct from the doctrine of informed consent. In the particular doctor-patient relationship which arose in these emergency circumstances it is apparent that the doctor could not inform the patient of the risks involved in her prior decision to refuse consent to blood transfusions in any circumstances. It is apparent also that her decision did not emerge out of a doctor-patient relationship. Whatever the doctor's obligation to provide the information needed to make an informed choice may be in other doctor-patient relationships, he cannot be in breach of any such duty in the circumstances of this relationship. The patient manifestly made the decision on the basis of her religious convictions. It is not for the doctor to second-guess the reasonableness of the decision or to pass judgment on the religious principles which motivated it. The fact that he had no opportunity to offer medical advice cannot nullify instructions plainly intended to govern in circumstances where such advice is not possible. Unless the doctor had reason to believe that the instructions in the Jehovah's Witness card were not valid instructions in the sense that they did not truly represent the patient's wishes, in my opinion he was obliged to honour them. He has no authorization under the emergency doctrine to override the patient's wishes. In my opinion, she was entitled to reject in advance of an emergency a medical procedure inimical to her religious values.

The remaining question is whether the doctor factually had reason to believe the instructions were not valid. On this question, the trial judge held that the doctor's "doubt about the validity of the card ... was not rationally founded on the evidence before him". I agree with that conclusion. On my reading of the record, there was no reason not to regard this card as a valid advance directive. Its instructions were clear, precise and unequivocal, and manifested a calculated decision to reject a procedure offensive to the patient's religious convictions. The instructions excluded from potential emergency treatment a single medical procedure well known to the lay public and within its comprehension. The religious belief of Jehovah's Witnesses with respect to blood transfusions was known to the doctor and, indeed, is a matter of common knowledge to providers of health care. The card undoubtedly belonged to and was signed by Mrs. Malette; its authenticity was not questioned by anyone at the hospital and, realistically, could not have been questioned. The trial judge found, "[t]here [was] no basis in evidence to indicate that the card [did] not represent the current intention and instruction of the card holder" [p. 268 O.R., p. 43 D.L.R.]. There was nothing to give credence to or provide support for the speculative inferences implicit in questions as to the current strength of Mrs. Malette's religious beliefs or as to the circumstances under which the card was signed or her state of mind at the time. The fact that a card of this nature was carried by her can itself be taken as verification of her continuing and current resolve to reject blood "fully realiz[ing] the implications of this position".

In short, the card on its face set forth unqualified instructions applicable to the circumstances presented by this emergency. In the absence of any evidence to the contrary, those instructions should be taken as validly representing the patient's wish not to be transfused. If, of course, there were evidence to the contrary — evidence which cast doubt on whether the card was a true expression of the patient's wishes — the doctor, in my opinion, would be entitled to proceed as he would in the usual emergency case. In this case, however, there was no such contradictory evidence. Accordingly, I am of the view that the card had the effect of validly restricting the treatment that could be provided to Mrs. Malette and constituted the doctor's administration of the transfusions a battery.

With respect to Mrs. Malette's daughter, I would treat her role in this matter as no more than confirmatory of her mother's wishes. The decision in this case does not turn on whether the doctor failed to follow the daughter's instructions. Therefore, it is unnecessary, and in my view would be inadvisable, to consider what effect, if any, should be given to a substitute decision, purportedly made by a relative on behalf of the patient, to reject medical treatment in these circumstances.

One further point should be mentioned. The appellant argues that to uphold the trial decision places a doctor on the horns of a dilemma, in that, on the one hand, if the doctor administers blood in this situation and saves the patient's life, the patient may hold him liable in battery while, on the other hand, if the doctor follows the patient's instructions and, as a consequence, the patient dies, the doctor may face an action by dependants alleging that, notwithstanding the card, the deceased would, if conscious, have accepted blood in the face of imminent death and the doctor was negligent in failing to administer the transfusions. In my view, that result cannot conceivably follow. The doctor cannot be held to have violated either his legal duty or professional responsibility towards the patient or the patient's dependants when he honours the Jehovah's Witness card and respects the patient's right to control her own body in accordance with the dictates of her conscience. The onus is clearly on the patient. When members of the Jehovah's Witness faith choose to carry cards intended to notify doctors and other providers of health care that they reject blood transfusions in an emergency, they must accept the consequences of their decision. Neither they nor their dependants can later be heard to say that the card did not reflect their true wishes. If harmful consequences ensue, the responsibility for those consequences is entirely theirs and not the doctor's.

Finally, the appellant appeals the quantum of damages awarded by the trial judge. In his submission, given the findings as to the competence of the treatment, the favourable results, the doctor's overall exemplary conduct and his good faith in the matter, the battery was technical and the general damages should be no more than nominal. While the submission is not without force, damages of $20,000 cannot be said to be beyond the range of damages appropriate to a tortious interference of this nature. The trial judge found that Mrs. Malette suffered mentally and emotionally by reason of the battery. His assessment of general damages was clearly not affected by any palpable or overriding error and there is therefore no basis upon which an appellate court may interfere with the award.

X

In the result, for these reasons I would dismiss the appeal and the cross-appeal, both with costs.

Should Living Wills Be Legalized?

Rory H. Fisher and Eric M. Meslin

Living wills allow patients to state their wish to die and not be kept alive through the use of medications, artificial means or "heroic" measures. They have been made legal documents in 38 states in the United States. Living wills permit advance expression of a patient's wishes, promote effective communication and demonstrate respect for the patient as a person. Problems with legal recognition of such wills include the need for agreement on fundamental terms, possible restriction of patients' rights, limitation of options in decision-making and possible negative effects on the physician-patient relationship. Before legislation is enacted,

R.H. Fisher and E.M. Meslin, "Should Living Wills be Legalized?" *Canadian Medical Association Journal* 1990; 142:23-26.

> public and professional attitudes toward the care of terminally ill patients should be assessed. All health care professionals should receive better education in this area, and palliative care services should be made more widely available. Only if these measures fail should living wills be made legal documents in Canada.

The emergence of advance directives, including living wills, can be traced to a societal concern that patients are not permitted to determine the type of care they would prefer to have begun or withdrawn during the process of dying.[1] This concern gained considerable prominence during the evolution of the patients' rights movement.[2] The underlying problem, therefore, is public concern that terminal illness is not well managed by physicians and that the process of dying is often unnecessarily prolonged by the use of overly aggressive interventions and technologic support.

Mentally competent patients are of course able to decide whether they wish to have aggressive treatment. However, there is a large number of patients with dementia who lack the capacity to make such decisions. In addition, there are smaller numbers of previously competent patients who are permanently mentally incapacitated by stroke, traffic accidents or failed resuscitative procedures. These groups are thought to benefit most directly from completion of a living will.

Many versions of a living will have been developed. One example is issued by Death with Dignity, Toronto. This document is directed to the patient's family, physician, lawyer and other concerned parties and is intended to act as an expression of the person's wishes and directions for the provision of health care while he or she is still of sound mind. It directs that in the event that there is no reasonable expectation of recovery the person be allowed to die and not be kept alive through the use of medications, artificial means or "heroic" measures. It is requested that medications be mercifully administered to alleviate suffering, even if this may shorten life. Although the living will is not legally enforceable, it is hoped that those to whom the will is addressed will regard themselves as morally bound by its provisions. Signators may add detailed statements to the document indicating particular treatments, medications or procedures they would want withheld or withdrawn.

Such living wills have been made legal documents through natural death acts in 38 states in the United States and the District of Columbia. The first such legislation was passed in California in 1976.[3]

ADVANTAGES OF A LIVING WILL

In principle there are several advantages of a living will.

- Permits advance expression of the patient's preferences: Like most advance directives for health care, a living will enables people to express their preferences about the withholding or withdrawal of life-sustaining procedures before such decisions are required. In particular, completion of a living will recognizes the importance of the patient's subjective, individual evaluation of well-being.
- Promotes communication: Completion of a living will allows people to discuss their wishes about medical care with family and friends. A living will also promotes more effective communication between patients and other caregivers. Discussion with physicians, nurses and other health care professionals can help clarify concerns about treatment.

- Demonstrates respect for the patient as a person: Following a directive fulfils an important value in medicine: it shows respect for the patient as a person.[4] The belief that patients have a right to self-determination is entrenched in law and medical ethics. This general right is often understood as the "right to die", which some physicians have difficulty recognizing or accepting. According to Fletcher,[5] "in actual practice, physicians often ignore, compromise, or even deny a patient's right to die, probably more commonly than we think. ... Physicians are less prone than some patients and ethicists to acknowledge that the patient has a moral right to choose to die."

PROBLEMS WITH LEGAL RECOGNITION OF A LIVING WILL

There are several problems with legal recognition of a living will. These are not equivalent to problems with a living will itself, however.

- Requires agreement on fundamental terms: Passage of legislation would require agreement on the definition of fundamental concepts such as "terminal illness" and "heroic measures" about which there is still disagreement. The US President's Commission for the Study of Ethical Problems in Medicine and Biomedical and Behavioral Research suggested that phrases such as terminal illness, which may be useful as general descriptions, are generally unacceptable as definitions because, among other things, "prognostication near the end of life is notoriously uncertain".[6] The term *heroic measures* also has been subjected to critical analysis. The commission concluded that distinctions between care that is ordinary/extraordinary, obligatory/optional, simple/complex or common/unusual have no moral significance.[7] An exception is when the distinction refers to usefulness or burdensomeness of treatments or procedures as perceived by the patient, who may appropriately decide not to undertake them.[7]

- May restrict patients' rights: Recent experience in the United States suggests that living will legislation has actually restricted rather than promoted or protected the rights of patients. At a recent meeting of the Canadian Bioethics Society it was learned that US legislation resulted in the provision of more rather than less care.[8]

Passage of living will legislation may also have a profound effect on patients who do not sign such a will, since physicians may feel compelled to use aggressive measures in the absence of a document requesting limitations on such measures. This poses an interesting problem in its own right. The legalization of living wills may suggest that the patient has to consent to *not* having medically and ethically inappropriate treatments. The provision of treatment unless a patient expressly refuses it represents a dangerous rationalism. We believe that an intervention that is not clinically indicated (or perceived as beneficial to a patient who is terminally and irreversibly ill) is also not ethically appropriate.

- Limits options available for decision-making: Living wills are said to limit the flexibility of physicians and patients in decision-making. For example, in some US jurisdictions (including those where living wills are legally recognized) it is mandatory to continue artificial hydration and nutrition.[9] In these circumstances a physician is obligated to carry on with procedures such as nasogastric tube feeding that may be medically inappropriate, as they may cause aspiration pneumonia, agitation and distress. The patient may have to be mechanically restrained; this adds to the discomfort and agitation while only prolonging the dying process. Such procedures may be ethically inappropriate because carrying them out in the face of a patient's expressed refusal violates patient autonomy.

• May affect physician-patient relationship: Legalizing living wills may negatively affect the physician-patient relationship. For example, physicians may feel compelled to adopt a legalistic or overly contractual relationship with patients. Although the contract model has advantages over other models of the health care relationship, particularly by empowering patients to play a greater role in decision-making,[10] it is also thought to reduce the physician-patient relationship to legalisms.[11]

INITIAL SOLUTIONS

It could be argued that there is no need at this time to take any legislative action at all. Maintaining the status quo presumes, however, that current mechanisms and sensitivities are sufficient to address the problem, and we do not take this to be the case. Therefore, we propose the following initial solutions.

• Assessment of public and professional attitudes: It would be precipitous to consider legal reform in the absence of empiric support demonstrating the need for such reform. Institutions, organizations and governments should be encouraged (individually or collaboratively) to assess public and professional attitudes toward the care of the dying. If past experience is any guide, professional attitudes will likely be markedly different from those of the public on matters of such gravity as the care of the dying patient. The interpretation of public opinion (including patients' attitudes) will depend on how the questions are framed.[12]

Public attitudes would be clarified if an evaluation tool were designed to assess people's values with respect to the care of the dying patient and the appropriateness of legislative reform. As an alternative to a potentially costly study the public should be made aware of the current discussion and their views solicited through public meetings. The CMA could consider striking a task force composed of public and professional members similar to the group convened to address the issue of allocation of health care resources.[13]

• Education: There is evidence to suggest that the public is interested in and informed about living wills. The President's Commission for the Study of Ethical Problems in Medicine and Biomedical and Behavioral Research reported that Concern for Living, a New York-based educational group, had distributed millions of living wills.[1]

However, public education alone is insufficient. Four additional approaches should be considered. There should be vigorous discussion and debate in scholarly journals about the medical, ethical and legal issues involved in enactment of living will legislation. A dialogue among health care professionals (not physicians exclusively) would ensure that a diversity of opinion is achieved. Much discussion has already occurred,[14,15] but this trend should continue.

Second, better education of all health care professionals is essential. There is a need for greater emphasis on the care of dying patients and the related medical and ethical issues in the undergraduate curriculum. Examples of the implementation of such teachings are available in other countries.[16] The importance of this area should be impressed on students through relevant examination questions. Physicians in acute care teaching hospitals need to act as role models for demonstrating skills in communicating with patients and families about issues related to terminal illness and its management. This presumes that such role models exist.

Third, medical students should be taught the attitudes, language and philosophy of palliative care. Preferably they should work in palliative care units during the clinical clerkship. Training should be incorporated in all postgraduate programs and made a requirement of training programs of the Royal College of Physicians and Surgeons of Canada and the College of Family Physicians of Canada. When these programs are surveyed such training should be assessed appropriately.

Finally, the increased interest in the field of bioethics has contributed to innovative institutional programs and structures within hospitals that can facilitate education. These developments should be pursued. Many hospitals now have institutional ethics committees whose responsibility it is to facilitate ethics programs within the hospital. More recently some hospitals have attracted bioethicists to assist in teaching medical ethics to all health care professionals. In addition to its Ethics Committee, our hospital has created a Clinical Ethics Centre to serve as an ethics resource for the hospital and the community.

- Use of quality assurance: Increased emphasis on quality assurance in hospitals should include assessment of the appropriate care of terminally ill patients and monitoring of the use of investigations and treatments in such cases. The Canadian Council on Hospital Accreditation should incorporate appropriate assessments in the accreditation process.
- Increased availability of palliative care services: More widespread services for the terminally ill are needed. Canada has provided leadership in this field in North America, with the pioneering work done by Dr. Balfour Mount at Royal Victoria Hospital, Montreal, in particular. Other palliative care services have been developed throughout the country, particularly in long-term-care institutions. Many acute care hospitals have instituted consultation teams, and there is an increasing number of community outreach teams and freestanding hospices. However, the availability of such services is still limited, and there is a serious need to extend them further. In addition, the entire approach to the care of dying patients in acute care hospitals must be changed for patients who are not transferred to specialized palliative care units.

CONCLUSION

In Canada there is no reason to precipitously introduce legislation to remedy what is at once a medical and an ethical problem. It may be a human trait to seek to remedy errors of medical judgement by passing legislation. However, such a solution may not correct future errors: this can be done only through education, experience and peer review.[17]

Living wills can serve as an important guide and a means of better communication of patients' wishes to physicians and families. Only if other measures fail should living wills be made legal documents.

NOTES

1. President's Commission for the Study of Ethical Problems in Medicine and Biomedical and Behavioral Research: *Deciding to Forego Life-Sustaining Treatment: Ethical, Medical, and Legal Issues in Treatment Decisions,* US Govt Printing Office, Washington, 1983: 139-141

2. Annas GJ: The emerging stowaway: patients' rights in the 1980s. *Law Med Health Care* 1982; 10: 32-45,46
3. California Natural Death Act, *Cal Health and Safety Code* sec 7185-7195(1976)
4. President's Commission for the Study of Ethical Problems in Medicine and Biomedical and Behavioral Research: *Deciding to Forego Life-Sustaining Treatment: Ethical, Medical, and Legal Issues in Treatment Decisions,* US Govt Printing Office, Washington, 1983: 136-137
5. Fletcher J: Medical resistance to the right to die. *J Am Geriat Soc* 1987; 35: 679-682
6. President's Commission for the Study of Ethical Problems in Medicine and Biomedical and Behavioral Research: *Deciding to Forego Life-Sustaining Treatment: Ethical, Medical, and Legal Issues in Treatment Decisions,* US Govt Printing Office, Washington, 1983: 25
7. Ibid: 87-88
8. Living will legislation in U.S. restricts citizens' rights. *Med Post* 1989; 25(1): 45
9. McCarrick PM: *Withholding or Withdrawing Nutrition of Hydration* (Scope Note 7), National Reference Center for Bioethics Literature, Kennedy Institute of Ethics, Washington, 1986
10. Veatch RM: *A Theory of Medical Ethics,* Basic, New York 1981: 108-138
11. Pellegrino ED, Thomasma DC: *For the Patient's Good: the Restoration of Beneficence in Health Care,* Oxford U Pr, New York, 1988: 102-104
12. Keyserlingk EW: Public opinion legalizing active euthanasia. *Humane Med* 1987; 3: 139-140
13. Task Force on the Allocation of Health Care Resources: *Health: a Need for Direction,* Can Med Assoc, Ottawa, 1984
14. Houston CS: Living wills: A solution to the prolonged act of dying? *Can Med Assoc J* 1988; 139: 241-243
15. Johnson D: Living wills: their interpretation depends on the situation. Ibid: 244-245
16. Stout RW: Teaching terminal care at Queen's University Belfast. *Br Med J* 1984; 289: 1604-1605
17. Gilligan JE, Lynn J: Natural death legislation [E]. *Med J Aust* 1980; 2: 473

Canadian Medical Association Policy, 1991: Advance Directives for the Resuscitation of Patients and Life-Saving or Sustaining Measures

A. PREAMBLE

In recent years, patient concern over decision-making in the medical setting has increasingly focused on advance directives for CPR, resuscitation in general and life-saving and/or sustaining measures. The Canadian Medical Association believes that the right to accept or reject any treatment or procedure ultimately resides with the patient or a duly empowered proxy. The Association also believes that this includes the right to accept or refuse resuscitative as well as life-saving and/or sustaining measures in general, should they become medically indicated. Furthermore, the Association believes that under certain circumstances it may be appropriate that a patient indicate to the physician and to other relevant persons, by means of an advance directive, whether the patient wants such resuscitative measures taken should the occasion for their use arise.

However, the Association is firmly convinced that the decision to accept or reject any medical treatment or procedure should only be made after an appropriate consultative process with a duly qualified health care professional. Furthermore, the Association maintains that in any case, such a decision should always be reviewed by the patient or the appropriate proxy decision-maker together with a physician at appropriate intervals. Finally, the Association believes that if a patient has made a decision in this regard, it is the responsibility of the patient to take all reasonable steps to make sure that this information is reasonably available to the attending physician and to other health care professionals who may be involved in the care of the patient.

Patients frequently believe that an advance directive to refuse life-saving and/or sustaining measures will be honoured under all circumstances. The reality of medical practice makes this impossible. If an advance directive is specific to a particular set of circumstances, the directive itself will have no force when these circumstances, or circumstances essentially similar to them, do not exist. On the other hand, if an advance directive is so general as to apply to all possible circumstances that could arise, it is usually so vague as to give no usable direction to the physician. In either case, physicians will have to rely on their professional judgement to reach a decision.

The Association therefore suggests that physicians who are involved in the consultative process surrounding such a decision make sure that patients understand the limits that are inherent in advance decision making. Furthermore, the Association suggests that physicians who are involved in such a consultative process encourage their patients to provide, in their directives, as much information as is

Canadian Medical Association, Policy: "Advance Directives for the Resuscitation of Patients and Life-Saving or Sustaining Measures." *Reports to the 1991 General Council.*

reasonable to enable a physician who is faced with implementing such a directive, to understand the directive in an appropriate fashion. The Association also suggests that any such advance directive be in writing.

Finally, the Association suggests that physicians who are involved in the consultative process surrounding advance directives encourage their patients to identify a specific person who will have the legal power to act as proxy decision-maker for the patient should the need for clarification of an advance directive arise. The Association also encourages physicians to inform their patients that in an emergency situation it is not always possible to get in touch with this duly appointed proxy to seek clarification about the advance directive should that prove necessary. Patients should therefore be encouraged to make these directives as clear as possible.

B. DECISION-MAKING

1. A patient has the right to accept or reject any treatment or procedure proposed by a physician.[1] This includes CPR or any other life-saving and/or sustaining measure.
2. When a competent patient informs the attending physician that such measures should not be undertaken, the physician shall make sure that the patient understands the nature and consequences of this decision.

   If, as a result of this communicative process, the patient reaffirms this decision, the physician shall record this decision on the patient's health record.
3. When a patient is incompetent and an appropriate proxy decision-maker[2] informs the attending physician of the decision not to engage in resuscitative or life saving and/or sustaining measures, the physician shall engage in the same consultative and communicative process with the proxy as though it were the patient him/herself. If, as a result of this, the proxy still insists on the request not to employ resuscitative and/or sustaining measures, the physician shall record this decision an the patient's health record.
4. When the clinical picture of a patient indicates to the attending physician that resuscitation is inappropriate and the patient (or appropriate proxy) has not raised the issue with the physician, the attending physician shall discuss the matter with the patient (or the appropriate proxy). The exception would be when in the estimation of the physician, the patient would be harmed by such a discussion. In that event, the physician shall turn to the appropriate proxy who shall assume the patient's decision-making role in this matter, having due regard to the previously expressed wishes of the patient.

C. IMPLEMENTATION

5. If a patient has competently refused life-saving and/or sustaining measures, or if a duly empowered patient proxy has refused such intervention, the physician shall honour such wishes. All other patient care measures should be employed as appropriate and required, especially those measures that involve comfort care and pain relief.
6. If there are unexpected changes in the person's condition, a nurse or another physician may rescind a "no resuscitation" order until the persons's

condition can be reassessed by the attending physician. Such a rescinding should be communicated to the attending physician immediately.

D. ADVANCE DIRECTIVE

7. A physician should assist a patient in a consultative capacity in the preparation of an advance directive for life-saving and/or sustaining measures if the patient requests such assistance. In the course of this consultative process, the physician should try to make sure that the patient understands the limits of advance directives. The physician should also impress on the patient the need to make this advance directive reasonable, accessible against need.
8. A patient's duly executed advance directive shall be honoured by the attending physician unless there are reasonable grounds to suppose that it no longer represents the wishes of the patient or that the patient's understanding was incomplete at the time of making the directive.

E. HEALTH CARE PROXY DECISION-MAKER

9. Sometimes patients are concerned about who will make health care decisions for them when they are no longer in a position to do so themselves but at the same time the patient may not wish to execute an advance directive. Physicians who become aware of this in their are encouraged to explore with these patients the possibility of identifying a specific person who will have the legal power to make health care decisions on their behalf in such an eventuality.
10. Physicians whose patients wish to draw up an advance directives are encouraged to explore with these patients the possibility of identifying a specific person who will have the legal power to act as appropriate proxy decision-maker for the patient should the need for clarification of an advance directive arise.

NOTES

1. The Canadian Medical Association, *Code of Ethics,* clause 5: "An ethical physician will recognize that a patient has the right to accept or reject any physician and any medical care recommended."
2. Whether a particular individual is an "appropriate proxy" depends on provincial legislation, regulations or guidelines as and where these exist. Examples of "appropriate proxy decision makers" would be next-of-kin (in the order of priority indicated in the legislation or guidelines), someone who has been given durable power of attorney (cf. Nova Scotia), or a relevant other who is otherwise identified. In some cases, the proxy may be someone other than the next-of-kin of the patient. See *Mawdsley v. Austin,* [1985] 1 W.W.R. 369 (B.C.S.C.). Health care facilities have an obligation to ensure that health care professionals under their jurisdiction are familiar with and follow the order of appropriate proxy authority as thus provided for.

FURTHER READINGS

Childress, James F., *Who Should Decide? Paternalism in Health Care.* (Oxford and New York: Oxford University Press, 1982).

Emanuel, Ezekiel J. and Linda L. Emanuel, "Living Wills: Past, Present and Future," *Journal of Clinical Ethics* 1:1 (Spring 1990) 9-19.

Hackler, C., R. Moseley and D.E. Vawter, eds., *Advance Directives in Medicine.* (New York: Praeger, 1989) 141-145.

Kuhse, Helga *The Sanctity of Life Doctrine in Medicine: A Critique.* (Oxford: Clarendon Press,1987).

Law Reform Commission of Canada, Working Paper 46, *Omission, Negligence and Endangering.* (Ottawa: Law Reform Commission, 1985).

Law Reform Commission of Canada, Report 20, *Euthanasia, Aiding Suicide and Cessation of Treatment.* (Ottawa: Minister of Supply and Services, 1983).

Maguire, Daniel, *Death by Choice.* (New York: Doubleday, 1974).

Nova Scotia Medical Consent Act, 1988, c.14, s.1.

Picard, Ellen, *Legal Liability of Doctors and Hospitals in Canada.* (Toronto: Carswell, 1984).

Rosner,F., *Modern Medicine and Jewish Law.* (N.Y.: Yeshiva University, 1972).

Schmeiser, Douglas A., "Living Wills and Medical Treatment of the Terminally Ill," *Health Management Forum* 2:3(Fall 1989) 32-37.

Society for the Right to Die, *Handbook of Living Will Laws.* (New York: Society for the Right to Die, 1987).

CHAPTER 13 ABORTION AND RELATED ISSUES

INTRODUCTION

Abortion is generally defined as the deliberate termination of a pregnancy prior to foetal viability.[1] While this definition makes no reference to killing or bringing about the death of the foetus, the usual reason for performing an abortion is not simply to terminate the pregnancy by removing the foetus from the uterus, but also to kill the foetus. Therefore in actual fact, in most cases the death of the foetus is precisely what is intended by performing the abortion. Since a human foetus is a human being, abortion is really an act of deliberate death. Abortion is therefore appropriately dealt with in this chapter.

Historically, abortions have been approached in a variety of ways. In Roman and Greek times they were not considered ethically reprehensible, because an unborn foetus was not a person in the eyes of the law.[2] Even early Christian writers such as St. Augustine and St.Thomas Aquinas more or less shared this view. In more recent times, abortion became a criminal misdemeanour and ultimately was considered an act of murder. It was considered defensible only under exceptional circumstances: specifically, when the life of the pregnant woman was threatened and the only way to save it was through an abortion. This exception was enshrined in Section 251 of the *Criminal Code of Canada,* which was struck down in 1988 by the Supreme Court of Canada in the famous case of *R. v. Morgentaler*. Excerpts from that case are reproduced below. Since 1988, Canada has not had any statute law specifically dealing with abortion.

Wayne Sumner presents a philosopher's perspective on abortion. In a classic Canadian discussion, he depicts the issue of abortion as involving a complex series of questions that deal with personhood, autonomy and a balance of social and individual rights.

Cefalo and Engelhardt deal with another issue that has risen to prominence over the last few years: the question of whether it is ethically acceptable to use foetal tissue (and tissue from anencephalics) to help others. The question is important because it centres around a difficult problem in bioethics: Is it ever ethically acceptable to kill human beings, no matter what their state of development, to help other humans? To some, how we answer this question will determine whether we can ethically use medical data obtained from experiments and research that was conducted in an ethically unacceptable fashion.

NOTES

1. See Canadian Medical Association, Policy Statement on Abortion.
2. Roman civil law recognized the fiction that an unborn child *en ventre sa mère* is a person in the sense that it will inherit property left to it while still unborn. However, that status did not carry over into the criminal sphere, which defined legal personhood. In Canada, the fiction was first introduced into civil proceedings in *Léveillé v. Montreal Tramway*.

R. v. Morgentaler

Supreme Court of Canada

The Chief Justice — The principal issue raised by this appeal is whether the abortion provisions of the Criminal Code, R.S.C. 1970, c. C-34, infringe the "right to life, liberty and security of the person and the right not to be deprived thereof except in accordance with the principles of fundamental justice" as formulated in s. 7 of the Canadian Charter of Rights and Freedoms.

...

RELEVANT STATUTORY AND CONSTITUTIONAL PROVISIONS

Criminal Code

251. (1) Every one who, with intent to procure the miscarriage of a female person, whether or not she is pregnant, uses any means for the purpose of carrying out his intention is guilty of an indictable offence and is liable to imprisonment for life.

(2) Every female person who, being pregnant, with intent to procure her own miscarriage, uses any means or permits any means to be used for the purpose of carrying out her intention is guilty of an indictable offence and is liable to imprisonment for two years.

(3) In this section, "means" includes

R.v.Morgentaler, [1988] 1 S.C.R. 30, 63 O.R.(2d.)281, 26 O.A.C. 1, 44 D.L.R.(4th) 385, 82 N.R. 1, 3 C.C.C.(3d)449, 62 C.R.(3d)1, 31 C.R.R.

(a) the administration of a drug or other noxious thing,
b) the use of an instrument, and
(c) manipulation of any kind.

(4) Subsections (1) and (2) do not apply to

(a) a qualified medical practitioner, other than a member of a therapeutic abortion committee for any hospital, who in good faith uses in an accredited or approved hospital any means for the purpose of carrying out his intention to procure the miscarriage of a female person, or

(b) a female person who, being pregnant, permits a qualified medical practitioner to use in an accredited or approved hospital any means described in paragraph (a) for the purpose of carrying out her intention to procure her own miscarriage, if, before the use of those means, the therapeutic abortion committee for that accredited or approved hospital, by a majority of the members of the committee and at a meeting of the committee at which the case of such female person has been reviewed,

(c) has by certificate in writing stated that in its opinion the continuation of the pregnancy of such female person would or would be likely to endanger her life or health, and

(d) has caused a copy of such certificate to be given to the qualified medical practitioner.

(5) The Minister of Health of a province may by order

(a) require a therapeutic abortion committee for any hospital in that province, or any member thereof, to furnish to him a copy of any certificate described in paragraph (4) (c) issued, by that committee, together with such other information relating to the circumstances surrounding the issue of that certificate as he may require, or

(b) require a medical practitioner who, in that province, has procured the miscarriage of any female person named in a certificate described in paragraph (4) (c), to furnish to him a copy of that certificate, together with such other information relating to the procuring of the miscarriage as he may require.

(6) For the purposes of subsections (4) and (5) and this subsection

"accredited hospital" means a hospital accredited by the Canadian Council on Hospital Accreditation in which diagnostic services and medical, surgical and obstetrical treatment are provided;

"approved hospital" means a hospital in a province approved for the purposes of this section by the Minister of Health of that province;

"board" means the board of governors, management or directors, or the trustees, commission or other person or group of persons having the control and management of an accredited or approved hospital;

"qualified medical practitioner" means a person entitled to engage in the practice of medicine under the laws of the province in which the hospital referred to in subsection (4) is situated;

"therapeutic abortion committee" for any hospital means a committee, comprised of not less than three members each of whom is a qualified medical practitioner, appointed by the board of that hospital for the purpose of considering and determining questions relating to terminations of pregnancy within that hospital.

(7) Nothing in subsection (4) shall be construed as making unnecessary the obtaining of any authorization or consent that is or may be required, otherwise than under this Act, before any means are used for the purpose of carrying out an intention to procure the miscarriage of a female person.

A. The Canadian Charter of Rights and Freedoms

1. The Canadian Charter of Rights and Freedoms guarantees the rights and freedoms set out in it subject only to such reasonable limits prescribed by law as can be demonstrably justified in a free and democratic society.

7. Everyone has the right to life, liberty and security of the person and the right not to be deprived thereof except in accordance with the principles of fundamental justice.

...

III

...

B. Security of the Person

The law has long recognized that the human body ought to be protected from interference by others. At common law, for example, any medical procedure carried out on a person without that person's consent is an assault. Only in emergency circumstances does the law allow others to make decisions of this nature. Similarly, art. 19 of the Civil Code of Lower Canada provides that "The human person is inviolable" and that "No person may cause harm to the person of another without his consent or without being authorized by law to do so". "Security of the person", in other words, is not a value alien to our legal landscape. With the advent of the Charter, security of the person has been elevated to the status of a constitutional norm. This is not to say that the various forms of protection accorded to the human body by the common and civil law occupy a similar status. "Security of the person" must be given content in a manner sensitive to its constitutional position. The above examples are simply illustrative of our respect for individual physical integrity.

... Nor is it to say that the state can never impair personal securities interests. There may well be valid reasons for interfering with security of the person. It is to say, however, that if the state does interfere with security of the person, the Charter requires such interference to conform with the principles of fundamental justice.

... The case law leads me to the conclusion that state interference with bodily integrity and serious state-imposed psychological stress, at least in the criminal law context, constitute a breach of security of the person. It is not necessary in this case to determine whether the right extends further, to protect either interests central to personal autonomy, such as a right to privacy, or interests unrelated to criminal justice.

... Parliament could choose to infringe security of the person if it did so in a manner consistent with the principles of fundamental justice. The present discussion should therefore be seen as a threshold inquiry and the conclusions do not dispose definitively of all the issues relevant to s. 7. With that caution, I have no difficulty in concluding that the encyclopedic factual submissions addressed to us by counsel in the present application establish beyond any doubt that s. 251 of the *Criminal Code* is *prima facie* a violation of the security of the person of thousands of Canadian women who have made the difficult decision that they do not wish to continue with a pregnancy. At the most basic, physical and emotional level, every pregnant woman is told by the section that she cannot submit to a generally safe medical procedure that might be of clear benefit to her unless she meets criteria entirely unrelated to her own priorities and aspirations. Not only does the removal of decision-making power threaten women in a physical sense; the indecision of knowing whether an abortion will be granted inflicts emotional stress. Section 251 clearly interferes with a woman's bodily integrity in both a physical and emotional sense. Forcing a woman, by threat of criminal sanction, to carry a foetus to term unless she meets certain criteria unrelated to her own priorities and aspirations, is a profound interference with a woman's body and thus a violation of security of the person. Section 251, therefore, is required by the Charter to comport with the principles of fundamental justice.

... [T]he operation of the decision-making mechanism set out in s. 251 creates additional glaring breaches of security of the person. The evidence indicates that s. 251 causes a certain amount of delay for women who are successful in meeting its criteria. In the context of abortion, any unnecessary delay can have profound consequences on the woman's physical and emotional well-being.

More specifically, in 1977, the *Report of the Committee on the Operation of the Abortion Law* (the Badgley Report) revealed that the average delay between a pregnant woman's first contact with a physician and a subsequent therapeutic abortion was eight weeks (p. 146). Although the situation appears to have improved since 1977, the extent of the improvement is not clear. The intervener, the Attorney General of Canada, submitted that the average delay in Ontario between the first visit to a physician and a therapeutic abortion was now between one and three weeks. Yet the respondent Crown admitted in a supplementary factum filed on November 27, 1986 with the permission of the Court that (p. 3):

> ... the evidence discloses that some women may find it very difficult to obtain an abortion: by necessity, abortion services are limited, since hospitals have budgetary, time, space and staff constraints as well as many medical responsibilities. As a result of these problems a woman may have to apply to several hospitals.
>
> If forced to apply to several different therapeutic abortion committees, there can be no doubt that a woman will experience serious delay in obtaining a therapeutic abortion...

The entire process [of obtaining an abortion] was found to be protracted with women requiring three to seven contacts with health professionals. ... but in the case of abortion, the implications of any delay, according to the evidence, are potentially devastating. The first factor to consider is that different medical techniques are employed to perform abortions at different stages of pregnancy. The testimony of expert doctors at trial indicated that in the first twelve weeks of pregnancy, the relatively safe and simple suction dilation and curettage method of abortion is typically used in North America. From the thirteenth to the sixteenth week, the more dangerous dilation and evacuation procedure is performed, although much less often in Canada than in the United States. From the sixteenth week of pregnancy, the instillation method is commonly employed in Canada. This method requires the intra-amniotic introduction of prostaglandin, urea, or a saline solution, which causes a woman to go into labour, giving birth to a foetus which is usually dead, but not invariably so. The uncontroverted evidence showed that each method of abortion progressively increases risks to the woman.

... The second consideration is that even within the periods appropriate to each method of abortion, the evidence indicated that the earlier the abortion was performed, the fewer the complications and the lower the risk of mortality.

... It is no doubt true that the overall complication and mortality rates for women who undergo abortions are very low, but the increasing risks caused by delay are so clearly established that I have no difficulty in concluding that the delay in obtaining therapeutic abortions caused by the mandatory procedures of s. 251 is an infringement of the purely physical aspect of the individual's right to security of the person.

... The above physical interference caused by the delays created by s. 251, involving a clear risk of damage to the physical well-being of a woman, is sufficient, in my view, to warrant inquiring whether s. 251 comports with the principles of fundamental justice.

However, there is yet another infringement of security of the person. It is clear from the evidence that s. 251 harms the psychological integrity of women seeking abortions. A 1985 report of the Canadian Medical Association, discussed in the *[Report on Therapeutic Abortion Services in Ontario]* Powell Report, at p. 15, emphasized that the procedure involved in s. 251, with the concomitant delays, greatly increases the stress levels of patients and that this can lead to more physical complications associated with abortion.

... I have already noted that the instillation procedure requires a woman actually to experience labour and to suffer through the birth of a foetus that is usually but not always dead ... The psychological injury caused by delay in obtaining abortions, much of which must be attributed to the procedures set out in s. 251, constitutes an additional infringement of the right to security of the person.

... [T]he evidence demonstrates that the system established by the section for obtaining a therapeutic abortion certificate inevitably does create significant delays. It is not possible to say that delay results only from administrative constraints, such as limited budgets or a lack of qualified persons to sit on therapeutic abortion committees. Delay results from the cumbersome operating requirements of s. 251 itself. ... Although the mandate given to the courts under the Charter does not, generally speaking, enable the judiciary to provide remedies for administrative inefficiencies, when denial of a right as basic as security of the person is infringed by the procedure and administrative structures created by the law itself, the courts are empowered to act.

... In summary, s. 251 is a law which forces women to carry a foetus to term contrary to their own priorities and aspirations and which imposes serious delay causing increased physical and psychological trauma to those women who meet its criteria. It must, therefore, be determined whether that infringement is accomplished in accordance with the principles of fundamental justice, thereby saving s. 251 under the second part of s. 7.

C. The Principles of Fundamental Justice

... A pregnant woman who desires to have an abortion must apply to the "therapeutic abortion committee" of an "accredited or approved hospital". Such a committee is empowered to issue a certificate in writing stating that in the opinion of a majority of the committee, the continuation of the pregnancy would be likely to endanger the pregnant woman's life or health. Once a copy of the certificate is given to a qualified medical practitioner who is not a member of the therapeutic abortion committee, he or she is permitted to perform an abortion on the pregnant woman and both the doctor and the woman are freed from any criminal liability.

... As is so often the case in matters of interpretation, however, the straightforward reading of this statutory scheme is not fully revealing. In order to understand the true nature and scope of s. 251, it is necessary to investigate the practical operation of the provisions.

... [T]he seemingly neutral requirement of s. 251(4) that at least four physicians be available to authorize and to perform an abortion meant in practice that abortions would be absolutely unavailable in almost one quarter of all hospitals in Canada.

Other administrative and procedural requirements of s. 251(4) reduce the availability of therapeutic abortions even further. For the purposes of s. 251, therapeutic abortions can only be performed in "accredited" or "approved" hospitals.

... [Furthermore t]he requirement that therapeutic abortions be performed only in "accredited" or "approved" hospitals effectively means that the practical availability of the exculpatory provisions of subs. (4) may be heavily restricted, even denied, through provincial regulation.

... A further flaw with the administrative system established in s. 251(4) is the failure to provide an adequate standard for therapeutic abortion committees which must determine when a therapeutic abortion should, as a matter of law, be granted. Subsection (4) states simply that a therapeutic abortion committee may grant a certificate when it determines that a continuation of a pregnancy would be likely to endanger the "life or health" of the pregnant woman. It was noted above that "health" is not defined for the purposes of the section.

... Various expert doctors testified at trial that therapeutic abortion committees apply widely differing definitions of health. For some committees, psychological health is a justification for therapeutic abortion; for others it is not. Some committees routinely refuse abortions to married women unless they are in physical danger, while for other committees it is possible for a married woman to show that she would suffer psychological harm if she continued with a pregnancy, thereby justifying an abortion. It is not typically possible for women to know in advance what standard of health will be applied by any given committee.

... It is no answer to say that "health" is a medical term and that doctors who sit on therapeutic abortion committees must simply exercise their professional judgment. A therapeutic abortion committee is a strange hybrid, part medical committee and part legal committee.

... The combined effect of all of these problems with the procedure stipulated in s. 251 for access to therapeutic abortions is a failure to comply with the principles of fundamental justice.

... The Crown argues in its supplementary factum that women who face difficulties in obtaining abortions at home can simply travel elsewhere in Canada to procure a therapeutic abortion. That submission would not be especially troubling if the difficulties facing women were not in large measure created by the procedural requirements of s. 251 itself. If women were seeking anonymity outside their home town or were simply confronting the reality that it is often difficult to obtain medical services in rural areas, it might be appropriate to say "let them travel". But the evidence establishes convincingly that it is the law itself which in many ways prevents access to local therapeutic abortion facilities. The enormous emotional and financial burden placed upon women who must travel long distances from home to obtain an abortion is a burden created in many instances by Parliament. Moreover, it is not accurate to say to women who would seem to qualify under s. 251(4) that they can get a therapeutic abortion as long as they are willing to travel.

... I conclude that the procedures created in s. 251 of the Criminal Code for obtaining a therapeutic abortion do not comport with the principles of fundamental justice.

...

V

... The appellants contended that the sole purpose of s. 251 of the Criminal Code is to protect the life and health of pregnant women. The respondent Crown submitted that s. 251 seeks to protect not only the life and health of pregnant women, but also the interests of the foetus. ... In my view, it is unnecessary for the purpose of deciding this appeal to evaluate or assess "foetal rights" as an independent constitutional value. Nor are we required to measure the full extent of the state's interest in establishing criteria unrelated to the pregnant woman's own priorities and aspirations. What we must do is evaluate the particular balance struck by Parliament in s. 251, as it relates to the priorities and aspirations of pregnant women and the government's interests in the protection of the foetus.

Section 251 provides that foetal interests are not to be protected where the "life or health" of the woman is threatened. Thus, Parliament itself has expressly stated in s.251 that the "life or health" of pregnant women is paramount. The procedures of s. 251(4) are clearly related to the pregnant woman's "life or health" for that is the very phrase used by the subsection.

... I think the protection of the interests of pregnant women is a valid governmental objective, where life and health can be jeopardized by criminal sanctions. ... I agree that protection of foetal interests by Parliament is also a valid governmental objective. It follows that balancing these interests, with the lives and health of women a major factor, is clearly an important governmental objective.

... I am equally convinced, however, that the means chosen to advance the legislative objectives of s. 251 do not satisfy any of the three elements of the proportionality component of *R. v. Oakes*. The evidence has led me to conclude that the infringement of the security of the person of pregnant women caused by s. 251 is not accomplished in accordance with the principles of fundamental justice.

... I conclude, therefore, that the cumbersome structure of subs. (4) not only unduly subordinates the s. 7 rights of pregnant women but may also defeat the value Parliament itself has established as paramount, namely, the life and health of the pregnant woman. ...

CONCLUSION

Section 251 of the Criminal Code infringes the right to security of the person of many pregnant women. The procedures and administrative structures established in the section to provide for therapeutic abortions do not comply with the principles of fundamental justice. Section 7 of the Charter is infringed and that infringement cannot be saved under s. 1.

... Having found that this "comprehensive code" infringes the Charter, it is not the role of the Court to pick and choose among the various aspects of s. 251 so as effectively to re-draft the section. The appeal should therefore be allowed and s. 251 as a whole struck down under s. 52(1) of the Constitution Act, 1982. ...

Beetz J.:

... "Security of the person" must include a right of access to medical treatment for a condition representing a danger to life or health without fear of criminal sanction. If an act of Parliament forces a person whose life or health is in danger to choose between, on the one hand, the commission of a crime to obtain effective and timely medical treatment and, on the other hand, inadequate treatment or no treatment at all, the right to security of the person has been violated.

... With the greatest of respect, I cannot agree with the view that the therapeutic abortion committee is a "strange hybrid, part medical committee and part legal committee" as the Chief Justice characterizes it ... The committee is not called upon to evaluate the sufficiency of the state interest in the foetus as against the woman's health. This evaluation of the state interest is a question of law already decided by Parliament in its formulation of s. 251(4).

... The wording of s. 251(4)(c) limits the authority of the committee. The word "health" is not vague but plainly refers to the physical or mental health of the pregnant woman. ...The standard is further circumscribed by the word "endanger". Not only must the continuation of the pregnancy affect the woman's life or health, it must endanger life or health, so that a committee that authorizes an abortion when this element is not present or fails to authorize it when it is present exceeds its authority. Finally, the expression "would or would be likely" eliminates any requirement that the danger to life or health be certain or immediate at the time the certificate is issued.

... Just as the expression of the standard in s. 251(4)(c) does not offend the principles of fundamental justice, the requirement that an independent medical opinion be obtained for a therapeutic abortion to be lawful also cannot be said to constitute a violation of these principles when considered in the context of pregnant women's right to security of the person. ... [B]y requiring that a committee state that the medical standard has been met for the criminal sanction to be lifted, Parliament seeks to assure that there is a reliable, independent and medically sound opinion that the continuation of the pregnancy would or would be likely to endanger the woman's life or health. ...

... [Although] the current mechanism in the Criminal Code does not accord with the principles of fundamental justice [, this] does not preclude, in my view, Parliament from adopting another system, free of the failings of s. 251(4), in order to ascertain that the life or health of the pregnant woman is in danger, by way of a reliable, independent and medically sound opinion.

Parliament is justified in requiring a reliable, independent and medically sound opinion in order to protect the state interest in the foetus. This is undoubtedly the objective of a rule which requires an independent verification of the practising physician's opinion that the life or health of the pregnant woman is in danger. It cannot be said to be simply a mechanism designed to protect the health of the pregnant woman ... Parliament requires this independent opinion because it is not only the woman's interest that is at stake in a decision to authorize an abortion. The Ontario Court of Appeal alluded to this ... when it stated that "One cannot overlook the fact that the situation respecting a woman's right to control her own person becomes more complex when she becomes pregnant, and that some statutory control may be appropriate". The presence of the foetus accounts for this complexity. By requiring an independent medical opinion that the pregnant woman's life or health is in fact endangered, Parliament seeks to ensure that, in any given case, only therapeutic reasons will justify the decision to abort. The amendments to the *Criminal Code* in 1969 amounted to a recognition by Parliament, as I have said, that the interest in the life or health of the pregnant woman takes precedence over the interest of the state in the protection of the foetus when the continuation of the pregnancy would or would be likely to endanger the pregnant woman's life or health.

... I do not believe it to be unreasonable to seek independent medical confirmation of the threat to the woman's life or health when such an important and distinct interest hangs in the balance.

... I am of the view that there would still be circumstances in which the state interest in the protection of the foetus would require an independent medical opinion as to the danger to the life or health of the pregnant woman. Assuming without deciding that a right of access to abortion can be founded upon the right to "liberty", there would be a point in time at which the state interest in the foetus would become compelling. From this point in time, Parliament would be entitled to limit abortions to those required for therapeutic reasons and therefore require an independent opinion as to the health exception.

... Some delay is inevitable in connection with any system which purports to limit to therapeutic reasons the grounds upon which an abortion can be performed lawfully... Furthermore, rules promoting the safety of abortions designed to protect the interest of the pregnant woman will also cause some unavoidable delay. It is only in so far as the administrative structure creates delays which are unnecessary that the structure can be considered to violate the principles of fundamental justice... A fair structure, put in place to decide between those women who qualify for a therapeutic abortion and those who do not, should be designed with a view to efficiently meeting the demands which it must necessarily serve.

... Does the objective of protecting the foetus in s. 251 relate to concerns which are pressing and substantial in a free and democratic society? ... I am of the view that the protection of the foetus is and, as the Court of Appeal observed, always has been, a valid objective in Canadian criminal law. ... I think s. 1 of the Charter authorizes reasonable limits to be put on a woman's right having regard to the state interest in the protection of the foetus.

... The Crown must show that the means chosen in s. 251 are reasonable and demonstrably justified... [N]ot only are some of the rules in s. 251 unnecessary to the primary objective of the protection of the foetus and the ancillary objective of the protection of the pregnant woman's life or health, but their practical effect is to undermine the health of the woman which Parliament purports to consider so important. Consequently, s. 251 does not meet the proportionality test ...

... The gist of s. 251(4) is, as I have said, that the objective of protecting the foetus is not of sufficient importance to defeat the interest in protecting pregnant women from pregnancies which represent a danger to life or health. I take this parliamentary enactment in 1969 as an indication that, in a free and democratic society, it would be unreasonable to limit the pregnant woman's right to security of the person by a rule prohibiting abortions in all circumstances when her life or health would or would likely be in danger. This decision of the Canadian Parliament to the effect that the life or health of the pregnant woman takes precedence over the state interest in the foetus is also reflected in legislation in other free and democratic societies.

... Finally, I wish to stress that we have not been asked to decide nor is it necessary,... to decide whether a foetus is included in the word "everyone" in s. 7 so as to have a right to "life, liberty and security of the person" under the Charter.

The reasons of McIntyre and La Forest JJ. were delivered by
McIntyre J. (dissenting)

... The charge here is one of conspiracy to breach the provisions of s. 251 of the *Criminal Code*. There is no doubt, and it has never been questioned, that the appellants adopted a course which was clearly in defiance of the provisions of the Code and it is difficult to see where any infringement of their rights, under s. 7 of the Charter, could have occurred. There is no female person involved in the case who has been denied a therapeutic abortion and, as a result, the whole argument on the right to security of the person, under s. 7 of the Charter, has been on a hypothetical basis. The case, however, was addressed by all the parties on that basis and the Court has accepted that position.

... In considering the constitutionality of s. 251 of the *Criminal Code,* it is first necessary to understand the background of this litigation and some of the problems which it raises. Section 251 of the *Code* has been denounced as ill-conceived and inadequate by those at one extreme of the abortion debate and as immoral and unacceptable by those at the opposite extreme. There are those, like the appellants, who assert that on moral and ethical grounds there is a simple solution to the problem: the inherent "right of women to control their own bodies" requires the repeal of s. 251 in favour of the principle of "abortion on demand". Opposing this view are those who contend with equal vigour, and also on moral and ethical grounds, for a clear and simple solution: the inherent "right to life of the unborn child" requires the repeal of s. 251(4), (5), (6) and (7) in order to leave an absolute ban on abortions. The battle lines so drawn are firmly held and the attitudes of the opposing parties admit of no compromise.

... [Parliament has made an] attempt... to balance the competing interests of the unborn child and the pregnant woman. Where the provisions of s. 251(4) are met, the abortion may be performed without legal sanction. Where they are not, abortion is deemed to be socially undesirable and is punished as a crime.

... The values we must accept for the purposes of this appeal are those expressed by Parliament which holds the view that the desire of a woman to be relieved of her pregnancy is not, of itself, justification for performing an abortion.

... It is not for the Court to substitute its own views on the merits of a given question for those of Parliament... [I]ts role is confined to deciding whether the solution enacted by Parliament offends the Charter. If it does, the provision must be struck down or declared inoperative, and Parliament may then enact such different provisions as it may decide

... The Court must not resolve an issue such as that of abortion on the basis of how many judges may favour "pro-choice" or "pro-life". To do so would be contrary to sound principle and the rule of law affirmed in the preamble to the Charter which must mean that no discretion, including a judicial discretion, can be unlimited.

... It is said that a law which forces a woman to carry a foetus to term unless she meets certain criteria unrelated to her own priorities and aspirations interferes with security of her person.... All laws, it must be noted, have the potential for interference with individual priorities and aspirations. In fact, the very purpose of most legislation is to cause such interference. It is only when such legislation goes beyond interfering with priorities and aspirations, and abridges rights, that courts may intervene.

... In my view, it is clear that before it could be concluded that any enactment infringed the concept of security of the person, it would have to infringe some underlying right included in or protected by the concept. For the appellants to succeed here, then, they must show more than an interference with priorities and aspirations; they must show the infringement of a right which is included in the concept of security of the person. The proposition that women enjoy a constitutional right to have an abortion is devoid of support in the language of s. 7 of the Charter or any other section. While some human rights documents, such as the *American Convention on Human Rights*, 1969 (Article 4(1)), expressly address the question of abortion, the Charter is entirely silent on the point. It may be of some significance that the Charter uses specific language in dealing with other topics, such as voting rights, religion, expression and such controversial matters as mobility rights, language rights and minority rights, but remains silent on the question of abortion which, at the time the Charter was under consideration, was as much a subject of public controversy as it is today.

... Governmental action for the due governance and administration of society can rarely please everyone. It is hard to imagine a governmental policy or initiative which will not create significant stress or anxiety for some and, frequently, for many members of the community.

... To invade the s. 7 right of security of the person, there would have to be more than state-imposed stress or strain ... The mere fact of pregnancy, let alone an unwanted pregnancy, gives rise to stress. The evidence reveals that much of the anguish associated with abortion is inherent and unavoidable and that there is really no psychologically painless way to cope with an unwanted pregnancy.

It is for these reasons I would conclude, that save for the provisions of the *Criminal Code,* which permit abortion where the life or health of the woman is at risk, no right of abortion can be found in Canadian law, custom or tradition, and that the Charter, including s. 7, creates no further right. Accordingly, it is my view that s. 251 of the *Code* does not in its terms violate s. 7 of the Charter.

... The solution to th[e abortion] question in this country must be left to Parliament. It is for Parliament to pronounce on and to direct social policy. This is not because Parliament can claim all wisdom and knowledge but simply because Parliament is elected for that purpose in a free democracy and, in addition, has the facilities — the exposure to public opinion and information — as well as the political power to make effective its decisions...

I would dismiss the appeal.

...

Wilson J.

At the heart of this appeal is the question whether a pregnant woman can, as a constitutional matter, be compelled by law to carry the foetus to term. The legislature has proceeded on the basis that she can be so compelled.

... A consideration as to whether or not the procedural requirements for obtaining or performing an abortion comport with fundamental justice is purely academic if such requirements cannot as a constitutional matter be imposed at all. If a pregnant woman cannot, as a constitutional matter, be compelled by law to carry the foetus to term against her will, a review of the procedural requirements by which she may be compelled to do so seems pointless. Moreover, it would, in my opinion, be an exercise in futility for the legislature to expend its time and energy in attempting to remedy the defects in the procedural requirements unless it has some assurance that this process will, at the end of the day, result in the creation of a valid criminal offence. I turn, therefore, to what I believe is the central issue that must be addressed.

... I agree with the Chief Justice that we are not called upon in this case to delineate the full content of the right to life, liberty and security of the person. ... What we are asked to do ... is define the content of the right in the context of the legislation under attack. Does section 251 of the *Criminal Code* ... violate her right to life, liberty and security of the person within the meaning of s. 7?

Leaving aside for the moment the implications of the section for the foetus and addressing only the s. 7 right of the pregnant woman, it seems to me that we can say with a fair degree of confidence that a legislative scheme for the obtaining of an abortion which exposes the pregnant woman to a threat to her security of the person would violate her right under s. 7

... The Charter is predicated on a particular conception of the place of the individual in society. An individual is not a totally independent entity disconnected from the society in which he or she lives. Neither, however, is the individual a mere cog in an impersonal machine in which his or her values, goals and aspirations are subordinated to those of the collectivity. The individual is a bit of both. The Charter reflects this reality by leaving a wide range of activities and decisions open to legitimate government control while at the same time placing limits on the proper scope of that control. Thus, the rights guaranteed in the Charter erect around each individual, metaphorically speaking, an invisible fence over which the state will not be allowed to trespass. The role of the courts is to map out, piece by piece, the parameters of the defence.

The Charter and the right to individual liberty guaranteed under it are inextricably tied to the concept of human dignity. ... The idea of human dignity finds expression in almost every right and freedom guaranteed in the Charter ... Thus, an aspect of the respect for human dignity on which the Charter is founded is the right to make fundamental personal decisions without interference from the state. This right is a critical component of the right to liberty ... Liberty in a free and democratic society does not require the state to approve the personal decisions made by its citizens; it does, however, require the state to respect them.

... The question then becomes whether the decision of a woman to terminate her pregnancy falls within this class of protected decisions. I have no doubt that it does. This decision is one that will have profound psychological, economic and social consequences for the pregnant woman. The circumstances giving rise to it can be complex and varied and there may be, and usually are, powerful considerations militating in opposite directions. It is a decision that deeply reflects the way the woman thinks about herself and her relationship to others and to society at large. It is not just a medical decision; it is a profound social and ethical one as well. Her response to it will be the response of the whole person.

It is probably impossible for a man to respond, even imaginatively, to such a dilemma not just because it is outside the realm of his personal experience (although this is, of course, the case) but because he can relate to it only by objectifying it, thereby eliminating the subjective elements of the female psyche which are at the heart of the dilemma.

... Given then that the right to liberty guaranteed by s. 7 of the Charter gives a woman the right to decide for herself whether or not to terminate her pregnancy, does s. 251 of the *Criminal Code* violate this right? Clearly it does. The purpose of the section is to take the decision away from the woman and give it to a committee. ... The fact that the decision whether a woman will be allowed to terminate her pregnancy is in the hands of a committee is just as great a violation of the woman's right to personal autonomy in decisions of an intimate and private nature as it would be if a committee were established to decide whether a woman should be allowed to continue her pregnancy. Both these arrangements violate the woman's right to liberty by deciding for her something that she has the right to decide for herself.

... I agree with my colleague ... the present legislative scheme for the obtaining of an abortion clearly subjects pregnant women to considerable emotional stress as well as to unnecessary physical risk. I believe, however, that the flaw in the present legislative scheme goes much deeper than that. In essence, what it does is assert that the woman's capacity to reproduce is not to be subject to her own control. It is to be subject to the control of the state. She may not choose whether to exercise her existing capacity or not to exercise it. This is not, in my view, just a matter of interfering with her right to liberty in the sense (already discussed) of her right to personal autonomy in decision-making, it is a direct interference with her physical "person" as well. She is truly being treated as a means — a means to an end which she does not desire but over which she has no control. She is the passive recipient of a decision made by others as to whether her body is to be used to nurture a new life. Can there be anything that comports less with human dignity and self-respect? How can a woman in this position have any sense of security with respect to her person? I believe that s. 251 of the *Criminal Code* deprives the pregnant woman of her right to security of the person as well as her right to liberty.

... I believe, therefore, that a deprivation of the s. 7 right which has the effect of infringing a right guaranteed elsewhere in the Charter cannot be in accordance with the principles of fundamental justice.

In my view, the deprivation of the s. 7 right with which we are concerned in this case offends s. 2(a) of the Charter. I say this because I believe that the decision whether or not to terminate a pregnancy is essentially a moral decision, a matter of conscience. I do not think there is or can be any dispute about that. The question is: whose conscience? Is the conscience of the woman to be paramount or the conscience of the state? I believe, for the reasons I gave in discussing the right to liberty, that in a free and democratic society it must be the conscience of the individual. Indeed, s. 2(a) makes it clear that this freedom belongs to "everyone", i.e., to each of us individually.

... The Chief Justice sees religious belief and practice as the paradigmatic example of conscientiously-held beliefs and manifestations and as such protected by the Charter. But I do not think he is saying that a personal morality which is not founded in religion is outside the protection of s. 2(a). Certainly, it would be my view that conscientious beliefs which are not religiously motivated are equally protected by freedom of conscience in s. 2(a). In so saying I am not unmindful of the fact that the Charter opens with an affirmation that "Canada is founded upon principles that recognize the supremacy of God ..." But I am also mindful that the values entrenched in the Charter are those which characterize a free and democratic society.

... It seems to me ... that in a free and democratic society "freedom of conscience and religion" should be broadly construed to extend to conscientiously-held beliefs, whether grounded in religion or in a secular morality. Indeed, as a matter of statutory interpretation, "conscience" and "religion" should not be treated as tautologous if capable of independent, although related, meaning. Accordingly, for the state to take sides on the issue of abortion, as it does in the impugned legislation by making it a criminal offence for the pregnant woman to exercise one of her options, is not only to endorse but also to enforce, on pain of a further loss of liberty through actual imprisonment, one conscientiously-held view at the expense of another. It is to deny freedom of conscience to some, to treat them as means to an end, to deprive them ... of their "essential humanity". Can this comport with fundamental justice?

... In my view, the primary objective of the impugned legislation must be seen as the protection of the foetus. It undoubtedly has other ancillary objectives, such as the protection of the life and health of pregnant women, but I believe that the main objective advanced to justify a restriction on the pregnant woman's s. 7 right is the protection of the foetus. I think this is a perfectly valid legislative objective. ... I think s. 1 of the Charter authorizes reasonable limits to be put upon the woman's right having regard to the fact of the developing foetus within her body. The question is: at what point in the pregnancy does the protection of the foetus become such a pressing and substantial concern as to outweigh the fundamental right of the woman to decide whether or not to carry the foetus to term? At what point does the state's interest in the protection of the foetus become "compelling" and justify state intervention in what is otherwise a matter of purely personal and private concern?

... It would be my view ... that the value to be placed on the foetus as potential life is directly related to the stage of its development during gestation. The undeveloped foetus starts out as a newly fertilized ovum; the fully developed foetus emerges ultimately as an infant. A developmental progression takes place in between these two extremes and, in my opinion, this progression has a direct bearing on the value of the foetus as potential life. It is a fact of human experience that a miscarriage or spontaneous abortion of the foetus at six months is attended by far greater sorrow and sense of loss than a miscarriage or spontaneous abortion at six days or even six weeks. This is not, of course, to deny that the foetus is potential life from the moment of conception. ... It is simply to say that in balancing the state's interest in the protection of the foetus as potential life under s. 1 of the Charter against the right of the pregnant woman under s. 7 greater weight should be given to the state's interest in the later stages of pregnancy than in the earlier. The foetus should accordingly, for purposes of s. 1, be viewed in differential and developmental terms ... A developmental view of the foetus ... supports a permissive approach to abortion in the early stages of pregnancy and a restrictive approach in the later stages. In the early stages the woman's autonomy would be absolute; her decision, reached in consultation with her physician, not to carry the foetus to term would be conclusive. The state would have no business inquiring into her reasons. Her reasons for having an abortion would, however, be the proper subject of inquiry at the later stages of her pregnancy when the state's compelling interest in the protection of the foetus would justify it in prescribing conditions. The precise point in the development of the foetus at which the state's interest in its protection becomes "compelling" I leave to the informed judgment of the legislature which is in a position to receive guidance on the subject from all the relevant disciplines. It seems to me, however, that it might fall somewhere in the second trimester.

... One final word. I wish to emphasize that in these reasons I have dealt with the existence of the developing foetus merely as a factor to be considered in assessing the importance of the legislative objective under s. 1 of the Charter. I have not dealt with the entirely separate question whether a foetus is covered by the word "everyone" in s. 7 so as to have an independent right to life under that section. The Crown did not argue it and it is not necessary to decide it in order to dispose of the issues on this appeal.

I would allow the appeal.

...

Appeal allowed, McIntyre and La Forest JJ. dissenting.

Toward a Credible View of Abortion

L. W. Sumner

As little as a decade ago most moral philosophers still believed that the exercise of their craft did not include defending positions on actual moral problems. More recently they have come to their senses, one happy result being a spate of articles in the last few years on the subject of abortion.[1] These discussions have contributed much toward an understanding of the abortion issue, but for the most part they have not attempted a full analysis of the morality of abortion.[2] Such an analysis is too large a task for a single paper, but a sketch of it will be undertaken here, the details to be filled in elsewhere.[3]

The moral problem which abortion poses results from some familiar biological and social contingencies. Because *homo sapiens* is a mammal the young of the species are carried by the female during the period of initial development. The weight of reproduction itself is therefore divided unequally between the sexes. Social practice ordinarily enhances this unequal division of labour by arranging that the woman will rear the children as well as bearing them. Her fertility is therefore no small matter for a woman, affecting as it does her opportunity to plan the course of her own life. Thus in the first instance she seeks to control whether (or when) she will conceive. But once conception has occurred its normal outcome is avoidable only by terminating the pregnancy, that is to say by

L.W. Sumner, "Toward a Credible View of Abortion," *Canadian Journal of Philosophy* 4 (September 1974) 163-181.

killing the developing fetus. Such an intentional interruption of the gestation process is an abortion. And so the issues are drawn. Were one or another of these contingencies otherwise abortion might create no moral problem. But as matters now stand the liberty of the woman may conflict directly with the life of the fetus. Such is the stuff of the abortion issue.

The temporal boundaries of abortion are conception and birth: abortion is necessarily post-conceptive and pre-natal. Therein lies its ambiguous moral status. Contraception functions by preventing pregnancy rather than interrupting it. For this reason it does not destroy life and only a small minority persists in objecting to it (or to some particular contraceptive method) on moral grounds. At the other extreme, infanticide involves killing the newborn child. Only an even smaller minority is able to accept infanticide on moral grounds, except perhaps in some extreme cases. Contraception and infanticide are relatively clear moral cases precisely because they are located on either side of pregnancy. Abortion is a difficult case precisely because it occupies this uncertain middle ground. Pro-abortionists tend to assimilate it to contraception while anti-abortionists tend to assimilate it to infanticide. An analysis of the morality of abortion must properly locate it on this continuum between the clear cases.

To speak of the morality of abortion may obscure the fact that there are at least two distinct moral problems concerning abortion. The first requires developing and defending a moral evaluation of abortion itself. We may assume that it will answer the question: When is an abortion morally permissible and when is it not? The second problem requires developing and defending a state policy on abortion. We may assume that it will answer the question: When should an abortion be legally permissible and when should it not? These questions are both moral ones, since they both ask for evaluations from the moral point of view, but they are different moral questions, since evaluating abortion is not the same as evaluating abortion policies. Once we have decided on the moral status of abortion, it is a further issue how it should be treated by the law.[4]

To be complete, positions on the morality of abortion must speak to both problems and most have done so. Two such positions are worth outlining as material for discussion. The first, which may be called the liberal position, is a defense of abortion and of a woman's right to have an abortion if she so chooses. It has at its heart the contention that abortion is a matter private to the woman because it does not substantially affect the welfare of any other person. As such, it raises no moral issues whatsoever, although it may, because of its potential hazards, raise prudential ones. As in the case of other medical procedures, we need to ensure only that the operation is carried out safely, efficiently, and with consent. Any further legal regulation of abortion is incompatible with the principle that the state has no right to interfere in the private activities of the individual. Laws which prohibit or restrict abortion constitute an illegitimate tampering with individual liberties. A woman has the right to decide for herself whether to bear children, a right which is already recognized when the state refrains from regulating contraception. The availability of abortion is simply a further guarantee of this right for cases in which an unwanted pregnancy has already occurred. Furthermore, prohibitive or restrictive abortion policies have the defect of enforcing the moral views of some (anti-abortionists) against the rest. Indeed, in the light of the traditional Catholic position on abortion, such policies establish the moral beliefs of a particular religious sect, thus undermining the separation of church and state. A permissive policy, or no policy at all, leaves each woman free to decide the matter for herself.

What may by contrast be called the conservative position rests upon the view that abortion is not a private matter because it involves the killing of the fetus. It is generally agreed that the taking of human life is in most circumstances wrong. But the fetus is a human life and so abortion is always homicide. As such, it is morally justifiable only in very special circumstances, such as when the continuation of pregnancy would endanger the life of the woman. The welfare or liberty of one person is not in general sufficient to justify the killing of another. It is also usually agreed that protection of human life is one of the legitimate functions of the law. Prohibitive or restrictive laws are therefore not to be seen as the enforcement of private morals or as the establishment of a church but rather as a proper extension of laws forbidding homicide. While it may be true that more permissive laws would produce benefits for women, and perhaps for others as well, these benefits must always be balanced against the toll in human life which abortion necessarily exacts.

These two positions are the ones most commonly heard in discussions of the morality of abortion. Each is internally coherent, each has a venerable tradition behind it, and each is now promoted by vocal and organized pressure groups. The two positions are also diametrically opposed and between them they define the opposite poles in the abortion debate. Nevertheless, it is likely that each position commands the allegiance only of a minority among persons aware of the abortion problem. Many, perhaps most, find themselves somewhere in the middle ground between the two sides. To such persons neither position as it stands seems very credible, because each represents an extreme among available possibilities. The one focuses entirely on the rights of the woman and ignores the fate of the fetus; the other just as resolutely fastens on the welfare of the fetus and subordinates the problem of the woman. The one entirely assimilates abortion to contraception, while the other simply identifies it with infanticide. Each position attaches itself too thoroughly to one of the two ingredients whose conjunction creates the moral issue in the first place. Surely abortion is not just a private matter but is also not always a fullblown case of homicide. Surely there are less crude and less simplistic alternatives available than either of these.

So goes the view from the middle. This paper is an attempt to vindicate this view. It will argue that neither of the standard positions is acceptable because each is too extreme. It will also outline a more credible, because more moderate, alternative. The first step involves a closer look at the two given positions. Out of each can be distilled the basic argument around which the position as a whole is built.

PRIVACY ARGUMENT

P1 Actions which cause no harm are never morally wrong.

P2 The law may not legitimately prohibit actions which cause no harm.

P3 The fetus is not a human individual.

P4 Abortion is never morally wrong.

P5 The law may not legitimately prohibit abortion.

HOMICIDE ARGUMENT

H1 It is always morally wrong to kill a human individual.

H2 The law may legitimately prohibit the killing of human individuals.

H3 The fetus is a human individual.

H4 Abortion is always morally wrong.

H5 The law may legitimately prohibit abortion.

Neither of these arguments is here formulated so as to be logically tight, although the missing steps could be easily supplied, and each argument is presented in a particularly strong and unqualified form. The arguments are therefore more extreme even than the positions from which they were extracted, and it may be that few would defend them in their present form. As stated, however, they will serve as excellent reference points for discussion. Ultimately it will be clearer to what extent, and in what manner, they must be weakened in order to be acceptable.

The arguments plainly have a common structure. Each contains two conclusions which speak to the two moral questions about abortion. Analogous conclusions in the two arguments (P4 and H4, P5 and H5) are mutually incompatible. Each argument derives its conclusions from three premises, of which the first two (P1 and P2, H1 and H2) are moral principles. The third premise in each case (P3 and H3) seems to be a statement of fact about the fetus which serves as the hinge between principles and conclusions. Further, the real differences between the arguments, in virtue of which they yield incompatible conclusions, do not seem to lie in the moral principles to which they appeal. These principles form a mutually compatible set and when put in a somewhat more qualified manner might all have considerable appeal. The point of departure would appear to lie in the third premise. There the homicide argument seems to flatly affirm what the privacy argument just as flatly denies, namely that the fetus is human.

This question about 'the status of the fetus' is obviously in one way or another at the heart of the abortion debate.[5] It cannot be true that abortion is homicide unless the fetus is to be accounted a human person, and it cannot be true that abortion is a private matter unless the fetus is not to be so accounted. Doubts about abortion are above all doubts about how to classify, and therefore treat, the fetus. Sooner or later this question must be confronted. The larger part of this paper will be spent confronting it.

It will be convenient to organize the discussion as a commentary on the privacy and homicide arguments, but particularly on the latter. It is natural to begin by examining the contention that the fetus is human. The structure of the argument suggests that this is the crucial fact about the fetus whose acceptance will pave the way to acceptance of the argument's conservative conclusions. If this is so then one implication follows immediately. It cannot be that the humanity of the fetus is a matter of theological tenet or religious dogma. It is sometimes argued that an individual is human in virtue of possession of a soul, or perhaps a distinctively human soul, and thus that the fetus is human from the moment that it acquires such a soul. The history of controversy about abortion within the Catholic Church consists largely of disagreement over when to locate this moment of 'ensoulment'.[6] Whereas Aquinas seems to have believed that the event occurred sometime during the gestation period, the weight of official opinion now is that it accompanies conception. The role of this opinion within the homicide argument will be obvious.

Whatever the merits of contrary positions within this theological debate, its outcome cannot affect our evaluation of the homicide argument or of abortion. The one characteristic of the event of ensoulment which seems to be universally accepted is that, whenever it occurs, it is not observable or open to any sort of empirical test. There exists no empirical method of confirming that, or when, an individual is ensouled. But if the premise concerning the fetus is to play its role within the homicide argument it must be open to confirmation or disconfirmation. Otherwise the argument as a whole is undecidable and will carry no weight whatever for anyone who rejects the theology on which it rests. Sectarian dogmas based upon faith, revelation, or scriptural authority can have no place in public moral discussion of abortion. They may of course be used to reinforce the consciences of the faithful, but the homicide argument, if it is to carry any weight whatever for the unfaithful, must be able to stand free of theological props.

However, once we have agreed that whether an individual is human is an empirical fact about that individual, we encounter an intractable problem. The argument cannot just stipulate what it will mean by this word 'human' for that again would be to abandon its aim of widespread acceptance. It must show that in some common and ordinary sense of the word the fetus is clearly human. But therein lies the problem: there are too many such common and ordinary senses. Like all predicates the word 'human' is a tool of classification; when we use it we distinguish the category of things human from things not human. But different categories suit different purposes and different contexts, and so the word comes to be used in different senses. For example, in saying that a person is human we may mean that he is particularly warm, or gentle, or loving (as opposed to inhuman, i.e. cold, callous, unfeeling), or we may mean that he is fallible or imperfect (as opposed to superhuman or divine). As a classificatory term 'human' in this respect somewhat resembles the word 'real', which can be opposed to any of 'artificial', 'counterfeit', 'fake', 'forged', 'synthetic', 'imitation', 'illusory', and so on, depending on the sort of object being described and on the context. Like 'real', 'human' admits of a variety of meanings. No doubt there are some common threads running through these meanings, but the fact remains that deciding whether the fetus is human is rather like deciding whether the wax apple is real. It may or may not be, depending on the categories one has in mind.

The nature of the term 'human' makes things at once easy and difficult for the proponent of the homicide argument. It is easy to show that in some ordinary sense the fetus is human, but it is difficult to show either that it is human in all such senses or that one particular sense is privileged. The nature of the problem will be clearer if we restrict our attention, as proponents of the homicide argument tend to do, to senses of 'human' which are biological in nature. It is sometimes claimed that advances in biology (and especially in genetics and embryology) in the past two centuries or so have shown beyond any doubt that the fetus is human from conception.[7] Biologists and other professionals have agreed that the fetus is human, and there's an end to it. We must be wary of arguments of the form "the professionals all agree ..." For one thing the professionals seldom do all agree, and the existence of many prominent pro-abortionist biologists and obstetricians would seem to indicate that they do not all agree in this instance. But even if they did, it is surely not a matter for them to decide. They will of course be expert in a number of facts which are relevant to deciding whether a fetus is human, but these may not be the only relevant facts and anyway scientific professionals have no license to tell us how to construct our categories. It will be apparent presently how deciding that a fetus is human is not making a simple statement of fact about it but rather drawing a particular conclusion from accepted facts or organizing these facts in a certain manner. Professionals are not notably better qualified than the rest of us to draw such conclusions or to decide how the facts are best organized.

If we explore what biology can tell us that is relevant to classifying individuals as human we find again more possible categories than we want. There are at least three distinct senses of the word 'human', each of which is derived from and therefore consonant with the biological facts. The first and simplest of these may be called the *specific* sense, because it pertains to the distinction of animal species. Certainly one thing we can mean by saying that an individual is human is that it is not a baboon or a tuna or a woodpecker. The category of human individuals which is generated by this sense of the word has the undoubted virtue of being quite sharp at the edges: it includes all and only members of the species *homo sapiens.* We would be uncertain only of hybrids or mutations, and these are rare.

This specific sense of 'human' can be used as the basis of two other, still biological, senses of the term. Each of these further senses generates a narrower category of human individuals, since it includes only a subset of the members of the species. When biologists do animal classification (taxonomy) they tend to describe the characteristics of a given species in terms of a model individual of the species which satisfies two conditions: it is structurally and functionally normal and it is mature. This procedure is a simplifying device which involves describing the model individual first and then allowing for variations displayed by members of the species which are either abnormal (runts and albinos, for example) or immature and not fully developed. Species are compared primarily in terms of the properties of their standard or model members. Thus *homo sapiens* is identified, and differentiated from other primate species, in terms of the height range, weight range, posture, skeletal and muscular structure, brain size, and so on, of the normal and mature individual.[8] What is interesting for our purpose is that normality and maturity can themselves serve as criteria which generate quite different, though overlapping, categories of human individuals.

Consider first normality. If a member of our species is abnormal enough in physiology then he is liable to be described as a freak, or a monster, or a vegetable, or an animal. Even staid medical science continues to use the term 'monster' to describe a specified set of gross abnormalities or anomalies.[9] Since fetal growth proceeds so rapidly from such a small beginning, even minor deviations from normal development early in pregnancy can produce gross malformations in the later fetus. No part of the human physiology is immune. The most extreme fetal malformations affect the central nervous system: total absence or extreme underdevelopment of the brain, nonclosure of the spinal column, and so on. Other major organ systems are however also susceptible to gross malformations. When we refer to such malformed individuals as monsters it certainly seems that we are denying that they are completely or fully human, despite the fact that they may be genetically quite normal and that they are unquestionably members of our species. They fail of being fully human because they are so abnormal, because they fall so far short of the paradigm or model member of the species. It is only at the margin, only in the extreme cases, that we are likely to describe members of the species, on physiological grounds, as monsters or to say that they are less than human. But to the extent that we do so we are employing a sense of the word 'human' other than the specific one. It is appropriate to call it the *normic* sense.

Finally, a member of the species can fail to exhibit the characteristics of the model individual not because it is abnormal but because it is immature. Thus if we follow the adult backward through the developmental process we sooner or later reach a stage when the individual is so undeveloped or immature that we begin to speak of its potential, or what it will become, rather than what it is. Thus the chicken is at the earliest stage an egg, the oak an acorn, the plant a seed. It is proper to say that the egg, acorn, or seed will grow into, develop into, or become the chicken, oak, or plant and also that they are not yet these things. Likewise, in our species, at the earliest stage of development the individual is a single cell (zygote), the result of the union of sperm and ovum. It is common and natural to say that this cell is a potential human individual, or that it will grow into, develop into, or become a human individual but that it is not yet a human individual. Again we tend to use this classification only at the margin; the child or infant is a human individual, but the zygote will become one. And again the operative consideration seems to be the degree to which the individual fails to exhibit the properties of the model member of the species. The zygote is microscopic in size, spherical in shape, and contains no organ systems whatsoever. When we react to this difference in degree by saying that the zygote is not yet a human individual we are once more employing a sense of the term other than the specific sense. Since level of development is now central it seems suitable to call this third sense of the word 'human' the *developmental* sense.

There may well be other ways in which categories of human individuals are constructed out of raw biological data, but these three will suffice for the present discussion. It seems that even the hard facts of biology generate no unique and privileged category of human individuals. In the specific sense all members of the species are human, however abnormal or undeveloped. In the normic sense only those members of the species are human who display, or will come to display, to a sufficient degree the physiological characteristics of the normal individual. In the developmental sense only those members of the species are human who have reached some minimal stage of development. It should be stressed that each of these senses of the word is quite legitimate. Each is grounded in the biological data, though each organizes these data differently. Each picks out one of the strands of meaning in the ordinary word 'human', and each of the resulting categories appears in common speech. Each is internally coherent and each enables us to distinguish tolerably well between what is human and what is not. Finally, each corresponds to analogous distinctions for other animal species.

If we bring these categories to bear on the fetus we derive divergent answers to the question whether the fetus is human. We must remember that "the fetus" is a developmental stage in the history of the individual. Technically, the fetal stage does not occupy even all of the individual's pre-natal history, since it is preceded by the zygotal stage (first five weeks) and embryonic stage (next four weeks). If we use the term 'fetus' loosely to cover all developmental stages prior to birth, then it is clear that the class of fetuses contains individuals very different in many important ways. A newly fertilized ovum or zygote is a tiny dot barely visible to the naked eye, while the full-term fetus is usually 18-22 inches long and 5-10 pounds in weight, with almost all major bodily systems in working order. Given the sheer quantity of development in the first nine months of life, the fetal category *must* contain very different sorts of individuals. We should of course be wary of attributing to all fetuses characteristics pertaining only to a particular stage of development.

In the specific sense of the word all fetuses conceived of human parents are human, regardless of normality or developmental stage. In the normic sense most fetuses are human, gross abnormalities being rare. In the developmental sense the zygote is clearly not yet human and the full-term fetus is just as clearly human, while the fetus at some stages in between will not be easily classifiable. We will return later, from a slightly different perspective, to both the extreme and the middle cases. For the present we need only note that in the developmental sense of the word some fetuses are human while others are not and that the difference between them lies only in their level of development.

We are now back where we started. The deceptively simple question "Is the fetus a human individual?" has no unique answer, even when only biological data are admitted. We can perhaps now see why many biologists shy away from this category of humanity. It is not itself a ground-floor biological category, but rather a way of organizing ground-floor data. Unfortunately, there are a number of alternative ways of organizing and presenting these data, none of which is privileged *so long as we consider only the facts themselves.* Even though our question certainly looks like a factual one, there seems no way to answer it satisfactorily by appeal even to a limited range of facts. The substance of premise H3 of the homicide argument is that all fetuses conceived of human parents are human. This contention is true of the specific sense of the term 'human' and only of that sense. Thus the homicide argument requires this sense of the word, but there is so far no way of showing that this sense is privileged or that it should be preferred. The status of the homicide argument is thus far undecidable. The privacy argument, however, fares less well. The substance of its premise P3 is that no fetus, regardless of stage of development, is human. We have located no common biological sense of the word 'human' in which this claim is true. Unless some viable candidate has been overlooked, which is certainly possible, we are entitled to suspect that the privacy argument rests its conclusions on a highly implausible premise.

It is an attractive strategy to consider the homicide argument piecemeal, and to begin with that premise which looks like a straightforwardly empirical one. It can now be seen why the strategy must fail. In the absence of a specific context the question of the humanity of the fetus is undecidable. But the homicide argument itself, through its first two premises, provides just such a context. Once these premises are given (and it should be remembered that each of them appears a familiar and attractive moral principle) then only one step remains to generate the argument's conclusions. In this context to concede that the fetus is human is to concede that it is to be included within the scope of the two moral principles and therefore to concede the conclusions. Conversely, if the conclusions are to be avoided, given the principles, then the humanity of the fetus must be denied. This surely is why debates about whether the fetus is human are so heated: each side knows the moral issue at stake, namely when it is morally permissible for the fetus to be killed. The assumption common to both sides is that if the fetus is human it is wrong to kill it. Against this assumption the question of the humanity of the fetus is no longer a neutral and empirical one, which is how it has so far been treated in this discussion. Now the fate of the fetus turns on the answer to this question alone. Suddenly all of the moral passion which is part of the abortion debate is infused into this supposed question of fact, and a decision on it, one way or the other, becomes itself a moral decision. It ought to be obvious that some basic and hard moral decisions must somewhere be involved in either accepting or rejecting the homicide argument. This fact is concealed when we are first asked to accept some moral principles which appear quite reasonable and then, because of the "facts" of the matter, shown that we are thereby committed to some strong conclusions about abortion. The facts will simply not bear this weight and the underlying moral disagreement will show itself as a preference for one or another interpretation of the word 'human'. Our assessment of the homicide argument will be much more clearheaded if the moral decisions involved are clearly located and carefully identified.

The homicide argument must be evaluated as a whole and not piecemeal. It is a requirement of logic that in order for the argument to be sound it must not equivocate on this word 'human': the sense of the term which is employed in one part of the argument must be employed throughout. We have seen already that H3 requires the specific sense of the term; this sense must therefore be employed as well in the two moral principles H1 and H2. When interpreted in this manner the principles include in their scope all members of the species, including the fetus. To assent to the principles is to agree that the fetus, regardless of its level of development, is to be treated from the moral point of view in just the same manner as the child or the adult. It is now obvious just how much is being conceded in making even the first two moves in the argument, and how short the distance is from there to its conclusions. If H3 is rendered uncontroversially true by use of the specific sense of 'human' the moral issue simply shifts to the two principles. In no way can this issue be evaded: Does the fetus belong within the scope of H1 and H2? Can we devise moral principles concerning homicide which are plausible for both the fetus and the adult? Should the fetus be accorded the same treatment, and therefore the same protection of life, as the adult? This surely is the moral crux in the abortion debate: not whether the fetus is human but how it is to be treated.

The homicide argument makes the moral claim that the fetus is to be treated in the same way as the adult and it does this by including the fetus within the scope of its principles concerning homicide. These principles state that it is wrong to take human life and that human life should have legal protection. In this somewhat stark form they are probably too strong for most moral tastes; surely killing is sometimes morally justifiable and should be sometimes legally justifiable. Still, if the argument is to yield suitably conservative conclusions about abortion, such as that abortion is justifiable only to save the life of the mother, the principles must be given a strong formulation. Proponents of the homicide argument speak sometimes of human life as possessing a uniquely high or absolute value, where this seems to mean that nothing but the preservation of life can compensate the loss of life. If we incorporate this valuation into the two principles we derive the result that it is wrong to kill except to preserve life and that in all cases save this one killing must be prohibited by law. Even in this somewhat weakened form these principles are not easy to live by. They suffice to condemn killing in almost every instance, since it is only rarely that killing is necessary to preserve life. Virtually all warfare and political terrorism, along with such practices of the state as the death penalty and firing upon criminal suspects would be unjustifiable. We would also need to question such technological advances as the automobile where we trade annually many thousands of lives for an increase in convenience. It is a fairly safe guess that few among us are really willing to carry such principles to their inevitable conclusions. But if not, then we cannot pretend to accept the principles. This burden weighs heavy upon proponents of the homicide argument. It is generally their purpose to show that abortion is permissible only to save the life of the mother and that in all other circumstances it should be proscribed by law. In order to generate these conclusions they require principles of the sort now under consideration. Once adopted, these principles must be applied to all cases and not just to that of abortion. The view that life can be sacrificed only for life is perhaps an admirable one, but it is a high ideal with radical implications. The acceptance of these implications, all of them, is the test of the anti-abortionist's sincerity.

Let us suppose, as the argument requires, that these are acceptable moral principles concerning human life. They are formulated for, and commonly applied to, post-natal life — infants, children, and adults. The question remains: Is the fetus to be included within their scope? In asking this question we place a severe strain on our moral principles. How far back in the life-history of the individual are we to take them to apply? To birth only? To conception? How different from the child or adult must the individual be before we will place him in a separate moral category? The point of the homicide argument is to extend these principles back to conception. To decide whether this extension is plausible we should look at the extreme case: the zygote, the individual at the point of conception, at the earliest stage in his life-history. If it is plausible to extend the principles to the zygote then it is plausible to extend them to all fetal stages; if it is not then the homicide argument must be rejected.

We must remember that at conception the zygote is a single cell, a tiny and barely visible entity. Consider now the following situation. Some experimental work has been done on a so-called 'morning-after' pill which is sometimes loosely referred to as a contraceptive but is in fact an abortifacient, since it causes the expulsion of the zygote should the woman conceive. What are we to think of a woman who regularly uses such a pill? She does so not knowing whether she will conceive, but knowing that if she does then the pill will cause the death of the zygote. Is she committing homicide? Her behaviour is structurally similar to that of someone who regularly leaves time bombs in randomly selected locations, set to explode at randomly selected times, not knowing whether anyone will be in the proximity when the bomb explodes, but knowing that if someone is then he will die. Is our moral attitude toward the two cases the same? Are we likely to condemn the woman, on moral grounds, as a probable killer? Would we consider her using the morning-after pill to fall into a different category from using an oral contraceptive? Would we insist that the pill be taken off the market, that all testing of it be curtailed? Would we support a law which made the use of the pill punishable with the severity usual to homicide statutes? The homicide argument requires affirmative answers to all of these questions.

There is as yet no morning-after pill in general use. But many women do now use the intrauterine device (IUD) which probably also works to expel the fertilized ovum by preventing its implantation in the wall of the uterus.[10] If so, it too is an abortifacient and all of the foregoing questions can be raised concerning it. Again the homicide argument requires that we regard women on the IUD as presumptively guilty of multiple homicide. Are we really ready to do so? Should we pass a law forbidding use of the IUD and begin arresting women who are using it? Is every such woman a public menace comparable to the setter of time bombs? If the homicide argument is correct then human life on a grand scale is at stake and innocent victims are dying every hour. But can we really accept this view of the matter?

Some laboratory experiments have united sperm and ovum in an artificial extrauterine environment. The resulting zygote does not long survive because of the absence of the sustaining uterine wall. Are experimenters who permit such conceptions murderers? Are their experiments comparable, morally speaking, to those Nazi medical experiments which cost the lives of their victims? Or consider the matter this way. Suppose that one experiment involves killing the sperm and ovum just before union while a second kills the resulting zygote immediately after union. Should we regard the two as radically different in their moral implications because conception occurred in the second but not in the first? The homicide argument requires that we do so. Finally, a large number of pregnancies end in spontaneous abortions. If the homicide argument is correct every such case costs a human life. Should we not take care that the abortion, while certainly accidental and unintended, was not in any way the result of negligence on the part of the woman? After all, we do take just such care to ensure that accidental death resulting from a highway accident was not the result of negligence on the part of the driver. A genuine desire to protect human life in the womb, however early its development, would surely require such steps. But are we really prepared to accept them?

The argument so far is simply an attempt to identify commonly shared moral intuitions. The homicide argument has certain unavoidable implications for the case of the zygote. If these implications are unacceptable then the argument must be rejected. I believe that most persons who reflect carefully on the situations described will be unable to accept these implications. I know that I cannot. Most persons, I suspect, regard the developmental stage of the individual as relevant to the morality of killing that individual. Killing the zygote does not strike us as homicide because developmentally the zygote is too primitive, too unlike the adult, child, or even the fetus in its later stages. It is precisely level of development which the homicide argument rules out as relevant. It tries to draw a firm and inflexible line at conception. Before that point no questions about homicide occur, while immediately after it the individual is to be regarded morally as the equal of a child or adult. Few will accept this hard and fast division of cases. The zygote for most will not seem to fall in a different moral category from the sperm or ovum, despite the fact that the zygote is, and the sperm and ovum are not, a genetically complete member of the species. Abortion at the earliest stage, through the agency of the morning-after pill or IUD, will be regarded by most as morally identical to contraception. At this extreme abortion is indeed assimilable to contraception for the purposes of morality.

Consider now the opposite extreme case, the full-term fetus. At term the fetus differs from the newborn (neonate) principally in its occupation of a quite different environment. Because this environment is both confined and fluid, the fetus is unable to breathe or to ingest food. Both oxygen and nourishment are received from the maternal blood supply through the medium of the placenta. All other organ systems which will be functioning just after birth are functioning just before it. The birth process transfers the individual to a new environment and severs the direct physical link between mother and child: the neonate must breathe and eat. In no other important respect does birth alter the individual. The process occupies only a few minutes and the individual is the same size, weight, and shape directly after it as before. Most of his bodily systems are unaffected by the process. In the light of these facts it seems difficult to accept the view that birth is of crucial importance from the point of view of the morality of killing. Assuming that it is wrong to kill the infant directly after birth, it would seem equally wrong, and for the same reasons, to kill it directly before birth. The differences between full-term fetus and neonate do not seem morally relevant, especially when we consider that the temporal point at which birth occurs varies widely and therefore that many full-term fetuses are older and more developed than many newborn infants. It would seem natural then to extend our moral principles concerning killing beyond the neonate to embrace the full-term fetus. At this extreme abortion is morally assimilable to infanticide. If this view of the matter is taken then the privacy argument as well cannot be accepted, since it implies that abortion at no stage of pregnancy, however late, is to be considered as an instance of homicide.

If I am right, then upon reflection most persons would be willing to include the full-term fetus, but not the zygote, within the scope of moral principles concerning homicide. They will therefore reject both the homicide argument and the privacy argument. Since attention has here been focused especially on the homicide argument, its fate should be described in detail. Its three premises must all employ the same sense of the word 'human'. The appeal to moral intuition implies that if the specific sense is chosen, so as to render H3 true, then H1 and H2 are both false. Conversely, if the developmental sense is chosen so as to render H1 and H2 true, H3 is false. There is no possible formulation of the homicide argument which preserves the truth of all three premises. In order to be acceptable, the homicide argument must be amended. There are two alternatives open:

AMENDED HOMICIDE ARGUMENT (1)

H1 It is always morally wrong to kill a human individual.

H2 The law may legitimately prohibit the killing of human individuals.

H3* Some fetuses are human individuals and some are not.

H4* Some instances of abortion are morally wrong and some are not.

H5* The law may sometimes legitimately prohibit abortion and sometimes not.

AMENDED HOMICIDE ARGUMENT (2)

H1* It is sometimes morally wrong to kill a human individual and sometimes not.

H2* The law may sometimes legitimately prohibit the killing of human individuals and sometimes not.

H3 The fetus is a human individual.

H4* Some instances of abortion are morally wrong and some are not.

H5* The law may sometimes legitimately prohibit abortion and sometimes not.

Formulation (1) employs the developmental sense of 'human' and therefore preserves H1 and H2 from the homicide argument, but not H3. Formulation (2) employs the specific sense of 'human' and so preserves H3 from the homicide argument, but not H1 and H2. It is now clear that the question of whether the fetus is human is not in itself crucial to the argument, since the same conclusions are derivable in either case. The considerations which would lead us to classify the fetus at different stages as human or not, in the developmental sense, are of course relevant since the developmental level of the fetus plays a large part in our moral decisions concerning abortion. But the ultimate questions at stake are moral ones.

The liberal and conservative positions, and the arguments on which they rest, are unacceptable because they entail conclusions which are too extreme. The case against these positions has been made entirely by appeal to commonly shared moral intuitions. It would be strengthened if these intuitions could be shown to cohere well with our considered views on moral issues other than, but related to, abortion.

It does not seem wrong to kill a zygote, even if the reason for doing so is simply that the woman does not wish to be pregnant, while it does seem wrong to kill a full-term fetus for this reason. The difference between the two cases seems to lie principally in the level of development of the fetus. This suggests a developmental approach to abortion in which the justifying conditions for an abortion will contract as the fetus develops. On this conception the fetus comes gradually to be treated as a moral person in the full sense.[11]

The question is why fetal development should be considered morally relevant in this way. As the fetus grows it changes in two main respects: globally (increase in size, alteration of shape) and systematically (acquisition of major body systems). Of these the latter seems the more important from the moral point of view. We should probably treat as moral persons individuals who were systematically identical to us, especially in the functioning of their central nervous systems, but who differed, even radically, in size, shape, or both. Even among organ systems many seem only marginally relevant. There is nothing distinctive about much of our bodies: other animals are swifter, stronger, better shielded, and keener of sense than we. In one respect alone are we pre-eminent, our brains having evolved to a point where we have the capacity for thought and the expression of thought (language). Emphasis on the development of the central nervous system is the physiological correlate of the ancient view that man is distinguished from other creatures by his rationality.

It seems plausible to suppose that we are willing to treat a fetus as a moral person only when it has come to possess a central nervous system developed at least to some minimal extent. Once this developmental view of abortion is taken it can be connected to views on cognate moral issues. A zygote and an embryo are distinguished by their relative lack of a central nervous system. A similar lack is rare, though possible, among other members of the species. An anencephalic is an individual in which the higher levels of the brain remain underdeveloped or totally absent. Such individuals rarely survive until birth and never long thereafter. In such cases abortion, or for that matter infanticide, does not seem morally objectionable. The condition is also approximated in those victims of disease or accident who have permanently lost the functioning of the higher levels of the brain but continue to live. In such cases euthanasia does not seem morally objectionable. An early abortion is therefore similar, from the moral point of view, to some cases of eugenic abortion (early or late) and to some cases of euthanasia, in that the individual who is killed lacks at the time a central nervous system functioning in more than a rudimentary manner. The cases are of course distinguished by the fact that the early fetus has not yet developed such a system while the anencephalic will never develop one and the accident victim has lost the functioning of a developed system. Thus in the former case but in neither of the latter one is preventing the evolution of an individual who otherwise would come to possess not only a highly developed central nervous system but also all of the characteristics typical of adult members of the species. But there seems nothing wrong with preventing the development of a human person (thus the moral innocuousness of contraception) while there seems much wrong with terminating the life of one which has already developed to a considerable degree. This single difference in the case of early abortion does not appear therefore to be morally relevant.

Somewhat further afield we encounter the treatment of other species. This issue is too complex to be discussed thoroughly but some broad features should be noted. Our attitudes toward other species are complicated by our need for a reliable food supply, by our love of killing for its own sake, and by our habit of keeping certain species of animals as pets. In general the protection of life we offer to other species is largely determined by our own needs: thus we may hunt mountain lions to extinction while supporting a burgeoning population of household cats and we may eliminate wolves while protecting poodles. But we do make a pervasive distinction between the value of human life and the value of the life of all other animal species, once again on the basis of what is considered distinctive in us. Thus through all the complicating factors we display a marked preference for the more intelligent and highly evolved species. The differences are, as always, most apparent at the extremes. We destroy insects when they are merely inconvenient for us while feeling a much closer kinship to those species of great apes who are our nearest living relatives. Here too we construct our moral categories in part around this most crucial of all human characteristics.

To mould these still scattered attitudes and practices into a single coherent system would require a thoroughgoing analysis of life and death and above all an account of when and why killing is wrong. This undertaking is too ambitious for the present but until it has been completed no view of abortion can be taken as firmly established. Once such an analysis is available, however, it is very likely that only a developmental view of abortion will be compatible with it.

It has thus far been left unspecified how abortion should be regarded between the extreme cases of the zygote and the full-term fetus. I will simply state my view of the matter with little supporting argument.[12] The major factors relevant to evaluating abortion are the situation and needs of the mother and the level of development of the fetus. The gradual and continuous nature of the latter renders the drawing of sharp lines out of the question. The attempt to draw such a line (whether at conception or both) is precisely the mistake common to the liberal and conservative positions. Any such line must make an arbitrary distinction between adjacent and similar cases. The developmental view must allow for the gradual acquisition by the fetus of the status of a moral person and the accompanying right to protection of life. It is customary to divide pregnancy (calculated at 40 weeks) into trimesters of approximately 13 weeks. Even by the end of the first trimester the fetus is well advanced in the development of its central nervous system, as well as other bodily systems. It has entered a transitional or threshold stage between its early undeveloped state and its later developed state. Likewise, the end of that trimester is the latest point at which the safest abortion procedures (dilatation and curettage, vacuum aspiration) can be employed, and by that time every woman has had an adequate opportunity to decide whether she wishes to continue her pregnancy. For all these reasons, during the early weeks of pregnancy an abortion is morally permissible whatever the woman's reason for wishing it, while during the final four or five months it is permissible only in very special circumstances analogous to those which justify killing in the case of post-natal persons. Between these relatively clear cases lies the borderline threshold period occupying a few weeks around the end of the first trimester. During this stage the morality of abortion is simply unclear.

This is so far only a sketch of a position, but when it is fully elaborated and properly defended we have a developmental view of abortion which is far more plausible than either the liberal or conservative position. While it lacks the elegant simplicity of the extreme views it makes up this lack by taking into account factors which they simply ignore. The morality of abortion is a difficult question in part because the fetus itself is so different at various stages of pregnancy. Only the developmental view allows us to attend to these differences in adopting a moral stance on abortion. It is for this reason that it both matches more closely our intuitions about abortion and coheres better with our views on related moral issues than does either of the more prominent positions.

The abortion policy appropriate to this view would permit abortion at the request of the woman before some fixed time limit, and would carefully screen abortions after that limit. Since the law must operate a workable policy, it cannot tolerate borderline cases and therefore must establish a clear and definite time limit. It is reasonable to set this limit around the end of the third month of pregnancy. Such a limit lies within the threshold period, coincides with the latest stage at which the safest abortion methods can be used, allows every woman sufficient time to discover that she is pregnant and decide whether to terminate the pregnancy, and captures the majority of abortions actually performed even where there is no time limit. After the third month the law will consider abortion as homicide and will specify the grounds on which it will be permitted. We may assume that these grounds will be narrow and strictly medical in nature and that some screening apparatus will be established. Again the details of the policy and of its justification cannot be considered here.

NOTES

1. R. B. Brandt, "The Morality of Abortion," *The Monist,* LVI, No. 4 (October 1972); B. A. Brody, "Abortion and the Law," *Journal of Philosophy,* LXVIII, No. 12 (June 17, 1971), and "Thomson on Abortion," *Philosophy and Public Affairs,* I, No. 3 (Spring 1972); R. J. Gerber, "Abortion: Parameters for Decision," *Ethics,* LXXXII, No. 2 (January 1972); Judith Jarvis Thomson, "A Defense of Abortion," *Philosophy and Public Affairs,* I, No. 1 (Fall 1971); Michael Tooley, "Abortion and Infanticide," *Philosophy and Public Affairs,* II, No. 1 (Fall 1972); Mary Anne Warren, "On the Moral and Legal Status of Abortion," *The Monist,* LVII, No. 1 (January 1973); Roger Wertheimer, "Understanding the Abortion Argument," *Philosophy and Public Affairs,* I, No. 1 (Fall 1971); B. A. Brody, "Abortion and the Sanctity of Human Life", *American Philosophical Quarterly,* X, No. 2, (April 1973).
2. The exceptions are the articles by Tooley and Warren (see note 1), each of which attempts to justify what I have classified as a liberal position on abortion. The present paper was completed before I encountered these articles and thus I have not commented on their arguments. Two of my purposes, however, are to discard this liberal view and to argue for an alternative to it.
3. A more thorough treatment of the matters discussed in this papers, and others pertinent to the abortion issue, is included in a book now in progress.
4. An answer to the first question is, however, an important step toward answering

the second. The close connection between a particular view of the morality of abortion and a particular sort of abortion law is stressed by Brody, *op. cit.*

5. The unavoidability of this issue is the main point of the discussion by Brody.
6. For an account of this history see John T. Noonan, Jr., "An Almost Absolute Value in History," in *The Morality of Abortion: Legal and Historical Perspectives,* ed. John T. Noonan, Jr. (Cambridge: Harvard University Press, 1970).
7. Catholic law professor Sergio Cotta, speaking for the Vatican against the 1973 U.S. Supreme Court decision on abortion: "By investigating the basic genetic structure of life, science has determined with unquestionable certainty that since the moment of conception the embryo is a living human being, entirely distinct from the parents." Reported in the *Toronto Star,* January 24, 1973.
8. For a typical taxonomical profile of our species see E. L. Cockrum, *et al., Biology* (Philadelphia: W. B. Saunders Company, 1966).
9. For a standard classification and description of fetal abnormalities see Edith L. Potter, *Pathology of the Fetus and Infant* (2nd ed.; Chicago: Year Book Medical Publishers, 1961).
10. See the discussion of the intrauterine device in Germain Grisez, *Abortion: The Myths, the Realities, and the Arguments* (New York and Cleveland: Corpus Books, 1970), pp. 106-109.
11. For the purpose of this discussion an individual is being treated as a full moral person when the conditions generally accepted as justifying the killing of that individual are those and only those which are generally accepted as justifying killing members of the species in general. In the language of the earlier discussion, he must be included within the scope of general moral principles concerning homicide.
12. A full defense of this view is made in the book referred to in footnote 3.

The Use of Fetal and Anencephalic Tissue for Transplantation

Robert C. Cefalo and H. Tristram Engelhardt, Jr.

ABSTRACT

Advances in transplantation have extended the life and relieved the suffering of thousands of individuals. The prospect of being able to use tissues from embryos, as well as from anencephalic newborns, offers the promise of further relief of suffering. However, these possibilities raise significant moral and public policy issues. The question arises of the extent to which those who disapprove of abortion may make use of tissues

Robert C. Cefalo and H.T. Engelhardt, Jr., "The Use of Fetal and Anencephalic Tissue for Transplantation," *The Journal of Medicine and Philosophy* 14:1(1989) 25-43.

derived from abortion in order to treat serious diseases. This essay argues that, with proper safeguards, such tissue can be used without cooperating in abortion. That is, even those who oppose abortion can benefit from the use of tissue procured during abortion. Questions also arise regarding the probity of maintaining a pregnancy in order to produce an anencephalic newborn whose biological existence will be maintained so as better to secure organs once death is declared. It is argued that, since no harm can be done to a being that has neither a sense of self or the capacity to feel pain, and since women have a right to forego abortions, there is no legitimate ground for opposing women's seeking meaning in their pregnancy through maximizing the opportunity of others to use the organs of their anencephalic newborn once death has been declared. Finally, it is argued that, since the capacities for sentience, a minimal condition for personhood, are never realized by an anencephalic, the entity has never been alive as a person. Therefore, there should be no opposition in principle to aborting anencephalics nor, after proper declaration, to making their organs available as one would after whole-brain death, despite the continued functioning of the brain stem.

The transplantation of organs and tissues is one of the major contributions of modern high-technology medicine. However, the use of transplantation as a treatment modality is not without controversy (Engelhardt, 1984). The expectation of new advances has raised serious moral and public policy questions. Recent results from neuronal and adrenal medulla grafts in humans and monkeys with spontaneous or chemically induced Parkinsonism suggest, despite some contrary evidence (Kolata, 1988b), that cell transplantation may provide a useful therapy. Hematopoietic stem cells (HSC) from fetal marrow and liver have been used to treat genetic diseases and radiation sickness. Also, developments in surgical techniques for organ transplantation from anencephalics may establish a lifesaving source of organs for infants and children dying of heart, liver, and kidney disease. These new technological prospects for controlling diseases and extending life raise special moral and legal issues that must be addressed in order to develop responsible public policy in these areas.

The morality of harvesting fetal tissues depends on the status of the fetus at the time the tissue is taken. The moral and legal issues are fairly clear if the fetus meets current definitions of death. Still, a moral problem arises for those who hold that elective abortion is immoral. There is the question whether individuals may in good conscience, without having cooperated in an immoral action, participate in securing such tissue or in using it in treatment of diseases. The use of anencephalics as organ donors also raises the issue of the status of the donor. There may be some technical and philosophical difficulties in applying whole-brain criteria for death to an anencephalic newborn, while optimally maintaining the organs for subsequent transplantation (American Academy of Pediatrics, 1987; Coutler, 1987; Volpe, 1987; Harrison, 1986; Capron, 1987; Holzgreve *et al.,* 1987). In addition, there are hesitations regarding the propriety of maintaining a pregnancy simply to produce a child who will be an organ donor, or of postponing death only in order to find a suitable recipient (Arras and Shinnar, 1988).

The most fundamental question is the one we will treat last: should anencephalics have the legal and moral status of brain-dead but otherwise alive human beings?

Unlike most whole-brain-dead individuals, anencephalics do not possess a past history of mental life. They have never experienced, felt, or acted upon the world, nor will they ever. Should they be considered to be living persons if they have never had and will never have the capacity for sentience? This essay addresses the general problem of fashioning morally justified public policy regarding the transplantation of organs from fetuses and anencephalic infants. The final accent will be on the use of anencephalics as donors: we close by offering a set of proposals for refashioning public policy regarding the status of anencephalics.

BACKGROUND — MEDICAL ISSUES

Currently there are no curative modalities and few palliative therapies for degenerative neurological disorders such as Parkinson's disease, Huntington's chorea disease, and senile dementia of the Alzheimer's type. Preliminary research in reversing the deficits these patients experience involves the grafting of neuroblastic tissue in hopes of selective functional reconstruction of the brain. A few patients with Parkinson's disease have demonstrated transient clinical improvement after autologous adrenal medullary tissue from adults was transplanted into specific parts of their brains (Merz 1987; Madrazo *et al.*, 1987). In 1986, the survival of transplanted fetal monkey neurons suggested that fetal neuron grafting may have an application in the treatment of Parkinson's disease (Redmond *et al.*, 1986). In monkeys with chemically induced Parkinsonism, behavioral and functional improvement continued for ten weeks after cell grafts were performed. Nervous tissue obtained from viable and nonviable fetuses (very early gestational age) in primates demonstrated survivability and growth. Most animal transplantation studies have involved graft and host tissue of identical genetic background to avoid immune rejection of the graft. Homologous grafting of fetal neuroblasts yields the best results for brain repair or reconstruction (Smith *et al.*, 1986). Human fetal nervous system tissues have the advantage that after grafting, the fetal cells function in an environment without the adverse immunological reactivity. Currently, use of human fetal neural tissue for transplantation is experimental and must stand the rigors of scientific reviews.

The transplantation of HSC from fetal bone marrow and fetal liver have recently been investigated in the treatment of genetic defects in the hematopoietic system, leukemia, and aplastic anemia (Barranger, 1984; Simpson and Globus, 1985). Fetal liver HSC are derived when the liver is the primary organ of hematopoiesis. Animal experimentation since the late 1950s has shown that fetal liver hematopoietic cells are better accepted by the recipient as compared to adult bone marrow HSC. In humans, fetal HSC have been used successfully for transplantation when a matched donor was not available.

The rapidly improving technical ability to transplant fetal organs such as kidney, liver, heart, bone marrow, and pancreatic islet cells may offer the possibility of saving the lives of a significant number of children. Approximately 7,500 children are born annually with a fatal cardiac disorder. Of these approximately 500 are born with fatal hypoplastic left heart syndrome that may benefit from a neonatal heart transplant (Walters, 1987; Bailey *et al.*, 1985; Penkoske, 1984). If organs were available for renal transplantation, 400 to 500 children with fatal renal disease could be removed from dialysis each year in the United States (So *et al.*, 1985). Fetal liver and thymus transplantation has been utilized in children born with fatal combined immunodeficiencies (Buckley, 1976). There are some 800 children born each year with liver failure or metabolic defects who could survive through liver transplantation (Lloyd-Still, 1985; Iwasuki, 1984; Schmind, 1983). There are other children who die secondary to immunologic, hematologic and endocrine deficiencies who potentially could be saved by various tissue transplants. Of all the children under two years of age who are awaiting organ transplantation, 40% to 70% will die before suitable organs can be found. Continued experimental development of tissue transplantation techniques is dependent upon the availability of fresh human tissue from voluntary interruption of pregnancy. Material from spontaneous abortions is not adequate to fulfill these needs (Buckley, 1976).

One possibility for increasing the donor pool for neonatal tissue and organs involves using anencephalics as an organ source. In the United States approximately 2,000 to 3,000 anencephalics are born each year, 50% of which are born alive. Of these, approximately two-thirds will die in the first 24 hours, with the additional one-third expiring within one week. Most die from respiratory failure after repeated episodes of bradycardia and asphyxia. Anencephaly is a uniformly fatal disease.

Anencephaly is characterized by the absence of most of the forebrain consisting of frontal, occipital, and parietal cerebral lobes and the cranium and skin covering these areas. This defect is regarded as resulting from nonclosure of the neural tube. Although the possibility exists that this condition may arise by secondary disruption of a closed neural tube (Gardner, 1973), studies of experimental animals support a primary nonclosure hypothesis (Kallen, 1973; Lemire, 1988; Smith, 1982). The human neural folds from which the brain forms normally complete their closure by the 24th day post-conception in the human, when the embryo is less than 4.5 mm long (Muller, 1986); the malformation is considered to arise prior to this time. After the 36th day post-fertilization, the neural folds develop the forebrain, midbrain, and hindbrain structures. Cerebral hemispheres do not develop until the 100th day post-fertilization. Animal models have shown that the damage that results in nonclosure of the neural tube, in fact, may occur much earlier than the actual closing process; i.e., 24 days post-fertilization (Kallen, 1973). Animal models of anencephaly have illustrated that the neural tissue that is exposed to the exterior at the site of nonclosure degenerates. Degeneration is evident in experimental animals at stages that correspond to those in the human embryo at seven to eight weeks post-fertilization (Peters, 1979). Overall, anencephaly includes lack of development of both cerebral hemispheres and hypothalamus, an incompletely developed pituitary and cranium (skull), altered facial features rendering a grotesque appearance, and abnormalities of the cervical vertebrae. The eyes may appear grossly normal, but the optic nerve, if present, does not extend to the brain. There is, however, hindbrain stem function that can stimulate various reflexes, such as heart and lung function for a short period of time.

Some anencephalics have grasping, sucking, and vestibular activity and respond to "painful" stimuli (Swaiman, 1982, p. 410). However, the latter is best understood as a reflex pain response mediated by the brain stem. This terminological choice depends on a distinction among several factors: 1) mere reflex responses to "painful" stimuli, which are analogous to the knee-jerk (patella) reflex and require no more than an intact reflex arc, but no sentient appreciation of the stimuli; 2) the pure sensation of pain, which requires more than the presence of the brainstem (e.g., the thalamus); and 3) suffering, which requires the neural substrate necessary for perceiving the sensation of pain as threatening (i.e., the neocortex of the frontal lobes). Because ablating crucial areas of the thalamus makes the experience of pain impossible, and since anencephalics do not possess a thalamus, they lack a neural substrate necessary for the experience of pain, as well as lacking the neural substrates required for reasoning, communication, cognition, and sentience generally (Casey, 1980, p. 186; Adams, 1980, p. 116).

Because the combination of antenatal maternal serum and amniotic fluid alphafetoprotein open neural tube screening programs and ultrasound can establish the diagnosis of anencephaly with certainty in the great majority of cases, many cases end in elective termination of pregnancy. This has decreased the number of usable organs by reason of immaturity or fetal demise associated with the termination of pregnancy. If an anencephalic child is born, the physicians would not generally attempt to prolong life. The 'Baby Doe' regulations allow withholding treatment other than appropriate "comfort care" of warmth and nutrition to infants when reasonable medical judgment dictates that additional treatment would be futile in terms of biological survival or that the child will be permanently comatose. The Department of Health and Human Services does not, however, provide a definition of the state of being comatose. Anencephalics qualify for withholding treatment on either score (i.e., if this state is understood as the permanent loss of consciousness). (Department of Health and Human Services, 1985).

Autopsy findings have substantiated that anencephaly is primarily a disease of the brain and that other vital organs are normal. Still, the suitability of organs from anencephalics for transplantation is not fully established because little data and experience exist. In addition, during the time necessary for whole-brain oriented criteria of death to be met, organs may suffer damage, making them less than optimally useful for transplantation. However, successful heart and kidney transplantations have been reported from anencephalic newborns to children and adults (Holzgreve *et al.,* 1987; American Medical News, 1987; Kinnaert *et al.,* 1981; Ohshima *et al.,* 1984; Kinnaert, 1984; Goodwin *et al.*, 1963).

BACKGROUND — LEGAL ISSUES

Upon valid consent of the parents, the donation of tissues from dead fetuses is regulated in all states and the District of Columbia under the Uniform Anatomical Gift Act (UAGA), whereby family members are permitted to donate organs from a deceased individual for research and possible therapy (Uniform Anatomical Gift Act, 1983). Federal regulations appear not to restrict the use of fetal tissue or cell transplants from abortuses that are delivered with the intent of using their organs for donation: 1) if the tissue and organs are obtained from fetuses after death; 2) the fetus is a donor of biological material and not a research subject; and 3) the use of the fetal material is not part of federally funded research (Capron, 1987). For a review of some of the laws bearing on fetuses and embryos which may apply to the retrieval of cells and tissues from dead embryos and fetuses, see U.S. Congress, Office of Technology Assessment (1988). In addition, the removal of organs from living, albeit non-viable fetuses-ex utero may be grounds for prosecution as an act of murder or mayhem. Further, it is unlikely that the removal of organs, tissues, or cells from living fetuses could meet the requirements of federally funded research under the United States Health Research Extension Act of 1985 (42 USC, Sec. 289g), by which the use of fetuses must be a part of projects: "(1)

that may enhance the well-being or meet the health needs of the fetus, (2) that may enhance the probability of the fetus's survival to viability, or (3) whose purpose is to develop important biomedical knowledge that cannot be obtained by other means and that will pose no added risk of suffering, injury, or death to the fetus." One must also note that a temporary moratorium has been declared on federally funded therapeutic cell-transplant experiments that involve the use of tissues from intentionally aborted fetuses (Blue Sheet, 1988; Kolata, 1988a). Still, there appear to be no special restrictions on the non-federally funded therapeutic use of organs, tissues, and cells validly donated after the death of a fetus.

The organs from anencephalics who have been declared dead after brain stem activity ceases may or may not be adequate for transplantation. However, under current statutory definitions of death, organs cannot be taken from a person who does not meet the currently accepted whole brain definition of death, which requires irreversible cessation of all functions of the entire brain, including the brain stem. Thus, the removal of a vital organ for transplantation purposes from an anencephalic prior to death could be interpreted as homicide, if death results from organ removal. Even if removing tissues, organs or cells does not cause death, such may be considered criminal acts of mayhem.

There appear, however, to be few legal restrictions on the therapeutic use of organs from dead anencephalics or on the decision of a woman to carry an anencephalic to term so that it can be used as an organ donor. When an anencephalic dies, after a spontaneous or induced delivery, the UAGA allows the parents to donate organs and tissues for purposes of research or transplantation (Pittsburgh Transplant Foundation). Also, the woman is likely to have a constitutionally based legal right to refuse an abortion for whatever reason, including the reason of seeking some meaning from her pregnancy by having the organs of her anencephalic fetus contribute to the life of another child. One might ask whether the mother has or should have the legal right to subject her child to medical treatment, if that treatment will not be of benefit to the child. Maintaining a pregnancy involving an anencephalic in order to deliver the child so as to harvest organs is somewhat similar to postponing the death of a deeply comatose adult in order that organs can be secured after death. In the case of both the anencephalic and the comatose adult, the individual involved is not capable of sensing, feeling pain, or suffering. Treating to postpone death does not cause pain or suffering. Moreover, though treatment interventions are employed that are extraordinary in terms of the life being sustained, they may be justified in terms of the benefit to the recipient(s) of the organs to be transplanted. But there are also dissimilarities. In the case of the deeply comatose adult, there may have been a previous wish not to have life prolonged or to be an organ donor. The difference between an anencephalic infant and a dying comatose adult is that anencephalics have never formed views as to how they would wish to be treated, nor could they ever. When the choice to treat

1) has an altruistic, beneficent end,
2) will cause no pain and suffering,
3) nor violate past wishes, then
4) public policy will be served when surrogate decision-makers are free to make altruistic and beneficent choices that competent individuals may make for themselves. That is, it would surely be in concert with good public policy to support the decision of competent individuals to have the dying of their wards postponed, if as it can

be one without pain and suffering, so as to benefit third parties by increasing the likelihood of successful transplantation of organs after death. In allowing such choices, public policy permits altruistically motivated actions, which have demonstrable benefits (i.e., saving the lives of children), and which involve at best only theoretical risks (e.g., possible exploitation of a woman's altruism or an undermining of the value of the life of children by allowing anencephalics to be used in such circumstances).

In summary, there appear to be few legal barriers to the non-federally funded acquisition and therapeutic use of tissues derived from dead fetuses. In particular, the UAGA for the Donation of Organs makes it easy to provide the tissues of dead fetuses for non-federally funded therapeutic purposes. The same can be said with regard to tissues and organs derived from anencephalic infants who are declared dead in accordance with usual and customary criteria. Beyond that, the privacy-based constitutional right of women to refuse an abortion should allow women to carry an anencephalic fetus to term so that its organs can be transplanted.

ETHICAL ISSUES

The use of fetal tissues and the organs of anencephalics for transplantation engenders controversy because of 1) a concern not to be involved in the immorality associated with abortion, 2) a concern that prolonging the lives of anencephalics simply to increase the opportunity to transplant their organs is to use humans as means merely, and 3) a suspicion that anencephalics should not be considered to be alive as other children are. The first issue involves the time-honored moral issue of cooperation in the immoral acts of another. Traditionally, moral theology has distinguished between formal and material cooperation where in formal cooperation one wills the evil and in material cooperation one cooperates without an evil intention. Though formal cooperation has traditionally been regarded as morally forbidden, material cooperation is considered licit as long as there is no evil intention, there is a sufficient reason for cooperation, and the act of cooperation itself is not morally evil. At stake in this analysis is an application of the moral theological doctrine of double-effect (Slater, 1908, vol. 1, pp. 203-208). However, when the decision to ask permission to transplant fetal tissue is not associated with the decision to procure an abortion, there may be neither formal nor material cooperation. The acquisition of fetal tissue can be structured so there is no participation in nor obvious encouragement of abortion. Procedures, for example, can be established so that women are never asked for permission to use tissue from their fetuses until after the abortion has been completed. In this way, there is no endorsement of abortion. In fact, the use of fetal tissue secured from abortion for transplantation is compatible with vigorously condemning abortion so as to counterbalance any unintended, indirect encouragement. As medicine can learn from the trauma of the battlefield without approving of war, so, too, physicians and patients can benefit from the use of fetal tissues without approving of the method of acquisition. Still, individuals may be concerned that the benefits drawn from the use of the tissues of aborted fetuses may indirectly imply approval of abortion or subtle encouragement of the practice. Here the issue of balancing benefits with harms will be the key. As long as there is no formal cooperation, one can oppose abortion and still make use of fetal tissues derived from abortion, when the good derived from the use of the fetal tissue outweighs the evil of any indirect, unintentional encouragement of abortion. In the end, it is an empirical matter as to whether the benefits will outweigh the harms. In short, opposition to abortion should not in principle preclude the use of tissues derived from abortion.

As suggested above, there appears to be little legal ground to oppose women foregoing abortion in order to produce an anencephalic child as an organ donor. For opponents of abortion, the concern not to encourage the evil of abortion should provide an argument in favor of bringing the fetus to term, even if the purpose is the acquisition of organs for donation. Once birth has occurred, postponing death neither causes suffering to the anencephalic, nor does it violate past wishes. Under such circumstances, it is difficult to understand how prolonging life would be a harm to the anencephalic. Moral suspicion regarding such a practice must be grounded either in consequentialist concerns regarding the possibility that such use will undermine the moral regard for human individuals, or in a view that one should on principle never use a human being as a means in this fashion. It seems implausible that foregoing abortion in order to deliver anencephalics and keep them alive until a recipient can be found will undermine respect for persons or the sympathetic regard of suffering human life. The permission from the parents required for death-postponing treatment and for the acquisition of organs under the UAGA for the Donation of Organs underscores the importance of respecting the wishes of competent individuals, albeit surrogate decision-makers. Consent in both cases also acknowledges the need to set limits to the pursuit of even beneficent goals. Finally, the concern to save the lives of those children who can be saved accents a commitment to human life generally. In short:

1) where no pain is involved;
2) where the interventions to sustain life are not considered by most to be gruesome or horrifying;
3) where the anencephalic plays a central role in an altruistic project; and
4) where the consent of guardians is required, there is an underscoring of the important human values of respect and beneficence and an honoring of the rights of those involved. When one cannot determine actual wishes (as with an anencephalic who has never had and can never have a wish), it is not misguided to impute beneficent wishes when that imputation will not cause harm. The practice of postponing the death of anencephalics until an appropriate recipient can be located does not appear to threaten the practice of respecting persons or having sympathy for suffering humans.

The issue of the morality of using anencephalics as means is more complex. First, one cannot use them as means merely in the sense of violating their actual or past wishes. Anencephalics can neither give nor withdraw authority. They cannot be used contrary to goals they themselves endorse. A second interpretation of using persons as means merely is the use of them contrary to what a rational human being would choose. For example, Immanuel Kant's injunction against using others as means merely was set in a framework of moral analysis that did not interpret autonomy as capricious choice but as choice on moral grounds that can be justified in terms of its universalizability. "There is, therefore, only one categorical imperative. It is: Act only according to that maxim by which you can at the same time will that it should become a universal law" (Kant, p. 39, AK IV, 421). The use of anencephalics as organ donors, when it causes them no harm and benefits others, can without difficulty be willed as a universal law of nature. Nor will it violate the second formulation of the categorical imperative (Kant, p. 50, AK IV, 431), which must be understood not as using a person against that person's inclinations or desires, but rather as using the person in ways incompatible with the notion of that person as a moral agent, as "a will giving universal law", i.e., "Act so that you treat humanity, whether in your own person or in that of another, always as an end and never as a means only" (Kant, p. 47, AK IV, 429). In postponing the death of anencephalics in order to use them as organ donors, one will be using them as means merely neither in a Kantian sense nor in the voluntaristic sense of using them against their actual wishes. Nor will one be using them in a way that would violate what a rational being would choose for itself. Unable to be harmed or benefited as an anencephalic, the hypothetical choice of a rational moral agent should be in favor of beneficence, however that might be defined (McCormick, 1974).

The last issue, the moral status of anencephalics, may undermine the legitimacy of moral concerns regarding aborting anencephalics in order to make use of their cells and tissues or regarding postponing their death in order to secure an appropriate recipient. In the case of anencephalics, nothing more than parts of the vegetative portions of the brain develops. As a consequence, it is tempting to hold that anencephalics have never become alive as persons and therefore can never die as persons. There is already, one should note, some hesitation regarding the whole-brain definition of death (Zaner, 1988). On the one hand, the President's Commission for the Study of Ethical Problems in Medicine and Biomedical and Behavioral Research argued against a higher-brain-center-oriented definition of death (1981, No. 13, pp. 31-43). On the other hand, in the 1983 report, 'Deciding to Forego Lifesaving Treatment', the President's Commission argued that all treatment, including artificial hydration and nutrition, may be discontinued for permanently unconscious individuals, given the consent of the next-of-kin (1983, No. 12, p. 6). This development in policy may in part reflect implicitly the view that individuals who have permanently lost all capacity to sense the world or act in the world are in fact dead. If one holds that a minimal necessary condition for presence in this world is the capacity to perceive the world, however minimally, then it makes no sense to speak of permanently unconscious human beings as living persons; the physical basis for all sentience has been destroyed. This can be put in traditional theological terms. There must be appropriate matter for the soul to inform, for the soul to be in the world, embodied as a human. Where such appropriate matter is destroyed, one must conclude that the person is dead. Where there has never been an appropriate embodiment, one must conclude there has never been a person alive.

This can be approached in a somewhat commonsensical fashion by reflecting on the distinction between human personal and human biological life, which has been introduced by the whole-brain definition of death. If, for instance, one were to develop a degenerative neurological disease that would destroy all of one's brain, but one were offered the possibility of artificial respiratory and other support so that one could continue to live a full life expectancy, and one rejected that option, not just because such an intervention would fail to secure a life of quality or because the costs would be extraordinary, but because one did not hold that one would still be alive, one would have embraced the ontological presuppositions of the whole-brain-oriented definition of death. One would recognize that one's life as a person in the world would be over, though the human biological life of one's body would continue and be available for transplantation. Would matters change if the brain stem could be saved? If one regards the life of human persons as requiring a minimal level of sentience, then the person as a sentient being is no longer in the world, even if the brain stem is saved (Engelhardt, 1986, p. 210). If one regards the brain as the sponsor of sentience, and sentience as the necessary condition for being in the world, then that necessary condition has been removed when the higher centers of the brain are destroyed. Even if one puts this argument in a more organismic fashion, focusing on the integration of the body as a whole, that integration in sentience has ceased even if brain-stem functions remain.

The difficulty in appreciating the status of anencephalics lies, perhaps, in a failure to see the full implication of conceptual and empirical understandings that were already forged in the 19th century (Engelhardt, 1975). Traditionally, the soul was seen not only as the essential unity of the person as a sentient moral agent, but it was also regarded as a sort of catalyst or principle of organic functions. The work of individuals such a Friedrich Woehler, who synthesized urea in vitro in 1828, led to a distinction between the biological integrative functions of the body and those that are conditions for the integrated sentient unity of life. The first has come to be fully accountable and understandable in physical terms. Biological functions are open to biological explanation and mechanical substitution. The mere reflex actions of the brain stem are part and parcel of those biological activities and are not a part of the sentient integrative life of a human person. One can see why this is the case by imagining the development of an implantable, artificial replacement for the brain stem. Under such circumstances, the mere integrative, biological unity of the human body could be maintained. Technically, a human body would then not meet the whole-brain criteria for death, even if the whole brain had been destroyed. But insofar as a plausible definition of death should indicate when life in this world of sentient moral agents has ceased, such individuals should be recognized as dead.

The foregoing reflections strongly support revising definitions of death so that individuals can be recognized as having died when the destruction of the brain is so extensive as to preclude any further sentient presence in the world. These reflections also have implications regarding the status of anencephalics: they support an alternative interpretation of brain-absent (except for the brain stem), anencephalic monsters. Michael Harrison (1986) has suggested that the anencephalic be termed "brain absent," with "brain absent" having the same legal and moral implications as "brain dead". Under those circumstances, life support could be withdrawn and organs retrieved. However, not all the brain is absent, and some parts of the brain continue to function. It is also true that the anencephalic is non-viable and is in the act of dying (Mahowald, 1987). Fletcher *et al.* view the removal of organs from a brain-dead anencephalic as similar to the removal of organs for transplantation from a brain-dead body (Fletcher *et al.*, 1986). The argument has also been made that, since post-natal non-treatment of anencephalics is allowable, removal of a vital organ prior to cessation of brain-stem activity is morally acceptable. As Fletcher *et al.* point out, this conclusion would require endorsing a sentience-oriented view of personhood. This last issue is the central and fundamental one (Fletcher *et al.*, 1986).

If a human body has never been organized so that it has become a sentient, responsive whole, then it has never become the body of a person (Engelhardt, 1973). It has never become alive as a person is alive in the world. It is, rather, more analogous to the body of a brain-dead but otherwise living human being. Therefore, when it determined that an anencephalic has been delivered, there should be a formal declaration of brain absence analogous to the declaration of whole-brain death. Even if criteria for the whole-brain definition of death are not revised with regard to permanently unconscious individuals generally, where there may still be concerns (however poorly founded) regarding false positive determinations of death, and where in the past a human person was alive, none of these concerns applies to the anencephalic. Therefore, a declaration of brain absence, even in the presence of a functioning brain stem, should in the case of anencephalics signal that there has been a failure in development so that no person has ever been alive in the body of the anencephalic. After such a formal declaration (consequent on appropriate changes in applicable law), the organs of the anencephalic should be available for donation, as they would from a body after the declaration of whole-brain death, even though there is in this case persistent brain-stem function.

Arguments have been made that, upon the prenatal diagnosis of anencephaly, parents should be free to choose to continue or to terminate the pregnancy. Whether one decides to induce labor at term or upon diagnosis prior to term, the anencephalic remains non-viable in the sense that anything more than a brief life is impossible without massive artificial support. If the woman chooses to terminate the pregnancy, some have argued that she is acting in a manner similar to a physician who with legal and moral propriety prescribes only comfort care the anencephalic after its birth (Daniels, 1984). However, the most decisive argument turns on the ontological status of the fetus. If the anencephalic never develops the neurological substrate that is necessary for even minimal human sentience, then the anencephalic lacks the necessary condition for human personhood (Ashley, 1978). Given its developmental history, the anencephalic should not be described as one who has lost the use of human personal capacities, but as an entity that has never had them, that has never been alive as a person. As a consequence, in aborting an anencephalic, one is not killing anyone, for there has been no person present. This point has been suggested by Richard McCormick (1974, p. 175) in his argument that one is not obliged to give full respect to instances of human life that are incapable of any future relationships. One here draws a distinction between human biological and human personal life. Just as one currently recognizes whole-brain dead but otherwise living human bodies as not being persons, though they are genetically human, so too should one recognize anencephalics. This has immediate implications both for the abortion of anencephalics and for their use as organ donors.

SOME RECOMMENDATIONS

The following are proposed as a summary of the last section. They are offered as an encapsulation of a set of reflections that we believe must in the end lead to the revision of public policy regarding the status of anencephalics. We do not claim to have stated here or even to know all of the necessary and sufficient conditions for an entity's being a human person. That remains an important ethical and legal question. But the nature of anencephalics is now clearly enough understood, and there is sufficient clarity regarding the nature of persons as moral agents, so that the following considerations should apply:

1. To have a right to the full enjoyment of the moral protections provided to those who are persons, an entity must have the minimal biological substrate, which

is the basis for sentience, a necessary condition for being alive as a person.

2. In the absence of the biological conditions for the possibility of any capacity for sentience, it is appropriate to declare a person dead or to declare that a person has never developed. Law and public policy should be developed in order better to take account of these realities.
3. Therefore, those who advise or choose to terminate a pregnancy in which anencephaly has been clearly established cannot be said to be acting in a way that is morally wrong.
4. Furthermore, the use of anencephalics, after delivery, as a source of organs and tissues for transplantation, is not a violation of personal dignity.

REFERENCES

Adams, R.D.: 1980, 'Coma and related disturbances of consciousness', in R. D. Adams, E. Brownwald, R. Petersdorf, and J. Wilson (eds.), *Principles of Internal Medicine,* McGraw-Hill Book Company, New York, N.Y. p. 116.

American Academy of Pediatrics: 1987, 'Guidelines for the determination of brain death in children: Report of the task force', *Pediatrics,* 80, 298-300.

American Medical News: November 6, 1987, p. 47.

Arras, J.D., and Shinnar, S.: 1988, 'Anencephalic newborns as organ donors: a critique', *Journal of the American Medical Association* 259 (15), 2284-2285.

Ashley, B.M., and O'Rourke, K.D.: 1978, *Health Care Ethics,* Catholic Hospital Association, St. Louis.

Bailey, L.L., Jang, J., Johnson, W. *et al.*: 1985, 'Orthotopic cardiac xenografting in the newborn goat', *Cardiovascular Surgery,* 89, 242-247.

Barranger, J.A.: 1984, 'Marrow transplantation in genetic disease', *New England Journal of Medicine,* 311, 1629-1630.

'Blue Sheet, the NIH transplantation of human fetal tissue obtained from abortions prohibited pending committee review'. Leber R, Windom R, Wyngaarden, April 20, 1988, p. 7.

Buckley, R.H.: 1976, 'Correction of severe combined immunodeficiency by fetal liver cells', *New England Journal of Medicine,* 294, 1076-1081.

Capron, A.M.: 1987, 'Anencephalic donors: separate the dead from dying', *Hastings Center Report,* 17 (February), 5-9.

Casey, K.L. 1980, 'Supraspinal mechanisms in pain: the reticular formation,' in H.W. Kosterlitz and L.Y. Terenius (eds.), *Pain and Society,* Verlag Chemie, Weinbein, West Germany, pp. 183-200.

Coulter, D.: 1987, 'Neurologic uncertainty in newborn intensive care', *New England Journal of Medicine,* 316, 870-874.

Daniels, W.: 1984, 'The anencephalic fetus and termination of pregnancy', *The Australian Catholic Record,* 65-74.

Department of Health and Human Services: 1985, *Federal Register* 50, 14878-14890.

Engelhardt, Jr., H.T.: 1975, 'John Hughlings Jackson and the mind-body relation', *Bulletin of the History of Medicine,* 49 (Summer), 137-151.

Engelhardt, Jr., H.T.: 1973, *Mind-Body: A Categorical Relation,* Martinus Nijhoff, The Hague.

Engelhardt, Jr., H.T.: 1984, 'Allocating scarce medical resources and the availability of organ transplantation', *New England Journal of Medicine,* 311, 66-71.

Engelhardt, Jr., H.T.: 1986, *The Foundations of Bioethics,* Oxford University Press, New York.

Fishman, D.S.: 1986, 'Neural transplantation: scientific gains and clinical perspectives', *Neurology,* 35, 389-392.

Fletcher, J.C., Robertson, J.A., and Harrison M.: 1986, 'Primates and Anencephalics as sources for pediatric organ transplants: medical, ethical, and legal issues', *Fetal Therapy* **1,** 150-164.

Gardner, W.J.: 1973, *The Dysraphic States from Syringomyelia to Anencephaly,* Exerpta Medica Foundation, Amsterdam.

Goodwin, W.E. *et al.* : 1963, 'Human renal transplantation: clinical experiences with sex cases,' *Journal of Urology,* 89, 13-24.

Harrison, M.R.: 1986, 'The anencephalic newborn as organ donor', *Hastings Center Report,* April, 21-23.

Holgreve, W. *et. al.*: 1987, 'Kidney transplantation from anencephalic donors', *New England Journal of Medicine,* 316, 1069-1070.

Iwatsuke, S., Shaw B.W., and Starzl T.E.: 1984, 'Liver transplantation for biliary atresia', *World Journal of Surgery,* 8, 51-56.

Kallen, B.: 1973, 'Errors in the differentiation of the central nervous system', in P.J. Vinken and G.W. Bryn (eds.), *Handbook of Clinical Neurology,* 30, 41-83.

Kant, I.: 1976, *Foundations of the Metaphysics of Morals,* transl. L.W. Beck, Bobbs-Merrill, Indianapolis.

King, P. and Areen, J.: 'Fetal tissue transplantation: legal issues', unpublished paper.

Kinnaert, P., Vereerstraeten, P., Van Asperen de Boer, F. *et al.:* 1981, 'Transplantation of both kidneys of an anencephalic newborn to a 23-year-old patient', *European Urology,* 7, 373-376.

Kinnaert, P., Persijn, G., Cohen, B. *et al.*: 1984, 'Transplantation of kidneys from anencephalic donors', *Transplant Procedures,* 16, 71-72.

Kolata, G.: 1988a, 'Federal agency bars implanting of fetal tissue', *New York Times,* April 16, 1,2.

Kolata, G.: 1988b, 'Parkinson procedures fervor turns to disillusion', *New York Times,* April 21, A1, A24.

Lemire, R.J.: 1988, 'Neural tube defects', *Journal of the American Medical Association,* 259, 558-562.

Lloyd-Still, J.D.: 1985, 'Mortality from liver disease in children: implications for hepatic transplantation programs', *American Journal Disc Child,* 139, 381-384.

Madrazo, I. *et al.*: 1987, 'Open microsurgical autograft of adrenal medulla to the right caudate nucleus in two patients with intractable Parkinson's disease', *New England Journal of Medicine,* 316, 831-834.

Mahowald, M.B., Silver, J., and Ratcheson, R.A.: 1987, 'The ethical options in transplanting fetal tissue', *Hastings Center Report,* 17 (February), 9-15.

McCormick, R.A.: 1974, 'To save or let die: the dilemma of modern medicine', *Journal of the American Medical Association* 229, 172-176.

Merz, B.: 1987, 'Adrenal-to-brain transplants improve the prognosis of Parkinson's disease', *Journal of the American Medical Association,* 257, 2691-2692.

Muller, F. and O'Rahilly, R.: 1986, 'The development of the human brain and the closure of the rostral neurospore at stage 11', *Anat Embryo,* 175, 205-222.

Ohshima, S. *et al.*: 1984, 'Kidney transplantation from an anencephalic baby: a case report', *Journal of Urology,* 132, 546-547.

O'Reilly, R.J., Pollack, M.S., Kapoor, N. *et al.*: 1983, 'Fetal liver transplantation in man and animals', in R.G. Gale (ed.), *Recent Advances in Bone Marrow Transplantation,* Alan R. Liss, New York, pp. 799-830.

Penkoske, P.A., Freidman, R.M., Rowe, R.D. *et al.*: 1984, 'The future of heart and heart-lung transplantation in children', *Heart Transplant,* 3, 233-238.

Peters, P.W.J., Dormans, J.A.M.A. and Geelen, J.A.G.: 1979, 'Light microscopic and ultrastructural observations in advanced stages of induced exencephaly and spina bifida', *Teratology* **19,** 183-196.

Pittsburgh Transplant Foundation: 1987, *Postmortem Organ Procurement Protocol* 1038 J Scaife Hall, Pittsburgh, PA 15261.

President's Commission for the Study of Ethical Problems in Medicine and Biomedical and Behavioral Research: 1983, *Deciding to Forego Life-Sustaining Treatment,* U.S. Government Printing Office, Washington, D.C.

President's Commission for the Study of Ethical Problems in Medicine and Biomedical and Behavioral Research: 1981, *Defining Death,* U.S. Government Printing Office, Washington, D.C.

Redmond, D.E.: 1986, 'Fetal neuronal grafts in monkeys given methylphenyltetrahydropyridine', *Lancet,* 1, 1125-1127.

Schmind, R., Berwick, D.M., Combes, B. *et al.*: 1983, *Liver transplantation,* National Institutes of Health Consensus Development Conference Summary, Vol. 4, No. 7.

Simpson, T.S., and Globus, M.S.: 1985, 'In utero hematopoietic stem cell transplantation', *Seminars in Perinatology,* 9, 68-74.

Slater, T.: 1908, *A Manual of Moral Theology, Benziger Brothers,* New York.

Smith, G.M.: 1986, 'The changing role of forebrain astrocytes during development, regeneration failure, and induced regeneration upon transplantation', *Journal of Comparative Neurology,* 251, 23-43.

Smith, M.T., Wood, L.R., and Honig, S.R.: 1982, 'Scanning electronmicroscopy of experimental anencephaly development', *Neurology,* 32, 992-999.

So, J.K.S. *et al.*: 1985, 'Preliminary results of renal transplantation', *Transplant Procedures,* 17, 182-183.

Swaiman, K.R., and Wright, F.S.: 1982, *The Practice of Pediatric Neurology,* vol. 1, The C.V. Mosby Co., St. Louis.

Uniform Gift Act: 1983, 'Table of jurisdictions wherein act has been adopted', *8 A Unif Laws Annot,* 15-16.

U.S. Congress, Office of Technology Assessment: 1988, *Infertility: Medical and Social Choices,* U.S. Government Printing Office, Washington, D.C., pp. 324-325.

Volpe, J.J.: 1987, 'Brain death determination in the newborn', *Pediatrics,* 80, 293-297.

Walters, J.: 1987, 'Should the law be changed?', *Loma Linda University Ethics Center Update,* 3(4), 3-6.

Zaner, R., *et al.*: 1988, *Death: Beyond Whole-Brain Criteria,* Kluwer, Dordrecht.

FURTHER READINGS

Borowski v. Canada (Attorney General), [1989] 1 S.C.R. 342, affirming on other grounds (1987) 33 C.C.C. (3d) 402.

Engelhardt, Jr., Tristam,
The Foundations of Bioethics. (Oxford: Oxford University Press, 1986), 301-317.

Feinberg, Joel, ed.
The Problem of Abortion. (Belmont, Calif.: Wadsworth, 1973).

Foot, Philippa
"The Problem of Abortion and the Principle of Double Effect," *Oxford Review* 5.

Kluge, E.-H.W.
The Ethics of Deliberate Death. (Port Washington, N.Y.: Kennikat Press, 1981).

Kluge, E.-H.W.
"St. Thomas, Abortion and Euthanasia," *Philosophical Research Archives*, 1981/82.

Makdur, I.
"Sterilization and Abortion from the Point of View of Islam," in *Islam and Family Planning*, vol. 2 (271).

Murphy v. Dodd et al., 70 O.R. (2d) 681.

Ney, P.G. and A.R. Wickett
"Mental Health and Abortion: Review and Analysis," *Psychiatric Journal of the University of Ottawa* 14: 4 (Nov., 1989).

Overall, Christine
Ethics and Human Reproduction: A Feminist Analysis. (Bristol: Allen and Unwin, 1987).

Overall, Christine
"Selective Termination of Pregnancy and Women's Reproductive Autonomy," *Hastings Center Report* 20:3 (1990) 6-11.

Sacred Congregation for the Doctrine of the Faith
Declaration on Procured Abortion (Rome: Vatican, 1985).

Shaw, M. and A. Doudera, eds.
Defining Human Life: Medical, Legal and Ethical Implications. (Ann Arbor: AUPHA Press, 1983).

Tooley, Michael
Analysis of Abortion and Infanticide. (Oxford: Clarendon Press, 1983).

Tremblay v. Daigle, 62 D.L.R. (4th) 634.

PART 4 HUMAN REPRODUCTION

CHAPTER 14 THE RIGHT TO HAVE CHILDREN

INTRODUCTION

Advances in knowledge never take place in isolation. They occur in a social setting that lays the conceptual foundations for their development and provides the technical basis for their realization. The social setting also furnishes the economic base for their application, and in that sense provides them with pragmatic significance. The social context therefore has tremendous influence on their development and, in the end, is what makes them possible.

However, the influence of the social context goes further. It also surrounds our knowledge with value-associations that colour how it is perceived. The development of knowledge is therefore never value-neutral.

This is especially true in the area of reproductive technology. That this should be so is not surprising. Reproduction is the normal way in which societies regenerate their membership. Therefore, societies have an inherent interest in ensuring that the reproductive practices that exist within their domain harmonize with the values that are characteristic of the societies themselves. To this end, reproduction is usually surrounded by a series of taboos and more or less formalized rituals, whose function is to define and control what is socially sanctioned. Consequently, it is not unexpected that developments in the domain of reproduction should immediately engage societal values that are fundamental to the world-views of the societies themselves. Therefore, unless these developments can somehow be integrated into or coordinated with the exiting societal value-framework, their introduction will be resisted.

Reproduction is also a fundamental aspect of individual biological existence. As people mature sexually, they undergo profound biological changes that affect how they relate to others as sexual beings. At the same time, as people grow up, they tend to internalize the value-system that characterizes the society in which they live, and to adopt it as their own. As a result, the societal values associated with reproduction tend to become an integral part of the value-system that the individual acquires in developing as a social being, and play an important role in defining the self-image of the individual person. And, just as developments that require a change in these areas may easily evoke a negative reaction from society as a whole if they are perceived as threatening to its fundamental values, so, too, such developments may be experienced as extremely threatening on the level of the individual and, evoke strong personal reactions.

The last few decades have seen profound developments in reproductive technology. Methods have been developed that allow many persons who would otherwise be childless to become biological progenitors; techniques have been invented that permit the identification and detection of congenital abnormalities while the foetus is still *in utero*; and procedures have been devised that allow us to interfere with the very genetic make-up of humanity. Even methods of reproduction that have been around for millennia, such as surrogacy, are being approached in an entirely novel fashion.

Many of these developments lie outside of the traditional realm of reproductive knowledge and practice. Consequently, they tend to challenge the traditional conceptual framework in which reproduction used to be approached, and put traditional values to the test. The government of Canada, struck by the tremendous implications of these technologies and their potential for social upheaval, has recently followed the example of several provinces[1] and other countries[2] and has struck a Royal Commission to consider the variety of ethical, social, legal and administrative issues raised by the development and use of the technologies themselves. The Commission is expected to make its report to Cabinet in the Fall of 1993.

The selections in this Chapter deal with a rather limited, but at the same time an exceedingly important, question: is there a right to have children? The issue has become important because it is generally assumed that there is a right to have children, and this right is often interpreted as a right to biological parenthood. Support for this assumption is often sought in the Universal Declaration of Human Rights, which states that

> Men and women of full age, without any limitation to race, nationality or religion, have the right to marry and found a family.

The development and application of much of the new reproductive technologies has therefore been presented as a means of ensuring that those who cannot otherwise have biological offspring will not be deprived of this right.

However, is this notion of a right to biological offspring of one's own really correct? Is there really a right in that sense? Of course, if there is such a right, it could then be argued that if society does not make reproductive technologies available to its citizens as a matter of principle, it will be treating those who cannot have children unfairly.

On the other hand, if there is no such right, does this mean that development of and access to the technologies should be a matter of private choice? Would it be entirely a matter of individual decision?

Finally, even if there is a right to have biological offspring of one's own, and even if that did entail a right of access to reproductive technologies as a matter of social policy, there would still be the fact that all rights have limits. What would be the limits in this case?

The excerpt from the Ontario Law Reform Commission's Report deals with some of these questions from the standpoint of a body charged to develop statutory policies. It focuses essentially on the issue of the right to procreate.

Kathryn Morgan, a feminist Canadian philosopher, adopts an entirely different approach. She suggests that the new reproductive technologies really bring to the fore a fact that has historically been ignored in all discussions of reproduction: the fact that the notion of a right to reproduce is really a male-centred perception. She maintains that in actual fact women have traditionally been seen as chattel whose sole, or at least primary, function was to reproduce, and that women have been traditionally acculturated into accepting a role as reproductive agents, as though biology was destiny. She argues that reproduction in general and the new reproductive technologies in particular should be re-examined from a woman-centred perspective.

Finally, the selection from the Canadian Medical Association is part of its policy position on the new reproductive technologies. The Association presented it to the Royal Commission on New Reproductive Technologies as the perspective of organized Canadian medicine.

NOTES

1. Alberta, British Columbia, Manitoba, Ontario and Quebec.
2. Australia, New Zealand, Great Britain, France, Germany, etc.

The Prohibition of Artificial Conception Technologies: Is There a Right to Procreate?

Ontario Law Reform Commission

As with many questions concerning the Charter, no definitive answer can be given to the question whether it guarantees a right to procreate; clearly, the Charter makes no specific mention of such a right. While section 26 of the Charter states that the guarantee of certain rights and freedoms by specific Charter provisions "shall not be construed as denying the existence of any other rights or freedoms that exist in Canada", it appears appropriate to look primarily to section 7 for the basis of any procreative right. Section 7 provides:

> 7. Everyone has the right to life, liberty and security of the person and the right not to be deprived thereof except in accordance with the principles of fundamental justice.

Having regard to the language of section 7, it is useful to look to American constitutional law for some possible guidance concerning its scope and meaning. Over the last half century, the Supreme Court of the United States has evolved a qualified, constitutionally-based fundamental right of privacy,[32] which includes, *inter alia*, the right to procreate.[33] The right of privacy is based on the American equivalent of section 7 of the Charter — the due process clause — and a number of other Amendments to the United States Constitution. This right has manifested itself in various settings, in which the Supreme Court of the United States has held unconstitutional legislation requiring sterilization of some criminals,[34] prohibiting or restricting the availability of contraceptives,[35] and prohibiting abortions in the first trimester of pregnancy.[36]

Section 7 of the Charter does not expressly comprehend a right to procreate. But can it be said that section 7 may give rise to a broadly based right to privacy — a right that would include a right to procreate? In *The Queen v. Morgentaler*,[37] Parker A.C.J.H.C. discussed, *inter alia*, two models of interpretation respecting section 7.[38] One model views the provision as dealing narrowly with freedom from arrest and detention and protection from arbitrary interference with liberty. The second, broader model, which His Lordship favoured, sees section 7 "as providing broad protections for the individual against government interference, protections which permit substantive review of a wide variety of laws that purport to infringe or breach the privacy of the individual".[39] He went on to say that, "[u]nder this model, the word 'liberty' would include reproductive liberty ...".[40] At a later juncture, Parker A.C.J.H.C. returned briefly, and only in passing, to this theme:[41]

> This analysis would support the proposition that certain elements of the right to privacy may be protected by s. 7 of the Charter. The decision to marry and to have children might be granted constitutional protection because they are

Ontario Law Reform Commission, "Is There a Right to Procreate?" from Ontario Law Reform Commission, *Report on Human Artificial Reproduction and Related Matters*, 2 vols. (Toronto: Ministry of the Attorney General, 1985) 41-45.

> considered deeply rooted in our traditions, and fundamental to our way of life.

Since, however, the right to procreate was not in issue in the case, His Lordship did not elaborate on the point.

If, then, Canadian courts were prepared to read into the *Canadian Charter of Rights and Freedoms* a right to privacy, it might perhaps be argued that prohibiting resort to reproductive technologies in the case of infertile couples would be a violation of that right and, therefore, a contravention of the Charter. A comparable argument may be made regarding those whose natural reproduction would expose their children to the risk of transmission of deleterious genes.

But even if section 7 were interpreted to give rise to a right to procreate, it might be advanced that it guarantees only that the "right to life, liberty and security of the person" will not be denied without procedural due process. Accordingly, legislation prohibiting resort to the technologies altogether may not result in any infringement of any right enjoyed by virtue of section 7. In other words, it would be argued that, while section 7 guarantees procedural due process, it does not guarantee substantive due process, thereby denying to the courts under that provision the right to adjudge the reasonableness of the legislation. It should be pointed out, however, that in a number of cases courts have held that section 7 does, in fact, guarantee both procedural and substantive due process.[42]

In addition to relying on section 7 to dispute the constitutional validity of legislation prohibiting resort to the reproductive technologies under discussion, it may also be possible to found an argument to the same effect based on section 15 of the Charter, which will come into force on April 17, 1985. Section 15(1) of the Charter states as follows:

> 15.-(1) Every individual is equal before and under the law and has the right to the equal protection and equal benefit of the law without discrimination and, in particular, without discrimination based on race, national or ethnic origin, colour, religion, sex, age or mental or physical disability.

It might be contended that, if a right to procreate exists, for example under section 7 of the Charter, this right can be guaranteed to the infertile only if they are provided with equal opportunity, having regard to their physical disability. Thus, if the Charter guarantees a right to procreate to all, that right can be enjoyed by infertile couples only if the law does not impose any obstacles to the use of the new technologies.

One answer to this argument may be that, indeed, all citizens would be treated equally under a law that prohibits any resort to reproductive technologies. Both those who are fertile and those who are infertile would enjoy the same right or, rather, lack thereof, to the technologies. It may be granted that such a law would leave those who are fertile to their own devices, while potentially condemning the infertile to a childless future. Moreover, fertile couples seeking to avoid the transmission of genetic diseases by the use of artificial conception would also fall prey to the prohibition. However, the result would be no different in the case of any biological disadvantage that could be ameliorated only by certain allegedly undesirable practices outlawed by legislation.

State sanctioning of the technologies without any funding of resort to them may give rise to another section 15 line of argument. It may be contended that such an approach would discriminate against the infertile, at least in result: the state would be allocating resources for childbirth for the fertile, while denying resources to conceive in the case of the infertile, who, by definition, could not make use of state-supported childbirth facilities. Such a denial could be tantamount to prohibition for persons without adequate financial resources.

A somewhat similar problem has been considered by the United States Supreme Court. In *Harris v. McRae*[43] and *Williams v. Zbaraz*,[44] the Court held that the government's failure to provide Medicaid for medically necessary abortions did not violate the due process clause of the American Constitution. The Court stated that the right to an abortion in the first trimester of pregnancy, enunciated by the Supreme Court in *Roe v. Wade*,[45] was not infringed. All women were entitled to that right, but, as the Court in *Harris* said,[46] that right did not afford them

> a constitutional entitlement to the financial resources to avail [themselves] of the full range of protected choices. The reason why was explained in [*Maher v. Roe*[47]]: although government may not place obstacles in the path of a woman's exercise of her freedom of choice, it need not remove those not of its own creation. Indigency falls in the latter category.

Arguably, infertility also falls into the latter category and, although the Province perhaps cannot impede the enjoyment of the right to procreate, it need not facilitate access to the means to procreate.

It should be pointed out that the reasoning of the Supreme Court of the United States in the abortion funding cases has been criticized by some commentators. One of the grounds of criticism concerns the Court's opinion that the failure to fund medically necessary abortions did not create an obstacle to the right to an abortion, recognized by *Roe v. Wade*. It has been suggested by some that the government's allocation of resources was unconstitutional because it made a constitutionally forbidden classification: that is to say, the conferment of benefits for medically necessary procedures stopped at abortion. While the Court justified the line-drawing exercise on the basis of the state's interest in potential life, the critics argue that *Roe v. Wade* had rejected this rationale as the basis for restricting the right to an abortion in the first trimester of pregnancy.[48]

When we come to deal with the relevance of the Ontario *Human Rights Code, 1981*,[49] we shall consider the extent to which "constructive", unintended discrimination — discrimination arising from the effect of certain otherwise neutral actions — may be impugnable under the Code. While, unlike the Code, the Charter contains no provision directly relevant to this issue, the matter of constructive discrimination through the outright prohibition of artificial conception services at least ought to be mentioned in the present context. It remains to be seen whether and, if so, the extent to which, this issue will become relevant in Charter litigation.

Before we leave the issue concerning whether the Charter guarantees a right to procreate, we wish to emphasize again the limitation on the rights and freedoms enunciated by the Charter. As we have seen, section 1 provides that these rights and freedoms are guaranteed subject to "such reasonable limits prescribed by law as can be demonstrably justified in a free and democratic society". Accordingly, it might be argued that a total prohibition of resort to the new reproductive technologies is a reasonable and justifiable limit placed on any right to procreate, on the basis, for example, that all artificial means of conception are ethically unacceptable or, perhaps in the case of I.V.F. or *in vivo* fertilization and lavage, too fraught with medical risks.

NOTES

30. See, generally, abstracts of Charter decisions respecting s. 32, in Laskin *et al.* (eds.), *The Canadian Charter of Rights Annotated* (1984), at 27-4 et seq.
31. See Swinton, *supra*, note 24, at 49-59. See, also, Gibson, *supra*, note 24, at 517, where the author notes, in the course of argument, the "'governmental' quality" of public hospitals.
32. See, for example, *Griswold v. Connecticut*, 381 U.S. 479 (1965), and cases following it. Under American constitutional law, legislation interfering with a "fundamental right" — such as the right to privacy — would be upheld only if there was a "compelling state interest" served by the legislation: see Tribe, *American Constitutional Law* (1978), esp. at 1000-12, and 1019.
33. See, for example, *Skinner v. Oklahoma*, 316 U.S. 535 (1942). Compare *Buck v. Bell*, 274 U.S. 200 (1927).
34. *Ibid.*
35. *Griswold v. Connecticut, supra*, note 32; *Eisenstadt v. Baird*, 405 U.S. 438 (1971); *Carey v. Population Services*, 431 U.S. 678 (1977); and *Bolger v. Youngs Drug Products*, 103 S. Ct. 2875 (1983).
36. *Roe v. Wade*, 410 U.S. 113 (1973); *Planned Parenthood of Central Missouri v. Danforth*, 428 U.S. 52 (1976); *Belotti v. Baird*, 428 U.S. 132 (1976); *Belotti v. Baird II*, 443 U.S. 622 (1979); and *City of Akron v. Akron Reproductive Health Inc.*, 103 S. Ct. 2481 (1983).
37. (1984), 47 O.R. (2d) 353 (H.C.J.).
38. *Ibid.*, at 394 *et seq.*
39. *Ibid.*, at 394-95.
40. *Ibid.*, at 395.
41. *Ibid.*, at 407.
42. See, for example, *Reference re S. 94(2) of the Motor Vehicle Act (B.C.)* (1983), 42 B.C.L.R. 364, 147 D.L.R. (3d) 539 (C.A.), and *R. v. Carriere* (1983), 2 C.R.D. 850.60-10 (Ont. Prov. Ct. (C.D.)). Compare, for example, *Re Jamieson and the Queen* (1982), 70 C.C.C. (2d) 430, 142 D.L.R. (3d) 54 (Que. S.C.), and *R. v. Holman* (1982), 28 C.R. (3d) 378, 16 M.V.R. 225 (B.C. Prov. Ct.), aff'd on other grounds (1982), 2 C.C.C. (3d) 19, 143 D.L.R. (3d) 748 (B.C.S.C.).
43. 448 U.S. 297, 100 S. Ct. 2671 (1980) (subsequent reference is to 448 U.S.).
44. 448 U.S. 358, 100 S. Ct. 2694 (1980).
45. *Supra*, note 36.
46. *Supra*, note 43, at 316.
47. 432 U.S. 464 (1977).
48. See, for example, Goldstein, "A Critique of the Abortion Funding Decisions: On Private Rights in the Public Sector" (1981), 8 Hastings Const. L.Q. 313.

49 *Supra*, note 20.

Of Woman Born? How Old-Fashioned! — New Reproductive Technologies and Women's Oppression

Kathryn Pauly Morgan

Consider this passage:

> All human life on the planet is born of woman. The one unifying, incontrovertible experience shared by all women and men is that months-long period we spent unfolding inside a woman's body. Because young humans remain dependent upon nurture for a much longer period than other mammals, and because of the division of labor long established in human groups, where women not only bear and suckle but are assigned almost total responsibility for children, most of us first know both love and disappointment, power and tenderness, in the person of a woman. We carry the imprint of this experience for life, even into our dying.[1]

Now consider this one:

> ... if we continue in this framework, sex preselection, cloning and ectogenesis, combined with surrogate motherhood, will ensure that the fragility of woman's power is worn to gossamer and finally fades. Much as we turn from consideration of a nuclear aftermath we turn from seeing a future where children are neither borne nor born or where women are forced to bear only sons and to slaughter their foetal daughters.... The future of women as a group is at stake and we need to ensure that we have thoroughly considered all possibilities before endorsing technology which could mean the death of the female.[2]

Reproductive technologies are already with us and have become part of the fabric of everyday consciousness about childbearing. The media are filled with pictures of beaming heterosexual couples bearing their tender one (or, often, ones) in their arms. Their bliss is taken as unconditional testimony to and endorsement of the deeply humane, life-oriented motivations of the theorists and empirical scientists who make the exciting breakthroughs and discoveries which enable the reproductive technologists to bring into existence new life on their behalf.[3] While not wanting in any way to call into question the authenticity of the bliss — the anguish of infertility can be one of the deepest sources of pain to sear a woman's soul — I want to argue that this image calls for further analysis. While the technology, in principle, might make it possible for women to exercise collective and individual autonomy over their fertility, it is both described and carried out in ways whose misogynistic import cannot be mistaken. What women are exposed to are: illusory images of success which camouflage high rates of failure; iatrogenically induced disease and loss of life resulting from procedures allegedly done in the name of "safety"; and coercion and loss of control masquerading as "enhanced reproductive choice." Such mystification is central to the

---

Kathryn Paulyn Morgan, "Of Woman Born? How Old-Fashioned! — New Reproductive Technologies and Women's Oppression," from Christine Overall, ed., *The Future of Human Reproduction*. (Toronto: The Women's Press, 1989) pp. 62-79.

oppression of women in the area of reproductive technology.[4]

My purpose in this paper is to explore how internalizing the language, beliefs and values of the patriarchal reproductive technologists contributes to a profound experience of psychological oppression for women.[5]

In analyzing these forms of oppression, I propose to use the categories of institutional, systematic psychological oppression developed by Sandra Bartky in her paper, "On Psychological Oppression."[6] Three categories which apply to virtually all women in mediated forms are stereotyping, cultural depreciation and sexual objectification. Living under psychological oppression, women come to feel fragmented, devalued, infantilized, dehumanized, degraded, and rendered invisible. One dangerous effect of psychological oppression is that when these feelings have become internalized, other political and economic forms of oppression come to be seen as normal, justified, or our "problem," and fail to be identified as oppression.

STEREOTYPING

The stereotyping of women in the context of the new reproductive technologies is leading increasingly to the invisibility of motherhood. It may well lead to its very annihilation. As Rich argues, the complex history of symbols surrounding motherhood marks the conspicuous deterioration of the actual status of women as well as providing a mythic rendering of the male medical takeover of the entire process of human creation. Rich cites this passage from the work of Frieda Fromm-Reichman:

> ... there is a Persian myth of the creation of the World which precedes the biblical one. In that myth a woman creates the world, and she creates it by the act of natural creativity which is hers and which cannot be duplicated by men. She gives birth to a great number of sons. The sons, greatly puzzled by this act which they cannot duplicate, become frightened. They think, "Who can tell us, that if she can *give* life, she cannot also *take* life." And so, because of their fear of this mysterious ability of woman, and of its reversible possibility, they kill her.[7]

Even when a woman's creative power is seen as a magical force, the fears which fuel reigns of mysogynistic terror lead, wherever possible, to the controlling and harnessing of that power of fertility. Often, although the primary metaphors are naturalistic, it is assumed that Nature is there to be used, albeit with some respect. As Raymond points out, woman is seen as a fertile domain in need of seeding, ploughing and harvesting in order that her "fruit" may come forth from her womb.[8] While this cluster of metaphors clearly underscores the "incompleteness" of the reproductive process apart from the "seeder / plougher," it can carry with it a sense of affiliation with the growing child. The poet Erica Jong describes her growing baby as a "little rose blooming in a red universe," as "an avocado pit almost ready to sprout," as a "little swimming fish."[9] Obviously, these are metaphors of delight and pleasure for the future mother. Again, while it is important to resist the over-romanticization of an experience which leaves many women vomiting, weak, physically unbalanced, and facing potential death, it is just as important to listen to and fight for the right to use these metaphors; for they are endangered linguistic species. And they are not without merit in the sense that they are supportive of women as the bearers of children. That is what we are in danger of losing.

In many western cultures, in particular, the situation of women has been dominated by the psychological (if no longer legal) premise that women are chattel, that is, articles of personal moveable, animate property legitimately controlled by men. As Gena Corca points out, traditions and laws regarding the ownership, possession and control of women's reproductive and sexual powers continue to pervade the lives of many women.[10] But this is taking a new twist in the context of reproductive technologies, particularly in the context of in vitro fertilization, embryo transfer and "surrogate" motherhood. Instead of being the complex, powerful, natural setting in which the vulnerable seed can be nourished, protected and loved, a woman is coming to be seen as analogous to a kind of animate semi-precious mineral, the ovum. Women are no longer valued as biological mothers, as integrated (albeit inferior) human beings, but as ova caches and dubiously valuable receptacles. As Dworkin and Corea have noted, this is fundamentally a continuation of the chattel premise transformed by modern technological advances in the aptly named field of animal "husbandry."[11]

In "Egg Farming and Women's Future," Julie Murphy argues that in the context of the new reproductive technologies, women are seen as egg farms and men as the egg farmers.[12] Here it is imperative to understand the term "farm" as referring to the modern farm, a highly technologized form of livestock exploitation rather than the notion of the cosy "family farm" of wintry greeting cards. In this context women are seen as agricultural "primitives," as a kind of vast, natural resource to be exploited since each woman stores virtually two million ova at the onset of menstruation.[13] According to this way of looking at things, the only process that affects a woman (and which is virtually outside the domain of her agency as an active subject, unless she is taking ovulatory drugs), is this ripening of the eggs. Where the language of agency occurs, it is in reference to the men who describe the *removal* of eggs as the "recovery" of the eggs. As Murphy points out, this term is a complete misnomer for women.[14] On the one hand, the woman herself isn't recovering anything; she is losing something. The agent and recipient here must be identified: he is male. Secondly, one can only "recover" what one has lost, misplaced or lost control of. What are we to think about men who take ova from women and describe it as their "recovery"? Only some objectifying notion such as the chattel assumption allows us to make sense of this.

Further linguistic usage that is documented by Murphy includes the following: the description of spontaneous abortion as "embryonic wastage" and the description of the ovaries of a mature woman as a "production line" of eggs. It is men who remove eggs; men who fertilize eggs; men who transplant embryos; and men who are the primary recipients of the harvest in the context of "surrogate" motherhood. As Murphy notes, women are increasingly coming to be seen through the dominant ovarian ideology as egg storers, egg layers and egg hatchers in a larger eugenicist context of genetic engineering.[15] Where women are referred to at all, they are referred to by such terms as "the uterine environment," "the maternal milieu" or "the embryo carrier." Such metaphors are, of course, consistent with the somewhat older metaphor applied to women entering menopause, viz. "the empty nest."

What is the import of these new metaphors? It is the psychologically oppressive reduction of biological motherhood to a genetic primitive coupled with a mediocre incubator function. It is the annihilation of anything recognizable as an integrated, human, woman-focused experience of conception and maternity. Seen in the light of the patriarchal hope for complete ectogenesis, I believe it is a crucial ideological step in the direction of destroying the desirability and powerful symbolism of biological motherhood altogether.

CULTURAL DOMINATION

In this context, cultural domination takes place in at least three major ways: (1) through the direct devaluing and dehumanization of women, (2) through the transformation of reproduction as a patriarchal artefact, and (3) through the experience of coerced voluntariness.

Devaluation of Women

Direct devaluing of women is most graphic in the context of sex predetermination / sex selection procedures. Whether it takes the form of using sex-targeted douches, refusing to implant female embryos in the context of in vitro fertilization, electively aborting female embryos after chorionic villi sampling or amniocentesis, or killing healthy female embryos in the context of anticipated multiple births so as to give male fetuses a greater chance of survival, the message is clear: females are not wanted. While there may be particular genetic medical conditions where knowing the sex of the fetus is crucial in one's decision-making, these are not the situations I am speaking about. I am speaking about the elimination of healthy future women. Future daughters, sisters or mothers are not as valued as future sons, brothers or fathers. Raymond describes this as the "previctimization" of women.[16] Powledge refers to this as "... one of the most stupendously sexist acts in which it is possible to engage. It is the original sexist sin ..."[17] I agree.

Further evidence of the devaluing of women comes from the testimonies of women who undergo the invasive procedures associated with infertility testing, in vitro fertilization and the monitoring of "surrogate" mothering. As one woman put it, "You feel like a piece of meat in a meat-works." Another remarked, "Our generation were guinea pigs for the Dalkon Shield and now we're guinea pigs for a new form of modern technology."[18] In addition to the lack of respect represented by the absence of explanations, counselling, discussion and political analysis of the social construction of motherhood by the reproductive technologists, I believe it is fair to say that, as in the discussion of ova importance, women are valued primarily in this context as raw experimental data. A number of medical ethicists and feminists have noted that no proper primate studies have been carried out prior to the implementation of the new reproductive technologies. *It is my conviction that women are the primate studies,* that actual practice between technologists and women does not support a perception of this as a genuinely reciprocated human encounter. "Egg farms," "guinea pigs," "piece of meat" — these are the terms the women use to describe their experience. These are deeply oppressive terms and reflect oppressive practices.

Fears about women's capacity to bear children are also translated into misogynistic language which strengthens the reproductive technologists' program to take motherhood out of the bodies of women.[19] In the influential book, *Birth Without Violence,* Dr Frederick Leboyer says,

> One day, the baby finds itself a prisoner ... the prison comes to life ... begins, like some octopus, to hug and crush ... stifle ... assault ... the prison has gone berserk ... with its heart bursting, the infant sinks into this hell ... the mother ... she is driving the baby out. At the same time she is holding it in, preventing its passage. It is she who is the enemy. She who stands between the child and life. Only one of them can prevail. It is mortal combat ... not satisfied with crushing, the monster ... twists it in a refinement of cruelty.[20]

While other theorists do not characterize biological mothers as monsters engaged in mortal combat with their babies, the central sentiment is still there albeit in somewhat muted form. Consider the remarks of Edward Grossman who, in an article entitled "The Obsolescent Mother. A Scenario" remarks that among the advantages of a "glass womb" would be the "fact" that the environment would be safer than a woman's womb, that women could be "spared the discomfort" of childbirth, and that women could be permanently sterilized.[21] Similarly, in 1983, world-famous geneticist Jerome Lejeune discussed the possibility of men being pregnant. He "told the court human embryos rely on their mother only for shelter and sustenance. He said a fetus is so independent it could be implanted in a man's abdominal cavity and grow to maturity."[22] Again, whether one considers the biological mother to be a monster, or to be an unsafe environment, or dispensable altogether, it is impossible to experience any feeling of being valued as a woman. Women are oppressed by the frame of reference, by the descriptions of birthing, and by the negative assessment of our normal ability to be healthy childbearers.

Further devaluing of women can take place in two ways. First, when our stories, our myths, our descriptions of our bodily and emotional feelings, and our preferences are undermined through ridicule and pathological labeling (for example, as "neurotic," "hysterical" and "masochistic") and disregarded, we feel and are silenced by the power of the patriarchal medical establishment. Secondly, we are not only silenced in the present. We are silenced with respect to the past. We are encouraged to think of the time when maternity and birthing was a woman-centred experience controlled by the birthing mother, her sisters, her woman friends and her midwives as a time of irresponsible, risky and primitive practices much scorned by contemporary technical practitioners. As a consequence our individual reproductive lives, our experiences of our fertility and our collective history are subordinated to the constructions of the dominant patriarchal culture.

Reproduction as Patriarchal Artefact

A second important form of cultural domination takes place when the "natural pathology" assumption regarding women's bodies is used to transform conception, maternity and birthing into a technologized artefact that, optimally, takes place outside women's bodies altogether. While woman's reproductive power is redefined in primitive reductionistic ways, her power to create and give birth to life (which could, in principle, be enhanced by some of the new technologies) is seen as dangerously mediocre when compared with the promises attached to the development of an artificial womb. Gena Corea entitled her influential book *The Mother Machine* to underscore the double meaning of that phrase: on the one hand, the mechanization of conception, maternity and birthing in the actual lives of women so that more and more of what seems to be happening in and to a woman's body and through her agency is controlled, monitored, stimulated and deadened by machines and technicians; and, two, the complete appropriation of human reproduction by men in the form of fertility experts and "fetologists" whose ultimate goal is to breed children outside of the caring bodily presence of women altogether in the artificial "mother machine," that is, the artificial womb. When Grossman says, "Natural pregnancy may become an anachronism ... the uterus would become appendixlike," it is difficult not simply to substitute the word "woman" for "natural pregnancy" since woman is *defined* in heterosexual erotic and reproductive terms under patriarchy.[23] Clearly, then, this is the limiting case of cultural domination: a complete population of sterilized women whose reproductive powers have simultaneously been stolen and destroyed in the same act of political violence.

I believe that what we have in this context is parallel to what happened during the persecution of women as witches. Allegations of insanity, neurosis and bizarre sexual tendencies were made against women by men who tortured them to make "confessions" and who themselves took pleasure both in the narration and in the torture. The judgement of patriarchal history is that the women were largely crazy and their persecutors normal. The judgement of feminist history is just the reverse.[24] Similarly, I hold that with respect to the reproductive technologists, the technologists themselves should be the target of distrust, critique and subordination, and not those women who are fighting to hang on to some goal of reproductive integrity and who are resisting the fragmentation, the reductionism and the messages of pathology.

Coerced Voluntariness

A third form of cultural domination takes place when women struggle to exercise what they are told is "free" choice in a context of coerced voluntariness. In her discussion of Rowland's article, Raymond points out that often the aspects of coercion and control are camouflaged by language and practice that is characterized as benevolent, therapeutic and voluntaristic.[25] She notes that the technologists will either report that their patients want access to technology or insist on some principle of liberal individualism (for example, parents have the right to choose the sex of their child) without examining the social and political context which, as she puts it, "... not only conditions a woman's choices but her motivation to choose as well. This is what one might want to call a voluntaristic means of behaviour control and modification."[26]

What is the importance of focusing on the context? I argue that it is twofold: one, it brings into prominence the extent to which many women continue to live under and are dominated by a situation we might call "obligatory fertility" or "compulsory motherhood"; and, two, it renders visible the extent to which women act in accord with a powerful technological imperative from the moment of conception through birthing itself.[27] If we add to these two coercive aspects of women's lives the struggle to maintain a sense of self in the light of the already discussed aspects of psychological oppression, it is not difficult to make the case that the experience of appearing to make a choice is, at best, only partially real. And in many cases, material, psychological, economic and political forms of coercion are explicit.

The ideology of obligatory fertility and the definition of women in terms of reproductive destiny and fulfilment is one of the most powerfully oppressive psychological forces bearing down on married heterosexual women of childbearing age (particularly if they are white in a white supremacist culture such as Canada).[28] Moreover, as conception, maternity and birthing are brought further and further into the domain of productive activity (as contrasted with natural "happening"), reproduction becomes conceptualized as an area of potential "achievement" for women (and its absence a domain of blameworthy "failure" rather than a sad but natural event). For those women for whom opportunities for achievement are severely limited, fertility and childbearing continue to be seen as forms of achievement. As more and more achievement is expected from women and broader opportunities for achievement are fought for by women, biological motherhood continues to be seen as obligatory by the liberated or independent woman as well. Under patriarchy, pronatalist maternal ideology makes the conceiving and bearing of children definitional of the "true" woman, the "complete" woman, the "good" woman and, now, the "Superwoman." Like success at heterosexual romantic affiliation, childbearing is bound up with and defined by the culture as the proper form of power, the locus of identity and the guarantee of a woman's womanliness.

For a woman who has internalized that message and whose life manifests the material construction of that ideology so that her childbearing is the key both to her survival and her sense of social identity and place, fighting the pressures of obligatory fertility may lead to her feeling and being desexualized, devalued and identityless in relation to her social world.[29] Often, internalization of the assumption of obligatory fertility expresses itself more clearly in feelings of emptiness, lack of identity and worthlessness associated with not bearing a child than in the desire to have a child, a desire which has many varied and deep roots. In both cases, however, it is clear that the psychological and socioeconomic pressures associated with obligatory fertility are lived out by virtually all women and that whatever choice is made here is affected by these pressures.[30]

A second way in which the voluntary aspect of reproductive choices by women is eroded is through submission to the technological imperatives of the medical establishment.[31] This argument has been convincingly made with respect to the medical technologizing of birthing. It is important to make it in this context as well since the technology is often ordered or recommended in the name of enhanced choice. In one sense, the advance of the technologies is making more choices possible. A woman can now choose the sex of her child, can choose to abort a baby with spina bifida, can choose to have a Caesarean section if indicated by the fetal monitor and so on. The technologies would seem to hold out the promise of greater control, greater options and avoidance of painful, unliveable consequences: in short, greater promise for a genuinely human life of social mothering. In some ways this cannot be denied.

However, as Rothman, Rowland and Hanmer have all argued, much of this freedom is illusory.[32] In reality, actual participation in the patriarchal technologies leads to the consequence that although one's own inner experience feels like that of autonomous choice, the reality of one's world is that one becomes increasingly dependent on a veritable empire of medical experts which may include fetologists, gynecologists, endocrinologists, psychiatrists, anesthesiologists, research scientists and pharmacologists.[33] And it is this group of experts who will create, monitor and bring into existence the desired child, the new life, not the biological mother. Parallel to the medicalizing of birthing as a "crisis event," both informal pressure on women to seek out the reproductive technologies and expert pressure to submit to every invasive procedure of infertility testing, in vitro fertilization experimentation and pregnancy monitoring support the patriarchal cultural domination of the experience. Thus, while women are encouraged to think that this is a choice-maximizing situation, it often turns out to be precisely the reverse. Women are devalued and infantilized, and knowledge and fear are used as coercive levers to bring about the submission of women to the technologies controlled by men.

The upshot of these experiences of devaluation, these allegations of pathology, and these illusory promises of reproductive choice is that women are coming under further psychological oppression as the patriarchal control of women's reproduction takes on more radical and complete forms.

SEXUAL OBJECTIFICATION

Bartky defines sexual objectification as a mode of fragmentation which takes the "... form of an often-coerced and degrading identification of a person with her body".[34] Just as women have to fight against the degrading identification of themselves with parts of their body in the area of sexuality (for example, as "cunt," "piece of ass," etc.) so, too, must women fight against the psychologically oppressive objectifications of themselves in the area of reproduction.

Embodied women have a right to bodily integrity. The first way in which sexual objectification is oppressive to women is through loss of integrity. This integrity is threatened by often repeated procedures such as superovulation, surgical interventions requiring anesthetics, puncturing with needles to search for eggs that are ripening, invasion of the uterus with canulas in the case of chorionic villi sampling and embryo implantations, and other diagnostic tests including amniocentesis and multiple ultrasounds. These processes often culminate in further surgical intervention and anesthetics through Caesarean section births. The experience of women who undergo these dangerous, potentially traumatizing invasions of their bodies is reflected in feelings of manipulation, assault, personal infantilization, physical pain, anxiety and failure. Values of autonomy, bodily integrity, reproductive control and choice are destroyed as the medical conglomerate, family, friends, spouses, and often the woman herself, become increasingly fixated on the achievement of fertility. Humiliation, subordination and sadistic medical practices are often camouflaged as altruistic treatment and therapy.[35]

The second way in which sexual objectification is oppressive is in the personal and collective dissection, dismembering and marketing of women's reproductive powers.[36] An individual woman experiences the fragmentation of the integrated experience of fertility as she, personally, comes to be seen as a "difficult" assemblage of organs and processes, some of which may be malfunctioning.[37] This fragmentation takes place not only at the individual level. At the collective level the new reproductive technologies are conceptualizing conception, maternity and birthing as separable stages of reproduction as they already are in the context of animal husbandry. The process of biological motherhood is literally being dismembered as one woman comes to be valued for her "high quality" ova; a second for her usefulness as a temporary incubator during the early stages of the pregnancy; yet a third for her utility as the long-term incubator subsequent to embryo flushing and transfer. And a fourth woman may be targeted as the appropriate social rearer of the child. The psychological upshot of this is that women, medical researchers and technical practitioners are coming to motherhood in a radically different way: it becomes a collective noun, a collective experience that is intrinsically socially contructed so as to "optimize" the outcome for the child.

As we move more towards this Fragmentation Model of biological motherhood, we can see that the potential for the biological, economic and political exploitation of women and women's bodies is enormous. What is psychologically oppressive about this process is that we are losing any sense of integrity with respect to our own bodies as childbearing bodies; we are simultaneously becoming more reproductively defined at the same time as that definition becomes more dangerously anatomized.[38] We are losing the individual sense of creativity and power that can accompany chosen motherhood, and are being regarded as, at best, fragmentary or partial breeders.

The final scenario of a reductionist nightmare is already with us. I am not speaking here of future scenarios such as ectogenesis and cloning which involve the elimination of biological motherhood altogether. I am speaking of the cases of pregnant brain-dead women who have been kept alive until the fetus was sufficiently mature to be delivered. In one case the woman was kept alive for over two months while the fetus matured.[39] She was kept on support systems until a Caesarean section could be performed, then the life-support systems were removed. In commenting on the case, Dr. Russell Laros of the Department of Obstetrics, Gynecology and Reproductive Sciences at the University of California School of Medicine in San Francisco said, "The experience left me with real confidence that this can be done without any great difficulties.... In the future, I'll suggest to family members that the option is there."[40] Again, whether we consider the prospect of partial ectogenesis through removing mature ovaries from women or through raising female embryos for ova, or whether we consider using the bodies of dead women as (albeit expensive) incubators, the twisted annihilation of the reality of biological motherhood is such that both women who are yet to be born and women who are dead may be politically preferable to women who wish to become independent mothers with a sense of integrity and choice.

This picture is a terrifying one but one we must look at. Otherwise we may fail to see how profoundly these technologies are altering our feelings, our hopes, and the very way we think about motherhood. As conception and maternity move out of the patriarchal categories of the prehuman, the instinctual, the uncontrollable and unpredictable into the domain of technological artefact, patriarchal science is radically reconceptualizing not only the process itself but also the nature of woman and mother in such a way that a patriarchal exclusively male utopia becomes increasingly realizable within the domain of science.

Throughout the world, feminists are calling for the reempowerment of women and the importance of women generating both the knowledge and the political and material control of our own fertility. As I have argued, it is also crucial to fight for psychological control so that we are able, as Adrienne Rich points out, "to recognize the full complexity and political significance *of the woman's body,* the full spectrum of power and powerlessness it represents, of which motherhood is simply one — though a crucial — part."[Emphasis added.][41] Women are central to the fight for choice and the right to reproductive self-determination, women who are dreaming, speaking and creating new visions, perhaps technological in nature, so that we can "...release the creation and sustenance of life into the same realm of decision, struggle, surprise, imagination, and conscious intelligence, as any other difficult but freely chosen work."[42] Without such struggles, we and our daughters may well be the silenced victims of the coming gynocide.[43]

NOTES

1. Adrienne Rich, *Of Woman Born: Motherhood as Experience and Institution* (New York, W.W. Norton and Co., 1976), p. 11.
2. Robyn Rowland, "Motherhood, Patriarchal Power, Alienation, and the Issue of 'Choice' in Sex Pre-Selection" in Gena Corea *et al.*, eds., *Man-Made Women* (Bloomington, Indiana, Indiana University Press, 1987), p. 75.
3. Rona Achilles distinguishes reproductive technologies on the basis of their function in relation to life. She categorizes three kinds: those that inhibit new life, those that monitor new life, and those involved in the creation of new life. See Rona Achilles, "What's New about the New Reproductive Technologies?" Discussion Paper, Ontario Advisory Council on the Status of Women, 1988, p. 1.
4. For a disturbing account of how patriarchal mystification is engineered through the media, see the paper by Ana Regina Gomez Dos Reis, "IVF in Brazil: The Story told by the Newspapers" in P. Spallone, D. Steinberg, eds., *Made to Order: the Myth of Reproductive and Genetic Progress* (New York, Pergamon Press, 1987).
5. This analysis is, of course, only part of a much larger collective feminist critique. Many of the other central moral and political issues are discussed by Susan Sherwin in this volume: the (over-)medicalization of contraception, conception and childbirth and the medical risks involved; the inequity of access and distribution of reproductive technological benefits; the form of political coercion and economic exploitation of women that are generated by the new technologies; and dangerous eugenicist implications involved along with the correlative social intolerance toward the disabled and those women who choose not to use the technologies.
6. Sandra Bartky, "On Psychological Oppression" in S. Bishop, M. Weinzweig, eds., *Philosophy and Women* (Belmont, California, Wadsworth Publishing Co., 1979), pp. 33-41. I am, of course, not denying that there can be individual, soul-destroying personal forms of psychological oppression sometimes referred to as "mental cruelty."
7. Rich, op. cit., p. 110.
8. Janice Raymond, "Fetalists and Feminists" in *Made To Order,* op. cit., p. 62.
9. Erica Jong, *Ordinary Miracles* (New York, New American Library, 1983). Phrases are taken from the following poems: "The Birth of the Water Baby" and "For Molly."
10. Corea, "The Reproductive Brothel" in *Man-Made Women,* op. cit., pp. 42-43.
11. *Cf.* Ibid.; Gena Corea, *The Mother Machine* (New York, Harper and Row, 1985); and Andrea Dworkin, *Right-Wing Women* (New York, G. P. Putnam's Sons, 1982).
12. Julie Murphy, "Egg Farming and Women's Future" in Rita Arditti, Renate Duelli Klein, Shelley Minden, eds., *Test-Tube Women: What Future for Motherhood?* (London, Pandora Press, 1984).
13. This is the figure cited by Murphy. Ibid.

14. Ibid., p. 70.
15. Ibid., p. 73.
16. Janice Raymond, "Preface" to *Man-Made Women,* op. cit.
17. Tabitha Powledge, "Unnatural Selection: On Choosing Children's Sex" in Helen B. Holmes, Betty B. Hoskins, Michael Gross, eds., *The Custom-Made Child: Woman-Centered Perspectives* (Clifton, New Jersey, The Humana Press, 1981).
18. Robyn Rowland, "Of Woman Born, But For How Long? The Relationship of Women to the New Reproductive Technologies and the Issue of Choice" in *Man-Made Women,* op. cit., p. 75.
19. In her discussion of this issue in *The Mother Machine,* op. cit., Corea entitles her chapter "The Artificial Womb: an Escape from the 'Dark and Dangerous Place.' "
20. Frederick Leboyer, *Birth Without Violence* (New York, Alfred A. Knopf, 1975). This passage is discussed both by Adrienne Rich in "The Theft of Childbirth" in C. Dreifus, ed., *Seizing Our Bodies* (New York, Vintage Books, 1977) and in *OurBodies, OurSelves,* 3rd edition (New York, Simon and Schuster, 1984).
21. Reported by Robyn Rowland in "A Child at ANY Price?" *Women's Studies International Forum,* vol. 8, no. 6 (1985), pp. 542-543.
22. Reported by Connie Clement, "Science Fiction / Science Fact," *Healthsharing,* vol. 6, no. 4 (Fall 1985), p. 18.
23. Rowland, op. cit.
24. See Mary Daly, *Gyn-Ecology: The Metaethics of Radical Feminism* (Boston, Beacon Press, 1978), pp. 211-212.
25. Raymond, op. cit., p. 11.
26. Ibid.
27. I am adopting Achilles' use of the notion of a "technological imperative." See Achilles, op. cit., p. 28.
28. Clearly, reverse forms of coercion, ones forbidding fertility, are often experienced by women whom a racist, heterosexist, patriarchal culture marginalizes and stigmatizes in some way: lesbians, disabled women, unmarried teenage women (and unmarried women in general), women who are "too old," Native women, Women of Colour, and so on. From within their own communities, however, such women may experience equally intense pressures to bear children.
29. This thesis is brilliantly analyzed in a paper by Martha Gimenez, "Feminism, Pronatalism, and Motherhood" in J. Trebilcot, ed., *Mothering: Essays in Feminist Theory* (Totowa, New Jersey, Rowman and Allanheld, 1984). Similar points are made by Sandra Bartky in relation to femininity in Bartky's paper, "Foucault, Femininity, and the Modernization of Patriarchal Power" in I. Diamond, L. Quinby, eds., *Femininity and Foucault* (Boston, Northeastern University Press, 1988); and by Kathryn Morgan in relation to romantic love in "Romantic Love, Altruism, and Self-Respect," *Hypatia,* vol. 1, no. 1 (1986), reprinted in G. Nemiroff, ed., *Women and Men* (Toronto, Fitzhenry & Whiteside, 1986).

30. For a spirited and moving defence by a feminist who lives in a situation of class and race privilege, see Margaret Simons' paper "Motherhood, Feminism, and Identity," *Women's Studies International Forum,* vol.7, no. 5 (1984), pp. 349-360.
31. Achilles, op. cit., p. 28.
32. *Cf.* Jalna Hanmer, "A Womb of One's Own" and Barbara Katz Rothman, "The Meanings of Choice in Reproductive Technology" in *Test-Tube Women,* op. cit., and Robyn Rowland, "Motherhood, Patriarchal Power ..." in *Man-Made Women,* op. cit.
33. I am grateful to Janice Raymond for making this point in relation to the aspirations for transcendence and the undermining conditions of dependence in the context of transsexual surgery. See Raymond, *The Transsexual Empire: The Making of the She-Male* (Boston, Beacon Press, 1979).
34. Bartky, "On Psychological Oppression," op. cit., p. 34.
35. Raymond, "Fetalists and Feminists ..." in *Made to Order,* op. cit., p. 61.
36. Renate Duelli Klein, "What's 'New' about the 'New' Reproductive Technologies?" in *Man-Made Women,* op. cit., p. 65.
37. Of course, this isn't always true. In cases of sex preselection and in vitro fertilization, perfectly healthy women may be involved in submitting to these dangerous procedures.
38. For a terrifying "fictional" account of this see Margaret Atwood's *The Handmaid's Tale* (Toronto, McClelland and Stewart, 1985).
39. This case is described by Rowland in "Motherhood, Patriarchal Power ..." in *Man-Made Women,* op. cit.
40. Russell Laros, *Obstetrics, Gynecology News,* vol. 18, no. 11 (1983).
41. Rich, op. cit., p. 283.
42. Ibid., p. 280.
43. I am adopting this phrase from Andrea Dworkin's essay by that name in *Right-Wing Women* (New York, G.P. Putnam's Sons, 1983).

The Right to Have Children

Canadian Medical Association

THE MEANING OF THE PHRASE

Once these questions are asked, they entrain a series of still more fundamental questions: What does the notion of a right to have children amount to? Does it mean that everyone has the right to biological offspring of their own? That everyone has the right to be a parent? A combination of these? Or is there something else entirely that is here at stake? These are not questions of mere lexicography. Depending how the notion of a right to have children is understood, different consequences follow.

The Right to Parent

If it is understood as the right to be a parent, then nothing in principle would bar society from interfering in the reproductive capabilities of its citizens. So long as people were provided with children to parent, their right would be fulfilled. Involuntary sterilization for reasons unrelated to the health of the individual person would, therefore, not be ruled out. The capacity to parent would not thereby be affected. Furthermore, as long as society provided anyone who wanted it with the opportunity to parent, society would not have an obligation to investigate and correct the causes of infertility.

For medicine, this would mean that investigations into infertility would not have to rank high on any list of research priorities. Although infertility might well be a health issue and might be of interest to physicians from a scientific perspective, this would not necessarily be the case. Nor would physicians' obligation to their patient, whether that be understood in an individual or in a global sense, include the duty to assist in the fulfilment of parental aspirations.

The Right to Have Biological Offspring of One's Own

On the other hand, if the right to have children were to be understood as the right to have biological offspring of one's own, the situation would be entirely different. Then society would have an obligation to try to prevent or, failing prevention, to cure infertility. It would also have a *prima facie* obligation to fund those areas of research that are directed toward improving the chances of biological parenthood.

However, by the same token, it would not follow that society had an obligation to assist or even encourage biological parents to keep their offspring. In other words, it would be gratuitous to assume that biological progenitors had an automatic right to parent the children that carried their genetic heritage. This would become particularly important in the contemporary context, where surrogate motherhood has become a reality.[94]

For medicine, this interpretation would entail an obligation to assist those who are unable to have biological offspring of their own. That obligation, in turn, would affect

The Canadian Medical Association, "The Right to Have Children," from *The New Reproductive Technologies: A Preliminary Perspective of the Canadian Medical Association*. (Ottawa: Canadian Medical Association, 1991) 42-49.

the orientation that the profession would have to adopt in this matter. Among other things, it would mean that investigations into the causes of infertility from a preventive perspective would become as much a priority item for the profession as would investigations into other preventable health problems, and research projects aimed at ways of curing infertility and infertility-associated problems would be mandated. The profession might even be faced with an obligation to develop new techniques of reproduction for those who are inherently incapable of having children. Furthermore, because equity and justice would demand that the right to have children could not be confined only to women, research into such things as artificial placentas, male pregnancies, etc., would become entirely appropriate.

The Right to Reproduce and to Parent

Finally, if the right to have children is understood to include both the right to have biological offspring of one's own and the right to be a parent to them, the picture would shift once again. Not only would society have an obligation to fund research aimed at eradicating or curing infertility, it would also have an obligation to help everyone in their efforts to function as parents — even if they have difficulties doing so.

This would assume considerable significance in the case of mentally or otherwise handicapped people. A whole domain of social support services would be implicated. It should also be clear that the orientation of these services could not be directed solely toward the prospective parents. It would be coloured by an admixture of the obligation that the state has toward children independent of any other duty.[95] The difficulties inherent in reconciling the two duties might well create a difficult situation.

Not only would the medical profession have an obligation to assist patients in their efforts to have biological offspring of their own, it would also have an obligation to delve into the psychology of parenting, to provide psychiatric assistance to those who need it to realize their right to parent. In other words, the profession would have to address and deal with medically based social implications of and requirements for parenting.

A Modified Social Notion

The Association suggests that there is a fourth way to understand the notion: a way that combines some of the features of the interpretations just canvassed. The right to have children should be seen as the right to take advantage of the opportunity to function in parental capacity, where it is an underlying assumption of this notion that in the normal course of events, this opportunity will arise because of the exercise of normal biological functions.

The Argument The Association favours this interpretation for several reasons. First, it places the right firmly where it belongs: into the overall social context. It thereby recognizes that this right is not absolute. It is subject to those concerns and considerations that motivate society when dealing with any other right. It may be overruled when it conflicts with a more fundamental right or with a deeper social obligation. Furthermore, it means that like any right, the right to have children has certain preconditions. In the present case, these preconditions would centre in the capability of individuals to make reasoned choices and to function in a parental role.[96]

Second, it means that considerations of equity can be grounded in an appeal to equal opportunity. It therefore requires society to act whenever there is an inequity of opportunity, whether that be for people in general or for specific groups. This is particularly important for handicapped people who have the capacity to parent, but who may exercise that capacity only with societal assistance.

Third, it recognizes that society has a *prima facie* obligation to try to alleviate any impediments to the exercise of the reproductive biological functions that are normally found in human beings. Therefore, society would have a *prima facie* obligation to fund research into the causes of and cures for non-voluntary infertility and to make the results of that research available on an equitable basis.

Fourth, it would cast the medical and associated health care professions in an appropriate role in this matter: as providing assistance with the fulfilment of this right to have children, but not as judges of who should and who should not have that right. In other words, it would deny control in this matter to all but the individuals themselves.

Supporting Arguments This interpretation finds support in arguments that are intended to show that there is a right to have children. The Association hastens to add that it does not support all such arguments.

The Association does not support the argument that is based on the biological nature of the human species. This argument begins with the observation that unless human beings reproduce, the species will disappear. From this it deduces that the right to reproduce — that is, the right to have children — is grounded in the biological nature of humanity itself.[97]

Although the Association is conscious that the biological facts referred to are beyond doubt, it contends that they do not support the conclusion. The fact that a species will disappear unless its members reproduce entails neither a right nor a duty to reproduce. Any such inference would require the premise that the species should continue to exist in the first place. However, the very biological facts that form the underpinning of this reasoning cast doubt on the tenability of such a premise.

More important, the Association wishes to dissociate itself from this sort of approach for another reason: it would have pernicious consequences. It would mean that not every person has the right to reproduce. It would follow that all and only those people who could reasonably be expected to contribute to the survival of the species would have that right. That, however, would exclude all who carry identifiable dominant lethal genes or who carry genes that would not be advantageous in a changing global environment. In fact, it would deny the right to everyone whose reproduction would in any way compromise the survival of the species as a whole. Instead of grounding a universal right to have children, the argument would entail a right governed by the most rigorous eugenic and evolutionary standards. The Association cannot support such a position.

Another argument for the right to have children that the Association cannot accept derives from the contention that most people want to have children. Using this as a premise, the argument then concludes that people do have a *prima facie* right. Although the argument admits that this right may be overruled on certain occasions, it contends that it could never be overruled as a matter of social whim.[98]

Although the Association applauds some aspects of this argument — in particular the thesis that the right to have children should not be overruled as a matter of societal whim — it cannot attach itself to the reasoning as a whole. The Association believes that the premise on which the argument is based is ethically unacceptable. More specifically, the Association rejects the premise that the desire to have children creates a *prima facie* right. The Association contends that, to accept that premise, it would have to accept the more general thesis that the existence of a desire in itself creates a right. In the eyes of the Association, a desire does not secure a right — not even a *prima facie* right. If it were otherwise, pathological murderers would have a *prima facie* right to their victims simply because they desire to kill them, kleptomaniacs would have a *prima facie* right to the goods of others, and so on.

The Association also notes with alarm that acceptance of the underlying premise would spell disaster for health care funding. It would mean that as soon as any member of society desired to be treated in a certain fashion, or to have access to a certain treatment modality, society had a *prima facie* obligation to provide it.

The entire practice of medicine would also be hamstrung by such an assumption. It would put the practising physician into the position of having to justify the refusal of a medically inappropriate treatment against the *prima facie* right of the patient. Although the wishes and desires of members of society are relevant when considering the extent of health care services, and although they are of central importance in the physician-patient relationship, they cannot be seen as determining.

A third argument is based on the fact that human beings have the potential to grow as persons in the context of a family. It is this context that provides an opportunity to develop qualities like empathy and compassion. It is here, also, that they can develop as nurturers, providers of security and so on. Without children, however, these potentials will never be fulfilled.[99]

The Association is sympathetic toward the sentiment expressed in this argument. It accepts the thesis that the realization of human potential may be a good in itself, and that its development might appropriately be encouraged. However, the Association cannot accept in its unconditioned form the premise that is associated with this sentiment. On a pragmatic level, in some instances the insistence on the realization of such a potential may predictably lead to dysfunctional families. Furthermore, the realization of a potential is ethically acceptable only for those potentials whose realization should be encouraged. Not all potentials fall into this category. The potential for psychotic dysfunctions falls under this rubric. Finally, and in any case, the Association would argue that the right to realize a potential is a *prima facie* right at best. The considerations that were alluded to in the previous discussion of the argument from desire are here apropos as well.

Another argument centres in the thesis that society offers its members the opportunity to have biological offspring as a matter of general and socially sanctioned expectation through an expression of their sexuality in a socially acceptable fashion. This expectation is so fundamental and so universal that it amounts to a right.

It strikes the Association that this line of reasoning is persuasive. At the same time, the Association is conscious that this line of reasoning does not stand alone. If it is accepted, its consequences would be as immediate as they would be powerful. They would include the conclusion that the right to have children is fundamental to membership in society itself, and that it may be limited or conditioned only by the circumstances in which a society may find itself and by the competing rights of others.

This would have important consequences for how the right to have children would manifest itself in practice, as well as for the obligations that it would impose on society in general and the profession of medicine in particular.

Societal implications would include society's perception of normalcy with respect to the exercise of a given right. For example, it is a normal expectation of society that people will not unnecessarily and irresponsibly expose others to harm. Therefore, the right to freedom of reproduction would be limited by this expectation.

This in turn would mean that society would have the right, and indeed the duty, to interfere with those expressions of sexuality that put other members of society at risk. The duty to control the spread of sexually transmitted diseases would here be implicated.

It would also mean that society would not be derelict in its duty if it did not develop and provide techniques of reproductive technology that went beyond ameliorating inequities of opportunity in this regard. In other words, this perspective would allow society to exercise its discretion in funding those techniques of reproductive technology whose primary function is personal convenience.

For the profession of medicine, it would mean that the refusal of individual physicians to provide what thus could be called elective reproductive services would not stand in contravention of their ethical mandate.

These implications notwithstanding, the Canadian Medical Association is inclined to accept this perspective. The Association is of the opinion that the right to have children is indeed a socially guaranteed right that finds its basis in the fact of social membership itself. However, the Association also believes that for that very reason, this right is not absolute. It is subject to the limiting conditions that affect all other socially grounded rights. The conditions that normally attend the expectation of opportunity for sexual expression and the opportunity for having children are here crucial. They may shift as the resources and abilities of society change. However, the fact remains that the right is conditioned.

SOME CONSEQUENCES

As has already been indicated, the perception of the right to have children, and the reasoning in support of it, have certain important consequences. One of these consequences centres in the expectation of normalcy referred to above. The predominant expectation of people who want children is that the children they have will meet the social norm in terms of natures and abilities. People may be aware that there is a statistical possibility that this expectation may not be met, that is, their biological offspring may suffer from some congenital disease or condition.[100] This awareness is sometimes expressed in terms of the fears that they might not have children that will be normal and healthy. Nevertheless, because people's expectations tend to be shaped by the norm of experience, their usual expectations are that their children will be normal.

The expectation in Canadian society, therefore, as a matter of perceived right, is not simply for a child as such. It also contains as a strong undercurrent the expectation that the child will be normal and healthy. This undercurrent forms part of the overall framework in which the notion of the right to have a child is at home. That in turn leads to the expectation — again as a matter of right — that if either the expectation of having a child in the first instance, or of having a normal child in the second, is unlikely to be met, then society has an obligation to assist those who cannot share in these expectations.

If this inference is granted, then the assistance that society may legitimately be expected to provide may take various forms, depending on the reason why the initial expectation is unlikely to be met. If the reason lies in infertility, then society may be seen to have an obligation to try to overcome it. The various medical techniques of assisted reproduction would then be implicated.

If the reason lies in a defect in the genetic endowment of the parents, society may be expected to try to remedy the relevant defects, or at least to ameliorate their impact. Techniques of genetic screening for carrier status and the development of techniques of germ line therapy would here have their place. So would programs designed to assist the parents of children suffering from congenital anomalies, and to assist the children themselves.

Finally, if the reason lies in the conditions that contribute to the offspring's development *in utero,* then it would seem appropriate to say that society should address the situation. The development and funding of intra-uterine screening technology, methods of intra-uterine therapy, gene therapy, etc., would here become relevant. So would efforts to provide a salubrious environment for the possibility of conception and for the gestational development of a fetus.[101]

There are only two conditions under which society would be freed from an obligation in these matters: when the reason for action is the convenience of members of society; and when it would be impossible to provide a remedy. In the former case, social actions would be at the discretion of the general will and would be subject to the availability of resources. In the second case, society would have a *prima facie* obligation to attempt to provide a remedy in some other fashion. For instance, by developing appropriately structured adoption laws, or by exploring other approaches to child bearing. Surrogate motherhood would provide a recent, albeit controversial, example.

However, the Association wishes to emphasize that in its opinion, if the reason why certain people cannot have children is by its nature irremediable, then society cannot be expected to attempt to provide a remedy. The law has an expression that applies in this context: "Equity does not require the impossible." Ethics accepts a similar principle.

A second consequence that would seem to follow is: if, under the circumstances, and despite society's best efforts, prospective parents carry such a severe and irremediable genetic load that the quality of life of any children they might have would be irremediably impaired, then these prospective parents should be counselled to exercise responsibility and not to have children. The reason lies not so much in the burden that such children would impose on society, but in the fact that the children themselves would be the recipients of harm.[102]

To reiterate, if there is a right to have children, and if that right is derivable from the fact of social existence and the expectations that normally are legitimated by such existence, then such a right is neither absolute nor unconditioned. It is conditioned by the competing rights of others. If others have rights that are more basic or more fundamental, then these rights will overrule the right to have children.

On this assumption, the right to have children is conditioned and not absolute. It presupposes that certain requirements are met. For example, it presupposes that society is materially capable of providing the opportunity for sexual expression and for supporting the children that foreseeably will result from it. It also presupposes that the other members of society are willing to subordinate their relevant and competing rights if and when the need arises. Finally, it presupposes that those who claim the right are themselves able to treat as persons the children that might result from their sexual activities.

The last point is crucial: the right to have children is not like the right to have an object or an animal. Children are persons and must be treated as persons. The right to have children is, therefore, better understood as the right to take advantage of opportunities that are open to everyone as a matter of course. When those opportunities are not present, then society has an obligation to assist those who lack the opportunities. When such a lack can be remedied by the development or application of reproductive technologies, then society has an *prima facie* obligation to develop and apply them. However, any societal action in this regard must always be with an eye to the fact that children are persons.

NOTES

94. For a discussion of surrogate motherhood, see *infra.*
95. For a fuller discussion of this from a legal perspective, see the discussion of parens patriae powers of the courts by Supreme Court Justice LaForest in *Eve.*
96. Compare *Re B (a minor),* [1987] All E R 206, 219, at 213; Lord Halsham:

    > ... whilst I find La Forest J.'s history of the *parens patriae* jurisdiction of the Crown... extremely helpful, I find, with great respect, his conclusion... that the procedure of sterilization "should *never*[sic] be authorised for non-therapeutic purposes" totally unconvincing and in startling contradiction to the welfare principle.... To talk of the "basic right" to reproduce of an individual who is not capable of knowing the causal connection between intercourse and childbirth, the nature of pregnancy, what is involved in delivery, unable to form maternal instincts or to care for a child appears to me wholly to part company with reality.

    Lord Oliver's position, although focused on the ability to make a choice, was essentially similar:

    > [In the case of D], Heilbron J declined to sanction an operation which involved depriving [D] of the right to reproduce. That, if I may say so respectfully, was plainly a right decision. But the right to reproduce is of value only if accompanied by the ability to make a choice.

    For a similar position, see Alberta Institute of Law Research and Reform: *Competence and Human Reproduction,* Report no. 52, Edmonton, Alta, 1989: 13:

    6(1) In addition to the matters referred to in section 5, before determining whether an order authorizing the performance of an elective sterilization would be in the best interests of the person in respect of whom the order is sought, the judge shall consider (j) the ability of the person to care for a child at the time of application and any likely changes in that ability.
97. For a discussion of this, see Vaux K: *Birth Ethics: Religious and Cultural Values in the Genesis of Life,* Crossroads, New York, NY, 1989, chapter 3, "Biologic ethics of attraction and affection."

98. This current is reflected in *re Eve* as well as most other Canadian and UK cases dealing with non-consensual sterilization of incompetents.
99. See *re Eve* for judicial recognition of this strand.
100. The awareness of such a possibility may be the result of a family history, genetic screening, etc. Huntington's chorea, thalassaemia, Tay-Sachs, etc., are here implicated. At present, the list of diseases or conditions extends to well over 200.
101. For discussion of research funding, see also Québec, Ministère de la Santé et des Services sociaux: *Rapport du Comité de Travail sur les Nouvelles Technologies de Reproduction Humaine,* Quebec, 1988: 92.
102. For a discussion of this position, see Purdy LM: Genetic diseases: can having children be immoral? In Buckley JJ (ed), *Genetics Now: Ethical Issues in Genetic Research,* Univ Press of America, Washington, DC, 1978.

FURTHER READINGS

Arras, J.D.
"HIV and Childbearing," *Milbank Memorial Quarterly* 68:3 (1990) 353-382.
Bayles, Michael D.
Reproductive Ethics. (Englewood Cliffs, N.J.: Prentice Hall, 1984).
McLean, S.
"The Right to Reproduce," in T. Campbell et al, eds., *Human Rights: From Rhetoric to Reality.* (New York: Basil Blackwell, 1986).
Ryan, M.A.
"The Argument for Unlimited Reproductive Liberty: a Feminist Critique," *Hastings Center Report* 20:4 (1990) 6-12.
Stefan, S.
"Whose Right is it Anyway? Reproductive Rights of Incarcerated, Institutionalized and Incompetent Women," *Nova Law Review* 13:2(1989) 405-456.

CHAPTER 15 STERILIZATION OF THE MENTALLY HANDICAPPED

INTRODUCTION

The selections in the preceding chapter suggest that if there is a right to have children, then any interference with someone's reproductive processes and abilities immediately becomes problematic. Involuntary sterilization is especially implicated in this regard.

However, the issue of involuntary sterilization has wider relevance. It brings into prominence the general question of how far society may go in interfering with the personal autonomy of its members and with the security of their persons.

The issue also highlights one of the most difficult concerns in all applied ethics: are the rights that we have as social beings absolute and unconditional, or are these rights based on certain presuppositions? If they are based on certain presuppositions, what happens when these presuppositions are not met? Does that mean that the rights lapse completely? Alternatively, does society have a duty to remedy the situation? Are there limits to societal obligations in this regard? And if there are, how could they be identified?

The case of *Eve*, excerpts from which are presented below, indicates the position of Canada's highest court on the subject. It adopts the position that there is "a great privilege" to give birth, and that this privilege cannot be non-consensually interfered with unless such interference redounds to the benefit of the person whose body is being interfered with. Therefore, while the judgment in *Eve* does not assert a right to biological parenthood, it sets very narrow limits to the state's right of interference. It is ironic that one of the major cases on which the Supreme Court rested its argument was struck down by a subsequent ruling of the House of Lords in the UK a short time later, in the case of *re B (a minor)*.[1]

The article by Kluge takes a look at the underlying principles used by the court in the *Eve* case. Kluge argues that the Court ignored the balancing that must attend the right to autonomy and integrity of the person. Gillon, who addresses the general issue of non-consensual sterilization in his article, adopts a different, more practically oriented approach to the matter.

NOTE

1. *Re B (a Minor)*, [1987] All E R 206, 219.

Eve v. Mrs. E

Supreme Court of Canada

On Appeal from the Court of Appeal for Prince Edward Island

BACKGROUND

... [Mr. Justice McQuaid, the trial judge, on the basis of the evidence before him, found that the following description summed up Eve's situation:]

> The evidence established that Eve is 24 years of age, and suffers what is described as extreme expressive aphasia. She is unquestionably at least mildly to moderately retarded. She has some learning skills, but only to a limited level. She is described as being a pleasant and affectionate person who, physically, is an adult person, quite capable of being attracted to, as well as attractive to, the opposite sex. While she might be able to carry out the mechanical duties of a mother, under supervision, she is incapable of being a mother in any other sense. Apart from being able to recognize the fact of a family unit, as consisting of a father, a mother, and children residing in the same home, she would have no concept of the idea of marriage, or indeed, the consequential relationship between, intercourse, pregnancy and birth. Expressive aphasia was described as a condition in which the patient is unable to communicate outwardly thoughts or concepts which she might have perceived. Particularly in the case of a person suffering from any degree of retardation, the result is that even an expert such as a psychiatrist is unable to determine with any degree of certainty if, in fact, those thoughts or concepts have actually been perceived, or whether understanding of them exists. Little appears to be known of the cause of this condition, and even less of its remedy. In the case of Eve, this condition has been diagnosed as extreme.

From the evidence, he [Mr. Justice McQuaid] further concluded:

> [t]hat Eve is not capable of informed consent, that her moderate retardation is generally stable, that her con-

Re Eve (1987), 31 D.L.R.(4th) 1 (S.C.C.).,[1987] 2 S.C.R. 388 (S.C.C.).

> dition is probably non-inheritable, that she is incapable of effective alternative means of contraception, that the psychological or emotional effect of the proposed operation would probably be minimal, and that the probable incidence of pregnancy is impossible to predict.

Mrs. E. wanted to be sure she had a right to consent to the sterilization of Eve, so she applied ... for the following remedies:

(a) that Eve be declared a mentally incompetent pursuant to the provisions of the Mental Health Act;

(b) that Mrs. E. be appointed the committee of the person of Eve;

(c) that Mrs. E. be authorized to consent to a tubal ligation operation being performed on Eve.

... Having reviewed the Canadian and English case law and found no governing authorities, McQuaid J. considered whether the court should, in the exercise of its *parens patriae* jurisdiction, intervene on behalf of Eve. He had no doubt that the court could authorize a surgical procedure necessary to health even though a side-effect might be sterilization, and he postulated that it could also do so where the public interest clearly required it, though he found it difficult to come up with an example. However, McQuaid J. was of the view that Eve, like other individuals, was entitled to the inviolability of her person, a right that superseded her right to be protected from pregnancy. That this might result in inconvenience and even hardship to others was irrelevant. The law must protect those who are unable to protect themselves; it must ensure the protection of the higher right. He, therefore, concluded that the court had no authority or jurisdiction to authorize a surgical procedure on a mentally retarded person, the intent and purpose of which was solely contraceptive. It followed that, except for clinically therapeutic reasons, parents or others similarly situated could not give a valid consent to such a surgical procedure either, at least in the absence of clear and unequivocal statutory authority. He, therefore, denied the application.

An appeal to the Supreme Court of Prince Edward Island, *in banco*, was launched, and an order was then made appointing the Official Trustee as Guardian ad litem for Eve. The appeal was allowed. The general view of the court is set forth in an addendum to its notes of judgment as follows:

> In rendering judgment in this matter, we are unanimously of the opinion that the Court has, in proper circumstances, the authority and jurisdiction to authorize the sterilization of a mentally incompetent person for non-therapeutic reasons. The jurisdiction of the Court originates from its *parens patriae* powers towards individuals who are unable to look after themselves and gives the Court authority to make the individual a ward of the Court.

The court, however, differed on the evidence. A majority (Large and Campbell JJ.) was of the view, MacDonald J. dissenting, that there was sufficient evidence to warrant the sterilization of Eve. The court therefore ordered that:

> (a) "Eve" be appointed a ward of the Court pursuant to the *parens patriae* jurisdiction for the sole purpose of facilitating and authorizing her sterilization;
>
> (b) the Court authorizes the sterilization of "Eve" by a competent medical practitioner;
>
> (c) the Court reserves its approval of the method of sterilization to be

followed pending further submissions of counsel as to the medically preferred surgical procedure.

... Leave to appeal to this Court was then granted to Eve's Guardian *ad litem* by the Prince Edward Island Supreme Court, Appeal Division. The major issues raised in this appeal are substantially as follows:

1. Is there relevant provincial legislation that gives a court jurisdiction to appoint a committee vested with the power to consent to or authorize surgical procedures for contraceptive purposes on an adult who is mentally incompetent?
2. In the absence of statutory authority, does the court's *parens patriae* jurisdiction allow the court to consent to the sterilization of an adult who is mentally incompetent?
3. What is the appropriate standard of proof to be applied in a case where an application is made to the court for its substituted consent to a non-therapeutic procedure on behalf of a mentally incompetent adult? Upon whom is the onus of proof?
4. If the court has jurisdiction to provide substituted consent for a non-therapeutic procedure on behalf of a mentally incompetent adult, did the Supreme Court of Prince Edward Island, *in banco*, properly exercise its jurisdiction in granting an order authorizing the sterilization of Eve?
5. Does the Canadian Charter of Rights and Freedoms protect an individual against sterilization without that individual's consent?
6. If the Charter provides such protection, when will it permit the non-therapeutic sterilization of a mentally incompetent who is incapable of giving consent?
7. Does the Charter give an individual the right to choose not to procreate, and if so does the court have jurisdiction to make that choice on behalf of an individual who is unable to do so?

GENERAL CONSIDERATIONS

Before entering into a consideration of the specific issues before this Court, it may be useful to restate the general issue briefly. The Court is asked to consent, on behalf of Eve, to sterilization since she, though an adult, is unable to do so herself. Sterilization by means of a tubal ligation is usually irreversible. And hysterectomy, the operation authorized by the Appeal Division, is not only irreversible; it is major surgery. Eve's sterilization is not being sought to treat any medical condition. Its purposes are admittedly non-therapeutic. One such purpose is to deprive Eve of the capacity to become pregnant so as to save her from the possible trauma of giving birth and from the resultant obligations of a parent, a task the evidence indicates she is not capable of fulfilling. As to this, it should be noted that there is no evidence that giving birth would be more difficult for Eve than for any other woman.

A second purpose of the sterilization is to relieve Mrs. E. of anxiety about the possibility of Eve's becoming pregnant and of having to care for any child Eve might bear.

... [Mr. Justice LaForest then discusses the history and rationale of proxy decision-making in the UK and the roles of the courts. He then turns to the US and discusses two approaches to proxy decision-making that have been used there.]

... While many state courts have, in

recent cases, been prepared to recognize an inherent power in courts of general jurisdiction to authorize sterilization of mentally incompetent persons, they differ on the standard of review. Two distinct approaches have emerged: the "best interests" approach and the "substituted judgment" approach. In five of the nine states in which equitable jurisdiction to authorize the non-consensual sterilization of a mentally incompetent person is recognized, that jurisdiction is based on the inherent equitable power of the courts to act in the best interests of the mentally incompetent person; ... The test necessarily leads to uncertainties ... and in an effort to minimize abuses, American courts have developed guidelines to assist in determining whether the best interests of the affected person would be furthered through sterilization....

.... As noted these facts indicate that the courts of the United States in acting under the best interests test have a very wide discretion.

The second approach, the substituted judgment test, raises Charter implications.

... The primary purpose of the substituted judgment test is to attempt to determine what decision the mental incompetent would make, if she were reviewing her situation as a competent person, but taking account of her mental incapacity as one factor in her decision. It allows the court to consider a number of factors bearing directly upon the condition of the mental incompetent. Thus the court may consider such issues as the values of the incompetent, any religious beliefs held by her, and her societal views as expressed by her family. In essence, an attempt is made to determine the actual interests and preferences of the mental incompetent. This, it is thought, recognizes her moral dignity and right to free choice. Since the incompetent cannot exercise that choice herself, the court does so on her behalf. The fact that a mental incompetent is, either because of age or mental disability, unable to provide any aid to the court in its decision does not preclude the use of the substituted judgment test.

The respondent submitted that this test should be adopted in this country. As in the case of the best interests test, various guidelines have been developed by the courts in the United States to ensure the proper use of this test.

... [I]t is easy to understand the natural feelings of a parent's heart. ...[However] a court ... must exercise great caution to avoid being misled by this all too human mixture of emotions and motives. So we are left to consider whether the purposes underlying the operation are necessarily for Eve's benefit and protection.

The justifications advanced are the ones commonly proposed in support of non-therapeutic sterilization ... Many are demonstrably weak. The [Law Reform] Commission dismisses the argument about the trauma of birth by observing at p. 60: [Working Paper 24, Sterilization: Implications for Retarded and Mentally Ill Persons. Ottawa: Minister of Supply and Services, 1978.]

> For this argument to be held valid would require that it could be demonstrated that the stress of delivery was greater in the case of mentally handicapped persons than it is for others. Considering the generally known wide range of post-partum response would likely render this a difficult case to prove.

The argument relating to fitness as a parent involves many value-loaded questions. Studies conclude that mentally incompetent parents show as much fondness and concern for their children as other people; see *sterilization, supra,* p. 33 et seq., 63-64. Many, it is true, may have difficulty in coping, particularly with the financial burdens involved. But this issue does not relate to the benefit of the incompetent; it is a social problem, and one, moreover, that is not limited to incompetents. Above all it is not an issue that comes within the limited powers of the courts, under the *parens patriae* jurisdiction, to do what is necessary for the benefit of persons who are unable to care for themselves. Indeed, there are human rights considerations that should make a court extremely hesitant about attempting to solve a social problem like this by this means. It is worth noting that in dealing with such issues, provincial sterilization boards have revealed serious differences in their attitudes as between men and women, the poor and the rich, and people of different ethnic backgrounds.

As far as the hygienic problems are concerned, the following view of the Law Reform Commission (*[Sterilization]* at p. 34) is obviously sound:

> ... if a person requires a great deal of assistance in managing their own menstruation, they are also likely to require assistance with urinary and fecal control, problems which are much more troublesome in terms of personal hygiene.

Apart from this, the drastic measure of subjecting a person to a hysterectomy for this purpose is clearly excessive.

The grave intrusion on a person's rights and the certain physical damage that ensues from non-therapeutic sterilization without consent, when compared to the highly questionable advantages that can result from it, have persuaded me that it can never safely be determined that such a procedure is for the benefit of that person. Accordingly, the procedure should never be authorized for non-therapeutic purposes under the parens patriae jurisdiction.

To begin with, it is difficult to imagine a case in which non-therapeutic sterilization could possibly be of benefit to the person on behalf of whom a court purports to act, let alone one in which that procedure is necessary in his or her best interest. And how are we to weigh the best interests of a person in this troublesome area, keeping in mind that an error is irreversible? Unlike other cases involving the use of the parens patriae jurisdiction, an error cannot be corrected by the subsequent exercise of judicial discretion. That being so, one need only recall Lord Eldon's remark, *supra,* that "it has always been the principle of this Court, not to risk damage to children which it cannot repair" to conclude that non-therapeutic sterilization may not be authorized in the exercise of the parens patriae jurisdiction. McQuaid J. was, therefore, right in concluding that he had no authority or jurisdiction to grant the application.

Nature or the advances of science may, at least in a measure, free Eve of the incapacity from which she suffers. Such a possibility should give the courts pause in extending their power to care for individuals to such irreversible action as we are called upon to take here. The irreversible and serious intrusion on the basic rights of the individual is simply too great to allow a court to act on the basis of possible advantages which, from the standpoint of the individual, are highly debatable. Judges are generally ill-informed about many of the factors relevant to a wise decision in this difficult area. They generally know little of mental illness, of techniques of contraception or their efficacy. And, however well presented a case may be, it can only partially inform. If sterilization of the mentally incompetent is to be adopted as desirable for general social purposes, the legislature is the appropriate body to do so. It is in a position to inform itself and it is attuned to the feelings of the public in making policy in this sensitive area. The actions of the legislature will then, of course, be subject to the scrutiny of the courts under the Canadian Charter of Rights and Freedoms and otherwise.

... The foregoing, of course, leaves out of consideration therapeutic sterilization and where the line is to be drawn between therapeutic and non-therapeutic sterilization. On this issue, I simply repeat that the utmost caution must be exercised commensurate with the seriousness of the procedure. Marginal justifications must be weighed against what is in every case a grave intrusion on the physical and mental integrity of the person.

... I cannot agree that a court can deprive a woman of that privilege [of giving birth] for purely social or other non-therapeutic purposes without her consent. The fact that others may suffer inconvenience or hardship from failure to do so cannot be taken into account. The Crown's *parens patriae* jurisdiction exists for the benefit of those who cannot help themselves, not to relieve those who may have the burden of caring for them.

I should perhaps add ... that sterilization may, on occasion, be necessary as an adjunct to treatment of a serious malady, but I would underline that this, of course, does not allow for subterfuge or for treatment of some marginal medical problem.

The foregoing remarks dispose of the arguments based on the traditional view of the *parens patriae* jurisdiction as exercised in this country. Counsel for the respondent strongly contended, however, that the Court should adopt the substituted judgment test recently developed by a number of state courts in the United States. That test, he submitted, is to be preferred to the best interests test because it places a higher value on the individuality of the mentally incompetent person. It affords that person the same right, he contended, as a competent person to choose whether to procreate or not.

There is an obvious logical lapse in this argument. I do not doubt that a person has a right to decide to be sterilized. That is his or her free choice. But choice presupposes that a person has the mental competence to make it. It may be a matter of debate whether a court should have the power to make the decision if that person lacks the mental capacity to do so. But it is obviously fiction to suggest that a decision so made is that of the mental incompetent, however much the court may try to put itself in her place. What the incompetent would do if she or he could make the choice is simply a matter of speculation. The sophistry embodied in the argument favouring substituted judgment has been fully revealed in *Eberhardy* ... where ... the court stated:

> The fault we find in the New Jersey case is the ratio decidendi of first concluding, correctly we believe, that the right to sterilization is a personal choice, but then equating a decision made by others with the choice of the person to be sterilized. It clearly is not a personal choice, and no amount of legal legerdemain can make it so.
>
> ...
>
> We conclude that the question is not choice because it is sophistry to refer to it as such, but rather the question is whether there is a method by which others, acting in behalf of the person's best interests and in the interests, such as they may be, of the state, can exercise the decision. Any governmentally sanctioned (or ordered) procedure to sterilize a person who is incapable of giving consent must be denominated for what it is, that is, the state's intrusion into the determination of whether or not a person who makes no choice shall be allowed to procreate.

Counsel for the respondent ... argued that there is what he called a fundamental right to free procreative choice. Not only, he asserted, is there a fundamental right to bear children; there is as well a fundamental right to choose not to have children and to implement that choice by means of contraception. ... [H]e appears to base this argument on s. 7 of the Charter. But assuming for the moment that liberty as used in s. 7 protects rights of this kind (a matter I refrain from entering into), counsel's contention seems to me to go beyond the kind of protection s. 7 was intended to afford. All s. 7 does is to give a remedy to protect individuals against laws or other state action that deprive them of liberty. It has no application here.

Another Charter related argument must be considered. In response to the appellant's argument that a court-ordered sterilization of a mentally incompetent person, by depriving that person of the right to procreate, would constitute an infringement of that person's rights to liberty and security of the person under s. 7 of the Canadian Charter of Rights and Freedoms, counsel for the respondent countered by relying on that person's right to equality under s. 15(1) of the Charter, saying "that the most appropriate method of ensuring the mentally incompetent their right to equal protection under s. 15(1) is to provide the mentally incompetent with a means to obtain non-therapeutic sterilizations, which adequately protects their interests through appropriate judicial safeguards." A somewhat more explicit argument along the same lines was made by counsel for the Public Trustee of Manitoba. His position was stated as follows:

> It is submitted that in the case of a mentally incompetent adult, denial of the right to have his or her case presented by a guardian ad litem to a Court possessing jurisdiction to give or refuse substituted consent to a non-therapeutic procedure such as sterilization, would be tantamount to a denial to that person of equal protection and equal benefit of the law. Such a denial would constitute discrimination on the basis of mental disability, which discrimination is prohibited by Section 15 of The Canadian Charter of Rights and Freedoms.

Section 15 of the Charter was not in force when these proceedings commenced but, this aside, these arguments appear flawed. They raise in different form an issue already dealt with, i.e. that the decision made by a court on an application to consent to the sterilization of an incompetent is somehow that of the incompetent. More troubling is that the issue is, of course, not raised by the incompetent, but by a third party. The court undoubtedly has the right and duty to protect those who are unable to take care of themselves, and in doing so it has a wide discretion to do what it considers to be in their best interests. But this function must not, in my view, be transformed so as to create a duty obliging the court, at the behest of a third party, to make a choice between the two alleged constitutional rights — the right to procreate or not to procreate — simply because the individual is unable to make that choice. All the more so since, in the case of non-therapeutic sterilization as we saw, the choice is one the courts cannot safely exercise.

... Since, barring emergency situations, a surgical procedure without consent ordinarily constitutes battery, it will be obvious that the onus of proving the need for the procedure is on those who seek to have it performed. And that burden, though a civil one, must be commensurate with the seriousness of the measure proposed. In conducting these procedures, it is obvious that a court must proceed with extreme caution; otherwise ... it would open the way for abuse of the mentally incompetent.... I would allow the appeal and restore the decision of the judge who heard the application.

Sterilisation of the Mentally Severely Handicapped: A Violation of the Right to Have Children?

Eike-Henner W. Kluge

INTRODUCTION

The Universal Declaration of Human Rights (1948) stated, and the Declaration of Teheran (1968) reiterated, that every person 'of full age' has the right to have children and 'found a family'. The right thus enunciated is usually interpreted as being universal, inalienable and indefeasible: and it is at least in part on this basis that many jurisdictions have rejected the non-consensual sterilisation of the mentally severely handicapped as being both discriminatory and unethical when performed for reasons other than to safeguard the health and welfare of the handicapped person. It is on this basis also that most commentators have rejected such sterilisation.

However, both the general thesis, as well as its application to the mentally severely handicapped, may be challenged. The general claim may be challenged on three grounds: the nature of the right claimed, as well as its legitimacy, is extremely dubious; the grounding of the alleged right presents severe ontological problems; and the claim that such a right is indefeasible ignores the contextual nature of all rights. As to the particular claim as advanced for the mentally severely handicapped, three further arguments may be raised against it: the mentally severely handicapped cannot meet the basic precondition for such a right; insistence on such a right would violate the rights of children; and, finally, it would also violate the rights of other people.

While none of these considerations, even if successful, entail that the mentally severely handicapped should be sterilised as a matter of course, they do entail that under circumstances where conception and procreation of the mentally severely handicapped can reasonably be prevented only in this fashion, sterilisation is ethically permissible.

THE NATURE OF THE CLAIM

To begin with the nature of the claim itself: what precisely does the alleged right to have children amount to? Several possibilities come to mind, but one is generally taken to be central: the right to have biological progeny of one's own. In the interest of clarity, however, it should be noted that such an interpretation is rather simplistic. In the first place, one cannot have a right to what it is impossible to provide. Many persons are irremediably sterile and cannot have biological progeny. In their case, therefore, the alleged right would fail for want of its logical precondition. Whence it would follow that, contrary to the initial claim, the alleged right would not be universal (unless, of course, it were to be argued that the right is universal after all, and that in cases such as these, society has an obligation to develop and employ techniques of artificial reproduction that would overcome this problem. We shall not pursue the issue here.)

E.-H.W. Kluge, "Sterilisation of the Mentally Severely Handicapped: A Violation of the Right to Have Children?" *Ethical Problems in Reproductive Medicine* 1989; 1:1, 12-15.

Second, the right, no matter how construed, centrally involves children. Children, however, are not objects. They are persons. Therefore it follows that if there is a right to have progeny at all, it could not ethically be interpreted in a proprietary or dispositionary fashion. It would have to be understood in some other way. But how?

Finally, the right to have biological progeny of one's own would not ordinarily be considered to be satisfied by the mere existence of such progeny without any contact and association on part of the progenitor. A direct and personal interaction of an ongoing and formative sort is also taken to be implicated. An acceptable interpretation of the right claim, therefore, must include this associative parameter.

How to combine all this into a reasonable whole? The Universal Declaration of Human Rights, in its insistence on the right to 'found a family', points the way. Whatever its cultural idiosyncracies of constitution, the family context is one of nurturing, of education, and of raising children. In short, insofar as the person context is concerned, it is one of parenting. Therefore in keeping with the preceding considerations we suggest that the claim of a universal right to have children amounts to this: everyone has the right to (attempt to) have biological progeny and parent without undue state interference.

GROUNDING THE RIGHT

If we assume that this is an appropriate interpretation, the next question is, 'How could such a right be grounded?' The literature, and indeed pure reasoning itself, suggest several possibilities: in the biological survival needs of the human species, the fact of individual desire, the requirements for the realisation of a truly human potential, and the fact of social policy. We shall not here examine these possibilities in detail but merely sketch some consideration.

No purely material fact, and *a fortiori* no fact of biology, can establish an ethical right. That requires an ethical premise, which is here not given. Less abstractly, it is one thing to say that the human species will not survive unless its members reproduce; but is another to say that it ought to reproduce, or that it has the right to do so. Furthermore, even if the right were granted, it would not follow that every member of the species therefore had a right to progeny. Logically, such an inference would commit the fallacy of division because materially, the facts of biology would deny it. At best, what would follow from this basis would be that all and only those whose progeny could reasonably be expected to advance species survival would have such a right. The biological argument, therefore, would only allow for a limited right conditioned by evolutionary considerations.

The argument from individual desire fares no better. To put it bluntly, the connection between desire and right must be shown. It cannot merely be assumed. Otherwise it begs the question. As to the argument from the realisation of personal potential, it faces the same problem. The existence of a fact, in this case, personal potential, does not establish a right. As it stands, the argument assumes that the connection between the fact (desire) and the right is established independently, in some other fashion; but that is not the case. The argument requires that children be considered as objects, as entities whose function it is to assist in the development of others. That, however, is ethically anathema. What one can argue is that *if* there is a particular potential and *if* there is a child, then *ceteris paribus* whoever has that potential has a *prima facie* right to use the child's existence to realise the potential. But *only if* the child will not be treated as an object. That, however, is quite different from the right claimed in the first instance. It is not the right to bring about a child for that purpose.

The argument from social existence has two versions, one legally oriented, the other ethical. The former focuses in the law extant in a given society. We shall not deal with it here. The latter is based on the thesis that society, whether it recognises this explicitly in its laws or not, *de facto* guarantees each of its members certain fundamental rights as a condition of membership, and that the right to procreation and to parenting is one of these. However, while we may grant that society does indeed guarantee certain fundamental rights to its members, this does not establish that the right in question is one of them.

Furthermore, even if we did allow that there was such a right and that it was grounded in the fact of social existence, this would not show that it was absolute and unconditioned. The very fact that it was grounded in the social context would entail that like all other rights thus grounded, it would be subject to conditioning constraints. For one thing, it would be conditioned by the competing rights of others. Therefore if the exercise of this right interfered with the exercise of another person's more fundamental right e.g., the right to life, then the right would become ineffective. For another, it would be conditioned from the perspective of society as a whole. That is to say children, both as persons and as biological organisms, have needs. Providing for these, however, is not simply a parental function. No matter how wealthy, well-endowed or positioned, no set of parents can meet these conditions alone. Directly or indirectly, meeting them involves whole social institutions such as health, education and welfare which no-one is wholly able to defray. The coming-into-being of a child, therefore, is a social affair; and society, by allowing someone to claim the right to have a child, acquires the obligation to provide for its needs if, when and as it becomes necessary. Justice, however, entails that no one can have an obligation unilaterally thrust upon him or her. There must be some ethically acceptable way for the individual to escape the obligation. This means that it must be possible for society to avoid being locked into the relevant obligations vis-à-vis the new child. This would be possible only by preventing the child from coming into existence in the first place. It therefore follows that although there may be a socially guaranteed right to have children, that right is not absolute but defeasible from the side of society itself.

Finally, the right also is defeasible from the side of the child. That is to say, there are situations in which the conditions governing the genesis of a child are the beginning of a causal chain which predictably will eventuate in such a qualitative state for the child that, were it imposed *de novo* upon a person who is already present, it would constitute the infliction of harm. To procreate under such circumstances would be tantamount to a temporally protracted infliction of harm. Therefore while the act of procreation *per se* may be morally blameless, the act *under such circumstances* would be blameworthy and constitute an injury. Under such circumstances, therefore, the right to have a child fails.

THE MENTALLY SEVERELY HANDICAPPED

The right to have a child, therefore, even if it is granted, is neither universal, absolute nor unconditioned. So far, we have only argued this for persons in general. How does it apply to the mentally severely handicapped?

To avoid confusion, we shall define a mentally severely handicapped person as someone who is congenitally so severely impaired that he or she cannot look after his or her needs as an independent and autonomous being but requires continuous supervision and assistance in order to allow him or her to survive and function; and furthermore as someone who cannot grasp the nature of a child as a person, and who fails to comprehend the requirements inherent in providing for a child. Does such an individual have a right to have a child, in the sense discussed above? And is there a right on the part of society to sterilise such an individual in order to prevent him or her from having children?

If our preceding analysis is correct, then the answer to the first question is negative. There are two reasons for this: one logical, the other ethical. *Ex hypothesi,* the mentally severely handicapped cannot perceive, relate to or otherwise treat children as persons. Consequently, they cannot fulfil the requirements of a parenting role. Since the ability to fulfil such a role is a precondition of the right to have children, it follows that the right itself fails from a purely logical perspective. As to the ethical reason for its failure, the very nature of the handicap entails that a child born into such a situation would play the role of an object of personal development and self-gratification for the severely handicapped. However, as we said before, no right can involve the use of persons purely as objects in an instrumental fashion. The right, therefore, fails once again.

It might be argued that while the inabilities of the handicapped to parent and to see children as persons may be admitted, this does not entail that they do not have a right to have children. Instead, it entails that society has an obligation to provide for the services of someone who will take over those areas of parenting which the severely handicapped are constitutionally unable to provide: to act, as it were, *in loco parentis* towards the children. The inability of the handicapped thus being made up, their right is preserved and they will be able to benefit from and enjoy the remainder of the parenting experience.

But such an argument would fail. The central precondition ineluctably associated with the right to have a child is that the individual who claims the right must be able to experience, relate to and otherwise interact with the child as a person. The proposal at hand would not allow the mentally severely handicapped to meet this precondition. It would be the parent-proxy, the individual who is provided by society to act *in loco parentis,* who would relate to the children in the requisite manner. Short of changing his or her nature, nothing can be done for or to the mentally severely handicapped that would allow him or her to meet this condition. For him or her, the children will still remain objects. In more formal terms, if a's having quality ϕ is a necessary precondition of having right R, then the fact that b has quality ϕ does not establish that therefore a has R after all. The only way in which a can acquire R is for a to acquire ϕ. In this case it would mean that the mentally severely handicapped would have to cease being mentally severely handicapped. If that were possible, there would be no ethical problem. As it stands, however, it is not the case.

STERILISATION

If the foregoing is correct, then the mentally severely handicapped do not have a right to have children in the sense we have developed. Society has both a right and a duty to step in. But in what fashion? Surely sterilisation is too restrictive?

Surely contraception and even abortion are less permanent, less irreversible and less intrusive alternatives?

As to abortion, it is almost as intrusive as tubal ligation and since it does not prevent future conceptions, it is a potentially repetitive procedure. Given that it does have an intrusive nature, it follows on the last count that any advantage it might have over sterilisation would have to be sought in the fact that it did not bring about an irreversible condition. That, however, prompts the following question: Under what circumstances would reversibility be a relevant consideration? The answer is only in those cases where the factor that mandated interference in the first place, the severe mental handicap, was not a permanent characteristic of the individual in question. However, instead of telling against sterilisation *per se,* this surely means that sterilisation is unacceptable *in those cases.* It does not mean that in cases where the severe mental handicap is permanent, sterilisation should also be withheld, in the expectation of a miracle, as it were.

Turning to contraception, since it is the least permanent and least intrusive alternative, it appears to be the method of choice. However, those methods of contraception which under the circumstances would be the most appropriate, subcutaneous implants, IUDs, etc, while they are indeed least intrusive in a mechano/physiological sense, emerge as quite intrusive when it is considered that they are biochemically active on the person as a whole. In any case they do have quantifiable risks of morbidity and mortality that exceed those of sterilisation. Their attractiveness on this count, therefore, wanes. As to their lack of permanence and irreversibility, not only do they also have long-term effects in that direction, but relevance of the criterion of reversibility should also be re-examined.

We suggest, therefore, that there are cases in which sterilisation is appropriate. All and only those, namely, where according to all appropriate standards of medical certitude the severe mental handicap is a permanent feature of the individual.

However, a fundamental question remains: Does the state have the right to breach the principle of inviolability and commit trespass to the person in the pursuit of its right and in order to prevent perceived harm to future persons?

There must be a proportion between a right/duty that is claimed and the method used to pursue it. And here the following consideration seems germane. Sterilisation by vasectomy or tubal ligation is currently being used by competent people on a voluntary basis to control their own fertility. Nor is sterilisation deemed ethically inappropriate or indefensible in this context. The method itself, therefore, is ethically acceptable *per se.* The only reason an objection might arise is that in the case of the mentally severely handicapped it would be imposed in a nonconsensual manner. Here, however, we should like to suggest the following as a particularisation of the principle of equality. If a particular method or procedure is unobjectionable when employed by a competent individual on a voluntary basis in order to control a particular activity or bodily function, then the fact that it is employed by a proxy decision-maker for an incompetent individual for reasons that are ethically defensible in their own right, does not render it ethically objectionable. If this principle is false, then nothing that a proxy decision-maker decides on the basis of comparison with normal situations will ever be ethically defensible. On the other hand if, as we have suggested, it is correct, then in many cases sterilisation will be an ethically appropriate way to proceed.

On Sterilising Severely Mentally Handicapped People

Raanan Gillon

At the time of writing, the House of Lords in England had not ruled in the case of Jeanette — a seventeen-year-old with allegedly the skills of at most a five- or six-year-old whose mother and gynaecologist wished to perform probably irreversible sterilisation by an operation to tie her fallopian tubes.[1] Whatever the legal decision, the ethical issues underlying decisions of this kind deserve analysis.

In the normal case the matter is settled by the decision of the woman and her gynaecologist — if she wishes to be sterilised, for example for the purposes of contraception, and a gynaecologist agrees to her request that is the end of the matter so far as the law in England is concerned.[2] The underlying ethical argument may presumably be simply but perhaps not inaccurately summarised along the lines that such sterilisation is an operation of sufficient potential benefit and sufficiently small likely harm to be justified if a patient understandingly and autonomously chooses it, and that there are no generally overriding considerations of justice, either in terms of people's rights or in terms of distribution of resources, to prevent such operations.

What changes the ethical argument in the case of a severely mentally handicapped person is of course the absence of sufficient autonomy in the potential patient to make possible her understanding and autonomous choice either to have or not to have the operation. We have developed, however, several apparently justifiable systems for dealing with cases of inadequate autonomy. In general the preferred approach is to try to approximate as closely as possible to what would be the autonomous decision of the person concerned (for instance by reference to earlier expressed autonomous preferences and decisions). That route is blocked however in the case of those people who have never developed sufficient autonomy, such as those who have been severely mentally handicapped from birth or early childhood. The second route is that commonly adopted in the case of children, where autonomous decisions are exercised by proxy on the child's behalf. The normally acceptable proxies are the parents (and there is argument as to whether they should exercise their proxy autonomy in the child's best interests or merely in the child's interests). The assumption that the parents are the appropriate proxies is however defeasible, certainly when there is reason to believe that they are unjustifiably acting against their child's interests and arguably even if they failing to act in their child's *best* interests.[3] What reasons are there to reject such an approach to proxy consent in the case of sterilisation of severely mentally handicapped people?

Three arguments are plausible candidates. The first is that it can never be in a mentally handicapped person's interests, let alone in his or her best interests, to be sterilised. The second is that it violates the rights of a mentally handicapped person to sterilise him or her without the person's understanding and autonomous consent. The third is that it is against the interests of society to permit it, either because of anticipated harm and/or because of some other anticipated injustice to others.

Raanan Gillon, "On Sterilising the Mentally Handicapped," *Journal of Medical Ethics* Na. 13 (2) 1987; 59-61.

So far as the first argument is concerned it is hard to see why it can *never* be in the best interests of a severely mentally handicapped person to be sterilised if it is accepted that it can sometimes be in the best interests of a mentally normal woman to be sterilised. The main benefit in the normal case is usually the virtually certain avoidance of pregnancy. Now of course there is a widespread countervailing presumption that pregnancy is a good thing. Doubtless this presumption is based on the evident truths that for many women pregnancy and the consequent nurturing of children are goods, fundamental to their flourishing, and moreover that the undergoing of pregnancy by at least *some* women is a necessary condition of the continued flourishing of humankind. But neither of those truths is sufficient for a conclusion that it is *never* in the best interests of a normal woman to be sterilised. If, as is widely accepted, it may for some women, whose beliefs permit such a choice, be beneficial, in their best interests and morally acceptable to be sterilised, why may not the same be true of some severely mentally handicapped women?

It could hardly be argued that the benefits of pregnancy justify such a ban for it is widely accepted even by those who absolutely oppose sterilisation of severely mentally handicapped women that great care should be taken to try to ensure that such women do not become pregnant. Nor can the argument that women flourish through the rearing and nurturing of their children be applied in such cases for almost inevitably severely mentally handicapped mothers will be unable to rear and nurture their children who will therefore be taken from them and placed elsewhere.

If the question of such women's best interests is pursued it becomes less and less clear that sterilisation is necessarily against their best interests. Given for example the pervasive assumption that pregnancy must if at all possible be avoided, women in such circumstances are likely to be subjected to considerably more repressive control over their contacts with men, and especially mentally handicapped men, in the hospitals, hostels and day centres where severely mentally handicapped people often spend much of their time. Indeed, only total sexual segregation can guarantee the avoidance of pregnancy. On the other hand if the possibility of pregnancy is eliminated by some effective means of contraception then ordinary mixed social intercourse becomes a much easier option.

Here people divide about the desirability of any form of contraception for the severely mentally handicapped. But suppose it is accepted that (a) ordinary social life, including the mixing of the sexes, is desirable for severely mentally handicapped too, and (b) that in the nature of mixed sex social life it is impossible to eliminate the possibility that sexually developed members of such a group will from time to time have sexual intercourse (some would argue that provided such intercourse was mutually desired and not exploitative it should not be prevented[4]) and (c) that it is important to ensure that no pregnancy results from any such intercourse, then the desirability of some form of effective contraception follows. However, even if contraception is accepted as desirable it may still be argued that other reversible and less dangerous forms of contraception are preferable to sterilisation which is usually irreversible and involves a surgical operation.

So far as the irreversibility is concerned this only seems to be important if there is some realistic chance that the severely mentally handicapped person will develop sufficiently to become capable of parenting and being allowed to parent a child. For it is surely the denial of possible parenthood and of the fulfilment that accompanies it which underlies such concern about the irreversibility of sterilisation. Where there is some realistic chance of such development then it does indeed seem in the best interests of the woman not to have an irreversible sterilisation. However, in many cases no such realistic chance of maturation to a state compatible with parenthood exists — and then the irreversibility of the operation seems to be irrelevant.

Undoubtedly other methods of contraception exist. Condoms and pills would probably be unsuitable for severely mentally handicapped people but intrauterine devices and long-acting injectable contraceptives could be suitable alternatives. Both, however, carry their own risks of harms (for example abdominal cramps, contraceptive failure, ectopic pregnancy, heavy and or irregular vaginal bleeding) and in particular cases may be unacceptable. Certainly sterilisation involves a surgical operation and probably a general anaesthetic — but such risks are regularly taken by the mentally normal in their own interests — again it is difficult to see how acceptance of such risks in preference to those of other methods of contraception could *never* be in the best interests of a mentally handicapped person.

The second type of argument favouring an absolute ban on sterilisation of severely mentally handicapped people is that it transgresses their rights. Such arguments must be taken very seriously but also need careful dissection. Precisely *which* rights are being protected? Proferred candidates seem to be a right to reproduce, a right not to be stopped from reproducing, a right to have sexual intercourse, a right not to be stopped from having sexual intercourse with a willing partner, and a right not to be surgically assaulted. The normal case again allows us to see these more clearly. Obviously there is no general right to reproduce — but there is a general *prima facie* right not to be stopped from reproducing and certainly in the normal case sterilisation without the person's understanding consent would be considered an outrageous transgression of his or her right not to be stopped from reproducing and his or her right not to be surgically assaulted. But again in the normal case these rights can be waived when it is in the interests of the person to waive them. One might even say that in the normal case people have a right to waive these rights.

As indicated above, we generally accept that where autonomous consent is unavailable (as is the case with severely mentally handicapped people) then the right not to have surgical intervention without consent can in some cases properly be waived, proxy autonomous consent for surgery be justifiably given and the surgery properly considered not to be an assault. So far as the right not to be stopped from reproduction is concerned we have seen that this is in general denied to severely mentally handicapped people; if this right were to justify a ban on sterilisation then it would equally require us not to prevent in other ways severely mentally handicapped people from reproducing. So far as the right not to be stopped from having sexual intercourse is concerned, sterilisation in no way infringes any such right, as the normal case makes clear. On the contrary reliable contraception makes its implementation easier, though there are few apart from those actually working on behalf of mentally handicapped people who show any concern to accommodate their sexual desires and the law while complicated tends to diminish any such sexual rights (though it by no means excludes them[4]).

Thus no absolute rights of the severely mentally handicapped are recognised either not to have surgery without consent or to be allowed to reproduce, and any right to have sexual intercourse would not be transgressed by sterilisation (on the contrary). Thus these rights-based arguments do not seem to justify an absolute ban on the possibility of proxy consent to sterilisation of a severely mentally handicapped person. The criterion for such consent would still have to be agreed — the weakest acceptable criterion presumably being that the action would not be against the person's interests, the next strongest being that it would be in his or her interests, and the strongest of all being that it would be in his or her best interests. Even with the last and strongest of these criteria (itself open to major objection for excluding any consideration of the interests of others) there seems no reason to assume that sterilisation could never be in such a person's best interests.

The third argument against sterilisation of a severely mentally handicapped person is that it would be against the interests of society to permit it, either because of harm to others or because of some other injustice to society or its members. In this context we have the appalling example of Hitler's reich in which mass sterilisation of the mentally incompetent was commonplace, by a variety of disgusting methods[5], and which is one of 'the ghosts that haunt the Jeanette file'[6]. Certainly if there were reason to believe that permitting of sterilisation in the interests of a mentally handicapped person would lead to the crimes of the third reich that would justify laws to ban it absolutely. This argument is an instance of the slippery slope argument, of which there are two types, the logical and the empirical. There is no logical slippery slope here if, unlike the case of the third reich, it is ensured that sterilisation is only permitted when it is not against the interests of the individual concerned (with mechanisms established to defend those interests). The problem with the second sort of slippery slope argument, the empirical, is that it can be used against *any* proposal that is capable of misuse. *Of course* if there were any realistic probability that sterilisation of the severely mentally handicapped when this was not against their own interests would lead to harm to others in society, let alone to the sort of repugnant society that characterised the third reich, then it should be prohibited. But there seems no reason to predict such developments if each case of proposed sterilisation of a mentally handicapped person is (a) not against the person's interests (and it might be safer to specify that it must be positively in his or her interests) and (b) decided in a way which explicitly protects that person's interests.

Given the worries involved, and given the peculiar vulnerability of the mentally handicapped, and given also the obvious conflicts between self-interest and the interests of the mentally handicapped which carers, parents and health care professionals alike, are likely to face, and given the irreversibility of sterilisation, it does seem wise to introduce a procedure for approval of proposed sterilisations which can be seen to defend the interests of the mentally handicapped person. One such procedure would be for all cases to obtain the approval of a court. Another might be to set up a committee to approve such proposals, of people with different backgrounds and independent of the mentally handicapped person's care, who would provide a backstop for protecting his or her interests, a system somewhat analogous to the approval now required under the Mental Health Act for certain sorts of irreversible treatments such as psychosurgery.[7]

Our attitudes to proposals for the sterilisation of mentally handicapped people are subject to powerful emotions — emotions that influence our responses to sexuality in general, emotions that influence our responses to mental handicap in general, and emotions that are heightened by our attitudes to a society whose morality functions as a dread warning of the depths to which human behaviour can sink. In such circumstances we must be even more than usually meticulous about subjecting our 'gut responses' to the searchlight of critical moral reasoning.

REFERENCES

1. Brahams D. Medicine and the law. *Lancet* 1987;i: 757-758.
2. Mason J K, McCall Smith R A. *Law and medical ethics.* London: Butterworths, 1983, 48.
3. Kennedy I, Dworkin G. Children and the law. In: Nicholson R H, ed. *Medical research with children: ethics, law and practice.* Oxford, New York, Tokyo: Oxford University Press, 1986, 125-139.
4. Dixon H, Gunn M. *Sex and the law — a brief guide for staff working in the mental handicap field (England and Wales only).* London: Family Planning Association Education Unit, 1985.
5. Ivy A C. Nazi war crimes of a medical nature. In: Reiser S J, Dyck A J, Curran W J. *Ethics in medicine — historical perspectives and contemporary concerns.* Cambridge Mass, London: MIT press, 1977: 267-272.
6. Acherson N. Ghosts that haunt the Jeanette file. *The Observer* 1987 Mar 22: 9.
7. Mental Health Act, 1983, s 57, 58, and regulations.

FURTHER READINGS

Alberta Institute of Law Research and Reform
Report for Discussion No. 6,"Sterilization Decisions: Minors and Mentally Incompetent Adults." (Edmonton, Alta, 1988).
Alberta Institute of Law Research and Reform
Report No. 52, "Competence and Human Reproduction," (Edmonton, Alta, 1989).
Chambers, D.
"The Right to the Least Restrictive Alternative," in M. Kindred et al, eds., *The Mentally Retarded Citizen and the Law.* (New York: Free Press, 1976).
Finch-Noyes, C.A.P.
"Sterilization of the Mentally Retarded Minor: the Re K. Case," *Canadian Journal of Family Law* 5:1 (1986) 277-99.
Great Britain, Department of Health and Social Services
Report of the Committee of Enquiry into Human Sterilization and Embryology. ed. by M. Warnock (London: HM Stationer's Office, 1984): "The Warnock Report".
Grubb, A. and D. Pearl
"Sterilization and the Courts," *Cambridge Law Journal* 46:3 (1987) 439-64.
Law Reform Commission of Canada
Working Paper 24, *Sterilization: Implications for Mentally Retarded and Mentally Ill Persons.* (Ottawa: Minister of Supply and Services, 1978).'
McLaren, Angus
"The Creation of a Haven for 'Human Thoroughbreds': Sterilization of the Feebleminded and the Mentally Ill in British Columbia," *Canadian Historical Review* 67:2 (1986) 127-50.

CHAPTER 16 THE NEW REPRODUCTIVE TECHNOLOGIES

INTRODUCTION

The development and application of new techniques of reproductive technology raises important philosophical questions. For instance, how should such technologies be viewed? What do they promise — and what is their price?

Christine Overall considers these issues from a feminist perspective. One of her most important claims is that the reproductive technologies should be considered essentially from a woman-oriented perspective, since it is women who do the child-bearing, and women's social roles that are affected by reproduction itself.

The second selection reflects the position of the medical profession, which of course is integrally involved in the development and providing of reproductive services. Its stance is less gender-oriented than that of Overall. It presents the new reproductive technologies as a medical modality that should be available only under certain conditions. However, it suggests that if they are to be offered at all, then they ought to be available on an equitable basis. It comes from the official position of the Canadian Medical Association, adopted by the Association in December of 1990 and presented to the Royal Commission on New Reproductive Technologies.

Ethics and Human Reproduction

Christine Overall

INTRODUCTION

Is the use of prenatal diagnosis a unique form of insurance for parents that their offspring will be healthy? Or is it a covert but potentially dangerous manifestation of eugenics?

Is the practice of surrogate motherhood a valuable service for men whose wives are infertile? Or is it a type of reproductive prostitution of women?

Is fetal sex preselection a benign process that enables people to have the precious son or daughter for whom they long? Or is it a form of gynecide — that is, wholesale slaughter of females?

Is the recovery of eggs from surgically removed ovarian tissue a good source of experimental material for use in reproductive research? Or is it an insidious type of egg snatching and egg farming?

These questions are examples of just a few of the ethical issues now being raised about reproduction and reproductive technology. They are part of a rapidly growing philosophical subdiscipline — reproductive ethics — that is concerned with the wide range of moral questions arising in connection with human reproduction. Although some reproductive issues, such as those pertaining to contraception, abortion, and birth, have always been of deep significance throughout human existence, the past ten years have witnessed the development of new reproductive technologies, such as in vitro fertilization, embryo transfer, and sex preselection, which have almost as great a capacity for affecting human lives.

They will affect human lives — but, in particular, they will affect *women's* lives, and that potential does not always receive the emphasis it deserves. In the current debates about issues in reproductive ethics there is a striking contrast in approach between, on the one hand, those which highlight women's experience, needs, and behavior in connection with reproduction and those which minimize, ignore, or deny the central relation between women and reproduction and instead profess concern for entities such as "society" or "the family." The latter approach is antifeminist or nonfeminist in nature; the former is feminist. This book develops a critique of antifeminist and nonfeminist approaches to reproductive ethics and offers in their place a feminist analysis of issues in reproduction.

Feminism: A Definition

Both historical and contemporary discussions show clearly that the term "feminism" encompasses a variety of meanings,[1] and not all of them are entirely consistent with one another. Nevertheless it is possible to outline the minimal but essential components of a feminist perspective.

First, a feminist perspective involves a commitment to understanding women's experience, beliefs, ideas, relationships, behavior, creations, and history. It stresses women's own perceptions; that is, how events, institutions, social groups, and individuals are apprehended and interpreted by women. It highlights those elements of

Christine Overall, "Introduction," from Christine Overall, *Ethics and Human Reproduction.* (Boston: Allen & Unwin, 1987) pp. 1-2 and 5-16.

women's personal and social experience which are common and shared as well as those which are distinct and diverse. This focus is justified by the fact that women's experience and history have for the most part been suppressed, ignored, manipulated, and exploited, both in the past and in the present. It is therefore necessary to recover what has been lost, to give recognition to what has been ignored, to revalue what has been depreciated in women's experience. This recovery process involves a variety of methods — from the informal and revelatory process of consciousness-raising to the more formal and scholarly research in women's studies. What they have in common is a determination to avoid duplicating those methods used in the past which, by treating women as, at most, objects to be studied, have misrepresented and misunderstood women's experience.

Second, a feminist perspective is founded upon and fully informed by an awareness that women as women have been and are the victims of oppression under patriarchy, the system of male dominance.[2] Such a claim does not necessarily imply that "men are the enemy" or that all men rule all women. But it does imply that although women are oppressed as women, men are not usually oppressed as men.[3] This awareness includes a conception of what oppression — unjust limitations and barriers — is and of its physical, psychological, social, and legal manifestations. And it is not complete without attention to the ways in which women's oppression can vary depending upon other variables such as age, race, class, religion, nationality, and sexual orientation.

Third, a feminist perspective includes some sort of theory about the origins of the oppression of women. Such a theory entails not necessarily a belief in one general "cause" of sexual oppression but, rather, attention to the ways in which that oppression is maintained and perpetuated, as well as attention to the agents — both individual and institutional — of oppression. It is on this aspect of feminism perhaps more than any other that feminists have disagreed; disputes about the sources of women's oppression have led to the development, particularly within the last two decades, of feminist political theories ranging from liberal feminism to socialist and Marxist feminism to radical feminism.[4]

Fourth, a feminist perspective is guided by a determination to avoid perpetuating or acquiescing in the oppression of women and to contribute, whenever possible, to the further understanding and dissolution of sexual inequality. In this respect feminism moves beyond the awareness of women's victimization to a vision of women's present and potential empowerment. Such a vision includes a concept of what the end of oppression would mean and would be like and of what the goal of feminist revolutionary change should be. Feminists have favored a variety of means to end oppression, including gradual reform, the production of alternate institutions and systems, and separatism of various sorts.[5]

Finally, a feminist perspective is characterized by the deliberate and self-conscious (in a positive sense) nature of its worldview. In its most developed form it fosters the creation of new or alternate epistemic, ontological, ethical, and cultural systems.[6] This is the most original aspect of feminism, and also its least developed.

Antifeminist and Nonfeminist Perspectives

In the preceding definition of feminism the first and second characteristics are most crucial; the third, fourth, and fifth follow from them. Hence antifeminist and nonfeminist perspectives can most easily be understood in terms of their relationship to the first and second characteristics of feminism.

A type of conservatism, antifeminism rejects the feminist commitment to understanding women's experience and denies the claim that women have been and are the victims of oppression.[7] The antifeminist believes that women are not oppressed, for such a term implies unjust treatment of women. Instead he (or she) maintains that differential treatment of women is justified, often on the grounds of innate differences between the sexes that lead to distinct social functions for women and for men. The antifeminist also tends to support the enforcement and elaboration of alleged sex differences through state-controlled mechanisms. In short, antifeminism champions a type of socially sanctioned biological determinism in which sexual and reproductive differences between the sexes are fundamental to their different roles.[8]

In speaking of a nonfeminist approach, on the other hand, I am grouping a variety of different views. They are not necessarily overtly and actively misogynistic. However, a nonfeminist perspective is one that, deliberately or not, tends to ignore rather than deny women's experience and to suspend belief about the claim that women are oppressed. In this perspective what is most noticeable is not a deliberately antifeminist or antiwomen stance but, rather, one that is simply unaware of the hard-won insights of feminist writings. A nonfeminist approach, then, is androcentric[9]: that is, it overlooks women's experience, taking male perceptions and interpretations as the norm. It lacks the deliberately self-conscious character of feminist discourse, which is aware that there is more than one possible framework for the discussion of social and moral issues. Such an approach shows little or no awareness or understanding of the past and present oppression of women, and as a result it fails to question — and even helps to reinforce — patriarchal control over women.

Antifeminist and Nonfeminist Approaches to Reproductive Ethics

Human beings are embodied beings, and an understanding of reproduction is essential to understanding human relationships and what it is to be human within the context of patriarchy. Broadly construed, reproduction includes not only the immediate biological processes of procreation and the social uses to which they are put but also sexual interactions and relationships, and childrearing. In this book the focus is primarily upon issues pertaining directly to procreation, but it is impossible to discuss them independently of a concern for questions about sexuality and child care.

To examine reproduction requires not just an understanding of nature, of what is biologically given; it requires also an understanding of the social construction and organization of sexual, procreative, and child care relationships. In fact, such an understanding calls into question the assumption that it is legitimate or even meaningful to speak of what is biologically given outside the context of the human interpretations put on it. As Zillah Eisenstein says,

> Women can sexually reproduce and they lactate. These are biological facts. That women are defined as mothers is a political fact and reflects a political need of patriarchy, which is based partially in the biological truth that women bear children. The transformation of women from a biological being (childbearer) to a political being (childrearer) is part of the conflict expressed in the politics of patriarchy. Patriarchy seeks to maintain the myth that patriarchal motherhood is a biological reality rather than a politically constructed necessity.[10]

Both antifeminists and nonfeminists, on the one hand, and feminists, on the other, have strived to understand human reproduction and to respond to the variety of issues raised by the social shaping of reproduction. The results of their investigations, however, have been very different.

Antifeminist and nonfeminist approaches to reproductive ethics are characterized by the tendency to concentrate on a few issues to the exclusion of others — which may in fact be equally or more important. *What* is overlooked, *that* it is overlooked, and *why* it is overlooked — all of this is as significant as what is actually discussed in reproductive ethics, but it is, of course, somewhat harder to recognize.

For example, contemporary philosophical discussions of reproduction have focused almost exclusively on the topic of abortion, and the literature on that subject is voluminous and complex. Moreover recent texts serving as general introductions to biomedical ethics or to contemporary social issues[11] almost always include a section on abortion but seldom on any other topics in reproductive ethics. This thanatological concentration is consistent with the general concern that philosophers have historically evinced for questions about death; it appears virtually to exclude any consideration of, for example, questions about birth.[12] It also entails lengthy and detailed discussions of the moral and metaphysical status of the embryo/fetus: for example, is it a person? If so, when does it become a person? If not, why is it not a person?[13] and so on. There is, however, relatively little discussion of the woman who is the co-creator and sole sustainer of the embryo/fetus, except insofar as she is treated as a container or "environment" for it. And on the rare occasions on which women are discussed within the context of abortion or birth, the fetus-woman relationship is most often seen as one of competition and antagonism rather than interaction and support.

Recent antifeminist and nonfeminist discussions of the uses of new reproductive technology have not done much to alter this myopic outlook. Once again, only a limited number of topics are considered to be worthy of discussion. In analyses of the implications of in vitro fertilization and surrogate motherhood, for example, we mainly find a concern for questions about so-called sexual ethics[14] (for example, is a surrogate mother committing adultery?),[15] about the security and sustenance of what is ambiguously referred to as "*the* family" (as if there were just one form of the family),[16] and about which woman is to be considered the "real mother" of the offspring produced through surrogacy.

Thus, in general an antifeminist or nonfeminist approach tends to avoid, overlook, or minimize what feminists would regard as crucial topics and issues in reproductive ethics and to concentrate on a rather small number of questions whose importance may, as a result, be exaggerated.

Second, antifeminist and nonfeminist approaches are characterized by a pervasive failure to examine or challenge certain underlying assumptions about reproduction that are widely held both by society in general and by the medical establishment in particular. The clearest example of this is found in discussions of infertility, its meaning, significance, and appropriate treatment. Infertility is an important topic because its growing incidence is usually offered as the main justification for the development of technologies of artificial reproduction. Antifeminist and nonfeminist experts from both medicine and the social sciences often assume that infertility is a legitimate problem only for women who are heterosexual and married[17]; that children are material commodities owned by their parents; that a family is incomplete, or not a family at all, if no children are present; and that a genetic link with one's children is psychologically and morally essential.[18]

These unexamined beliefs also have implications for what is assumed to be the appropriate and correct treatment of infertility. They suggest, for example, that people — especially men — have an inalienable right to be parents.[19] Yet it is also assumed that infertility should be treated only in women who are heterosexual and married[20]; that it should be treated so as to provide a child who is genetically related to the couple, and particularly to the father; and that therefore heroic measures, including in vitro fertilization, embryo transfer, and surrogate motherhood, may be preferable to adoption and to the less expensive, dangerous, and invasive procedure of artificial insemination by donor.[21] Finally, these beliefs are related to certain assumptions about women: that women are primarily dependent baby-making machines that, unfortunately, may threaten their offspring or fail to operate and therefore need a "technological fix."[22]

Are all of these beliefs true? The problem is not that antifeminist and nonfeminist writers *defend* them; in fact they usually offer virtually no justification whatsoever for holding them. The problem is that these ideas apparently are so self-evident to these writers that no one thinks to provide reasons for the ideas or that there could be any basis for questioning them.

Finally, antifeminist and nonfeminist approaches to reproductive ethics are characterized by a lack of insight into and concern for the implications of new reproductive technology for the well-being of women and children. One example is surrogate motherhood. Nonfeminist writers typically regard surrogate motherhood as, at best, a desirable, useful, and indeed necessary service that uncoerced women may offer for purchase by childless men. They believe that it is a relatively unproblematic social institution, requiring only careful legal regulation of its contractual aspects, as well as public scrutiny of its actual operation.[23] Little attention is paid in these discussions to the potential effects of the surrogate motherhood arrangement on children and on women, and there is no discussion of what the practice of buying reproductive services indicates about the social position of women.

Another example is fetal sex selection and preselection. Antifeminist and nonfeminist writers treat the use of these processes as inevitable and unproblematic. They seldom question the sexism implicit in a technology that would permit us to choose the human beings who will be our children on the basis of their sex alone. Such writers are remarkably undisturbed by the prospect of possible changes in the sex ratio that, given the almost universal parental preference for male offspring,[24] could be produced in some areas by widespread use of sex selection and preselection.[25] Instead most nonfeminist writers view fetal sex selection and preselection with great optimism as a potential cure for world population problems and a panacea for parents who would otherwise not get the kind of children they want.[26]

In general, then, as these examples show, antifeminist and nonfeminist discussions of reproductive ethics too often are almost oblivious to the possible consequences for children and women of the development and adoption of reproductive technology.

Feminist Approaches to Reproductive Ethics

Whereas much of patriarchal ideology defines women's "natural" function in terms of their capacities for sexual activity, procreation, and child-rearing, feminist analysis has recently begun to demonstrate that women's sexual, procreative, and child care abilities are manipulated, exploited, and appropriated to accommodate patriarchal interests.

This appropriation has been manifested historically through a variety of attitudes and behaviors.[27] In the arena of sexuality, for example, these include heterosexism and homophobia; pornography; contempt for women's bodies and women's sexuality; the institutions of incest, rape, sexual harassment, and prostitution; and sexual pressures and prohibitions of all types. In the arena of procreation the patriarchal appropriation of reproduction has produced compulsory motherhood — by means of contraception that is dangerous, unreliable, or often unavailable; abortion, which can be inaccessible or life-threatening; the prohibition of any life choices other than mothering, or the provision of work that mimics certain aspects of mothering; and the promotion of pronatalism and emphasis on fertility and fecundity, particularly in women. At the same time, not all women are judged suitable to be mothers. Some women have been the victims of involuntary sterilization; others have lost custody of and access to their children because of their sexual orientation. In the arena of child-rearing, patriarchal appropriation of reproduction takes the form of control over mothering, by means of an ideology of child-rearing that specifies what sort of mothers are desirable and what kind of children mothers should produce.[28] This is accompanied by a significant lack of support for mothering, evinced in the incompatibility of much productive labor and reproductive labor within patriarchy, and the absence of social mechanisms to support good child-rearing, such as paid maternity leave, adequate family allowances, and state-supported child care.

The most recent manifestation of the patriarchal appropriation of reproduction lies in the development and use of new reproductive technology. In contrast to the glorification of this technology by antifeminist and nonfeminist writers, feminists for the most part are not blinded by rosy visions of an approaching technological paradise, and generally adopt a more skeptical, sometimes even pessimistic stance toward issues in reproductive ethics. This is not, of course, uniformly true of all feminist theorists: Shulamith Firestone[29] is the exceptional example of a feminist who saw artificial reproduction as a liberating force for women. But more recent feminist writers who, unlike Firestone, have witnessed the implementation of the "technological fix" in reproduction have been less enthusiastic about the potential benefits of reproductive technology.[30]

In contrast to antifeminist and nonfeminist approaches, a specifically feminist approach to reproductive ethics fosters the recognition that there is a wide range of issues pertaining to human reproduction. For example, it helps us to see the significance of childbirth. The medicalization of the birth process, the usurpation of the role of midwives, and the place of birth (both in the sense of its physical location — in hospital, home, or clinic — and in the sense of its more general function in our society) are now recognized as genuine social and moral issues.[31] Feminist analyses have demonstrated that the way childbirth is handled reveals much about the status of women, as "patients" and as caregivers, and about the value we ascribe to infants and children.[32]

Furthermore, feminist discussions of reproduction have shown that there are other questions about abortion in addition to the undoubtedly important ones that center upon the fetus: questions having to do with reproductive freedom and choice, control of the body, and responsibility for one's actions.[33] Thus, in general a feminist approach transcends the often rather narrow range of issues recognized by antifeminist and nonfeminist writers and acknowledges the significance of women's experience in all areas of reproduction.

A feminist approach to reproductive ethics also challenges received opinions about reproduction. Feminist analysis has demonstrated that uncritical supporters of reproductive technology generally have narrow visions of what kind of family is "normal," what kind of children we should want, and especially what sort of responsibilities and roles women should have. Rejecting those visions, feminists examine critically the assumptions that underlie existing reproductive practices. For example, a feminist orientation to the problem of infertility asks: What are the pronatalist and pro-"family" pressures[34] that help to make infertility an almost unendurable burden, especially for women? In what ways is infertility a product of other interventions in the reproductive process? Why are women advised to endure the pain, uncertainty, and disappointments involved in in vitro fertilization, as a "treatment" for a low sperm count in their husbands, when artificial insemination by donor is easier, has a higher rate of success, and is pain-free?[35] How necessary is it, in fact, that one's child be one's own genetic product? Why is biological continuity especially important to men?[36] Feminism encourages the raising of questions about assumptions usually taken for granted in discussions of reproduction.

Finally, a feminist approach focuses attention upon what reproductive technology really is and upon its potential effects on children and women. For example, feminist writers have argued dramatically and effectively that surrogate motherhood is similar in some respects to prostitution,[37] that the surgical recovery of eggs and ovarian tissue from nonconsenting women is "egg-snatching,"[38] and that fetal sex selection may result in a sort of prenatal gynecide.[39] Thus the emphasis in feminist discussions is upon exploring in innovative ways all of the possible implications of the growing medical, legal, and social control of reproduction.

Feminism, Ethics, and Reproduction

It is clear that a feminist perspective contributes significantly to the reevaluation of issues in reproductive ethics and to the understanding of women and reproduction in patriarchy. So far, however, feminist discussions of reproduction and reproductive technology for the most part have been scattered and tentative. The aim of this book is to advance a cohesive feminist analysis of reproductive ethics.

For several reasons the analysis cannot claim to be complete. Not every possible issue is surveyed in detail; for example, contraception, reproductive hazards, and involuntary sterilization are discussed only briefly. And I do not discuss such related philosophical issues as population control and our obligations to future people. Moreover reproductive technology and the social structures of reproduction are subject to very rapid growth and change, which can overtake technical discussions of the subject. Finally, feminist theory itself is still at a stage of early development, and no contribution to the feminist discussion of reproduction can pretend to offer the final word on the subject.

Nevertheless, the book tries to extend and develop the feminist approach by incorporating the insights already achieved in feminist discussions of reproductive ethics and contrasting them with antifeminist and nonfeminist analyses. It examines some of the most important new technologies and their social uses and offers recommendations in regard to the formation of policy about reproduction. Most important, it attempts to highlight some significant ethical and social themes embedded within contemporary structures of reproduction: the manipulation of reproductive choices, the denigration of women's bodies, the overvaluing of fertility and a genetic link to one's offspring, and the commodification of reproduction.

To offer a feminist reassessment of reproductive ethics is, among other things, to make a claim for the inclusion — not the superiority — of women within moral decision making and policy. But the results of that inclusion are of such a magnitude that piecemeal alterations in morality and policy may no longer be adequate. According to Sandra Bartky, "feminists are not aware of different things than other people; they are aware of the same things differently."[40] This is partly right and partly wrong. For when feminists look at the "same things" differently, those things — issues, practices, values, behaviors, beliefs — cease to be the same.

NOTES

An earlier version of part of this chapter, entitled "Reproductive Ethics: Feminist and Non-Feminist Approaches," appeared in *Canadian Journal of Women and the Law / Revue juridique la femme et le droit* 1, no. 2(1986):271-278. The material is used here with the permission of the journal's editor.

1. See Alison M. Jaggar, *Feminist Politics and Human Nature* (Totowa, N.J.: Rowman & Allanheld, 1983); and Mary Midgley and Judith Hughes, *Women's Choices: Philosophical Problems Facing Feminism* (London: Weidenfeld and Nicholson, 1983), pp. 21-25.
2. For a discussion of the concept of patriarchy, see Zillah Eisenstein, *The Radical Future of Liberal Feminism* (New York: Longman, 1981), pp. 18-22.
3. Marilyn Frye, "Oppression," in *The Politics of Reality: Essays in Feminist Theory* (Trumansberg, N.Y.: Crossing Press, 1983), pp. 1-16.
4. These theories are ably discussed in Jaggar's book, and also in Catharine A. MacKinnon, "Feminism, Marxism, Method, and the State: An Agenda for Theory," in *Feminist Theory: A Critique of Ideology*, ed. Nannerl O. Keohane, Michelle Z. Rosaldo, and Barbara C. Gelpi (Chicago: University of Chicago Press, 1982), pp. 1-30.
5. See Sara Ann Ketchum and Christine Pierce, "Separatism and Sexual Relationships," in *Philosophy and Women*, ed. Sharon Bishop and Marjorie Weinzweig (Belmont, Calif.: Wadsworth, 1979), pp. 163-171.
6. Among many examples are the papers in *Discovering Reality: Feminist Perspectives on Epistemology, Metaphysics, Methodology, and the Philosophy of Science*, ed. Sandra Harding and Merrill B. Hintikka (Dordrecht, Holland: D. Reidel, 1983); and in *Beyond Domination: New Perspectives on Women and Philosophy*, ed. Carol C. Gould (Totowa, N.J.: Rowman & Allanheld, 1983).
7. My discussion of antifeminism owes much to Alison Jaggar's remarks about the conservative view of women. See her "Political Philosophies of Women's Liberation," in *Philosophy and Women*, pp. 258-259.
8. See Janet Sayers's discussion of biological arguments against feminism in *Biological Politics: Feminist and Anti-Feminist Perspectives* (London: Tavistock, 1982), pp. 7-104.

9. Jackie Davies, "Commentary on J. E. Bickenbach's 'The Empty Garage?: Recent Feminist Critiques of Scientific Methodology'," delivered at the Department of Philosophy Colloquium, Queen's University, Kingston, Ontario, 29 November 1984.
10. Eisenstein, *Radical Future of Liberal Feminism*, p. 15.
11. For example, see Wesley Cragg, ed., *Contemporary Moral Issues* (Toronto: McGraw-Hill Ryerson, 1983); and Jan Narveson, ed., *Moral Issues* (Toronto: Oxford University Press, 1983).
12. Mary O'Brien, *The Politics of Reproduction* (Boston: Routledge & Kegan Paul, 1981), p. 20.
13. There are many instances of this approach. See, for example, John T. Noonan, Jr., "An Almost Absolute Value in History," Roger Wertheimer, "Understanding the Abortion Argument," and Michael Tooley, "A Defense of Abortion and Infanticide," in *The Problem of Abortion*, ed. Joel Feinberg (Belmont, Calif.: Wadsworth, 1973).
14. William J. Daniel, "Sexual Ethics in Relation to IVF and ET: The Fitting Use of Human Reproductive Power," in *Test-Tube Babies: A Guide to Moral Questions, Present Techniques and Future Possibilities*, ed. William Walters and Peter Singer (Melbourne: Oxford University Press, 1982), pp. 71-78.
15. Robert T. Francoeur, *Utopian Motherhood: New Trends in Human Reproduction* (Garden City, N.Y.: Doubleday, 1970), p. 104.
16. See John A. Henley, "IVF and the Human Family: Possible and Likely Consequences," in *Test-Tube Babies*, pp. 79-87; Herbert T. Krimmel, "The Case against Surrogate Parenting," *Hastings Center Report* 13 (October 1983): 35-39; and R. Snowden, G. D. Mitchell, and E. M. Snowden, *Artificial Reproduction: A Social Investigation* (London: George Allen & Unwin, 1983).
17. Leon R. Kass, "Babies by Means of In Vitro Fertilization: Unethical Experiments on the Unborn?" *New England Journal of Medicine* 285 (18 November 1971): 1176-1177, and Leon R. Kass, "Making Babies — The New Biology and the 'Old' Morality," *The Public Interest* 26 (Winter 1972): 20.
18. Robert Edwards and Patrick Steptoe, *A Matter of Life: The Story of a Medical Breakthrough* (London: Hutchinson, 1980), pp. 101-102; and Snowden et al., *Artificial Reproduction*, p. 43.
19. Edwards and Steptoe, *A Matter of Life*, pp. 101-102.
20. Snowden et al., *Artificial Reproduction*, p. 169.
21. R[obert] G. Edwards, "The Current Clinical and Ethical Situation of Human Conception In Vitro," in *Developments in Human Reproduction and Their Eugenic, Ethical Implications*, ed. C. O. Carter (New York: Academic Press, 1983), p. 95; and John A. Robertson, "Surrogate Mothers: Not So Novel After All," *Hastings Center Report* 13 (October 1983): 28.
22. A phrase taken from Hilary Rose and Jalna Hanmer, "Women's Liberation, Reproduction, and the Technological Fix," in *Sexual Divisions and Society: Process and Change*, ed. Diana Leonard Barker and Sheila Allen (London: Tavistock, 1976), pp. 199-223.

23. See Robertson, "Surrogate Mothers," pp. 28-34; Michael D. Bayles, *Reproductive Ethics* (Englewood Cliffs, N.J.: Prentice Hall, 1984), pp. 22-27; and Alan A. Rassaby, "Surrogate Motherhood: The Position and Problems of Substitutes," in *Test-Tube Babies*, pp. 97-109.
24. See Nancy E. Williamson, *Sons or Daughters: A Cross-Cultural Survey of Parental Preferences* (Newbury Park, Calif.: Sage Publications, 1976), and Nancy E. Williamson, "Sex Preferences, Sex Control, and the Status of Women," *Signs* 1 (1976): 847-862.
25. Amitai Etzioni, "Sex Control, Science, and Society," *Science* 161, no. 3846 (September 1968): 1109; John Postgate, "Bat's Chance in Hell," *New Scientist* 58, no. 840 (5 April 1973): 16.
26. Richard L. Meier, "Sex Determination and Other Innovations," in *Population in Perspective*, ed. Louise B. Young (New York: Oxford University Press, 1968), p. 410.
27. See MacKinnon, "Feminism, Marxism, Method and the State," pp. 15-19.
28. See, for example, Barbara Ehrenreich and Deirdre English, *For Her Own Good: 150 Years of the Experts' Advice to Women* (Garden City, N.Y.: Anchor Books, 1978); and Daniel Beekman, *The Mechanical Baby: A Popular History of the Theory and Practice of Child Raising* (Westport, Conn.: Lawrence Hill, 1977).
29. Shulamith Firestone, *The Dialectic of Sex* (New York: William Morrow, 1970), pp. 197-201.
30. See, for example, the papers in *Test-Tube Women: What Future for Motherhood?*, ed. Rita Arditti, Renate Duelli Klein, and Shelley Minden (London: Pandora Press, 1984); and *The Custom-Made Child? Women-Centered Perspectives*, ed. Helen B. Holmes, Betty B. Hoskins, and Michael Gross (Clifton, N.J.: Humana Press, 1981).
31. Adele E. Laslie, "Ethical Issues in Childbirth," *Journal of Medicine and Philosophy* 7 (1982): 179-195.
32. Barbara Katz Rothman, *Giving Birth: Alternatives in Childbirth* (Harmondsworth, England: Penguin, 1984); Ann Oakley, *Women Confined: Towards a Sociology of Childbirth* (New York: Schocken Books, 1980).
33. For example, Judith Jarvis Thomson, "A Defense of Abortion," *Philosophy and Public Affairs* 1 (Fall 1971): 47-66; Barbara Katz Rothman, "The Meanings of Choice in Reproductive Technology," in Arditti et al., *Test-Tube Women*, pp. 23-33; and Elizabeth W. Moen, "What Does 'Control over Our Bodies' Really Mean?" *International Journal of Women's Studies* 2 (March/April 1979): 129-143.
34. See Ellen Peck and Judith Senderowitz, eds., *Pronatalism: The Myth of Mom and Apple Pie* (New York: Thomas Y. Crowell, 1974); Martha E. Gimenez, "Feminism, Pronatalism, and Motherhood," in *Mothering: Essays in Feminist Theory*, ed. Joyce Trebilcot (Totowa, N.J.: Rowman & Allanheld, 1984), pp. 287-314; and Rebecca Albury, "Who Owns the Embryo?" in Arditti et al., *Test-Tube Women*, pp. 54-67.
35. Jalna Hanmer and Pat Allen, "Reproductive Engineering: The Final Solution?" in *Alice through the Microscope: The Power of Science over Women's Lives*, ed. The Brighton Women and Science Group (London: Virago, 1980), pp. 212-217; Jalna

Hanmer, "Reproductive Technology: The Future for Women?" in *Machina Ex Dea: Feminist Perspectives on Technology*, ed. Joan Rothschild (New York: Pergamon Press, 1983), pp. 184-188.

36. O'Brien, *Politics of Reproduction*, pp. 29-64; Mary Kay Blakely, "Surrogate Mothers: For Whom Are They Working?" *Ms.* 11, no. 9 (March 1983): 20.
37. Andrea Dworkin, *Right-Wing Women* (New York: Perigee Books, 1983), pp. 174-188.
38. Genoveffa Corea, "Egg Snatchers," and Julie Murphy, "Egg Farming and Women's Future," both in Arditti et al., *Test-Tube Women*, pp. 37-51 and 68-75, respectively.
39. Betty B. Hoskins and Helen Bequaert Holmes, "Technology and Prenatal Femicide," in Arditti et al., *Test-Tube Women*, pp. 237-255.
40. Sandra Bartky, "Toward a Phenomenology of Feminist Consciousness," in Bishop and Weinzweig, *Philosophy and Women*, p. 254.

Background Considerations

Canadian Medical Association

PERSPECTIVES OF RELEVANT PARTIES

The Canadian Medical Association is conscious that the topics that fall under the heading of new reproductive technology can be discussed from a variety of perspectives.

The Woman

First and foremost, there is the perspective of the woman. The majority of developments in the realm of reproductive technologies over the past few decades involve techniques or regimens that focus on the reproductive capacities of women. Implicated here are such techniques as of gamete retrieval, artificial insemination,[1] and intra-uterine monitoring. However, in all of this, the Association is concerned that society never lose sight of the fact that these technologies deal with people, that women are people first and foremost, and that any departure from this priority ranking is indefensible.

In some of the cultures that form the Canadian mosaic, the privilege of giving birth and nurturing a child is considered central to, and defining of, the role of a woman. The Canadian Medical Association is mindful that this perspective is not shared by all Canadian women. In fact, the Association is aware that the topic of new reproductive technologies has been perceived as an appropriate venue for advancing political and valuational perspectives opposed to this: values and perspectives that derive from what has been called a woman's perspective.

The Association would adopt a cautious approach in these matters. It would

Canadian Medical Association, "Background Considerations," from *The New Reproductive Technologies: A Preliminary Perspective of the Canadian Medical Association* (Ottawa: Canadian Medical Association, 1991)1-9.

suggest that any stance that is adopted by society in general and by this Commission in particular on the new reproductive technologies should not be driven solely by political agendas. The Association believes that, instead, it should be defensible in ethical terms, and that it should be based on moral principles that are respectful of the valuational and cultural diversity of the Canadian nation.

Furthermore, the Association believes that the very essence of an appropriate physician/patient relationship requires that physicians be respectful of the valuational perspectives of their patients. It does not believe that any body — least of all the medical profession — has the right to decide which value or cultural perspective is appropriate, or which should find recognition and which should not.

Therefore, so far as the Association is concerned, the appropriate way to approach the conflicting perspectives on the matter of female reproduction is to see them as distinct ends of a valuational scale where each part of the scale deserves consideration and respect. Consequently, the Association proposes that the following issues would constitute an appropriate focus for the deliberations of this Commission:

- education and counselling on the nature and role of female sexuality and on reproductive options available to women in the Canadian context, including adoption as a means of realizing parenthood;
- development of standardized approaches to such counselling;
- development and dissemination of information about causes and prevention of female infertility, and about possible means to alleviate it;
- standardization of the various techniques of new reproductive technology;[2]
- development and dissemination of information about the nature and success rates of techniques of new reproductive technology;
- informed consent in the use of the new reproductive technology;
- provision of access to the new reproductive technologies according to the principles of equality and justice;
- clarification of the legal status of female gamete donors with respect to ownership of gametes, rights of disposition and responsibilities;
- clarification of the legal status of women involved in various methods of new reproductive technology, as for instance surrogate and gestational motherhood;[3] and
- development of appropriate record-keeping.

The Child

A second major stakeholder in the development of techniques of reproductive technology is the child. In the eyes of the Association, it should never be forgotten that the primary reason for fertility-associated efforts and for the development of techniques of reproductive technology is the birth of a child. The Association also wishes to reiterate that a child is a person. The Association believes that a child is entitled to the same respect and to the same treatment as all other people. It, therefore, wishes to go on record as maintaining that if developments in the domain of reproductive technology cannot sustain such a perspective, if these developments reduce the child to the status of an object, or if they require that those who are involved adopt an instrumentalistic outlook toward children, then the Association opposes such developments fundamentally and unalterably. Furthermore, the Association wishes to stress that there should be no presumption that children who are "less than perfect," whatever their biological origin, are not deserving of the same respect as other people.

These considerations prompt the Association to suggest that this Commission pay particular regard in its deliberations to such matters as:

- clarification of the legal status of children born as a result of the use of new reproductive technologies;[4]
- record-keeping to allow appropriate tracing of children and their genetic parents;[5]
- screening programs for gamete donors;[6]
- quality assurance programs and standards for techniques of new reproductive technologies;[7]
- pre-natal screening programs;[8] and
- research programs involving the development of artificial gestational environments.[9]

The Association offers these suggestions, not in any order of priority, but with the underlying hope that all of them will be addressed. The Association also offers them with the firm conviction that no human being, whether it be a woman, a man or a child, should ever be viewed as a commodity.

The Man

A third perspective that should find reflection in any discussion of reproductive technologies is that of the man. In many of the cultures found in the Canadian setting, the status of a man is measured by his ability to be a progenitor, and his inability to be successful in that regard is considered a sign of personal failure. However, male infertility is not an uncommon phenomenon. Indeed, it is one of the major reasons why couples cannot have biological offspring of their own.[10]

As in the case of female infertility, it would strike the Association as inappropriate to pass judgment on culture-bound and personal values. As long as society accepts these values as legitimate, and as long as they are in keeping with the canons of medical ethics, the medical profession will accept them as they are relevant to the physician-patient relationship. The Canadian Medical Association, therefore, maintains that male infertility is an appropriate area of research and investigation, and that the male perspective on issues of infertility and reproductive technologies has an appropriate place in this discussion.

At the same time, the Association wishes to emphasize that, as in the case of a female perspective, although such views and perspectives have an appropriate place in the discussion of new reproductive technologies, they should not come to dominate the debate. There are other issues deserving of consideration. For example, men serve as gamete donors to a degree unparalleled by women. It strikes the Association that this role may well be a subject of investigation and standardization.

The Canadian Medical Association offers the following as a partial list of topics that this Commission might fruitfully consider under a male perspective:

- development and dissemination of information about the nature of, and reasons for, male infertility;
- development of standardized counselling services and of an informed consent process surrounding gamete donation;
- screening of gamete donors;[11]
- record-keeping;[12]
- clarification of the legal status of male gamete donors with respect to ownership of the gametes, rights of disposition and responsibilities;[13]
- clarification of the legal status of males involved in techniques of new reproductive technology;[14] and
- development and implementation of standardized counselling.[15, 16]

Society

A fourth perspective that should find consideration is that of society itself. Canada is a multicultural nation by history and by design. As such, it values the diversity of its various subcultures, it recognizes their importance to the make-up of the Canadian mosaic and cherishes their contribution to the richness and diversity of the nation as a whole.

This recognition and acceptance, however, does not come without a price. Each of the component subcultures has its own values and aspirations. Although innocent enough in the ordinary setting, and indeed something to be welcomed, this diversity presents special difficulties in the context of reproduction: difficulties that find their root in the distinct ways that the various cultures view reproduction itself. These distinct viewpoints must be balanced into an overall policy without being drowned in the sea of majority opinion. Only in that way will the character of Canada as a nation be preserved.

The social perspective must also reflect the unique nature of the partnership into which society enters with the medical profession and with the various sciences that are involved in the process of developing and applying the technologies themselves. It should view that process as a cooperative venture, rather than something that is controlled by the medical and scientific community.

The difficulty of reaching this goal is exacerbated by the fact that at present the distribution and strengths of these culturally determined values is not clear. There are few if any reliable data in this regard. In fact, not even the perspective of the Canadian majority, whether that be of the French- or of the English-speaking segment of the population, is understood in anything like a reliable fashion. To proceed appropriately and to do justice to all the views that go into shaping the Canadian societal perspective, these uncertainties will have to be remedied.

At the same time, a social perspective cannot exist in isolation from practical reality. The development of the new reproductive technologies has a financial component. In Canada, this development does not generally lie in private hands. It tends to take place in universities and hospitals. Both of these are dependent on societally generated funds, either directly through government grants or indirectly through various subsidies and funding mechanisms.

Because in Canada it is ultimately society that defrays most of the costs involved in the development of new reproductive technologies, it is legitimate that society should expect to have some input into the decision process about the nature of this development and that it should have some say over the direction that research and development should take.[17] To this end, the determination of societal opinion mentioned above might be a starting point.

However, the matter cannot be settled in this fashion. Society must do more than ask itself what it thinks about these issues when they are considered in isolation. It must also determine how it views the implications of, and the interrelations between, the various technologies. More specifically still, it must ask itself where, on balance, it stands with respect to the development and application of new reproductive stands vis-à-vis its other priorities. This is particularly important in the face of ever-increasing demands and a finite resource pool.

Furthermore, society cannot ignore the fact that once a technology has been developed, it is very difficult to interdict or even to limit its application. It is, therefore, legitimate for society to ask itself at the outset whether the development of these technologies is appropriate, or whether a different set of research priorities should prevail. It cannot afford to be trapped into a policy of development merely because the possibility exists.

The issue of resource allocation becomes even more important with respect to the application of the technologies. The required resources include not only materials but also personnel. In terms of personnel, there are two distinct parameters: education and manpower. On the level of education, society has to decide how many experts in the realm of new reproductive technology it considers to be necessary. This will assume increasing importance as fewer residency positions become available because of current funding cuts for obstetrical training.[18] Regional disparities in terms of practice patterns will also have to be addressed, and on a social scale. Society will have to decide how many technicians and support staff it is willing to fund in terms of actual service delivery, and how many clinics it is willing to fund to allow for service implementation. These considerations have to be balanced against each other and against an overall social goal of health care delivery.

Finally, the implications of the use this technology have repercussions on the very fabric of society. The perception of the social status of women and men, the definition of their roles within society, and the nature of their interrelationships as people are here at stake. The development of the new reproductive technologies presents the potential for divorcing the social destinies of both men and women from the dictates of their biology and of allowing an exploration of personal alternatives that would have a profound impact on the nature of social dynamics. Surrogate motherhood arrangements have excited public interest in this regard and have aroused public concern. The demand by homosexual couples for access to the techniques also has social implications, and may require a public process to determine the wishes of the community.[19] Single women who are not homosexual have also sought access to this technology.

Another reason for society's considerable interest in these matters is that the nature of the family unit is implicated. Anglo-American society has traditionally been predicated on the assumption that the nuclear family is the preferred and, indeed, normal type of familial relation.

The increasing representation of distinct cultures in the Canadian setting, already referred to above, and the growing awareness of different perspectives that are possible in this matter, have resulted in a re-examination of this assumption in the context of Canadian society. In fact, the Association feels that the Canadian perspective on this matter is in a process of evolution. The availability of the new technologies might well direct that process in important ways.

The Association believes that a whole host of issues should be examined from a societal perspective before any policy decisions are made in this arena: issues that also extend into the legal sphere. A partial list of the areas that deserve consideration includes such things as:[20]

- cultural variations in approaches to reproduction and the nature of personal choices that this entails;
- degree of socially guaranteed access to techniques of new reproductive technology;
- criteria for access to techniques of new reproductive technology;
- control of research on techniques of new reproductive technology;
- the balance that should be struck in matters of reproductive choice;
- establishment and enforcement of uniform standards of application of techniques of new reproductive technology on a national basis;

- clarification of the status of the human embryo;
- clarification of the legal status of children born as a result of techniques of reproductive technology;
- clarification of the legal definition of parenthood for those who have recourse to techniques of new reproductive technology;
- clarification of the legal status of parents understood in the terms of this new technology;
- enforceability of gestation contracts and the status of gestational as opposed to contractual and gamete mothers; and
- ownership of human gametes, zygotes and the right of disposition.

Despite the fact that this list is only partial, it will give some indication of the importance that the Association attaches to society's involvement in this arena.

NOTES

1. See CMA, *The New Reproductive Technologies* chapter III, "Artificial insemination," pp. 59-83.
2. See US Congress, Office of Technology Assessment: *Artificial Insemination: Practice in the United States: Summary of a 1987 Survey*, Washington, 1987. The Association benefitted from work done by several other organizations and bodies in developing its perspective. These include British Columbia: *Report of the Special Task Force Committee on Reproductive Technology of the British Columbia Branch, Canadian Bar Association*, June 1989; Ontario Law Reform Commission: *Report on Human Artificial Reproduction and Related Matters* (2 vols), Ministry of the Attorney General, Toronto, 1985; Saskatchewan: *Report on the New Reproductive Technologies to the Uniform Law Conference*, 1989; Australia, Family Law Council: *Creating Children: a Uniform Approach to the Law and Practice of Reproductive Technology in Australia*. Report of the Family Law Council incorporating and adopting the report of the Asche Committee on issues relating to AID, IVF, embryo transfer and related matters, 1985; New Zealand, Dept of Justice, Law Reform Division: *New Birth Technologies: An Issues Paper on AID, IVF, and Surrogate Motherhood*, 1985; Queensland: *Report of the Special Committee Appointed by the Queensland Government to Enquire into the Laws Relating to Artificial Insemination, In Vitro Fertilization and Other Related Matters*, 1984.
3. See ref. note 1 *ibid* pp. 109-116, 150-151, and Appendix, D. Rights of custody, control and disposition of gametes and embryos, and F. Parental status and family relationships.
4. See *ibid* Appendix, section F, for a discussion of some of the legal considerations involved.
5. See *ibid* pp. 76-84, 146, and Appendix, C. Record-keeping, sections on content of records, retention, confidentiality, and access, for further details of legal parameters that the Association believes are relevant in this regard.
6. See *ibid* pp. 68-70, 145-146.

7. See *ibid* pp. 77-78, 142-143, 146.
8. These should be offered in conjunction with appropriate counselling and gamete donor/recipient screening.
9. See *ibid* p. 20-21.
10. It is estimated that 16.67% of all couples are infertile, with male infertility accounting for about 40% of this infertility.
11. See *ibid* pp. 68-70, 145-146.
12. See *ibid* pp. 76-84, 143-145, 146.
13. See *ibid* Appendix, D. Rights of custody, control and disposition of gametes and embryos.
14. See *ibid* Appendix, F. Parental status and family relationships.
15. See *ibid* pp. 35, 88, 147-148.
16. The issue of male pregnancies has begun to surface in some of the more recent discussions. It is of interest because it goes straight to the heart of the philosophy of the new reproductive technologies. The Canadian Medical Association rejects the thesis that biology is destiny. That would condemn women to a biologically determined role just as much as it would condemn men to theirs. The Association also rejects the premise that what is not found in nature must be repudiated. That would mean that the practice of medicine itself would constitute an unacceptable interference in the natural course of events. The Association, therefore, finds itself unable to oppose as a matter of principle research into techniques of male pregnancy. However, the Association would suggest that this Commission should approach research into such matters with cxtreme caution, and that it should not allow itself to be lured into endorsing an undertaking merely because it is possible. The primary consideration in all aspects of human reproduction must always be the individual as a person.
17. See Québec, Ministère de la Santé et des Services sociaux: *Rapport du Comité de Travail sur les Nouvelles Technologies de Reproduction Humaine*, Québec, 1988: 92.
18. See Canada, Federal/Provincial Advisory Committee on Health Manpower: *Physician Manpower in Canada 1980-2000*, Ottawa, 1984; Wanatabe M (ed): *Physician Manpower in Canada,* Proceedings of the First and Second Annual ACMC Physician Manpower Conference, Association of Medical Colleges, Ottawa, 1988.
19. A British study indicates strong public rejection of this. See Walker A, Gregor S, McLaughlin E: Attitudes towards donor insemination — a post-Warnock survey. *Human Reproduction* 1987; 2: 745-750, which shows that 54% of those polled opposed AID for homosexual women and only 19% approved. In a US study of physicians' reasons for not accepting patients for AID, physicians gave no reason for rejecting 32% of applicants. In the context of that study (US Congress, Office of Technology Assessment, supra, note 2, Tables 2-5) it is possible to conjecture that homosexuality may have been a factor here as well.
20. See ref. note 1, Appendix, F. Parental status and family relationships.

FURTHER READINGS

Law Reform Commission of Ontario
"The Propriety of Artificial Conception Technologies," *Report on Artificial Human Reproduction.* (Ministry of the Attorney General, 1985), vol. 2, pp. 140-149.
Bayles, Michael D.
Reproductive Ethics. (Englewood Cliffs, N.J.: Prentice Hall, 1984).
Arras, J.D.
"HIV and Childbearing," *Milbank Memorial Quarterly* 68:3 (1990) 353-382.
Australia, Queensland
Report of the Special Committee Appointed by the Queensland Government to Enquire into the Laws Relating to Artificial Insemination, In Vitro Fertilization and Other Related Matters. (Brisbane, 1984).
Australia, Victoria, Committee to Consider Social, Ethical and Legal Issues Arising from In Vitro Fertilization
Report on the Disposition of Embryos Produced by In Vitro Fertilization. (Melbourne).
British Columbia Royal Commission on Family and Children's Law
Ninth Report of the Royal Commission on Family and Children's Law: Artificial Insemination. (Victoria: 1975).
Bryant, Heather
The Infertility Dilemma: Reproductive Technologies and Prevention. (Calgary: Canadian Advisory Council on the Status of Women, February, 1990) 4.
Cahill, Lisa Sowle
"Moral Tradition, Ethical Language, and Reproductive Technologies," *The Journal of Medicine and Philosophy.* 14: 5 (October, 1989) 497-522.
Ethical Considerations of the New Reproductive Technologies. A Report of the Combined Ethics Committee of the Canadian Fertility and Andrology Society and the Society of Obstetricians and Gynecologists of Canada (1990).
Gouvernement du Québec, Conseil du Statu de la Femme
General Opinion of the Conseil du Statu de la Femme in Regard to New Reproductive Technologies. (Quebec City, 1989).
Health and Welfare Canada
Report of the Advisory Committee on the Storage and Utilization of Human Sperm. (Ottawa: HWC, 1981).
Holmes, H., B. Hoskins and M. Gross
The Custom-Made Child: Woman-Centered Perspectives. (Clifton, NJ: Humana Press, 1981).
Lauritzen, Paul
"What Price Parenthood?" *Hastings Center Report* 20: 2 (March/April 1990) 38–46.
Law Reform Commission of Saskatchewan
Tentative Proposals for a Human Artificial Insemination Act. (Regina,1981).
Lenow, J.L.
"The Foetus as Patient: Emerging Rights as a Person?" *American Journal of Law and Medicine*, 9: 1 (Spring 1983), at 1-29.
Macklin, Ruth
"Artificial Means of Reproduction and our Understanding of the Family," *Hastings Center Report* 21:1 (1991) 5-11.

Ontario Law Reform Commission
Report on Human Artificial Reproduction and Related Matters (Toronto: Ministry of the Attorney General, 1985).
Report of the Commission of Enquiry of the German Bundestag, Prospects and Risks of Genetic Engineering, Parts I and II. (Deutscher Bundestag, 10. Wahlperiode: Bonn 1987; the so-called *Inquiry Commission*).
Rich, A.
Of Woman Born: Motherhood as Experiment and Institution. (New York, W.W. Norton and Co.: 1976).

CHAPTER 17 SURROGATE MOTHERHOOD

INTRODUCTION

In 1985, the Ontario Law Reform Commission defined surrogate motherhood as an arrangement involving a woman who is to bear the child and the persons who are to receive the child as their own. "...[T]he heart of any arrangement is a promise on the part of the surrogate mother to undergo the medical procedure necessary to achieve a pregnancy and to surrender custody of the child irrevocably upon birth, and a reciprocal promise on the part of the other party or parties to accept the child."[1] Since the time of the Commission's writing, reproductive technology has advanced both in its success-rates and in its sophistication. However, despite the technical advances, this definition still captures the essence of the matter. The only basic amendment one might add is that nowadays it is not necessarily correct to assume that the couple involved in the arrangement consists of a female and a male person — or indeed that the party who strikes the arrangement with the surrogate mother is a couple.

However, whatever the technical details, the idea of surrogacy raised and continues to raise several important ethical questions. For instance, should a woman have the right to bear a child for someone else, either for money or as a gesture of kindness and compassion? Does a pre-conception arrangement in which a woman undertakes to bear a child for someone else for a fee amount to "baby-selling?" Is entering into a pre-conception contract an ethically acceptable way of allowing others to have children — and for a woman to earn some money — or does it amount to a new form of servitude and degradation of the female person? Should the perspective of the people who seek a surrogacy arrangement predominate, or should surrogacy be evaluated from the perspective of the child? Should heterosexuality on the part of contracting parents be a requirement for surrogacy arrangements, or does the sexual orientation of the prospective parents matter? In fact, does it matter whether it is one person who seeks to become a parent by this means, especially in view of the evolution of the single-parent family?

Some of these issues are addressed in the selections below. The Law Reform Commission of Ontario was one of the first Canadian bodies to consider the issue. Its two-volume Report is still one of the classic discussions in the area. The Commission recommended legalization of surrogacy contracts, but under judicial supervision. The Commission also recommended that surrogacy contracts should be enforceable against the surrogate mother even if the surrogate mother changes her mind upon the birth of the child.

The Canadian Medical Association begins its discussion by distinguishing between surrogate mothers and gestational mothers. It understands the term "surrogate mother" as meaning a woman who agrees to bear a child where the ovum involved in the pregnancy is her own ovum, whereas it uses the term "gestational mother" to refer to a woman who has no genetic link to the child that will be borne. The Association suggests that there are important ethical and psychological differences between the two cases, and they should not be confused. However, the Association also maintains that surrogate motherhood should not be criminalized, but regulated. The right to act as surrogate or a gestational mother should be seen as an expression of the right of self-determination of a woman over her own body. However, to prevent abuses, surrogacy contracts should be subject to judicial review before their inception.

The positions of the Law Reform Commission of Ontario and of the Canadian Medical Association stand in opposition to the considerations and recommendations of the Council on the Status of Women of the Province of Quebec. The Council sees surrogacy as an unethical undertaking that involves a serious infringement of a woman's rights, and that leads to a dissociation of genetic and uterine bonds between women and their children. It recommends that preconception contracts be criminalized.

NOTE

1. Ontario Law Reform Commission, *Report on Human Artificial Reproduction and Related Matters*, 2 vols, (Toronto: Ministry of the Attorney General, 1985), vol 2, pp. 218-19.

The Surrogate Mother

Law Reform Commission of Ontario

THE SURROGATE MOTHER

Judicial approval of prospective surrogate mothers prior to performance of the artificial conception procedure is, in our view, absolutely crucial to the protection of the unborn child, the prospective parents, and indeed, the surrogate mother herself.

As far as the unborn child is concerned, whether the surrogate mother is to gestate an ovum supplied by another or her own fertilized ovum, her physical and mental state, both before and during pregnancy, will affect the health of the fetus. Where she is the genetic mother, her greater contribution to the child's development will increase the importance of assuring her health and, in particular, the absence of any deleterious genetically transmissible condition.

From the perspective of the social parents, the physical and mental state of the surrogate mother is important not only because it bears upon the health of the child whom they will raise, but because it affects whether she will be conscientious in adhering to her agreement. A prospective surrogate mother should appreciate fully the nature of the obligations she has undertaken so that her cooperation will be assured when it is time to transfer custody of the infant.

Judicial approval of the surrogate mother may also be of importance to the woman herself. Certain physical and psychological risks would appear to be associated with participating as a surrogate mother. The physical risks are those usually attendant upon pregnancy, which may involve various complications and may even have a long-term effect on a woman's health. While there have been no studies of psychological risks associated with the transfer of the newborn infant, this possibility must be acknowledged. Because of these risks, it would be advisable to exclude from participation in surrogate motherhood arrangements women who are demonstrably unsuited to the role, either because they are patently maladjusted or unstable, or because they clearly do not appreciate the nature of surrogate motherhood.

For these reasons, we recommend that, on the hearing of the application for approval of a surrogate motherhood arrangement, the court should be required to assess the suitability of the prospective surrogate mother.

We turn now to consider first, whether there should be any limits on eligibility to become a surrogate mother and, secondly, the criteria for assessment of prospective surrogate mothers.

a. Eligibility to Act as a Surrogate Mother

It has been suggested that the opportunity to participate as a surrogate mother should be restricted to certain categories of women. It has been argued, for example, that such participation should be limited to women who already have given birth to children, because only they can truly appreciate the

Law Reform Commission of Ontario, "The Surrogate Mother," *Report on Artificial Human Reproduction*. (Ministry of the Attorney General, 1985) pp. 239-260.

risks associated with pregnancy and the implications of surrendering a child upon birth. Alternatively, it has been said that women with children in their care should not be allowed to be surrogate mothers because these children may be traumatized upon surrender of the infant, fearing that they too will be given away. In addition, some commentators have suggested that married women are to be preferred, in the expectation that their husbands will be bulwarks of emotional support; others have taken an opposite view, in the belief that husbands will be potential sources of conflict.

We consider that there is no theoretical or empirical basis upon which to adopt a categorical approach to the eligibility of women to serve as surrogate mothers. This conclusion is, however, subject to a single exception. Under no circumstances whatsoever do we believe that a minor should be permitted to participate in a surrogate motherhood arrangement as a surrogate mother.

Earlier, we recommended that legal minors should be prohibited from acting as ovum donors because of the surgical risks involved and concerns about the genuineness of their consent.[347] In addition, in the case of *in vivo* fertilization and lavage, we were concerned that the ovum donor might become pregnant through the failure of the lavage technique. Similar concerns animate our rejection of minors becoming surrogate mothers. While this view may appear harsh in circumstances where, for example, a mature seventeen year old wishes to assist a close relative, we believe strongly that minors should not be exposed to the risks attendant upon surrogate motherhood.

It should be noted that, in order to prevent minors from applying for approval as surrogate mothers, it will be necessary to enact specific legislation. Pursuant to the regulations made under the *Public Hospitals Act,*[348] persons aged sixteen or over are legally competent to give autonomous consent to medical care;[349] accordingly, a minor could present herself for an artificial conception procedure.

Accordingly, we recommend that there should be no restriction on the eligibility of women to serve as surrogate mothers, so long as they have reached the age of majority at the date of the application for court approval of their participation in a surrogate motherhood arrangement.[350]

b. Assessment of Prospective Surrogate Mothers

Not surprisingly, there is virtually no scholarly writing about the qualities that are desirable in a surrogate mother. Reflecting the lack of experience with this phenomenon, empirical study of applicants and their motivations remains in a nascent stage of development.[351] Notwithstanding the absence of scientific guidance, we have confidence that this assessment can be left to the court, with its attention being directed to certain factors that, in our view, deserve special consideration.

We believe that the court should assess the physical and mental health of the prospective surrogate mother. It is envisaged that evidence respecting her condition, consisting, for example, of reports by doctors, psychologists, or other professionals, will be submitted by counsel for the prospective parents or by her own counsel.[352] Should the information appear incomplete, the court simply could withhold approval of the agreement until further satisfactory evidence is adduced.

Apart from considering the physical and mental state of the woman, the court should consider other matters, which may appear less obviously relevant. We believe that, where prospective surrogate mothers have partners in marital or nonmarital unions, the disposition of these partners to their participation in surrogate motherhood arrangements should be a factor to consider.[353] Where a partner is opposed to her participation, this may augur badly for the woman's state of mind during the pregnancy. This, in turn, may be harmful to the fetus and deleterious to the stability of the surrogate mother's family.

A further factor that should be considered is the effect of the arrangement on the children of the surrogate mother. If there are indications that they might be psychologically harmed by her participation and, in particular, by the planned transfer of custody, a court should not approve her involvement. It would be unconscionable to sacrifice knowingly the emotional stability of an otherwise secure child in the interests of creating another child.

We therefore recommend that, in assessing the suitability of a prospective surrogate mother, the court should consider, among other factors, her physical and mental health, her marital and domestic circumstances, the opinion of her spouse or partner, if any, and the likely effects of her participation in a surrogate motherhood arrangement upon existing children under her care.

THE COURT

For reasons discussed earlier,[354] we believe that the court should have the crucial responsibility for assessing the suitability of participants in a surrogate motherhood arrangement. While the role that we have assigned to the court may appear roughly similar to that of the court in the context of adoption, in fact the responsibility would differ substantially. In adoption, whether by a stranger or by a step-parent or close relative, the court gives legal finality to the relationship between the child and his or her new family *after* the child has been placed in the home. Moreover, even in the case of a stranger adoption, the court does not engage in detailed prior scrutiny of the prospective parent; that task is undertaken by social workers acting under the auspices of a children's aid society, a private adoption agency, or a licensed individual. Under our proposed scheme, by contrast, the court is to make the critical assessment before any action is taken lawfully to alter the *status quo*.

Notwithstanding this difference, we envisage that the general configuration of the hearing will be similar to adoption, in the sense that the proceedings will be non-adversarial in character. We anticipate that the parties represented will be the prospective social parents, the prospective surrogate mother and, as we shall explain shortly, [355] possibly a children's aid society...

b. The Prospective Surrogate Mother as a Co-Applicant

We have already discussed the importance of approving the participation of the prospective surrogate mother and the test for assessing her suitability.[358] Ancillary procedural issues relate to whether the surrogate mother should be a co-applicant in the proceeding, along with the prospective parents, and whether she should be required to attend the proceedings.

With respect to the first issue, the status of a surrogate mother as a co-applicant is necessary if the court order is to be binding on her. With respect to the second issue, the attendance of the prospective surrogate mother at the hearing would appear desirable as a matter of principle. It would allow the court better to consider her suitability and to ascertain her understanding of her contractual commitment. In particular, the court could attempt to determine whether she has received independent legal advice and counselling by professionals unconnected to the prospective social parents.

Requiring the attendance of the prospective surrogate mother at the hearing of the application, however, might involve her meeting the prospective social parents. Where both parties prefer that they should be unknown to each other, such a requirement would defeat their intentions. We see no reason to recommend a measure that might frustrate the legitimate wishes of the parties.

From our survey of the relevant literature, it is apparent that persons in the United States involved in these agreements choose various arrangements, depending on their individual and mutual preferences. While some agreements may involve disclosure of identity and personal meetings between the parties, others are negotiated and implemented in circumstances of mutual anonymity.

Based on the available literature, there is at present no basis for proposing normative guidelines concerning the nature of the relationship of the parties to a surrogate motherhood arrangement. We prefer to remain silent on this matter, allowing the parties and their lawyers to make their own determinations of what best suits their needs. Thus, while we are of the view that prospective surrogate mothers should be co-applicants in the proceedings, we do not wish to compel their attendance at the hearing as a rule. Should the court wish to receive testimony from the surrogate mother or to observe her in person, it could request her attendance and provide that the prospective social parents be absent.

We do wish, however, to emphasize the necessity of the prospective surrogate mother receiving separate legal representation at the hearing. Separate representation will accord a measure of protection to the surrogate mother and lessen the danger of exploitation, which justifiably has concerned those critical of unregulated surrogate motherhood arrangements.

Accordingly, we recommend that the surrogate mother should be a co-applicant in the proceedings, but that she should not be required to be in attendance at the hearing of the application in every case. We recommend also that the surrogate mother should receive separate legal representation.

c. Blood, Tissue and Other Testing of Parentage

Upon the birth of a child following judicial approval of a surrogate motherhood agreement, a question may be raised concerning whether the child is in fact the product of that arrangement. The biological paternity of the child may be contested by a prospective social father if the child is found to be affected by a genetic defect, or if his wife wants assurance that it is his child whom she is to be legally responsible for rearing. Similarly, a surrogate mother, perhaps seeking to resist surrender of the child, may deny the paternity of the prospective social father.

This issue would appear to be of special concern where a prospective surrogate mother is cohabiting with a husband or male partner. In such a case, the prospective parents will want assurance that the child has developed from the sperm of the social father or, where donated semen is used, from the sperm of the carefully selected, screened, and matched donor, and not from that of the surrogate mother's husband or partner. Accordingly, the surrogate mother will usually be asked to give undertakings that sexual relations will be avoided at the time of insemination, in order to ensure that the sperm then used will account for any pregnancy that ensues.

The issue could also arise, although much less frequently of course, in the context of a maternity dispute, where, for example, a donated ovum is used. Indeed, the ovum might be donated by the prospective social mother.

Disputes respecting the parentage of a child, which will be accompanied inevitably by disagreements over custody, obviously are detrimental to all concerned, especially the child, whose parentage and future will be cast in doubt.

Scientific means are available to avoid unnecessary disputes about parentage. Blood tests, tissue tests and similar methods of genetic diagnosis may establish the child's biological parents with reliable accuracy.[359] Acquisition of blood or tissues for such a diagnosis from the surrogate mother and the prospective social parents should cause no special problem, since the physicians involved would be expected to establish their respective blood groups and similar characteristics. Where anonymous donor gametes are used, the gametes may be required to carry documented information of the donor's blood group and similar biological status. Conscientious screening of donors should make the data readily available.

A disadvantage of testing is that it may require a newborn child to suffer blood-drawing or a biopsy. The risk and discomfort of these procedures are normally considered acceptable.[360] Moreover, it should be emphasized that the *Children's Law Reform Act*[361] permits blood testing of infants.

We believe that the available technology should be used to avoid, or at least reduce, unnecessary uncertainty respecting the parentage of a child, and to limit the opportunity of a surrogate mother to refuse to surrender the child on the ground that it is not the child of the approved arrangement. As the testing of children and adults to determine parentage after birth is permitted now under the *Children's Law Reform Act,* there is no need for specific legislation to address this matter. In order to require that the blood groups and other relevant biological characteristics of the adults involved — the surrogate mother, her husband or male partner, if any, and the persons who produced the gametes involved — are reliably and accessibly recorded prior to birth, legislation would have to be enacted.[362]

We believe that the responsibility for ensuring that this information is compiled should rest with the court as part of its supervisory function. Accordingly, we recommend that, in order to minimize uncertainty concerning a child's parentage upon birth, prior to the approval of a surrogate motherhood arrangement the court should require to be placed before it information relating to blood type and other relevant biological characteristics of the surrogate mother, her husband or partner, if any, and the persons who produced the gametes involved.

d. Participation of the Children's Aid Society

While we have recommended that the important responsibility for vetting prospective parties be assigned to the court, we believe that children's aid societies may play a useful role in the process. We have indicated already that the hearing of the application will be non-adversarial in nature, since the interests of the prospective parents and the surrogate mother will coincide. Neither party will have an interest in adducing evidence tending to demonstrate the unsuitability of the other. We believe, therefore, that there is good reason to provide for the involvement of a reliable source of information independent of the parties, whose participation can avoid the approval of the patently unsuitable.

In our view, children's aid societies are well suited to undertake this responsibility. We should emphasize, however, that we do not favour involvement similar to that in the context of stranger adoption, where a homestudy of the prospective parents is required in every case. Rather, we believe that children's aid societies should have standing to intervene in the proceedings only where their records disclose information demonstrating the unsuitability of either the surrogate mother or the prospective parents for participation in the proposed arrangement. Where the information available does not disclose any reason to be concerned about the parties, participation in the proceedings would not be necessary.

We realize that the introduction of this additional precaution may cause some discomfort to the parties, whose confidentiality will be compromised through the unavoidable disclosure of their identities to a children's aid society.[363] One response to concerns about the disclosure of parties' planned participation in a surrogate motherhood arrangement is that the staff of children's aid societies do observe proper confidentiality. In our view, however, the decisive consideration is that the applicants are seeking judicial approval of an arrangement that will culminate in the birth of a child, whose best interests are the overriding factor. To that factor, all others are subordinate, including concerns about possible embarrassment or vulnerability attendant upon revelation of admittedly sensitive information.

Accordingly, we recommend that notice of an application to the court for approval of a surrogate motherhood arrangement should be served upon the appropriate children's aid society, and that the society should have standing to attend at the hearing of the application. However, a children's aid society should intervene only where its records disclose information demonstrating the unsuitability of either the surrogate mother or the prospective social parents for participation in the surrogate motherhood arrangement.

TERMS OF THE AGREEMENT

In this section, we turn to discuss whether our legislative scheme should require that specific matters be addressed in every surrogate motherhood agreement. In the course of reviewing the literature, it soon became evident that certain difficult issues were seen as more important, and capable of having a substantial impact on the persons affected. This led to the question whether these issues should be determined by legislation or whether the court, in approving the agreement, should be required to ensure that they have been confronted and resolved satisfactorily by the parties. As will be apparent from the following discussion, we are of the view that certain issues are so important that they should be addressed by legislation, rather than being left to be resolved by the parties.

In the ensuing discussion, we shall consider four of the most contentious issues — the surrender of the child, the question of payment to the surrogate mother, the possibility of a handicapped child, and the possibility of an abortion by the surrogate mother. We then shall review briefly a list of certain issues that, we believe, the parties to a surrogate motherhood agreement should be required to consider and resolve.

a. Surrender of the Child

Perhaps the most difficult issue that we have addressed in designing an appropriate regulatory scheme is whether, upon birth of the child, the surrogate mother should be under a legal compulsion to surrender the child in accordance with her promise to do so under the surrogate motherhood agreement. In its most stark incarnation, this question reduces to whether, in the face of a refusal by the woman to transfer custody of the newborn infant, a court should be obliged to issue an order to surrender the infant, which could be enforced against her will by seizure of the child.

Without elaborate discussion, it should be obvious that this is one of the most emotionally charged issues involved in surrogate motherhood. That a recalcitrant surrogate mother might be compelled through judicial process to surrender her newborn infant would seem to strike at the very heart of our shared values. For some, this possibility confirms the "unnaturalness" of this reproductive alternative.

We are acutely aware of the necessity of resolving this difficult and controversial issue if the parties to these arrangements, and through them the affected children, are to avoid uncertainty and conflict upon the birth of the child. In striving to arrive at the appropriate solution, we sought guidance in two distinct areas of the law.

First, we turned to contract law and, in particular, the law respecting specific performance. While we have yet to use this term in discussing the issue, the question can be cast in terms of whether the promise of the surrogate mother ought to be specifically enforceable. Although it may appear inappropriate to consider a problem respecting children by reference to contract law, it is useful to do so for analytical purposes.

Speaking generally, specific enforcement of a contract is a remedy available only where monetary compensation is inadequate.[368] For example, a strong argument can be made for specific performance if the contract concerns something that is unique, making it extremely difficult to assess the loss for which monetary compensation otherwise would be given. It also has been established that contracts for personal services are not specifically enforceable, in part because the courts cannot supervise the quality of the service to be rendered.

Applying these principles to a surrogate motherhood agreement, one might well argue that specific performance would be an appropriate remedy in the face of a refusal to surrender the child. Certainly the subject matter of the agreement is unique, and monetary compensation would not replace the loss to the social parents. And, while the entire surrogate motherhood agreement might be regarded as a contract for personal services, the enforcement of which would require judicial supervision — particularly in relation to a promise by the surrogate mother to maintain her health during pregnancy — the promise to transfer the child involves a discrete act that would not necessitate supervision.

While contractual principles may be applied for purposes of analysis, it bears emphasizing that, under the present law, these principles clearly are regarded as inappropriate for resolving disputes concerning the future of children. In an analogous context, the *Family Law Reform Act*[369] provides that "[i]n the determination of any matter respecting the support, education, moral training or custody of or access to a child, the court may disregard any provision of a domestic contract pertaining thereto where, in the opinion of the court, to do so is in the best interests of the child". This provision expressly requires the court to consider a principle — the best interests of the child — that is separate from, and superior to, the intentions evinced in the agreement. In deferring to this principle, the court is undertaking an inquiry very different from that undertaken in dealing with a commercial transaction.

For example, in a custody dispute, where custody is awarded to the parent who has been given custody under a separation agreement, the court is not truly enforcing the agreement. The agreement, along with various other factors, may be relevant to the court's view of the best interests of the child, but the contractual resolution of custody in no way circumscribes judicial discretion respecting this matter.

The other relevant area of the law that we have considered concerns adoption. Under the *Child Welfare Act,*[370] an adoption order can be made only with the written consent of both parents or the persons having lawful custody and control of the child,[371] except where the court has dispensed with this requirement.[372] Consent, however, cannot be given until after the child is seven days old.[373] Furthermore, any person who has given his or her consent can withdraw it as of right within twenty-one days after it has been given.[374] These measures recognize the importance and potentially traumatic nature of the decision to consent to adoption, and appear intended to ensure that the consent is in fact genuine and continuing. This is most evident in the limitation respecting consent to the adoption of newborn infants, which seeks to protect women in the particularly emotionally vulnerable period shortly after childbirth.

These two areas of the law suggest the only alternative resolutions to the question of surrender. Either the regulatory scheme should provide that the surrogate mother must honour her promise and surrender the child after birth, irrespective of any attitudinal change on her part in the intervening period, or the surrogate mother should be given a right, in effect, to rescind the agreement unilaterally within a period after birth. In the first case, the risk of disappointment and trauma rests on the surrogate mother, while, in the second, it is placed on the social parents.

The crucial question, however, is not where the risk of disappointment should lie, but which resolution will serve the best interests of the child. Unfortunately, the available scientific literature would appear to indicate no clear answer to this question. However, the Advisory Board that assisted the Commission, which included a child psychiatrist and a social worker, favoured requiring immediate surrender of the child to the approved social parents. It was thought that immediate surrender would serve to prevent bonding with the surrogate mother and to facilitate bonding with the person — the social mother — who, in the vast majority of cases, would be the ultimate recipient of the child and who, therefore, would be the primary influence in its life during the neonatal period and infancy.

We have been persuaded that, on balance, the legislation should provide for immediate surrender of the child. Hence, where a surrogate mother refuses to transfer custody, she could be compelled to do so by court order.

It may seem harsh and unfeeling to countenance a situation where, in the face of continuing recalcitrance, officers may be ordered to deliver the infant to the social parents. Yet physical seizure of a child may be effected under the present law in the context of a dispute over custody.[375] Further, there are judicial statements that infants may be taken from their mothers on birth by children's aid society workers where there has been a judicial finding that they are in need of protection.[376]

Accordingly, we recommend that a child born pursuant to an approved surrogate motherhood arrangement should be surrendered immediately upon birth to the social parents. Where a surrogate mother refuses to transfer the child, the court should order that the child be delivered to the social parents. In addition, where the court is satisfied that the surrogate mother intends to refuse to surrender the child upon birth, the court, prior to the birth of the child, should be empowered to make an order for transfer of custody upon birth.

Before leaving this issue, we wish to address a potential problem. In rare cases, in the intervening period between the judicial approval of the agreement and the birth of the child, circumstances may so change as to render undesirable the surrender of custody to the approved parents. While certain reasons why the social parents may become unsuitable to accept the child may be anticipated in the surrogate motherhood agreement, an event may occur that is beyond the reasonable expectations of the parties. Alternatively, information that was not available at the original hearing may come to light, indicating that the social parents are unsuitable. An extreme example might be the conviction of a social parent for commission of a serious offence, such as sexual assault of a child.

While the local children's aid society may intervene upon receiving credible evidence that the child would be in need of protection if delivered to the approved parents, we do not believe that the basis for preventing transfer should be restricted to the circumstances set out in the *Child Welfare Act*. In our view, it would be preferable to allow the surrogate mother, who presumably will have an interest in the welfare of the child, to apply to the court for a review of the approval of the arrangement, where circumstances indicate that the social parents are unsuitable to receive the child. In addition, where, subsequent to the approval of the surrogate motherhood arrangement, the children's aid society receives information indicating that the social parents are unsuitable, the children's aid society should be entitled to apply to the court for a review of the arrangement. On the hearing of the application, the court should be able to rescind the agreement even where the child would not be "a child in need of protection" within the meaning of the *Child Welfare Act*.[377] The custody of the child might be sought by the surrogate mother or by the local children's aid society.

Such a scheme would ensure that the welfare of the child is not sacrificed in the interests of certainty in the rare case where it becomes apparent that the social parents should not receive the child. Whatever dislocation necessarily is entailed in this position is preferable to placing the child at risk.

Accordingly, we recommend that, where there has been a change in circumstances, or where new information has become available, indicating that the approved social parents are unsuitable to receive the child, the surrogate mother or the children's aid society should be permitted to apply, at any time prior to the birth of the child, for a review of the approval of the surrogate motherhood arrangement. The judge should be empowered to rescind the agreement.

b. Payment to the Surrogate Mother

Among the most contentious issues that have arisen in connection with surrogate motherhood is that of payment to the surrogate mother by the persons to whom she will transfer custody of the child. As we have indicated,[378] the matter of payments has been the focus of much of the criticism of surrogate motherhood arrangements. Indeed, most arguments concerning the ethical impropriety of these arrangements are premised on the commercialization of the practice through the payment of a fee to the surrogate mother. Concerns have been expressed about the possibility of exploitation of disadvantaged women by the more affluent, and the dehumanization and debasement of both the surrogate mother and the child attendant upon payment for gestation and relinquishment of custody.[379]

In the course of our deliberations, we have considered four categories of payment. The first relates to the payment of a fee in the way of profit to the surrogate mother for her participation in the arrangement. Whether this fee is characterized as payment for a child, or merely as payment for services,[380] it is this controversial payment that raises the spectre of "baby-buying" and exploitation.

A second category of payment relates to the expenses incurred by the surrogate mother in the course of the arrangement. Our recommendation that the surrogate mother retain independent counsel necessarily will involve legal costs. In addition, a variety of medical and other expenses will be incurred. These will relate, for example, to medical screening and to the production of psychiatric, psychological, and social worker reports for submission to the court in relation to the assessment of the surrogate mother's suitability. Further costs will be incurred during pregnancy, relating to continuing medical supervision and maintenance of a sound diet. Finally, costs will be incurred in delivery and postnatal care, including counselling services for the mother. While the Ontario Health Insurance Plan may be expected to meet many of these costs, not all payments for services agreed between the mother and the social parents may be reimbursed by the Plan, and not all services may be conveniently available through medical practitioners who practice under the Plan or whose bills are limited to Plan fee schedules.

A third category of payment that has been suggested is payment for lost income and lost earning opportunities during the course of the pregnancy and the postpartum recuperative period. A fourth type of payment relates to compensation for pain and suffering, including, perhaps, postpartum grief for loss of the child.

All members of the Commission agree that no payment should be made in relation to a surrogate motherhood arrangement without the approval of the court. However, we are divided on which items of payment should be permitted by the legislation and the degree of discretion to be given the court.

One view is that the issue of payment should be left entirely to the court, without any legislative guidance as to which payments are to be permissible. A second view is that the court should be given a general power to approve payments, and should be expressly instructed that this power may extend, but is not limited, to payments for medical and similar costs, related out-of-pocket expenses, and lost income or earning opportunities. A third view is that the power of the court to approve payment should be confined to specified items only; however, there is a division respecting the items for which payment may be made. One Commissioner favours allowing the court to approve payments for medical and similar costs, related out-of-pocket expenses, and lost income or earning opportunities; the other[381] would restrict the list of items to medical and similar costs and related out-of-pocket expenses.

Notwithstanding this divergence of views, it bears emphasizing that we are in agreement respecting the fundamental principle that all payments relating to a surrogate motherhood agreement must receive the prior approval of the court. We believe that mandatory judicial control over payments is an effective answer to the concerns that have been voiced in connection with payment of the surrogate mother. In particular, we are of the view that this prophylactic measure will reveal any financial exploitation of a surrogate mother by the prospective social parents. Accordingly, we recommend that legislation should provide that no payment may be made in relation to a surrogate motherhood arrangement without the prior approval of the court.

NOTES

347. See *supra,* this ch., sec. 3(c)(ii).
348. *Supra,* note 165.
349. R.R.O. 1980, Reg. 865, ss. 50 and 51.
350. Dr. H. Allan Leal, O.C., Q.C., Vice Chairman of the Commission, dissents from the recommendation in favour of regulating surrogate motherhood arrangements: see Vice Chairman's Dissent, at page 287 of this Report. However, if such a procedure were adopted, Dr. Leal would require that surrogate mothers be married women or widows who have reached the age of majority and have had a child.
351. See Parker, "Motivation of Surrogate Mothers: Initial Findings" (1983), 140 Am. J. Psychiatry 170.
352. See *infra,* this ch., sec. 5(e)(iii)b.
353. See Parker, *supra,* note 351, and Parker, "Surrogate Motherhood: The Interaction of Litigation, Legislation and Psychiatry" (1982), 5 Int'l J. L. & Psychiatry 341.
358. See *supra,* this ch, sec. 5(e)(ii).
359. For a discussion of the efficacy of Human Leucocyte Antigen (H.L.A.) blood tissue testing, see Shaw and Kass, "Illegitimacy, Child Support and Paternity Testing" (1975), 13 Houston L. Rev. 41, and Lee, "Current Status of Paternity Testing" (1975), 9 Family L.Q. 615.
360. See *S. v. McC; W. v. W.,* [1972] A.C. 24 (H.L.).
361. *Supra,* note 122, s. 10.
362. Section 10(1) of the *Children's Law Reform Act, supra,* note 122, provides that, "[u]pon the application of a party in a civil proceeding in which the court is called upon to determine the parentage of a child, the court may give the party leave to obtain blood tests of such persons as are named in the order granting leave and to submit the results in evidence". This provision would allow blood testing to determine parentage only after the birth of a child. Our concern is to ensure that information pertaining to parentage is available prior to the birth of a child pursuant to a surrogate motherhood arrangement in order to avoid a parentage dispute or, where a dispute nonetheless occurs, to expedite its resolution.
363. Where, for example, a party is a member of the Roman Catholic community of Toronto, Hamilton or Windsor, the local Catholic Children's Aid Society will become involved. In view of the position of the Roman Catholic Church in relation to the artificial conception technologies and surrogate motherhood, this discomfort may be significant.
368. See, generally, Sharpe, *Injunctions and Specific Performance* (1983), and Waddams, *The Law of Contracts* (2d ed., 1984), at 507-27.
369. *Supra,* note 127, s. 55(1).
370. *Supra,* note 41.

371. *Ibid.*, s. 69(2). See the *Child and Family Services Act, 1984, supra,* note 41, s. 131(2).

372. *Child Welfare Act, supra,* note 41, s. 69(7). See the *Child and Family Services Act, 1984, supra,* note 41, s. 132.

373. *Child Welfare Act, supra,* note 41, s. 69(2). See the *Child and Family Services Act, 1984, supra,* note 41, s. 131(3).

374. *Child Welfare Act, supra,* note 41, s. 69(2). See the *Child and Family Services Act, 1984, supra,* note 41, s. 131(8).

375. Section 37(2) of the *Children's Law Reform Act, supra,* note 122, which deals with the enforcement of orders for custody and access, provides that, where a court is satisfied that there are reasonable and probable grounds for believing, *inter alia,* that any person is unlawfully withholding a child from a person entitled to custody of or access to the child, it may by order "direct the sheriff or a police force, or both ... to locate, apprehend and deliver the child to the person named in the order". Section 37(4) provides that, if such a direction is given, the "sheriff or police force ... shall do all things reasonably able to be done to locate, apprehend and deliver the child in accordance with the order". Section 37(5) provides further, that, for the purpose of locating and apprehending a child in accordance with an order under s. 37(2), "a sheriff or a member of a police force may enter and search any place where he has reasonable and probable grounds for believing that the child may be with such assistance and such force as are reasonable in the circumstances".

376. See *Re Children's Aid Society for the District of Kenora and J.L.* (1981), 134 D.L.R. (3d) 249 (Ont. Prov. Ct. (F.D.)) (*obiter dicta*), cited with approval in *Re Superintendent of Family and Child Service and McDonald* (1982), 37 B.C.L.R. 32, 135 D.L.R. (3d) 330 (S.C.).

377. *Supra,* note 41, s. 19(1)(b). The definition of "child in need of protection" has been revised in the new *Child and Family Services Act, 1984, supra,* note 41, s. 37(2).

378. See *supra,* this ch., sec. 5(b).

379. See discussion, *supra,* this ch., sec. 5(c).

380. See, for example, Note, "Surrogate Mothers: The Legal Issues" (1981), 7 Am. J. L. & Med. 323, at 331, and Keane, "Legal Problems of Surrogate Motherhood", [1980] S. Ill. U.L.J. 147, at 157-58.

381. Dr. H. Allan Leal, O.C., Q.C., Vice Chairman of the Commission, dissents from the recommendation in favour of regulating surrogate motherhood arrangements: see Vice Chairman's Dissent, at page 287 of this Report. However, if such a procedure were adopted, Dr. Leal would require that no payments be made to a surrogate mother without the prior approval of the court, and would limit the items for which payment may be made to medical and similar costs and related out-of-pocket expenses.

Surrogate and Gestational Motherhood

Canadian Medical Association

The terms "surrogate" and "gestational" motherhood refer to the practice where a woman volunteers to bear a child on the explicit understanding that once the child is born, she will relinquish her rights and responsibilities with respect to the rearing of that child to a second party, where that second party then assumes the status of legal parent to the child. This arrangement may be informal or it may be formalized in terms of a contractual agreement. In some instances, payment is made to the gestator for the services rendered; in other cases, no payment or consideration is involved.

As was noted before, there are several ways in which the phrase "surrogate mother" can be understood. In the most simple case, the so-called surrogate mother is artificially inseminated with the sperm of the male partner of the couple with whom the woman has struck the arrangement, and the ovum involved is her own. Variations include the fertilization of the woman's ovum in vitro with the sperm of the male partner of the couple or of a donor, and placement of the fertilized ovum into her uterus. ZIFT and TET are still further variations.[168]

On the other hand, a woman may agree to bear a child for another person or group of people, but the ovum involved may not be that of the woman herself. Here again, several variations are possible. For example, the ovum may be that of the woman who has arranged to raise the child. Alternatively, the ovum may be one that has been donated. Of course the various methods of ovum/zygote recovery and transfer referred to a moment ago may also be involved, as may ZIFT, TET and similar techniques.[169] Finally, in vivo fertilization in the woman who will ultimately be the social mother of the child, followed by lavage and implantation in the gestational mother, is also a possibility.

Both the concept of surrogacy and the concept of gestational motherhood have been criticized from several perspectives. One concern centres around the claim that when financial considerations are introduced into the notion of child-bearing for others, the practice amounts to a modern version of commerce in human beings.[170] Another concern is that both undertakings represent a threat to the nuclear family, which is the backbone of Western culture.[171] Some commentators have maintained that the consequences of these practices for women and women's relationship to their corporal autonomy, maternity and children is devastating,[172] and they have portrayed the practices as demeaning to women by turning them into walking incubators. The possibility has even been raised that surrogacy and gestational motherhood, if allowed, would prey on socioeconomically underprivileged women and lead to the development of two female classes: those who bear children, and those who can afford to raise them.[173]

Almost all jurisdictions in the world have begun to examine the issue. British Columbia, Ontario and Quebec have considered it already, as have several professional organizations.[174] Not all of the bodies who have considered the matter have

The Canadian Medical Association, "Surrogate Motherhood," from *The New Reproductive Technologies: A Preliminary Perspective of the Canadian Medical Association*. (Ottawa: Canadian Medical Association, 1991).

agreed. In Canada, the Ontario Law Reform Commission has recommended acceptance and legal recognition of surrogate motherhood arrangements, subject to certain conditions;[175] the Quebec Bar Association has suggested that surrogacy agreements should be banned altogether;[176] the British Columbia Bar Association has recommended that they should be permitted, but regulated.[177] In Great Britain, the Warnock Commission recommended rejection.[178] The Glover Report of the European Commission recommends acceptance, but control.[179] The American College of Obstetricians and Gynaecologists has expressed "significant reservations about this approach to parenthood," but has left its members free to decide whether to participate in such arrangements.[180] The American Medical Association has rejected it,[181] the Society of Obstetricians and Gynaecologists of Canada allows it at least in a research context under strictly monitored guidelines.[182]

The fact that there are a variety of opinions is not surprising. Surrogate motherhood presents many social, legal and ethical questions. Implicated are issues of legitimacy and economic coercion, the relationship between genetic parents and their offspring, autonomy, children as objects and so on. Given the differences in professional, legal and cultural perspective from which the issue has been approached, it would be surprising if there were unanimity, or even general agreement.

The Association cannot mention, let alone deal with, all of the issues that are raised by the topic. It has raised the issue because surrogate motherhood brings together several fundamental questions that are central to having children. One question is that of autonomy. All other things being equal, does a woman have the right to do with her body as she pleases? Equality and autonomy here move into the forefront. At first glance, at least, to interdict either surrogate or gestational motherhood would seem to limit a woman's personal autonomy severely. Both ethics and law recognize that autonomy may be curtailed under certain circumstances. However, before such a decision to curtail is made, the ethical and legal factors that outweigh the right to autonomy would have to be clearly spelled out and considered. In the eyes of the Canadian Medical Association, the case against a woman's autonomy in this matter has not been made.

Another argument against legitimizing surrogate and gestational motherhood is based on the contention that the way in which children would be brought into the world, and the reason for which they would be engendered, would constitute an ethical affront to these children as people.

In its deliberations on these and other issues, the Canadian Medical Association considered, among other things, the argument that, because of the affinity that a woman who bears a child may develop for that child, her custodial rights should be considered to be greater than the rights of any person other than herself even if the gametes of those other persons have been the genetic origin of the child. According to this line of reasoning, the claims of the birth mother should always take priority in cases of conflict. This would mean that exceptions would obtain only if the child could be shown to be in need of protection under the normal social service mechanisms. In such cases — so this reasoning has it — the courts should determine who should have custodial rights and obligations.

The Association can understand the thrust of these various positions. However, it is not convinced that all of them are valid. So far as the Association can see, all techniques of assisted reproduction are liable to this critique. In all of these instances, there is a deliberateness about the process, and there is someone who stands to gain materially from it. However, the Association does not believe that this should be seen as somehow degrading to the child that is born.

More specifically, the Association believes that the ethical status of a child has nothing to do with who engendered it or how it was brought about. Instead, the Association believes that its ethical status lies in the fact that it is a person. Nothing can take away from that fact. Furthermore, the Association would characterize any argument to the contrary as committing the fallacy of genesis; it confuses the origin or way that someone came about with the ethical status of the individual as a person.

The Association also believes that deliberately gestating a child to hand it to someone else need not constitute commerce in human beings. That would be true if some value or consideration were exchanged for the child that was handed over. However, the Association does not believe that this would be a correct way of characterizing either surrogate or gestational motherhood. Without holding any brief as to whether payment or consideration should change hands in the first instance, the Association believes that such an exchange might just as legitimately be described as an exchange of considerations for services rendered: namely the gestational service itself.

This last train of reasoning may be accepted in the case of gestational motherhood. However, it is possible to argue that it would not hold in the case of surrogate motherhood. Here, since the ovum involved is that of the surrogate mother, the latter is not merely a gestational parent, but a biological parent as well. That — so the argument goes — makes all the difference.

Although such an argument may be possible, the Association does not believe that it would establish the point at issue. The reason lies in the fact that ovum donation is accepted as an ethically praiseworthy act. It seems to the Association that surrogate motherhood may well be construed as an act of donation where what is donated — the ovum — does not leave the body of the donor. On that understanding, adding to the act of donation the service of a gestator does not turn the donation into the sale of a human being.

Finally, the issue of surrogate motherhood brings to a head one of the most fundamental issues that underlies all of the reproductive technologies: what should be the primary consideration in childbearing in general and in the use of reproductive technologies in particular? Should it be the welfare of the child, the position of the gestating woman, the feelings of prospective parents, or the expectations of society? The Association is in no position to give a definitive answer. However, it is always reminded that although the progenitors of children always have at least a modicum of choice in the matter, limited though it may be, the children that will result from that choice have none. Yet they are people.

After careful deliberation, the preceding considerations notwithstanding, the Association has come to the conclusion that, aside from medical problems of the sort already canvassed in the preceding discussion of AI, IVF and associated technologies, the issue of surrogate or gestational motherhood is not inherently medical in nature. It is ethical and legal. The Association looks forward to seeing an ultimate resolution of the question in social terms. However, it would like to offer the following observations.

First, the Association believes that the bond of biological or of gestational parenthood is not an indissoluble one. The generally accepted practice of adoption indicates how this is the case. It also points the way in which the bond of parenthood, as and where it exists, may be dissolved. Society accepts that it may be dissolved at the discretion of the parents and for reasons that are good and sufficient in the eyes of society itself.[183] If the Association understands the matter correctly, this process of dissolution attempts to balance the rights of the parents against the rights of the child. The

Association believes that such a balancing approach is not only ethically sound, but may also lead to a resolution of the issues surrounding surrogate and gestational motherhood.

Second, as far as the Association is concerned, there is nothing inherently unethical about a woman exercising her autonomy by volunteering to act as gestational mother, even though she may have no intention to act as social mother as well. The Association, therefore, endorses the notion of surrogacy. Consequently it rejects the claim that either surrogate or gestational motherhood amounts to "baby selling." Irrespective of whether they involve a transfer of financial or other considerations, the Association believes that to categorize them in that fashion is to misrepresent their nature as undertakings that allow others the privilege of becoming partners. This does not mean that the Association is blind to the emotional and personal implications of this procedure. It merely means that as far as the Association is concerned, to categorize the practice as "baby selling" is to introduce an emotional bias into the debate that falsifies the whole nature of the issue.

Third, the Association believes that informed consent is a necessary condition of such an undertaking. In the eyes of the Association, to fully understand the nature of the undertaking requires that the woman in question should have had the experience of motherhood. In no other way will she be able to estimate with anything approaching a reasonable degree of confidence, whether she will be able to carry through with the undertaking and give the child to the social parents. The Association, therefore, recommends that only women who have already had a child be allowed to volunteer as surrogate or gestational mothers.

Fourth, the Association is concerned that surrogate arrangements should operate according to certain guidelines, so as to avoid the possibility of coercion of the prospective surrogate or gestational mother or the introduction of other socially undesirable consequences. The Association, therefore, recommends that surrogacy arrangements be subject to prior legal screening, as was suggested by the Law Reform Commission of Ontario.[184] The Association is aware that this would mean judicial involvement in the process. However, it is convinced that such a review could be handled by appropriate adjustments to current adoption mechanisms. Such mechanisms include appropriate screening provisions for prospective adoptive parents. The Canadian Medical Association believes that the same criteria should be operative in the case of prospective social parents.

The Association is not prepared to go further than that at the present time. However, the Association recognizes that many issues of implementation remain unresolved. Consequently, it calls on this Commission to clarify the following issues:

- whether surrogacy and gestational arrangements should be enforceable against the surrogate or gestational mother;
- whether surrogate or gestational mothers should have the same amount of time to consider their decision to relinquish custody as they would have in normal adoption cases;
- whether in case of conflict between the surrogate or gestational mother and other parties (party) to the arrangement, the claims of the former should take priority over those of the latter; and
- whether, if the surrogate or gestational mother chooses to keep the child, contrary to the surrogacy agreement, the prospective social parents should have any rights of access to the child, or whether the surrogate or gestational mother, or

the child, should have any claim on the prospective social parents.

The Association can also envision situations where the child is appropriately adopted by the social parents, but these turn out to be unsuitable as parents according to current adoption standards. The Association believes that currently existing mechanisms embodied in child welfare legislation are sufficient to cover these cases.

As to the matter of payment to the surrogate mother, the Association believes that in itself, this would not be objectionable. It would be payment for an act, not payment for the child itself. The Association is aware that this opinion is not shared universally. Furthermore, the Association believes that to prevent any form of payment to surrogate or gestational mothers would be to treat them according to a standard whose stringency would exceed even that which is deemed appropriate in the case of gamete donation. Consequently the Association recommends that surrogate or gestational mothers be entitled to receive remuneration calculated to defray their gestation-related expenses and opportunity costs.

NOTES

168. The Ontario Law Reform Commission (*Report on Human Artificial Reproduction and Related Matters,* 2 vols, Ministry of the Attorney General, Toronto, 1985, vol 2, pp. 218-219) explains the notion of surrogate motherhood as follows: "A surrogate motherhood arrangement involves an agreement between the woman who is to bear the child and the persons who are to receive it to raise as their own. While a variety of terms may be agreed upon by the parties, the heart of any arrangement is a promise on the part of the surrogate mother to undergo the medical procedure necessary to achieve a pregnancy and to surrender custody of the child irrevocably upon birth, and a reciprocal promise on part of the other party or parties to accept the child." It will be clear that some refinements in the notion of surrogacy have occurred since the time of the Commission's writing.
169. For a somewhat similar discussion of the various possibilities, albeit one that does not include the more recent variations, see Ontario Law Reform Commission (*supra,* note 168) p. 218.
170. This view seems to underlie Brodribb S (*Women and Reproductive Technologies,* Status of Women Canada, Ottawa: May 1988, note 148): "The impact on the child of selling the child for money and on other children in the contract mother's family should also be studied" (p. 48).
171. Combined Ethics Committee of the Canadian Fertility and Andrology Society and the Society of Obstetricians and Gynaecologists of Canada: *Ethical Considerations of the New Reproductive Technologies,* Final Draft Copy, 1989, note 108) p. 27.
172. Brodribb (*supra,* note 148) p. 44.
173. See Brodribb (*ibid.,* pp. 44 and 46) for such a suggestion.
174. The British Columbia Bar Association, the Society of Obstetricians and Gynaecologists of Canada, the Christian Dental Association of Canada, etc.
175. Ontario Law Reform Commission: *Report on Human Artificial Reproduction* (note 168), pp. 41-45.

176. Barreau de Quebec: *Les Enjeux Ethique et Juridique des Nouvelles Technologies de Reproduction,* Quebec, April 1988: 33-34.
177. Canadian Bar Association, British Columbia Branch: *Report of the Special Task Force Committee on Reproductive Technology,* Vancouver, June 1989.
178. See Warnock M (ed): *Report of the Committee of Enquiry into Human Sterilization and Embryology,* Her Majesty's Stationer's Office, London, GB, 1984:
179. Glover J et al: *Ethics of New Reproductive Technologies: the Glover Report to the European Commission,* Northern Illinois Univ Press, DeKalb, IL, 1989.
175. Ontario Law Reform Commission: *Report on Human Artificial Reproduction* (note 168), pp. 41-45.
180. American College of Obstetricians and Gynecologists: *Ethical Issues in Surrogate Motherhood.* ACOG Statement of Policy, May 1983.
181. American Medical Association, Judicial Council report I-83 (1983). *Current Opinions* 1989; 2 (18).
182. Combined Ethics Committee (*supra,* note 108), Ethical Issue no. 7, Surrogacy.
183. The Association is aware that such a dissolution may also take place for socially sanctioned legal reasons. However, that does not alter the thrust of the present considerations.
184. See *supra,* note 168, vol. 2, chapter 6, section 5, Proposals relating to surrogate motherhood.

Preconception Contracts

Conseil du Statu de la Femme

The phenomenon of preconception contracts is closely tied to the growing use of the new human reproductive technologies of artificial insemination and in vitro fertilization. Formal preconception contracts have been in existence for about 15 years. It is estimated that, in the United States, nearly 25 agencies offer "contracting mother" services and there have been about 500 cases of "mothers under contract". In Québec, the practice is much less widespread and, although the existence of similar agencies cannot be confirmed, there have been many indications that this practice has existed for a few years, such as lawyers' testimony that they have drawn up such contracts and that of physicians who claim they are aware of 10 or so deliveries by "contracting mothers". Moreover, the report by the task force of the ministère de la Santé et des Services sociaux notes that advertisements are placed in daily newspapers by American agencies offering the services of "female Quebecers" in their catalogues, who provide "services at a lower price because expenses are covered by the Québec health care system".[1] Are

Conseil du Statu de la Femme, "Preconception Contracts," from Gouvernement du Québec, Conseil du Statu de la Femme, *General Opinion of the Conseil du Statu de la Femme in Regard to New Reproductive Technologies.* (Québec, 1989) pp.19-21.

uteruses being leased and children bought and sold? The problems raised must be studied, and the Conseil felt it should issue specific recommendations to eliminate the practice before it becomes more prevalent.

4.1 PRESENT SITUATION

4.1.1 Surrogate Mothers, Substitute Mothers or Preconception Contracts

The terms used must be clarified in order to better grasp the implications of this phenomenon. Feminist writers feel the commonly used expressions *surrogate mother* and *substitute mother* are misnomers. They claim that a mother under contract is not a "surrogate" or "substitute" for the social mother, but the true mother, since she conceives the child, carries it for nine months and brings it into the world. Furthermore, if the "contracting mother" is indeed a substitute for someone, it is not the mother of the child, but the spouse of the father, as the report by the task force of the ministère de la Santé et des Services sociaux points out.[2] This shift in meaning tends to minimize the role of the "contracting mother", reducing her to a surrogate, a mere "receptacle", and denying the important biological (she is the genetic and uterine mother) and emotional links she has with the child. The terms *preconception contract* and *contracting mother* are much more appropriate and the Conseil decided, after discussing the matter, to use them.

4.1.2 A Contract or the Leasing of Services? The Various Arrangements Possible

The phenomenon having been properly named, the various forms it takes should be described. At the International Forum on New Reproductive Technologies, Margrit Eichler listed the various arrangements possible:[3]

- **contracting parties:** on the supply side, there is always at least one "uterine mother", while on the demand side, the situation is not always clear. The contracting party may be (a) a man, (b) a man with a partner who is a beneficiary of the contract, although not a signatory to it, (c) a couple, (d) a woman or (e) a woman and a partner who is a beneficiary but not formally involved in the contract;
- **relations between the parties:** the contracting parties may be perfect strangers, they may be friends, in which case the contracting mother engages in the arrangement in order to render a service to a friend, or they may be relatives. Even in cases where the contracting parties are perfect strangers, a relationship of personal dependence is generally established since the contracting mother is subject to the contract and is often "under supervision";
- **fertilization methods employed:** the most commonly used fertilization methods are artificial insemination (the contracting mother is then the genetic and uterine mother of the child) and embryo transfer (if the couple wants to choose the genetic makeup of the child). The social and biological ties with the child may vary greatly according to the various methods used;
- **social and biological bonds with the child:** Eichler lists the following possible parenthood combinations: (1) if the "contracting mother" is inseminated with the sperm of the social father, the child has one uterine-genetic mother, one social

mother and one biological-social father (as in the case of Baby M); (2) if the mother is inseminated with the sperm of a donor, the child will have a uterine-genetic mother, a social mother, a biological father and a social father (if the donor is the uncle of the child, he may be both the biological father and the uncle); (3) if an egg fertilized by the contracting couple is implanted in the uterus of the "contracting mother", the child will have a uterine mother, a social-biological mother and a social-biological father; if the uterine mother is related to the couple (e.g. the South African case in which a grandmother gave birth to her grandchildren), the child will have a uterine mother who may be her grandmother, a social-genetic mother and a social-biological father. Other variations are possible, demonstrating the complexity of the resulting bonds of parenthood;

- **involvement of intermediaries or agencies:** private contractual arrangements are sometimes made by the parties (as in the South African case), or a third party or parties may be involved: a lawyer, who oversees the contract negotiations and who may or may not help in getting the two parties together, or an intermediary or agency specializing in matching contracting mothers with individuals or couples seeking one, where artificial insemination or embryo transfer is practised, medical personnel are also involved;
- **commercial aspects:** this practice does not always involve money (e.g. the South African grandmother). However, commercial transactions are common and may take the form of remuneration of the contracting mother or remuneration of an intermediary or agency or both. A contracting mother is said to receive about $10 000 to carry and give birth to a child. The intermediary or agency may receive an equal amount.

4.1.3 Legal Context

In Canada, preconception contracts are not legally recognized. These contracts are null and void according to the law as it now stands: "... the freedom and recognized rights or any pregnant woman during her pregnancy and delivery may not be limited by a third party and, after the birth, the only rights that may be asserted in regard to the child are those provided for in the Civil Code."[4]

4.2 CONSEIL CONCERNS AND POSITIONS

4.2.1 Legal Context in North America

Given the North American legislative and legal context, the Conseil feels it should alert the Québec government to the very serious implications that the creation of jurisprudence similar to that in the United States could have in this field.[4] The Conseil is also troubled by the recommendation of the Ontario Law Reform Commission that such contracts be recognized and that the various aspects be regulated.[5] The Commission goes so far as to suggest that restrictions on the mother's conduct during pregnancy (diet, prenatal diagnosis and therapeutic abortion, for example) be provided for in the contract. "The Conseil feels that these are extremely disturbing legal trends not only for women bound by such contracts, but for the status and rights of all women."[6]

4.2.2 Emotional and Human Implications

According to the Conseil:[7]

An agreement made before conception, binding the mother to renounce the child once and for all upon his birth could create traumatic situations if the mother becomes attached to the child through the physical and emotional experience of pregnancy and delivery; ... Moreover, not much is known, of course, about the longer term consequences for the psychological development of children conceived in this way, whether the children are told about their true origins or one tries to hide them. We also do not know enough about the long-term effects on the various parties concerned, or about the family relationships that ensue.

4.2.3 Buying and Selling of Human Beings

According to the Conseil:[7]

A woman's agreeing to the adoption of her child for monetary or other gain raises the problem of the buying and selling of children and the commercialization of human embryos (one American company, whose shares are quoted on the stock exchange, is already involved in this practice), even those removed from women who wish to interrupt their pregnancy. This also implies recognition of a new form of economic exploitation of women's bodies, on the basis of their reproductive capacities. Various surveys suggest that certain categories of women would be likely to agree to such contracts because of economic pressure or to abusive clauses in such contracts, while the biological fathers or contracting couples, who often have higher incomes, would be in a better position to impose their own conditions on the contracting mother and to defend their own interests in any subsequent dispute.

4.2.4 Alienation of Women's Rights During Pregnancy

According to the Conseil:[7]

Preconception contracts may entail the serious infringement of the rights and freedoms of pregnant women. For example, they may involve the waiving of the women's right to agree to or to refuse medical intervention during the pregnancy (examinations, drugs procedures, Caesarian section and so on), the waiving of their right to an abortion and a prior agreement to have an abortion when the biological father wishes one to be performed if a defect is diagnosed in the fetus, or any other form of constraint on the activities of the pregnant women (related to work, diet, travel and so on). Such constraints, if they were acknowledged to be justified for the welfare of the child or as legitimate rights of the biological father, could have dramatic consequences for the rights of any pregnant woman and for the concept of the inviolability of the human being.

4.2.5 Possible Effect on Perceptions of Motherhood and of the Reproduction of Life

According to the Conseil:[7]

Pregnancies resulting from an egg taken from the female partner of the contracting couple pose even more complex problems, partly because they lead to a dissociation and comparison of the genetic and uterine bonds with the child. The present trend according to a number of authorities, which has been confirmed by a recent American decision, is toward the merging of maternity and paternity by equating the genetic bonds created by the sperm with those created by the egg, thereby reducing pregnancy and delivery to a purely physiological process that establishes no significant link between the uterine mother and the child, and no significant right of the uterine mother to the child. This mentality reflects an androcentric perception reproduction and motherhood, which, if it gains adherents, will pave the way for the acceptance of completely extra-corporal human reproduction (artificial uteruses).

CONCLUSION

In its opinion regarding preconception contracts, the Conseil voiced its concern about the possibility of legislations to legalize such contracts, making them executory. It pointed out that, in civil law as it now stands, these contracts are null and void. The Conseil asked that no new legislation legitimizing preconception contracts be adopted.[8] This would mean that the freedom and recognized rights of all pregnant women could not be limited by a third party, and, after the birth, the only rights that could be exercised before the Court over the child would be those provided for in the Civil Code.

To prevent preconception contracts and curb their commercialization, the Conseil recommends:

- **that section 135.1 of the Youth Protection Act (R.S.Q., c. P-34.1) be amended so that any natural or artificial person involved directly or indirectly in a preconception contract may be found guilty of an offence and may be liable to a fine.**[9]

The Conseil is also disturbed by the media's part in the spread of the phenomenon in Québec through the publication of advertisements soliciting candidates for such arrangements. Considering the legal status of these contracts, it feels these advertisements should be prohibited.

Lastly, the Conseil reiterates its recommendation that children who are the result of contracted pregnancies have the right to know their origins, just as artificially conceived or adopted children have.

NOTES

1. *Rapport du Comité de travail sur les nouvelles technologies de la reproduction,* Direction générale de la planification et de l'évaluation, ministère de la Santé et des Services sociaux, Québec, 1988, 120 pp., pp. 65-66.
2. *Ibid.,* p. 65.
3. Conseil du statut de la femme, Margrit Eichler, "Preconception Contracts for the Production of Children — What are the Proper Legal Responses?", *Sortir la maternité du laboratoire,* Proceedings of the International Forum on New Reproductive technologies, 1988, 423 pp., pp. 187-204.
4. Conseil du statut de la femme, *Déclaration de principe sur la question des grossesses sous contract,* declaration in principle adopted by the Comité NTR on April 3, 1987.
5. Ontario Law Reform Commission, *Report on human artificial reproduction and*

related matters, Vol. I and II. Ministry of the Attorney General, Ontario, 1985, 390 pp.

6. Conseil du statut de la femme, *Déclaration, op. cit.*
7. *Ibid.*
8. Conseil du statut de la femme, *Les grossesses sous contrat,* opinion submitted to the Minister for the Status of Women, Québec, 1987, 6 pp., p. 5.
9. *Ibid.*, p. 6.

FURTHER READINGS

Alberta Institute of Law Research and Reform
Status of Children. (Report No. 20, 1976).

Anderson, E.S.
"Is Women's Labour a Commodity? *Philosophy and Public Affairs* 19:1 (Winter, 1990) 71-92.

Bartels, D.M., et al., eds.
Beyond Baby M: Ethical Issues in New Reproductive Techniques. (Clifton, NJ: Humana Press, 1990).

Brodrib, S.
Women and Reproductive Technologies. (Ottawa: Status of Women Canada, May 1989).

Corea, G.
The Mother Machine: Reproductive Technologies from Artificial Insemination to Artificial Wombs. (New York: Harper and Row, 1986) 6.

Ethical Considerations of the New Reproductive Technologies. A Report of the Combined Ethics Committee of the Canadian Fertility and Andrology Society and the Society of Obstetricians and Gynecologists of Canada (1990).

Field, M.A.
Surrogate Motherhood. (Cambridge and London: Harvard University Press, 1988).

Gostin, L., ed.
Surrogate Motherhood: Politics and Privacy. (Bloomington: Indiana University Press, 1990).

Merrick, J.
"Selling Reproductive Rights: Policy Issues in Surrogate Motherhood," *Politics and the Life Sciences* 8:2 (1990) 161-172.

Ontario Law Reform Commission
Report on Human Artificial Reproduction and Related Matters. (Toronto: Ministry of the Attorney General, 1985).

Raymond, J.C.
"Reproductive Gifts and Gift Giving: The Altruistic Woman," *Hastings Center Report* 20:6 (Nov/Dec 1990) 7-11.

Report of the Commission of Enquiry of the German Bundestag, Prospects and Risks of Genetic Engineering, Parts I and II. (Deutscher Bundestag, 10. Wahlperiode: Bonn 1987; the so-called *Inquiry Commission*).

Rich, A.
Of Woman Born: Motherhood as Experiment and Institution. (New York, W.W. Norton and Co.: 1976).
Shalev, C.
Birth Power: The Case for Surrogacy. (New Haven and London: Yale University Press, 1989).
Silver, L.M.
"New Reproductive Technologies in the Treatment of Human Infertility and Genetic Disease," *Theoretical Medicine* 11:2 (1990) 103-110.
Somerville, M.
"Weaving 'Birth' Technology into theValue and Policy 'Web' of Medicine, Ethics and Law: Should Policies on 'Conception' be Considered?" *Nova Law Review* 13:2 (1989) 515-608.
South Australia
Report of the Working Party on In Vitro Fertilization and Artificial Insemination by Donor. (1984).
The British Columbia Bar Association
Report of the Special Task Force Committee on Reproductive Technology of the British Columbia Branch, The Canadian Bar Association. (Vancouver: June 1989).
U.K., Department of Health and Social Security
Report of the Committee of Inquiry into Human Fertilization and Embryology. (Cmnd. 9314, 1984).

PART 5 THE GENETIC BASIS OF HUMAN LIFE

CHAPTER 18 GENETIC KNOWLEDGE

INTRODUCTION

Since time immemorial, people have known that the nature of living things depends not only on environmental influences, but also on the characteristics of the parents. People have put this knowledge to use in breeding livestock, developing food-crops and the like. They knew *that* selective breeding worked, but they did not know *why*.

Around the turn of the century, building on the pioneering work of Gregor Mendel, scientists began to unravel the mysteries of inheritance. With the discovery of the DNA molecule, the understanding of the nature of inheritance took a quantum leap forward. Subsequent decades saw the discovery of techniques for manipulating DNA by slicing it here and splicing there. With this, humanity acquired the ability to manipulate directly the blueprint of life.

Initially, this knowledge was applied only to animals and plants. However, right from the very start, some people argued that this knowledge should be applied not only to the breeding of animals and plants, but also to humans. After all, so they maintained, humans are also animals, and therefore are governed by the same laws of inheritance. Furthermore, if we take the trouble to improve animal and plant stocks — to remove hereditary diseases and provide them with beneficial characteristics — why shouldn't we take the same care for human beings? Surely human beings deserve the same amount of attention and care!

On the other side of the debate stand those who see this reasoning as specious. They contend that human beings have a dignity that transcends the merely material. They maintain that to treat human biological failings as defects that should be corrected by scientific means is to objectify human beings. They also see a danger in the fact that we do not know what the long-term effects of "correcting" so-called genetic defects would be. In fact, they maintain that what counts as a defect is very much a function of the conceptual framework we employ and the values by which we operate. In other words, it is culture-relative. Consequently, we cannot even define the notion of a genetic defect in any usable sense.

Finally, those who are opposed to the application of genetic technology and knowledge to the human sphere argue that humanity has worked for millennia to achieve a plateau of moral development that includes values like compassion, equality and the like. These values allow us to see beyond the handicap of the human body to the dignity of the human person. To apply the various genetic techniques to human beings is to erase this progress. Furthermore, applying this knowledge will result in an uncaring, callous and materialistic world. It will foster the attitude that it is appropriate to deal only with the material problem of a handicap, rather than trying to accommodate the handicap in agreement with the fundamental ethical principle of respect for persons and equality and justice.

The genetic knowledge we have gained and the mastery of techniques that we have acquired, in order to find out something about the genetic characteristics of persons, has important ethical implications. In a recent study paper prepared for the Law Reform Commission of Canada, Bartha Knoppers explores some of these. She suggests that, "while an ethical framework must form the basis for the construction of a theory of genetic justice, the formulation of a viable theory cannot be isolated from more pragmatic considerations." She proceeds to sketch, in broad terms, what she believes such a combined approach would have to take into consideration.

The selection by Lappé provides a somewhat different focus. His concerns are more issue-focused: What should be the limits of this drive to acquire knowledge? How should the knowledge itself be controlled, and by whom? How should it be used?

Towards Genetic Justice

Bartha Knoppers

INTRODUCTION

The advent of the year 2000, and of the next millennium, portends tremendous promise in the science of human genetics. Like the discovery of the atom and, more recently, the ability to conceive human life *in vitro,* advances in human genetics harbour the potential for good and for evil. The very essence of humankind is at stake. At the same time, the potential of this science lies in the knowledge it provides, knowledge that will finally force to the forefront a discussion of the nature, uniqueness and potential for change of the human species. Indeed, the era of genetics will provide us with the opportunity and the duty to give meaning to the inherent dignity of the human person.[1]

The lack of precise knowledge about where human genetics might take us raises false hopes in some and leads others to make wholesale denunciations. The latter group has applied such terms as "interfering with nature," "playing God" and the "slippery slope" to genetic engineering.[2] There is no doubt that the new tools of human genetics do, and will, affect the human being in the ultimate substratum, namely, the gene. Whether the result will be "good" or "evil" will depend on whether individuals, scientists and governments seek and apply genetic knowledge responsibly and discriminately. In order to understand the potential of this knowledge, we must understand first how the progress in molecular genetics has changed the practice of medical genetics.

In 1982, the Council of Europe, in its recommendation on Genetic Engineering, advocated that the right to life and to human dignity implied the right to an unaltered genetic pattern — one that had not been artificially altered.[3] It also proposed that this right should be made explicit in the European *Convention for the Protection of Human Rights and Fundamental Freedoms.*[4] However, no guidance was provided as to what was meant by a genetic pattern or heritage or how it could be protected from change by means of law.

Considering the advances in molecular biology affecting human genetics since that 1982 recommendation, we must now determine what genetic heritage is. Does it mean the collective gene pool or the individual genome?[5] Answers to this question are necessary to decide what is inherent to human dignity that merits legal protection.

Even though the inherent dignity of the human person is seen as fundamental, its interpretation in a human rights context is not yet clear. However, there is no doubt that respect for the human body, for one's genetic make-up and origins, is indivisible from respect for the person. Human cells, with their genetic information, are more than a temporary substrate for the existence of the human body; they are a constituent of human dignity. The Council of Europe linked the right to protection of the genetic heritage to the right to life and to human dignity. However, it

---

Bartha Knoppers, "Towards Genetic Justice," from *Human Dignity and Genetic Heritage*, Study Paper prepared for the Law Reform Commission of Canada, Protection of Life Series. (Ottawa: Law Reform Commission of Canada, 1991), pp. 1-4.

did not exclude therapeutic interventions. In fact, its preliminary report contains the startling suggestion that reproductive freedom of those persons at risk of transmitting certain serious genetic illnesses might be linked to their consenting to genetic therapy to reduce the probability of transmitting those illnesses to subsequent generations. Thus, assigning a right to a "healthy" genetic heritage to protect human dignity may do as much to undermine that human dignity by restricting freedom.

While the meaning of human dignity in international human rights law is not fully developed, the notion can serve as the foundation for the interpretation of human rights in the context of constitutional law. In particular, under the *Canadian Charter of Rights and Freedoms,* the rights to life, liberty and security of the person, the right to be free from unreasonable search and seizure and the right to equality and protection from discrimination have been seen as based on the recognition of that inherent dignity.[6] We may then ask whether such constitutional guarantees are directly applicable to the issues raised by the new human genetics in a free and democratic society such as Canada. Some examples of issues that may arise are: compulsory testing for disease or carrier status in particular groups of individuals; the obligation of parents to have their children tested for treatable diseases; and the use of DNA samples for unauthorized purposes.

Improving the capability to treat or alter the genome of an individual and genetic testing to identify the risk of future diseases may result in stigmatization. Indeed, "[f]rom a societal perspective, a gene probe for manic depression may be seen as akin to AIDS antibody testing: in both instances, testing leads to the uncovering of a marker."[7] The marker could predict (with varying degrees of accuracy) the onset of the disease. But attached to this prediction is a substantial risk of social stigmatization.

Such stigmatization and our reactions to the new genetics may be shaped by our view of human nature. If one sees genetic consequences as inevitable and certain, one may be inclined to look to the elimination of the genetically disabled rather than to the finding of ways to accommodate such persons within society. By adopting this view we are deciding what is "normal" and acceptable. We may, for example, screen workers and exclude them on the basis of their susceptibility genes, rather than looking to reduce the risk of disease by cleaning up the workplace. We may fail to examine our political system, which leaves those with genetic disabilities less insured than those without. We may exert pressure on individuals to control their reproductive outcome according to our view of normality, and promote the elimination of the handicapped by abortion rather than making the world a better place for them. If, on the other hand, we see the diversity of our genetic constitution as natural and as the essence of humanity, we may resist genetic intervention regardless of its moral justification.

Three ethical principles may be considered in an evaluation of the impact of modern science on the human being: autonomy, beneficence and non-maleficence. In the context of modern molecular biology and predictive genetics, as in medicine generally, the principle of autonomy may conflict with the principles of beneficence and non-maleficence. What framework do these principles provide for future legislative policy?

On a governmental level, the use of a cost-benefit analysis with its utilitarian rationale could lead to considerable pressure to test or be tested. It could force individuals to know about their genetic predispositions, to tell others and to act, so that the "proper choices" of those individuals would save society the long-term costs of disabling diseases. Such economic incentives could lead to a new eugenics based, not on undesirable characteristics, but rather on cost-saving, a form of economic social justice rather than "genetic justice." Considering those choices, genetic justice will require both greater communication of knowledge within the protection of the physician-patient relationship and civic responsibility on the part of the participant to share knowledge that will benefit his or her family.

The development of a theory of genetic justice will require an in-depth examination of human rights in the workplace, in matters of insurability and in the physician-patient relationship. Other issues that will need full elaboration in the future are: the individual's control of bodily tissues or cells and of the genetic information contained therein; control of the diffusion of genetic information to family members; and the availability and adequacy of genetic counselling services and genetic education.[8] However, the values and policy issues underlying such specific subjects require delineation now.

This study attempts to establish the basic, yet changing, philosophical and scientific knowledge underlying new developments in the science of human genetics. It looks at the impact that this understanding will have on the definition and legal protection of the human genetic heritage. The concept of genetic heritage and the legal means to protect it must be situated within an analysis of what is meant by the inherent dignity of the person. This will allow us to envisage a revised concept of genetic "abnormality" within a new concept of genetic justice.

The new genetics affects us individually and collectively, in our social, political and economic fabric. However, the inherent dignity of the human person, as recognized in the international covenants and national constitutions, has not yet been fully interpreted by the courts. It will be argued that the recognition of the dignity of each person, and of humanity as a whole, requires an approach to the protection of our genetic heritage that is based on medically oriented principles of respect for human life. It will be shown that human life in the genetic sense is not fixed in time, nor can it be reduced to one immutable gene pool. This study proposes that respect for the complexity, variability and uniqueness of the human being, and the recognition of equality through genetic difference, may be accomplished through the widespread genetic education of both the public and the medical profession. The failure to so educate could lead to the misuse of genetic knowledge for discriminatory purposes. It could also lead to the dangerous language of "genetic rights" with its accompanying legal claims and obligations. In short, the purpose of this study is to attach some meaning to the inherent human dignity of the person in the context of the new choices of human genetics, and to propose interpretations of human dignity that ensure the indivisible genetic nature of the human person within a common social ethic, that of genetic justice.

NOTES

1. *Universal Declaration of Human Rights,* G.A. Res. 217/A, Off. Doc. G.A., 3rd Session at 71, U.N. Doc. A/810 (1948):

   > *Whereas* recognition of the inherent dignity and of the equal and inalienable rights of all members of the human family is the foundation of freedom, justice and peace in the world ...
   >
   > *Whereas* the peoples of the United Nations have in the Charter reaffirmed their faith in fundamental human rights, in the dignity and worth of the human person and in the equal rights of men and women ... (Preamble).

2. Keith Boone, "Bad Axioms in Genetic Engineering" (1988) 18:4 *Hast. Cent. Rep.* 9.
3. Council of Europe, P.A., 33rd Sess., Pt III, *Texts Adopted, Recommendation 934 (1982) on Genetic Engineering,* s. 4(i).
4. (1955) 213 U.N.T.S. 221 [hereinafter European Convention on Human Rights].
5. See the Glossary, *infra* at 77 for the definitions of technical terms.
6. Part I of the *Constitution Act, 1982,* being Schedule B of the *Canada Act 1982* (U.K.), 1982, c. 11, ss. 7, 8 and 15.
7. Marc Lappé, "The Limits of Genetic Inquiry" (1987) 17:4 *Hast. Cent. Rep.* 5 at 7.
8. See generally Neil A. Holtzman, *Proceed with Caution: Predicting Genetic Risks in the Recombinant DNA Era* (Baltimore: Johns Hopkins University Press, 1989); Lori B. Andrews, *Medical Genetics: A Legal Frontier* (Chicago: American Bar Foundation, 1987).

The Limits of Genetic Inquiry

Marc Lappé

We are in the midst of an unprecedented explosion of knowledge in human genetics. Researchers armed with powerful new techniques are unstripping the secrets of three and a half billion years of molecular evolution. As recently as February 1987, scientists cautioned that an assault on the human genome was a daunting project, barely within the ambit of scientific feasibility.[1] Since then, an advisory committee of the Department of Energy has replaced this cautionary view with a glowingly optimistic one, unanimously recommending that $1 billion be spent over the next seven years to map and sequence the human genome.[2]

Within the next few years scientists will almost certainly have pieced together a broad map of the major gene locations on the twenty-three human chromosomes.

Marc Lappé, "The Limits of Genetic Inquiry," *Hastings Center Report* 17:4 (1987) 5-10.

Researchers are now able to break out whole segments of human DNA and "store" thousands of copies of each piece in clones of genetically identical bacteria. These veritable libraries of human genetic information can be loaned (or sold) to fellow researchers for more detailed analysis.

Indeed, the pace of discovery of key genes has accelerated geometrically in recent months, underscoring the revolutionary rate of acquisition of new knowledge in human genetics. At a minimum, these events suggest that we will be uncovering knowledge for which we are unprepared, and some that will challenge tightly held convictions about the predominance of nurture over nature. Certainly, the rapidity with which these findings are being made should give us pause.

As the new knowledge unfolds, how will it be shared? To believe that all the data on the human genome will be "public knowledge" is naive. Since anyone can decipher the genetic code, the sequence of bases that comprise any given segment can be used to construct complementary DNA molecules that can "probe" completely unknown sectors of a person's chromosomes for similar genes, or to construct the actual molecule encoded by the sequence. Since many of the sequences will code for valuable commercial products for diagnosing disease or preparing biologically active compounds, there are powerful incentives to "privatize" these data. Walter Gilbert of Harvard has founded the Genome Corporation from which he intends to offer for sale databases that contain sequences of key segments of the human genome.

This proposal, if it comes to pass, raises thorny questions about ownership of knowledge. Some of the uncovered genes will be of inestimable clinical value, allowing the early detection of biochemically based disorders. Awareness of such genes might enable clinicians to anticipate serious illness or chronic disorders and design remedial interventions accordingly. It would be ethically questionable to break with the tradition of open publication of such sequences to garner profit from their sale. Similar, but less pressing arguments apply to the large number of gene sequences that will have unknown functions and hence fall into the domain of pure research.

Other gene sequences are problematic for what they appear to foretell. A case in point could be the recently uncovered loci that seem to flag the presence of genes that predispose their carriers to manic depressive illness.[3] Should we use the knowledge of the likely presence of such "deviant" genes to abort affected fetuses? Such a program could conceivably reduce the genetic burden brought about by the presence of these genes in the human population, but it would also potentially deprive us of great poets like Sylvia Plath or politicians like Winston Churchill, each of whom may have suffered from bipolar manic depression.

Uncovering genes that regulate human vulnerability to grave illnesses such as Huntington chorea or Alzheimer's disease could increase the incidence of suicide as well as selective abortion. Given these possibilities, and the prospect of other abuses, it is prudent to examine such consequences now as we face the rapid arrival of these eventualities: What limits, if any, should be imposed on the acquisition of such knowledge? Who should control the wealth of resulting data? How should it be used?

THE TECHNOLOGY OF DNA PROBES

To appreciate the nature of these and relate first employed biochemical assays that identified the overproduction or deficiency of a protein produced by a specific gene. The second method utilized cytological studies to detect gross chromosomal abnormalities, such as those associated with Down syndrome.

With the advent of recombinant DNA technologies in the late 1970s, researchers could utilize various techniques to look directly at a person's DNA. This ability to manipulate genetic material spawned a wide variety of technologies, such as restriction fragment length polymorphisms (RFLP) analysis, chromosomal jumping libraries, and pulsed field gradient electrophoresis, all of which enable the researcher to analyze large stretches of DNA and subsequently identify small sections with techniques like in situ hybridization and gene probe analysis.[4,5]

The most powerful technique for clinical purposes is this last one. A DNA probe is a single strand of radioactively labeled or chemically "tagged" DNA. Each strand used as a probe has a known sequence of base nucleotides, the building blocks of the DNA molecule. Since these bases interlock only with their precise counterparts, a known sequence of DNA bases will always bind only with its complementary sequence.

An exact match of these bases will result in the formation of tight hydrogen bonds between the bases, linking the tiny probe to a DNA strand at a precise site. If the location of the site is not important, the fact that binding alone has occurred can be ascertained, and the probe can be considered to have made a "hit." A photographic emulsion will show such a hit by picking up the radioactivity of a bound DNA probe-unknown DNA composite.

A DNA probe of nineteen or more bases will almost certainly code for a unique length of DNA: a firm link or bond to a DNA strand by such a probe will unequivocably establish the existence of the sought-for DNA sequence.[6]

By the end of 1986, approximately 330 probes had been developed to detect human genetic variants; another 220 were available that detect genes with known functions.[7] This number will likely have doubled by the end of 1987. Some of the gene sequences studies have already been applied in the commercial sector. A probe reflecting the DNA sequence that codes for Factor VIII, the clotting factor deficient in hemophilia, has been used both to screen fetuses in utero at risk for this bleeding disorder and indirectly to assist in the rapid production of commercial quantities of human factor VIII.

THE MORAL USES OF SCIENCE

The rapid evolution of this field highlights the conflict between those who argue for the scientific imperative to acquire this new information en bloc and those who would monitor and temper its acquisition either to assure the utility of the data or minimize its adverse consequences.

The traditional maxim of scientific inquiry holds that researchers have a right of access to this "pure" knowledge unencumbered by considerations of how others might use it. But moral philosophers such as Daniel Callahan argue that researchers have a duty to use "moral imagination" to anticipate the full gamut of the most likely applications of their findings.[8] Failing to do so, argues Callahan, threatens to place agencies of potentially great power into the hands of less than wise users. At the heart of this issue is the question of free inquiry.

Some techniques will allow us to determine paternity, to discover the molecular fingerprinting of a felon, or to identify kidnapped children. More ominously, related techniques could be used to establish files of persons genetically at risk for acquiring AIDS following infection with the human immunodeficiency virus (HIV), knowledge which might be used to deny passports or employment. There are obviously a plethora of uses, and none is value neutral.

Some scientists have argued that the genome mapping enterprise is essentially an engineering problem and as such, is morally neutral. But consider that much contemporary research focuses on disorders with early onset. Cases in point include the genes associated with phenylketonuria (PKU), cystic fibrosis, polycystic kidney disease, sickle cell anemia, thalassemia, hemophilia B, Duchenne's muscular dystrophy, and familial retinoblastoma. Since uncovery of a genetic marker or probe for such disorders permits application in prenatal diagnosis, it is evident that moral as well as scientific considerations must attend the research.

Scientists can also argue that they have a fundamental obligation to unveil the 1,000 to 2,000 individual genes responsible for the structure of the major proteins that make up the building blocks and enzymes of the human form, without consideration of the consequences. They can reasonably insist that the good outweighs the possible abuses, and that no one can reasonably anticipate all of the potential benefits. For example, who could have predicted in the 1970s that our understanding of recombinant DNA would be an essential tool that led to the rapid progress in identifying the AIDS virus in the 1980s — or the genes that might confer susceptibility to its ravages?

Because scientific information usually precedes all but its most obvious uses, there will continue to be a struggle between those who want science to march forward without restraint and those who would monitor its direction in order to assure utility of the data acquired or to minimize its adverse consequences.

SETTING PRIORITIES

Some of these tensions can in theory be resolved by priority setting. Since an extremely large universe of individual DNA segments will need to be described to achieve the goal of sequencing the human genome (estimates run from 100,000 to 250,000 blocks of DNA fragments, each containing about 50,000 bases, which first need to be isolated before their actual genetic makeup can be deciphered[9]), many observers urge a more selective assault. If less than a complete picture is sought, scientists could choose those parts of the canvas they want to sketch in first, ones that concentrate broad regions of genetic material thought to carry genes of clinical importance. But this scheme is itself fraught with difficulties. Just how is it to be decided that priority be given to genes of medical importance, rather than to those of more fundamental biological interest? And given our state of ignorance, who is to say that a block of unknown sequences might not serve as the storehouse of some particularly unique and valuable data?

An argument for choosing knowledge for knowledge's sake could be made on the basis of the dramatic — and serendipitous — discoveries of the genetic heterogeneity underlying what we thought to be very simple *X*-linked disorders. Both classic (Duchenne) and Becker muscular dystrophy have been found to be complex but related disorders.[10]

Some genes might qualify on both basic and applied counts. The gene conferring risk of Alzheimer's disease, a progressive and fatal disorder that causes dementia in a substantial number of the elderly, is a case in point. Scientists have already mapped the general location of this gene to the same chromosome (No. 21) associated with Down syndrome. Since many of the symptoms of Alzheimer's mimic the late stages of Down syndrome, the genetic proximity may be more than fortuitous. Closer scrutiny of this chromosomal region could thus reasonably be given a high priority.

A partial solution to those who worry about priority setting so early in the game has been offered by Walter Gilbert: Go for the big picture, and worry about priorities later.[1] In this view, scientists would identify the major "cosmid" groups of the human genome and parse them out into analyzable sequencing. But such an approach might well be considered temporizing, since it simply postpones the question of assigning priorities.

ETHICAL DILEMMAS

How then should a tool to identify the causative gene in disease or susceptibility state candidates be developed? In what familial circumstances should related members of an affected individual be tested? For some disorders, such as cystic fibrosis, testing of family members is required to ascertain the likely genetic status of the fetus. Would family members then have a right to know the resulting information? Are there entities in our society other than the affected individuals themselves that have a bona fide "right-to-know" about such sensitive genetic data? Might not some persons legitimately wish neither the collection of genetic data nor its sharing even with family members?

These dilemmas faced the team that first discovered how to test for the presence of the gene for Huntington chorea. It took group leaders Nancy Wexler of New York University and James Gusella of Harvard over six years to develop an ethically acceptable plan to assist clinicians in handling the knowledge of risk status, particularly in the instance where minors or an extended family were going to be tested. Among the major ethical dilemmas were those posed by the uncovering of new at-risk persons among relatives, or the discovery of disease status in a young child. Some of these dilemmas were abrogated by denying testing to all but competent adults and assuring the confidentiality of testing of family members where requested.[11]

The remaining question of whether or not at-risk persons would in fact take the test if offered appears closer to resolution. Even with virtual certitude about Huntington chorea status, a recent survey of ninety-one at-risk persons in Pennsylvania revealed that only 74 percent would take the test,[12] a proportion comparable to the 56 to 84 percent previously reported to be willing to do so. But even with the test now available at two genetic centers, considerably fewer persons than the expected 60 to 75 percent of the at-risk persons in the general population expected to take the test have actually come forward. At the heart of this dilemma appears to be a lack of adequate counseling and concerns about confidentiality of the acquired data.

BANKING GENETIC KNOWLEDGE

This type of ethical issue — which I shall call the "locus of control question" — can be compared to those issues generated by developing any data bank that contains sensitive personal information, e.g., those created by the advent of computer-accessible records of financial and medical information. As so starkly illustrated by the acquisition of data about AIDS, a bank of human genetic information is potentially important both to the individual from whom it was collected and to others, such as health and life insurers, employers, and health maintenance organizations or group plans designed to underwrite health care for protracted periods.

A major difference between current repositories and projected genetic data banks is that financial and, to a lesser extent, medical data collections are subject to review, modification, or challenge by the identified individual. Computerized data sets also evolve over time and reflect financial or medical vicissitudes. A poor credit rating can become a good one (albeit not readily), a medical problem can be cured, a divorcée can remarry, and so on.

In contrast, a bank of genetic information will contain what may be perceived as immutable "facts" about a person. Except for technical errors, a genetic profile is likely to be a permanent fixture of one's biological legacy. Unlike a financial or medical catastrophe, a genetic one (say, a gene mutation for Huntington chorea) cannot usually be averted or restored. You cannot declare Chapter 11 on a flawed genome and start all over! In this sense, gene probing is qualitatively different from drug testing. In drug screening, a "positive" urinary test provides only a small window for discerning deviance. When a pattern of abuse is confirmed, presumably rehabilitation is possible, with greater or lesser social or medical sequelae. But a "positive" gene test, say, for manic depressive illness, provides an ineradicable marker of deviance with potentially lifelong social consequences to the affected individual.

From a societal perspective, a gene probe for manic depression may be seen as akin to AIDS antibody testing: in both instances, testing leads to the uncovering of a marker of varying prognostic value but substantial risk of social stigmatization.

MISUNDERSTANDING AND MISUSE OF GENETIC INFORMATION

Counselors have discovered that many affected persons perceive genetic information as both more personal and more revealing than a history of medical encounters or credit-worthy activities.[13] Even though classical geneticists have always insisted that genetic information is rarely final or conclusive and that genetic expression is strongly affected by interactive environmental forces, in the popular mind genes are widely perceived as emissaries of biological destiny.[14] Possibly because of a deep-seated need for diagnostic certainty, most people seem to view DNA probes as offering a virtually fail-safe diagnosis. Thus they make decisions not only on the basis of probabilities, but on a false sense of absolute predictability.

This tendency is underscored by a recent survey that indicates at-risk individuals are much more likely to act when given "certainty" of a particular fetal diagnosis than when given a slightly lesser probability. The willingness of mothers to abort an affected infant increases dramatically as the certainty of the diagnosis reaches 100 percent, even where prognosis is highly variable. When the diagnosis was presented as certain, but the severity of the prognosis variable (as in the case of a fetus with an unspecified neural tube defect) Johns Hopkins researchers have shown that almost 24 percent more married women would elect an abortion than when the diagnosis had a 95 percent probability (154 vs. 108 out of a sample of 193).[15]

In light of this dramatic finding, it is obvious that there is a gap between the stark genetic facts and a full understanding of their possible implications. If clinicians are to continue using gene probes as diagnostic tools (and all indications are that they will), it is essential to establish full-fledged education programs for their use.

DIAGNOSTIC AMBIGUITY

That this is more than an academic concern is underscored by the first indications that gene probe producers are aggressively seeking to market their products. Integrated Genetics of Framingham, Massachusetts, a self-described "genetic disease reference laboratory," has developed six test kits for genetic disorders, including cystic fibrosis, polycystic kidney disease, thalassemia, sickle cell anemia, retinoblastoma, and hemophilia B.[16] All are available to clinicians whether or not they can offer the recommended follow-up.

The readiness of these new tests for widescale clinical application is questionable. The recently uncovered gene for the enzyme deficiency thought to be responsible for Gaucher's disease illustrates the problem of over-precision. Actually a constellation of three related neurological disorders, the newly identified gene for Gaucher's had promised to be a "fail-safe" marker when present in a double dose for at least the most severe, early-onset form of the disease. Instead, the gene uncovered by a DNA probe was of little diagnostic value because it was associated with both the second and milder third forms of the disease. This uncertainty led a leading medical commentator to conclude that "we will be forced to look beyond the glucocerebrosidase gene to modifier genes or nongenetic factors to explain the differences" in manifestations of the Gaucher gene.[17]

Elsewhere, as with Integrated Genetics' test for cystic fibrosis, the assay is *not* for the gene itself, and comes with caveats from the company of the need for confirmatory testing. While the probability of successfully identifying an at-risk fetus in utero is likely to remain less than 100 percent until the gene itself is isolated, commercial companies may be expected to market increasing numbers of the most easily identified "flanking probes" for clinical use. Until consensus is reached in the medical community about what constitutes sufficient predictive value of such genetic tests, the potential for premature marketing and catastrophic medical error through false positive results will remain.

That this problem is imminent is underscored by the large investments of biotechnology firms in DNA probes. According to a Prudential-Bache Securities Firm employee, at least a $1 billion market in DNA probes will exist by 1995.[18] Neil Holtzman, a geneticist at Johns Hopkins University working for the Office of Technology Assessment, reported in 1986 that 43 of 86 biotechnology companies responding to a questionnaire survey are presently constructing DNA probes. An additional six plan to do so. Perhaps most interestingly, another twenty-two gave up plans to construct such probes. Seven said that they did so because the probe end uses were "too controversial." Of those who are developing probes, thirty-three plan to use them for diagnostic reagents. Twenty-eight (including some of the above thirty-three) plan to use the probes primarily as devices for making specific proteins.

Several of the companies reported to Holtzman that they intended to license probe tests from other companies. Focus Technology, an East coast biotechnology firm, intends to use the assembled probe battery as reagents for risk factor screening, with an eye toward the 100 to 200 diseases that have known biological markers or risk factors. According to Holtzman, major insurers such as Equitable Life Assurance Society have made substantial investments in developing such tests as part of potential screening programs. This "prognostic" probe market has already been entered by California Biotechnology of Mountain View, which has used five to seven RFLP-type tests to identify putative "risk status" of persons for atherosclerosis, diabetes and hypertension.

SUSCEPTIBILITY TESTING

Applications of such susceptibility testing are potentially unlimited. In addition to allowing rapid diagnosis for recurrent urethritis or periodontal disease, DNA probes could be used to assess which persons are most at risk for *developing* repeated bouts of bacterial infection. At least some of the underlying factors that determine such susceptibility are undoubtedly genetically determined, and given the large health costs of periodontitis, and recurrent urinary tract infection (UTI),[18] a screen to find high-risk persons would be medically attractive and no more controversial than current screening programs to find schoolgirls at risk for bacteria in their urine. Change the disease from UTI to AIDS and its implications for preemptive case finding becomes explosive.

In 1997 it might be common for a physician to give patients a battery of DNA probe tests as part of an intake procedure. Such a panel of tests would likely include susceptibility markers, since current panels include measurements of sentinel chemicals that are rough indicators of risk of heart or liver disease, and related problems. Predictive testing would almost certainly appeal to the physician charged with performing the intake screens on prospective applicants to an HMO — or to General Motors for that matter. What is at stake — in gathering some assurance of the long-term well-being of the clients or workers — is surely a powerful incentive to uncover genetically based deviance that indicates predisposition to disease.

A case in point is the widely touted development of susceptibility marker tests for autoimmune-associated arthritic conditions like ankylosing spondylitis. The gene for one such marker, the HLA B-27 allele, was cloned and used to develop a probe that presumably would detect increased susceptibility to back problems in the workplace. Like its monoclonal antibody counterpart developed by Cetusimmune, a biotechnology company in Palo Alto, California, this reagent promised to find at-risk workers and thereby enable the employer to take appropriate "remedial" measures — such as not employing them in the first place.

As with medical diagnostics that rely on DNA probes, a false sense of certitude colors the proposed applications of DNA probes for susceptibility testing. Unlike the problem of false positives in tests for specific, gene-directed diseases like cystic fibrosis, the higher precision of a susceptibility probe can do no more than reveal whether or not the sought-for gene is present — not that it will be responsible for causing a specific clinical problem later in life. Thus, the genes predisposing to heart disease that can now be "spotted" with a DNA probe,[19] are in fact substantially modifiable by environmental factors.

Clinicians and physicians may also be lulled into a false sense of security when they *fail* to uncover such a gene. Such an occasion could occur in the case of alpha-1-antitrypsin variants, a constellation of enzyme inhibitors associated with childhood cirrhosis of the liver and adult emphysema. Here, a probe for the Z variant most commonly linked to these pathological outcomes would *miss* the S variant also associated with a risk of liver or respiratory disease, since the probe would recognize the mutation leading to the Z variant, but not the different one giving rise to the S form.

A related but no less grave ethical dilemma arises from the characteristic variability of this recessive disorder. By age 4, only 3 percent of ZZ children deficient for alpha-1-antitrypsin will likely develop clinically evident liver disease — and a variable number of the remainder will develop emphysema, depending to a great extent on their smoking habits.[20] Yet, programs using high DNA technology to detect and abort the ZZ positive fetus have already begun[21] in spite of new evidence that this disorder is amenable to treatment.[22]

Thus, in the case of susceptibility markers, the gene is merely a statistical marker whose predictive value turns on the frequency with which gene-affected persons actually develop the expected disorder. Often, as in the case of ankylosing spondylitis, the arthritic condition linked to HLA B-27, many more of the persons positive for the gene remain disease-free than actually get ill.

MARKERS FOR TREATMENT OR DESTRUCTION

With their increasingly common application in prenatal diagnosis, DNA probes may be taken as an end to medical intervention itself. As defined by Lewis Thomas, such techniques might better be considered in the realm of "half-way technologies" that provide an intermediate "fix" for a condition. A gene probe for an affected fetus tells you it has found the defective gene. If you now abort that fetus, you are in effect negating the potential of the same genetic data to rescue that fetus. The identical gene sequence that can find an affected fetus can readily be modified to find the normal gene. The probe for the normal gene provides the instructions for making the gene product needed for its less fortunate mutant counterpart. With some imagination, genetic engineers have been able to use such "normal" probes to "reverse-engineer" the missing gene product, and to devise ways of putting that product, or instructions for its production, back into genetically deficient cells.

Such wholesome and patently useful applications of gene probes may be thwarted by their earlier — and easier — applications as simple markers of a fetus slated for abortion. This pattern may be happening in prenatal diagnosis for phenylketonuria and beta thalassemia. In both instances, DNA probes have permitted early diagnosis of affected fetuses. While abortion for PKU-positive fetuses (of which there are three variants of differing severity for this treatable disorder) has not yet been widely encouraged, the knowledge of the existence of the specific genes for such variants is currently not denied to prospective parents.[23]

If PKU probes are allowed into widespread use as prenatal diagnostic reagents, this will turn on its head the traditional end of previous PKU screening programs: the detection and successful treatment of a genetic disease.

A related dilemma exists for thalassemia. DNA analyses can be used to diagnose the group of blood disorders known as the thalassemias, in which the control of production of one or more of the chains of the hemoglobin molecule is disrupted.[24] Theoretically, the beta thalassemias are excellent candidates for genetic therapy. But the impetus for developing such therapies may now be blunted by the use of the gene probe (and other diagnostic technologies) to detect and abort affected fetuses — and to counsel at-risk adults against procreation.

THE FALLACY OF FAIL-SAFE DIAGNOSIS

The discovery of the means to preemptively detect *potentially* serious disease should not be taken to imply what we ought to do about those with the disorder. Nor should we blindly expand our net of DNA probes into the clinical arena without first reviewing how the resulting knowledge may be used or abused.

In a philosophical sense, the new wave of seemingly "fail-safe," precise DNA probe tests is colored with the optimism that reductionist biology can explain much if not most of the higher human capabilities or vulnerabilities. Indeed, this precision itself presents a dilemma. As indicators of the presence of gene sequences, DNA probes appear to offer a virtually fail-safe diagnosis. In fact, they can only reveal the presence of what is being sought — usually a *known* gene sequence. All probes will fail to correctly identify other defective variants of the gene, or a de novo mutation that differs in as little as one base pair from the DNA being sought.

It is well to remember that a *genetic* diagnosis also cannot fully account for the often variable phenotypic expression of the genes themselves. Nonetheless, because of a deep-seated need for certitude, many persons are likely to perceive a positive gene probe test as an indicator of biologic destiny. If this proves true, probes may acquire a misleading status in our medical armamentarium as indicators of a new kind of biological determinism. What can be done in the interim?

For a start, guidelines for the application of probes of varying predictive value could minimize the premature commercialization of imprecise diagnostic reagents. A second step would be to provide guidance to prospective parents using chorionic villi probes for prenatal diagnosis. Counseling here would detail the degree of *prognostic* as well as diagnostic uncertainty. A third would be to limit probes to clinicians' offices where trained counselors are available.

There is currently little, if any, justifiable application of DNA probes for rare untreatable metabolic or related disorders in population screening — either for newborns or mothers, since truly therapeutic interventions (unlike abortion) for newly targeted genetic diseases are still remote and without a family history of the disorder in question, the chance of finding an at-risk couple are infinitesimally low.

As illustrated by Gaucher's disease, certain genes are likely to be found that are indeed associated with complex and tragic medical disorders. But the gene is not the disease. We need to keep in mind that the final expression of the gene for any major human disorder requires interaction with other genes and/or provocative agents from the environment, a pattern that has been established for genes that predispose to coronary artery disease, diabetes, and high blood pressure.

Gene sequences are like the dots on a pointillist painting: without their context and interaction with other genes, the picture remains an abstraction. It is the interplay of genes among themselves and their external environment that shapes expression of ability and disability. If we fail to integrate this knowledge with our sensitivity to ethical principles, this new technology may fail to fulfill its true promise as an integral tool in detecting gene-based diseases and alleviating their concomitant suffering.

REFERENCES

1. Roger Lewin, "National Academy Looks at Human Genome Project, Sees Progress," *Science* 235 (1987), 747-48.
2. Joseph Palca, "Human Genome Sequencing Plan Wins Unanimous Approval in US," *Nature* 326 (1987), 429.
3. J.A. Egeland, D.S. Gerhard, and D.L. Pauls, "Bipolar Disorders Linked to DNA Markers on Chromosome 11," *Nature* 325 (1987), 783-87.
4. Francis S. Collins, Mitchell L. Drum, Jeffrey L. Cole et al., "Construction of a General Chromosome Jumping Library, with Application to Cystic Fibrosis," *Science* 235 (1987), 1046-49.
5. Anonymous, "Mapping the Human Genome," *Lancet* 1 (1987), 1121-22.
6. Lucy S. Tompkins, "Nucleic Acid Probes as Diagnostic Reagents," *APUA Newsletter* 4 (Summer 1986), 1-2.
7. Neil Holtzmann, "Susceptibility Conferring Genes," Paper presented at March of Dimes Bioethics Advisory Committee Meeting, September 21, 1986 (Tarrytown, New York).
8. Daniel Callahan, "Ethical Responsibility in Science in the Face of Uncertain Consequences," *Annals of the New York Academy of Sciences* 265 (1976), 1-12.
9. A. de la Chapelle, R.S. Sperkes, K. Berg, and H.P. Klinger, eds. *8th Annual Human Gene Mapping Conference,* (Basel: Karger, 1986).
10. H.M. Kingston, N.S.T. Thomas, P.L. Pearson et al., "Genetic Linkage between Becker Muscular Dystrophy and a Polymorphic DNA Sequence on the Short Arm of the X Chromosome," *Journal of Medical Genetics* 20 (1983), 255-58.
11. Nancy Wexler, personal communication, February 21, 1986.
12. Sandra G. Marchese and Robert Farrell, "The Attitudes and Limitations of Predictive Testing for Huntington's Disease," *Human Genetics* (Supp 1) A-175, December 1986.
13. Charles O. Leonard, Gary A. Chase, and Barton Childs, "Genetic Counseling: A Consumer's View," *New England Journal of Medicine* 287 (1972), 433-39.
14. Marc Lappé, *Genetic Politics* (New York: Doubleday Anchor Press, 1982).
15. Ruth R. Faden, A. Judith Chalow, Kimberly Quaid et al., "Prenatal Screening and Pregnant Women's Attitudes toward the Abortion of Defective Fetuses," *American Journal of Public Health* 77 (1987), 288-90.
16. Katherine K. Klinger. *Current Concepts in DNA Probe Analysis: Cystic Fibrosis* (Framingham, Mass.: Integrated Genetics, December 1986).
17. Arthur L. Beaudet, "Gaucher's Disease," *New England Journal of Medicine* 316 (1987), 619.
18. Jennifer Van Brunt and Arthur Klausner, "Pushing Probes to Market," *Bio/Technology* 5 (1987), 211-21.
19. R.A. Hegele, L. Huang, P.N. Herbert et al., "Apoliprotein B-gene DNA Polymorphisms Associated with Myocardial Infarction," *New England Journal of Medicine* 315 (1986), 1509-15.
20. T. Sveger and T. Thelin, "Four-year old children with alpha-1-antitrypsin deficiency," *Acta Pediatrica Scandinavia* 70 (1981), 171-77.
21. D.W. Cox and T. Mansfield, "Prenatal Diagnosis for Alpha-1-Antitrypsin Deficiency," *Lancet* 1 (1985), 230-32.

22. M.D. Weners, A. Casolavo, S.E. Sellers et al., "Replacement Therapy for Alpha-1-Antitrypsin Deficiency Associated with Emphysema," *New England Journal of Medicine* 316 (1987), 1055-62.
23. Savio Woo, Personal communication, March 12, 1987.
24. D.J. Weatherall, "Prenatal Diagnosis of Inherited Blood Disorders," *Clinics in Hoematology* 14 (1985), 747-74.

FURTHER READINGS

Bergsma, D., ed.
Ethical, Social and Legal Dimensions of Screening for Human Genetic Disease. Birth Defect Series, vol. 10. (New York: Stratton-Intercontinental).
Brown, J.
"Prenatal Screening in Jewish Law," *Journal of Medical Ethics* 16:2 (1990) 75-80.
Chadwick, D., et al., eds.
Human Genetic Information: Science, Law, Ethics. (New York: Wiley, 1990)
Clark, J.T.R.
"Screening for Carriers of Tay-Sachs Disease: Two Approaches," *Canadian Medical Association Journal*, 119 (1978), 450.
Kenen, R.H. and R.M. Schmidt
"Stigmatization of Carrier Status: Social Implications of Heterozygote Genetic Screening Programs," *American Journal of Public Health*, 68 (1978), 116-120.
Knoppers, B.M.
Human Dignity and Genetic Heritage. Study Paper for the Law Reform Commission of Canada (Ottawa: Law Reform Commission of Canada, 1991).
Murray, R.F.
"Problems Behind the Promise: Ethical Issues in Mass Genetic Screening," *Hastings Center Report* 2 (April 1979), 46-7.
Nelkin, D. and L. Tancredi
Dangerous Diagnostics: The Social Power of Biological Information. (New York: Basic Books, 1989).
Overall, C.
Ethics and Human Reproduction: A Feminist Analysis. (Boston: Allen and Unwin, 1987).
Powledge, Tabitha and Joseph Fletcher
"Guidelines for the Ethical, Social, and Legal Issues in Prenatal Diagnosis," *New England Journal of Medicine* 300: 4 (1979) 168-172.

CHAPTER 19 GENETIC COUNSELLING

INTRODUCTION

What should humanity do with the knowledge about genetics that it already has and that it is in the process of developing? One of the suggestions is that it should be used to tell people who carry so-called defective genes about their genetic make-up, and to inform them of the implications it has for their health and for the health of any offspring they might have. In other words, one possible use is genetic counselling.

Genetic counselling has become a standard aspect of reproductive medicine. However, such counselling is not without its own problems. For instance, what precisely is the role of the counsellor in this? Should the counsellor merely tell the patients of the nature of their genetic condition, and outline possible options? Or should the counsellor also give advice about such things as whether the patients should risk having children? In other words, should the counselling be only explanatory, or does the counsellor also have a right to try and influence the patients in their decision-making? These questions may be easy to answer, given current emphasis on patient autonomy. However, what about society? Does society have a role in this? Perhaps as guardian of future generations, or as the agency that will ultimately have to pay for any health care costs that might arise as a result of a decision by someone who carries deleterious genes?

The selection by West gives the perspective of a physician actively engaged in genetic counselling at St. George's Medical School, London (England). A particular focus of West's concern is another parameter that arises once we know something about the genetic make-up of a person: should the knowledge of this make-up be shared with the family of that person? After all, quite frequently the family will also be affected. West suggests that it may be reasonable to at least look at this.

Raanan Gillon, a physician and ethicist, focuses on the implications that West's suggestions would have for patient confidentiality, and places the issue into the wider context of confidentiality *per se*.

Genetic screening also carries with it the possibility of discrimination. For instance, Tay-Sachs disease is a progressive degenerative disease of the nervous system, which is inherited when both parents carry a defective gene governing the production of the enzyme hexosaminidase A. The disease is 100 times more frequent among Ashkenazi Jews than among non-Jews, and approximately one in 30 Ashkenazi Jews carries the gene. Some people have argued that not only would it cost too much to test the entire Jewish population but also that the result would be useless. One cannot ethically force people who carry the gene not to have children. That would be to discriminate against Jews in general, and Ashkenazi Jews in particular.[1] Similar arguments have been raised for a whole variety of heritable genetic conditions.

Purdy opposes this view. She argues that if we know that we carry a deleterious gene and that there is a good chance that our children will have a serious health problem as a result, we have an obligation to refrain from having children. This has nothing to do with ethnicity. It has to do with obligations to future persons. If we go ahead anyway, we are responsible for the injurious state in which they will live. Purdy believes that this is unethical.

NOTE

1. Goodman, M.J. and L.E. Goodman, "The Overselling of Genetic Anxiety," *Hastings Center Report* 12:5 (1982) 20-27.

Ethical Aspects of Genetic Disease and Genetic Counselling

Richard West

AUTHOR'S ABSTRACT

With the reduction in diseases due to nutritional deficiencies and infection, disorders which are wholly or partly genetic are becoming relatively more important in all branches of modern medicine.

Genetic counselling has developed in recent years from just explaining to an individual or a couple the risk of them producing a handicapped child, to the possibility in many cases of better diagnosis and active intervention to reduce the risks. At the same time antenatal screening programmes have

Richard West, "Ethical Aspects of Genetic Disease and Genetic Counselling," *Journal of Medical Ethics* 14:4 (1988) 194-197.

been introduced to detect women who may be carrying a fetus with a severe handicapping anomaly.

The ethical aspects of these advances are considered in this article. A practical approach to the resolution of any dilemmas is proposed which concentrates on the duties incumbent on doctors and other health care workers involved with patients who have or may carry genetic disorders.

INTRODUCTION

Genetic disorders are common and are seen in all medical specialties. Most are first manifest in childhood, and in developed countries the decline in importance of infective disease and nutritional deficiencies in childhood has led to congenital and genetic disorders becoming relatively more important. It is estimated that wholly or partly inherited disorders now account for between 11 and 27 per cent of hospital admissions of children, and are a major factor in 50 per cent of childhood deaths.[1]

In recent years there have been technological advances and growth in understanding of inheritance so that new practical applications have been and are being introduced into patient care in the management of genetic disease.

As genetic medicine and counselling can cover such topics as whether a couple should reproduce, the possibility of handicap in the offspring, and the investigation and possible termination of pregnancy they raise many ethical issues.[2, 3] The World Medical Association issued a brief statement of guidance on genetic counselling and genetic engineering in 1987 that highlights some of the issues they see as crucial,[4] and the King's Fund has recently held a consensus conference on screening for fetal and genetic abnormality which highlighted some of the ethical issues.[5] Genetic engineering is outside the scope of this article.

DOCTOR-PATIENT RELATIONSHIPS IN GENETIC DISEASE

There are three different types of doctor-patient relationship in genetic disease, each of which imposes different duties on the doctor.

Firstly, doctors in any specialty may care for patients whose disease is largely or wholly genetic. As with other patients the doctor's primary responsibility will be the diagnosis and management of the patient's medical condition. The doctor should explain to the patient the genetic aspects of the condition, and must point out if there are implications for other family members. Referral of the patient or relatives to a geneticist is appropriate where the doctor does not have the necessary knowledge or skills for giving genetic advice.

Secondly, doctors may be specifically involved in evaluating, from a genetic point of view, prospective parents before conception. This applies to individuals or couples who seek advice because they have had a child with an abnormality that may be genetic, or because such a disorder is in the family, or affects the individual seeking help. Couples who are consanguineous may also seek advice. When the doctor is involved in investigating a family in which there is a genetic problem he or she may have to take the initiative in seeking out family members who could be carriers of a genetic problem.

Thirdly, with the development of screening procedures for congenital and genetic disorders either before or during pregnancy doctors are involved in ensuring that there is informed consent to the procedure, and in meeting the need for skilled counselling if an abnormal condition is found.

STAGES IN GENETIC COUNSELLING

The aim of genetic counselling is to inform the patient or patients of the risks of genetic disease occurring in their offspring or those of other family members, and to advise them of the options for reducing that risk. This should have the effect of reducing the number of individuals being born with severe handicapping conditions of genetic origin.

Genetic diagnosis has to precede counselling, and consists of ascertaining both a full family history and as precise a diagnosis as possible of any congenital or genetic disease. An accurate diagnosis is important, as in some situations a given phenotype may have more than one genetic cause, or even not be genetic at all.

Counselling consists of a) giving information to an individual or a couple on the likelihood of them producing a child with a disease or abnormality, b) advising them on thc implications of producing such a child, including providing medical information about the severity and treatment of the condition, c) advising them of the ways the risk might be reduced, and d) helping them to understand and come to terms with this information, so that they can make informed decisions about whether to embark on a pregnancy.

REDUCING THE RISK OF HAVING A BABY WITH A HANDICAPPING CONDITION

The desire to have children of one's own can be very strong, and many couples will decide to have children even when they know the risk is high and the disease serious. The options available for lowering the risks of producing a child with a disability will depend both on the form of inheritance, and on the disease itself. The major options which are technically feasible are listed below. Many of them raise moral dilemmas for some couples and also for some doctors.

1) Discriminatory Pairing

In families where there is a serious recessive disorder the doctor should point out the risks inherent in cousin marriage. If it is possible to test for the carrier state it can be determined whether there is a risk for a particular pairing.

Screening adolescents to detect heterozygotes of serious recessive disorders has been practised for conditions such as Tay-Sachs disease, thalassaemia and sickle cell disease. Heterozygous individuals are counselled and advised to have prospective partners tested for carrier status before embarking on joint parenthood.

2) Not Having Children

Many couples who have had a child with a handicapping condition which could recur will opt not to have further children. Similarly some couples found to be carriers of genetic disease, either because of screening or a family study may make this decision.

3) Changing Partners

Marital breakdown sometimes occurs when a couple have produced a child with a handicapping condition. Genetically, for recessive disorders it may enable both partners to have other children without risk of recurrence. For an individual with a dominant disease, or carrying an x-linked condition or a balanced translocation the risk will remain high with any partner.

4) Minimising the Risk by Selective Abortion

With the use of chorionic villus biopsy, amniocentesis, fetoscopy, fetal blood sampling or ultrasound screening it is possible to detect many genetic disorders or serious abnormalities of the fetus in early pregnancy. If an abnormality is found to be present the woman could then be offered an abortion. For many x-linked disorders it is possible to determine by specific testing that a fetus is likely to be affected. Where this is not possible the abortion of all male fetuses prevents the birth of affected individuals, but not of carrier females.

Women not thought to be at particular risk may be found by ultrasound screening in early pregnancy to be carrying a fetus with a major abnormality such as anencephaly or spina bifida. Amniocentesis screening of older women for Down's Syndrome will also identify affected fetuses where the mothers were not at particular risk, apart from their age. Decisions on whether to consider abortion have then to be made quickly.

5) Artificial Insemination

Where a couple are both known to be carriers of a harmful recessive gene the use of artificial insemination from an unrelated donor can result in a pregnancy with minimal risk of handicap.

6) Ovum Transfer

Where a woman carries an x-linked harmful gene, ovum transfer (gamete intrafallopian transfer, GIFT) would be one way she could have a low-risk pregnancy.

7) Treatment of the Fetus In Utero

It seems probable that the incidence of spina bifida is lowered in high-risk families where mothers take vitamin and mineral supplements before conception.[6] In some conditions damage to a fetus can be prevented by medical treatment given to the mother. Dietary control of blood phenylalanine in mothers with phenylketonuria prevents mental handicap in the baby; steroids can prevent virilisation of the fetus in congenital adrenal hyperplasia. Surgical treatment of the fetus may also be possible. Fetal bladder catheterisation in urinary obstruction has been successful in preventing renal damage, and further developments of this approach are likely.

8) Genetic Manipulation of the Fetus

In the future it may be possible to implant into a fetus a missing gene, to prevent the development of a disease. Attempts have already been made at marrow and organ transplantation in some recessive conditions.[7] The use of specific gene clones may one day become possible.

AREAS OF ETHICAL UNCERTAINTY IN GENETIC COUNSELLING

Many of the steps listed above that necessitate active intervention and can be taken to alter the risk of producing a baby with a handicap are well recognised areas of moral uncertainty. Consensus does not exist over abortion, fetal rights, artificial insemination, ovum transfer or genetic manipulation. The arguments will not be restated here.

There is, however, general agreement that the doctor should respect the conscience and moral beliefs of the patient, and not impose his personal moral values. A doctor may choose not to give genetic advice where it conflicts with his own conscience, but in that situation he should alert the parents where there is a potential genetic problem, and advise them to seek genetic counselling.

Less well established are the issues of who should be given genetic advice, confidentiality and family information, which handicaps are severe enough to warrant intervention, and the particular problems of screening.

WHO SHOULD BE GIVEN GENETIC ADVICE AND WHO OWNS FAMILY INFORMATION?

A patient with a genetic disease and those seeking genetic advice should be given appropriate information and counselling. Indeed failure to do so, or giving wrong advice could be grounds for an action for negligence. Information given which is reinforced by writing to the patient goes some way to ensuring that the advice given is both understood and remembered.

Making a genetic diagnosis may have implications for some members of the extended family. For instance the sisters of a woman whose child has an x-linked disorder may also be carriers; a patient with a dominant disorder like Huntingdon's chorea may have first and second degree relatives who also carry the gene, and may pass it on, and in a family where consanguinity is common a recessive disorder may recur in other sibships. The doctor has a duty to other family members even if he has a special relationship with one family member.

The doctor also has a duty to the family to collect as much diagnostic information as possible. It may seem hard at a time when a family are distressed over a stillbirth or child death to recommend a post mortem, but it may be vital in establishing a precise diagnosis. Similarly the opportunity should not be lost to take photographs, x-rays, or blood and fibroblast specimens.

Not imparting relevant information that an individual might reasonably be expected to be told is difficult to justify. Sometimes imparting information could be thought as being potentially harmful, perhaps because of its effect on the mental state of a carrier of a harmful gene (particularly one with delayed effect like Huntingdon's chorea), or because it might disrupt a marriage. In most cases such paternalistic arguments are outweighed by the potential harm that could arise through not knowing.

A further difficulty in advising relevant members of the extended family may be the question of confidentiality. In most cases the family will readily share information amongst its members, and the relatives can then seek advice for themselves. When the index clients are reluctant to communicate with other family members every effort should be made by the doctor to persuade them. Where this approach fails the doctor must decide whether the need to know that one may be the carrier of a potentially harmful gene outweighs the duty of confidentiality to the index patient.

This will depend both on the severity of the condition and the likelihood of the person having affected offspring. For severe sex-linked disorders such as Duchenne muscular dystrophy or fragile-x syndrome the need of the sister of a carrier mother to know that she may also be a carrier outweighs the duty to preserve absolute confidentiality. If confidentiality is to be breached in this limited way the index patient should be informed, and the reasons explained.

As a general principle all members of a family should have a right of access to information about genetic disease within the family which might be of importance to them.

THE SEVERITY OF HANDICAP

One of the primary aims of genetic counselling is to reduce the numbers of babies born with serious handicap. In Britain conscientious objection to abortion on the grounds of fetal abnormality is only the viewpoint of a minority. However, difficulties can arise over a patient's perception of the severity of a handicap.

Few would disagree with a decision to terminate an early pregnancy where the fetus was shown to have anencephaly, or to have spina bifida, which it is known results in a poor quality of life for the child and serious problems for the family. For Down's Syndrome, where although the child is going to be mentally handicapped the quality of life for the individual can be very good, there might be less certainty. Termination of a fetus that has a surgically correctable abnormality cannot be rationally justified, although for some parents the detection of any abnormality may provoke a request for abortion.

PARTICULAR PROBLEMS OF ANTENATAL SCREENING

Apart from testing the fetus where there is known to be a familial risk of a handicapping condition, there are some screening procedures that are more widely used. Before undergoing these procedures women should be informed of the possibility of detection of fetal abnormality.

Ultrasound screening of the fetus is offered to all women in pregnancy to assess fetal maturity. At the same time the fetus is examined morphologically, and a severe fetal abnormality such as anencephaly or spina bifida may be detected. Screening for Down's Syndrome in older mothers by chromosomal analysis of fetal tissue obtained by amniocentesis or chorionic villous biopsy is offered in many centres.

Where an abnormality is discovered by antenatal screening the mother has to be informed and rapidly counselled about the implications of the discovery. A decision either to continue with the pregnancy or to have a termination has to be taken rapidly. The mother must be given enough information, support and counselling to enable her to make an autonomous decision, and she must decide on how much her partner should be involved in the decision-making.

An additional problem sometimes arises in chromosomal screening for Down's Syndrome, in that other chromosomal anomalies may be detected instead. Where these are known to be associated with severe handicap the woman can be appropriately counselled. More difficult are the chromosomal anomalies associated with less severe handicap or inconstantly associated with disease, such as Turner's syndrome, XXX and XYY. The doctor has a duty to inform the parents about the results of the test, but may not be in a position to say whether the baby is going to be seriously handicapped by the chromosomal anomaly. Included in the information given to a mother before screening for Down's Syndrome should be the possibility of the test detecting other anomalies and that if this happens she will be appropriately counselled about the possible significance of the anomaly.

DUTIES OF DOCTORS WHEN DEALING WITH GENETIC DISEASE

Many of the practical and ethical problems concerning genetic counselling and the management of genetic diseases are made easier for the doctor (or other health worker) by summarising the medical responsibilities. Inevitably some items included on such a list are debatable, but it is suggested that the following should be generally acceptable. They are in harmony with, and some are based on, the World Medical Association Statement on Genetic Counselling and Genetic Engineering.[4]

OBLIGATIONS AFFECTING ALL DOCTORS

Doctors have a duty to inform patients when they know of genetic factors that could lead to significant genetic or congenital disease in the offspring of the patient or other family members. The doctor should either give genetic advice himself, or offer referral to a geneticist for such advice.

The patient should be encouraged where appropriate to disseminate relevant genetic information within the family. The physician must be prepared to see other family members personally or refer them to an appropriate physician.

Doctors whose own moral values are opposed to abortion, sterilisation or contraception may choose not to give genetic advice. They must, however, inform prospective parents where a potential genetic problem exists, and advise that they seek the opinion of a clinical geneticist, and arrange such a referral.

Doctors should be aware that genetic diagnosis and screening is a field of rapid advance; the doctor has a duty to provide up-to-date information, or to refer to someone who can provide it.

When a genetic defect is found in a fetus prospective parents may or may not want an abortion. Doctors should avoid the substitution of their own moral judgement in place of that of the prospective parents.

A doctor should not breach his patient's confidentiality over genetic matters unless he has discussed the need to do so with the patient. If, in spite of encouragement the patient refuses to inform or involve other family members the doctor is entitled to limited breach of confidentiality to a third party where it is in the medical interest of that third party to know genetic information.

Special Obligations of Medical Geneticists

Doctors engaged in genetic counselling must provide prospective parents with the basis for an informed decision for childbearing.

Obligations Concerning Genetic Screening

Doctors should ensure that a woman is not to be a participant in a screening programme for genetic disease or congenital abnormality without her informed consent. A woman's access to a screening or diagnostic test should be independent of any decision she may make about the continuation of the pregnancy.

A woman's considered and informed decision not to participate in a screening programming must be respected. Appropriate care and support must be offered to her and the family.

ACKNOWLEDGEMENT

I would like to acknowledge helpful criticism from Dr M Patton.

REFERENCES

1. Emery A E H, Rimoin D L. Nature and incidence of genetic disease. In: Emery A E H, Rimoin D L, eds. *Principles and Practice of Medical Genetics.* Edinburgh: Churchill Livingstone, 1983:1-3.
2. Arnold A, Moseley R. Ethical issues arising from medical genetics. *Journal of Medical Ethics* 1976; 2:12-17.
3. Seller M J. Ethical aspects of genetic counselling. *Journal of Medical Ethics* 1982; 8:185-188.
4. World Medical Association. Statement on genetic counselling and genetic engineering. *IME Bulletin* 1987; 31:8-9.
5. King's Fund forum consensus statement. Screening for fetal and genetic abnormality. *British Medical Journal,* 1987; 295:1551-1553.
6. Smithells R W, Sheppard S, Schorah C J, *et al.* Possible prevention of neural-tube defects by periconceptual vitamin supplementation. *Lancet* 1980; 1:339-340.
7. Hobbs J R. Thirty-eight different metabolic errors (previously fatal) have been corrected by displacement bone marrow transplantation. *Archives of Disease in Childhood* 1985; 60:1097 (abstract).

Genetic Counselling, Confidentiality, and the Medical Interests of Relatives

Raanan Gillon

Following the World Medical Association's brief declaration on genetic counselling and genetic engineering,[1] Dr Richard West offers in this issue of the journal a resumé of areas of contemporary professional agreement about genetic counselling, at least so far as those health carers who accept the moral permissibility of abortion are concerned.

Thus the fundamental objectives of genetic counselling are seen to be the provision of information to those who are, or whose relatives are or will be, at risk of significant genetic or congenital disease, including information about such options as are available to reduce or eliminate such risks.

The issues which turn clearly on attitudes to abortion are not addressed — as Dr West says, the arguments have been well rehearsed. However, doctors are urged not to impose their own moral attitudes upon their patients and if they find themselves disagreeing with the moral stance of their patients over these issues they should explain their situation and advise the patient to consult a clinical geneticist. Such views are now sufficiently common within the medical profession, even among those members who strongly disapprove of abortion, to be properly described as consensus views.

Less agreement may be expected over Dr West's assertion that 'the doctor is enti-

Raanan Gillon, "Genetic Counselling, Confidentiality, and the Medical interests of Relatives," *Journal of Medical Ethics* 14:4 (1988) 171-172.

tled to limited breach of confidentiality to a third party where it is in the medical interest of that third party to know genetic information'; the underlying issues deserve some consideration.

The norms of medical confidentiality require doctors not to divulge information imparted to them by their patients which those patients wish to keep secret. Such medical confidentiality has been an obligation in medical practice at least since Hippocratic times and can be justified from a variety of moral standpoints — as a value in itself within the class of promise keeping, and/or within the class of respect for privacy; and/or as a manifestation of respect for autonomy; or simply as a value which conduces to the utilitarian ideal of welfare maximisation.[2] However, despite stalwart defences to the contrary[3] there seem to be no convincing moral defences for an *absolute* principle of medical confidentiality according to which confidences must in no circumstances be breached, no matter how harmful the consequences of maintaining confidentiality would be. Rather, the principle of medical confidentiality seems most firmly justifiable as a very strong *prima facie* principle, to be overridden only by even stronger moral claims.

A wide variety of such counterclaims are permitted as valid defences for breach of confidentiality by the General Medical Council (GMC) in Britain[4] and somewhat fewer by the British Medical Association (BMA)[5] — but neither organisation explicitly permits the medical interests of third parties to justify breach of medical confidentiality. However, perhaps the exceptions offered by the GMC and BMA do *implicitly* encompass the medical interests of third parties as being sufficient justification of breach of confidentiality? Seven of the eight proffered exceptions are clearly inapplicable. Thus by hypothesis the exception of patient consent does not apply and the transfer of information to other health care workers is not the relevant issue; the exception whereby doctors are permitted to inform relatives or close friends where it is medically undesirable to seek the patient's consent is clearly not relevant; nor is the exception of disclosure to a third party, other than a relative, in 'the best interests of the patient'; the exceptions based on statutory requirements to disclose and court directives to disclose do not apply, and nor does the dispensation to disclose medical information for the purpose of approved medical research. Only the remaining exception — overriding of confidentiality 'in the public interest' — seems to offer the possibility of support. However, as that exception stands at present it seems unlikely to encompass the medical interests of others, unless harm equivalent to 'grave or very serious crime' is caused or allowed to go unpunished by failure to disclose a medical confidence. Thus the possibly relevant GMC exception states: 'Rarely, disclosure may be justified on the ground that it is in the public interest which, in certain circumstances such as, for example, investigation by the police of a grave or very serious crime, might override the doctor's duty to maintain his patient's confidence'.[4] Similarly the BMA exception of 'the doctor's overriding duty to society' is also glossed in terms of 'a very grave crime where the security of the public is at risk'.[5]

Is disclosure of genetic information to other members of a patient's family, when the patient has refused to permit such disclosure and rejects the doctor's requests to pass on information given in medical confidence, justifiable under this exception as being 'in the public interest'? And if it is, is other information, apart from genetic information, disclosed in confidence by a patient also justifiably to be passed on to other members of the patient's family against the patient's will, provided that such disclosure is thought by the doctor to be in the third party's medical interests? And if so, why restrict such disclosure to family members? Presumably all third parties should then be entitled to be given confidential medical information if it is in their medical interests to have it? Thus the proposed exception to confidentiality of third party medical benefit would, for example, equally justify doctors breaking confidences and passing information about sexually transmitted disease on to sexual partners.

Such questions are not rhetorical, and arguments can be offered in support of disclosure — for example arguments based on the claim that doctors have a wide-ranging duty to all whose health is threatened to try to benefit them medically and to try to prevent or at least minimise their risk of being harmed by disease. Along such lines many will argue that if a doctor in the course of a consultation discovers that others are substantially threatened, whether by illness or anything else, then that doctor should ensure that the necessary steps are taken to minimise the threat, whether or not the patient gives permission. Similarly it could be argued that in some cases failure to inform about risks of severe genetic disease would result in sufficiently substantial harm to others to justify such overriding of a patient's confidences.

On the other hand with every additional erosion of medical confidentiality in the interests of others the principle itself becomes ever more suspect, more 'decrepit' in Siegler's memorable phraseology,[6] and presumably the medical profession becomes ever less trusted to keep its patients' secrets. Such reduction in trust is increasingly likely to stop patients from passing on any information to doctors which they wish to keep secret. As a result the general provision of good quality medical care is likely to suffer, to the detriment of the very public interest that is cited as justification for the breaking of medical confidentiality.

At present it seems likely that the norms of medical confidentiality as expressed in official guidelines favour the latter argument, and do not permit transgression of medical confidences in order to serve the medical interests of third parties, unless harm equivalent to grave or very serious crime is involved. Whether or not information about genetic disorders would 'officially' be thought to fall into this category is not stated in the GMC and BMA codes, but it seems unlikely. A recent King's Fund consensus statement on screening for fetal and genetic abnormality was more explicit, stating that 'if it is desirable to include relatives and partners in screening this must also be based on informed consent'.[7] However, in America the President's commission on bioethical issues argued that in limited circumstances confidentiality could justifiably be transgressed in the medical interests of relatives, where serious harm to relatives was likely to be prevented by so doing.[8]

In an area of such contention and uncertainty the case proposed by Dr West requires rigorous scrutiny not only by the medical professions but also by the public in whose interests such reform is offered. Whatever the outcome, the norms of medical confidentiality adopted by the profession should surely be widely and effectively publicised, so that patients can have a reasonably clear idea of the circumstances in which information which they give their doctors in confidence may nonetheless be passed on to others against their will.

REFERENCES AND NOTES

1. World Medical Association. Statement on genetic counselling and genetic engineering, 1987. Reprinted in: *IME Bulletin* 1987; 31: 8-9.
2. Gillon R. *Philosophical Medical Ethics.* Chichester: Wiley, 1986; 106-112.
3. Kottow M. Medical confidentiality: an intransigent and absolute obligation. *Journal of Medical Ethics* 1986; 12: 117-122.
4. General Medical Council. *Professional Conduct and Discipline: Fitness to Practise.* London: GMC, 1987: 19-22.
5. British Medical Association. *The Handbook of Medical Ethics.* London, 1984; 12-15.
6. Seigler M. Confidentiality in medicine: a decrepit concept. *New England Journal of Medicine* 1982; 307: 1518-1521.
7. King's Fund forum consensus statement: screening for fetal and genetic abnormality. *British Medical Journal* 1987; 295: 1551-1553.
8. President's commission for the study of ethical problems in medicine. *Screening and Counseling for Genetic Conditions.* Washington DC: US Government Printing Office, 1983: 42-45.

Genetic Diseases: Can Having Children Be Immoral?*

L. M. Purdy

I INTRODUCTION

Suppose you know that there is a fifty percent chance you have Huntington's chorea, even though you are still free of symptoms, and that if you do have it, each of your children has a fifty percent chance of having it also.

Should you now have children?

There is always some possibility that a pregnancy will result in a diseased or handicapped child. But certain persons run a higher than average risk of producing such a child. Genetic counselors are increasingly able to calculate the probability that certain problems will occur; this means that more people can find out whether they are in danger of creating unhealthy offspring *before* the birth of a child.

Since this kind of knowledge is available, we ought to use it wisely. I want in this paper to defend the thesis that it is wrong to reproduce when we know there is a high risk of transmitting a serious disease or defect. My argument for this claim is in three parts. The first is that we should try to provide every child with a normal opportunity for health; the second is that in the course of doing this it is not wrong to prevent possible children from existing. The third is that this duty may require us to refrain from childbearing.[1]

L.M. Purdy, "Genetic Diseases: Can Having Children Be Immoral?" in *Genetics Now: Ethical Issues in Genetic Research* ed. by J.J. Buckley, Jr. (Washington, DC: University Press of America, 1978) 6 pp.

One methodological point must be made. I am investigating a problem in biomedical ethics: this is a philosophical enterprise. But the conclusion has practical importance since individuals do face the choice I examine. This raises a question: what relation ought the outcome of this inquiry bear to social policy?[2] It may be held that a person's reproductive life should not be interfered with. Perhaps this is a reasonable position, but it does not follow from it that it is never wrong for an individual to have children or that we should not try to determine when this is the case. All that does follow is that we may not coerce persons with regard to childbearing. Evaluation of this last claim is a separate issue which cannot be handled here.

I want to deal with this issue concretely. The reason for this is that, otherwise, discussion is apt to be vague and inconclusive. An additional reason is that it will serve to make us appreciate the magnitude of the difficulties faced by diseased or handicapped individuals. Thus it will be helpful to consider a specific disease. For this purpose I have chosen Huntington's chorea.[3]

II HUNTINGTON'S CHOREA: COURSE AND RISK

Let us now look at Huntington's chorea. First we will consider the course of the disease, then its inheritance pattern.

The symptoms of Huntington's chorea usually begin between the ages of thirty and fifty, but young children can also be affected. It happens this way:

> Onset is insidious. Personality changes (obstinacy, moodiness, lack of initiative) frequently antedate or accompany the involuntary choreic movements. These usually appear first in the face, neck, and arms, and are jerky, irregular, and stretching in character. Contractions of the facial muscles result in grimaces; those of the respiratory muscles, lips, and tongue lead to hesitating, explosive speech. Irregular movements of the trunk are present; the gait is shuffling and dancing. Tendon reflexes are increased ... Some patients display a fatuous euphoria; others are spiteful, irascible, destructive, and violent. Paranoid reactions are common. Poverty of thought and impairment of attention, memory, and judgment occur. As the disease progresses, walking becomes impossible, swallowing difficult, and dementia profound. Suicide is not uncommon.[4]

The illness lasts about fifteen years, terminating in death.

Who gets Huntington's chorea? It is an autosomal dominant disease; this means it is caused by a single mutant gene located on a non-sex chromosome. It is passed from one generation to the next via affected individuals. When one has the disease, whether one has symptoms and thus knows one has it or not, there is a 50% chance that each child will have it also. If one has escaped it then there is no risk to one's children.[5]

How serious is this risk? For geneticists, a ten percent risk is high.[6] But not every high risk is unacceptable: this depends on what is at stake.

There are two separate evaluations in any judgment about a given risk. The first measures the gravity of the worst possible result; the second perceives a given risk as great or small. As for the first, in medicine as elsewhere, people may regard the same result quite differently:

> ... The subjective attitude to the disease or lesion itself may be quite at variance with what informed medical opinion may regard as a realistic appraisal. Relatively minor limb defects with cosmetic overtones are examples here. On the other hand,

> some patients regard with equanimity genetic lesions which are of major medical importance.[7]

For devastating diseases like Huntington's chorea, this part of the judgment should be unproblematic: no one could want a loved one to suffer so.

There may be considerable disagreement, however, about whether a given probability is big or little. Individuals vary a good deal in their attitude toward this aspect of risk.[8] This suggests that it would be difficult to define the "right" attitude to a particular risk in many circumstances. Nevertheless, there are good grounds for arguing in favor of a conservative approach here. For it is reasonable to take special precautions to avoid very bad consequences, even if the risk is small. But the possible consequences here *are* very bad: a child who may inherit Huntington's chorea is a child with a much larger than average chance of being subjected to severe and prolonged suffering. Even if the child does not have the disease, it may anticipate and fear it, and anticipating an evil, as we all know, may be worse than experiencing it. In addition, if a parent loses the gamble, his child will suffer the consequences. But it is one thing to take a high risk for oneself; to submit someone else to it without his consent is another.

I think that these points indicate that the morality of procreation in situations like this demands further study. I propose to do this by looking first at the position of the possible child, then at that of the potential parent.[9]

III REPRODUCTION: THE POSSIBLE CHILD'S POSITION

The first task in treating the problem from the child's point of view is to find a way of referring to possible future offspring without seeming to confer some sort of morally significant existence upon them. I will call children who might be born in the future but who are not now conceived "possible" children, offspring, individuals, or persons. I stipulate that this term implies nothing about their moral standing.

The second task is to decide what claims about children or possible children are relevant to the morality of childbearing in the circumstances being considered. There are, I think, two such claims. One is that we ought to provide every child with at least a normal opportunity for a good life. The other is that we do not harm possible children if we prevent them from existing. Let us consider both these matters in turn.

A. Opportunity for a Good Life

Accepting the claim that we ought to try to provide for every child a normal opportunity for a good life involves two basic problems: justification and practical application.

Justification of the claim could be derived fairly straightforwardly from either utilitarian or contractarian theories of justice, I think, although a proper discussion would be too lengthy to include here. Of prime importance in any such discussion would be the judgment that to neglect this duty would be to create unnecessary unhappiness or unfair disadvantage for some persons.

The attempt to apply the claim that we should try to provide a normal opportunity for a good life leads to a couple of difficulties. One is knowing what it requires of us. Another is defining "normal opportunity." Let us tackle the latter problem first.

Conceptions of "normal opportunity" vary among societies and also within them: *de rigueur* in some circles are private music lessons and trips to Europe, while in others providing eight years of schooling is a major sacrifice. But there is no need to consider this complication since we are here concerned only with health as a prerequisite for normal opportunity. Thus we can retreat to the more limited claim that every parent should try to ensure normal health for his child. It might be thought that even this moderate claim is unsatisfactory since in some places debilitating conditions are the norm. One could circumvent this objection by saying that parents ought to try to provide for their children health normal for that culture, even though it may be inadequate if measured by some outside standard. This conservative position would still justify efforts to avoid the birth of children at risk for Huntington's chorea and other serious genetic diseases.

But then what does this stand require of us: is sacrifice entailed by the duty to try to provide normal health for our children? The most plausible answer seems to be that as the danger of serious disability increases, the greater the sacrifice demanded of the potential parent. This means it would be more justifiable to recommend that an individual refrain from childbearing if he risks passing on spina bifida than if he risks passing on webbed feet. Working out all the details of such a schema would clearly be a difficult matter; I do not think it would be impossible to set up workable guidelines, though.

Assuming a rough theoretical framework of this sort, the next question we must ask is whether Huntington's chorea substantially impairs an individual's opportunity for a good life.

People appear to have different opinions about the plight of such persons. Optimists argue that a child born into a family afflicted with Huntington's chorea has a reasonable chance of living a satisfactory life. After all, there is a fifty percent chance it will escape the disease even if a parent has already manifested it, and a still greater chance if this is not so. Even if it does have the illness, it will probably enjoy thirty years of healthy life before symptoms appear; and, perhaps, it may not find the disease destructive. Optimists can list diseased or handicapped persons who have lived fruitful lives. They can also find individuals who seem genuinely glad to be alive. One is Rick Donohue, a sufferer from the Joseph family disease: "You know, if my mom hadn't had me, I wouldn't be here for the life I have had. So there is a good possibility I will have children."[10] Optimists therefore conclude that it would be a shame if these persons had not lived.

Pessimists concede these truths, but they take a less sanguine view of them. They think a fifty percent risk of serious disease like Huntington's chorea appallingly high. They suspect that a child born into an afflicted family is liable to spend its youth in dreadful anticipation and fear of the disease. They expect that the disease, if it appears, will be perceived as a tragic and painful end to a blighted life. They point out that Rick Donohue is still young and has not yet experienced the full horror of his sickness.

Empirical research is clearly needed to resolve this dispute: we need much more information about the psychology and life history of sufferers and potential sufferers. Until we have it we cannot know whether the optimist or the pessimist has a better case; definitive judgment must therefore be suspended. In the meantime, however, common sense suggests that the pessimist has the edge.

If some diseased persons do turn out to have a worse than average life there appears to be a case against further childbearing in afflicted families. To support this claim two more judgments are necessary, however. The first is that it is not wrong to refrain from childbearing. The second is that asking individuals to so refrain is less of a sacrifice than might be thought.[11] I will examine each of these judgments.

B. The Morality of Preventing the Birth of Possible Persons

Before going on to look at reasons why it would not be wrong to prevent the birth of possible persons, let me try to clarify the picture a bit. To understand the claim it must be kept in mind that we are considering a prospective situation here, not a retrospective one: we are trying to rank the desirability of various alternative future states of affairs. One possible future state is this: a world where nobody is at risk for Huntington's chorea except as a result of random mutation. This state has been achieved by sons and daughters of persons afflicted with Huntington's chorea ceasing to reproduce. This means that an indeterminate number of children who might have been born were not born. These possible children can be divided into two categories: those who would have been miserable and those who would have lived good lives. To prevent the existence of members of the first category it was necessary to prevent the existence of all. Whether or not this is a good state of affairs depends on the morality of the means and the end. The end, preventing the existence of miserable beings, is surely good; I will argue that preventing the birth of possible persons is not intrinsically wrong. Hence this state of affairs is a morally good one.

Why then is it not in itself wrong to prevent the birth of possible persons? It is not wrong because there seems to be no reason to believe that possible individuals are either deprived or injured if they do not exist. They are not deprived because to be deprived in a morally significant sense one must be able to have experiences. But possible persons do not exist. Since they do not exist, they cannot have experiences. Another way to make this point is to say that each of us might not have been born, although most of us are glad we were. But this does not mean that it makes sense to say that we would have been deprived of something had we not been born. For if we had not been born, we would not exist, and there would be nobody to be deprived of anything. To assert the contrary is to imagine that we are looking at a world in which we do not exist. But this is not the way it would be: there would be nobody to look.

The contention that it is wrong to prevent possible persons from existing because they have a right to exist appears to be equally baseless. The most fundamental objection to this view is that there is no reason to ascribe rights to entities which do not exist. It is one thing to say that as-yet-nonexistent persons will have certain rights if and when they exist: this claim is plausible if made with an eye toward preserving social and environmental goods.[12] But what justification could there be for the claim that nonexistent beings have a right to exist?

Even if one conceded that there was a presumption in favor of letting some nonexistent beings exist, stronger claims could surely override it.[13] For one thing, it would be unfair not to recognize the prior claim of already existing children who are not being properly cared for. One might also argue that it is simply wrong to prevent persons who might have existed from doing so. But this implies that contraception and population control are also wrong.

It is therefore reasonable to maintain that because possible persons have no right to exist, they are not injured if not created. Even if they had that right, it could rather easily be overridden by counterclaims. Hence, since possible persons are neither deprived nor injured if not conceived, it is not wrong to prevent their existence.

C. Conclusion of Part III

At the beginning of Part III I said that two claims are relevant to the morality of childbearing in the circumstances being considered. The first is that we ought to provide every child with at least a normal opportunity for a good life. The second is that we do not deprive or injure possible persons if we prevent their existence.

I suggested that the first claim could be derived from currently accepted theories of justice: a healthy body is generally necessary for happiness and it is also a prerequisite for a fair chance at a good life in our competitive world. Thus it is right to try to ensure that each child is healthy.

I argued, with regard to the second claim, that we do not deprive or injure possible persons if we fail to create them. They cannot be deprived of anything because they do not exist and hence cannot have experiences. They cannot be injured because only an entity with a right to exist could be injured if prevented from existing; but there are no good grounds for believing that they are such entities.

From the conjunction of these two claims I conclude that it is right to try to ensure that a child is healthy even if by doing so we preclude the existence of certain possible persons. Thus it is right for individuals to prevent the birth of children at risk for Huntington's chorea by avoiding parenthood. The next question is whether it is seriously wrong *not* to avoid parenthood.

IV REPRODUCTION: THE POTENTIAL PARENT'S SITUATION

I have so far argued that if choreics live substantially worse lives than average, then it is right for afflicted families to cease reproduction. But this conflicts with the generally recognized freedom to procreate and so it does not automatically follow that family members ought not to have children. How can we decide whether the duty to try to provide normal health for one's child should take precedence over the right to reproduce?

This is essentially the same question I asked earlier: how much must one sacrifice to try to ensure that one's offspring is healthy? In answer to this I suggested that the greater the danger of serious disability, the more justifiable considerable sacrifice is.

Now asking someone who wants a child to refrain from procreation seems to be asking for a large sacrifice. It may, in fact, appear to be too large to demand of anyone. Yet I think it can be shown that it is not as great as it initially seems.

Why do people want children? There are probably many reasons, but I suspect that the following include some of the most common. One set of reasons has to do with the gratification to be derived from a happy family life — love, companionship, watching a child grow, helping mold it into a good person, sharing its pains and triumphs. Another set of reasons centers about the parents as individuals — validation of their place within a genetically continuous family line, the conception of children as a source of immortality, being surrounded by replicas of themselves.

Are there alternative ways of satisfying these desires? Adoption or technological means provide ways to satisfy most of the desires pertaining to family life without passing on specific genetic defects. Artificial insemination by donor is already available; implantation of donor ova is likely within a few years. Still another option will exist if cloning becomes a reality. In the meantime, we might permit women to conceive and bear babies for those who do not want to do so themselves.[14] But the desire to extend the genetic line, the desire for immortality, and the desire for children that physically resemble one cannot be met by these methods.

Many individuals probably feel these latter desires strongly. This creates a genuine conflict for persons at risk for transmitting serious genetic diseases like Huntington's chorea. The situation seems especially unfair because, unlike normal people, through no fault of their own, doing something they badly want to do may greatly harm others.

But if my common sense assumption that they are in grave danger of harming others is true, then it is imperative to scrutinize their options carefully. On the one hand, they can have children: they satisfy their desires but risk eventual crippling illness and death for their offspring. On the other, they can remain childless or seek nonstandard ways of creating a family: they have some unfulfilled desires, but they avoid risking harm to their children.

I think it is clear which of these two alternatives is best. For the desires which must remain unsatisfied if they forgo normal procreation are less than admirable. To see the genetic line continued entails a sinister legacy of illness and death; the desire for immortality cannot really be satisfied by reproduction anyway; and the desire for children that physically resemble one is narcissistic and its fulfillment cannot be guaranteed even by normal reproduction. Hence the only defence of these desires is that people do in fact feel them.

Now, I am inclined to accept William James' dictum regarding desires: "Take any demand, however slight, which any creature, however weak, may make. Ought it not, for its own sole sake be satisfied? If not, prove why not."[15] Thus I judge a world where more desires are satisfied to be better than one in which fewer are. But not all desires should be regarded as legitimate, since, as James suggests, there may be good reasons why these ought to be disregarded. The fact that their fulfillment will seriously harm others is surely such a reason. And I believe that the circumstances I have described are a clear example of the sort of case where a desire must be judged illegitimate, at least until it can be shown that sufferers from serious genetic diseases like Huntington's chorea do not live considerably worse than average lives. Therefore, I think it is wrong for individuals in this predicament to reproduce.

V CONCLUSION

Let me recapitulate. At the beginning of this paper I asked whether it is wrong for those who risk transmitting severe genetic disease like Huntington's chorea to have "blood" children. Some despair of reaching an answer to this question.[16] But I think such pessimism is not wholly warranted, and that if generally accepted would lead to much unnecessary harm. It is true that in many cases it is difficult to know what ought to be done. But this does not mean that we should throw up our hands and espouse a completely laissez-faire approach: philosophers can help by probing the central issues and trying to find guidelines for action.

Naturally there is no way to derive an answer to this kind of problem by deductive argument from self-evident premises, for it must depend on a complicated interplay of facts and moral judgments. My preliminary exploration of Huntington's chorea is of this nature. In the course of the discussion I suggested that, if it is true that sufferers live substantially worse lives than do normal persons, those who might transmit it should not have children. This conclusion is supported by the judgments that we ought to try to provide for every child a normal opportunity for a good life, that possible individuals are not harmed if not conceived, and that it is sometimes less justifiable for persons to exercise their right to procreate than one might think.

I want to stress, in conclusion, that my argument is incomplete. To investigate fully even a single disease, like Huntington's chorea, empirical research on the lives of members of afflicted families is necessary. Then, after developing further the themes touched upon here, evaluation of the probable consequences of different policies on society and on future generations is needed. Until the results of a complete study are available, my argument could serve best as a reason for persons at risk for transmitting Huntington's chorea and similar diseases to put off having children. Perhaps this paper will stimulate such inquiry.

NOTES

1. There are a series of cases ranging from low risk of mild disease or handicap to high risk of serious disease or handicap. It would be difficult to decide where the duty to refrain from procreation becomes compelling. My point here is that there are some clear cases.

   I'd like to thank Lawrence Davis and Sidney Siskin for their helpful comments on an earlier version of this paper.

2. This issue is one which must be faced most urgently by genetic counselors. The proper role of the genetic counselor with regard to such decisions has been the subject of much debate. The dominant view seems to be that espoused by Lytt Gardner who maintains that it is unethical for a counselor to make ethical judgments about what his clients ought to do. ("Counseling in Genetics," *Early Diagnosis of Human Genetic Defects: Scientific & Ethical Considerations,* ed. Maureen Harris, [H.E.W. Publication No. (NIH) 72-25; Fogarty Center Proceedings No. 6]; p. 192.) Typically this view is unsupported by an argument. For other views see Bentley Glass "Human Heredity and Ethical Problems" *Perspectives in Biology & Medicine,* Vol. 15 (winter '72) 237-53, esp. 242-52; Marc Lappé, "The Genetic Counselor Responsible to Whom?" *Hastings Center Report,* Vol. 1, No. 2 (Sept. '71) 6-8; E. C. Fraser, "Genetic Counseling" *Am. J. of Human Genetics* 26:636-659, 1974.

3. I have chosen Huntington's chorea because it seems to me to be one of the clearest cases of high risk serious genetic disease known to the public, despite the fact that it does not usually manifest itself until the prime of life. The latter entails two further facts. First an individual of reproductive age may not know whether he has the disease; he therefore does not know the risk of passing on the disease. Secondly, an affected person may have a substantial number of years of healthy life before it shows itself. I do not think that this factor materially changes my case, however. Even if an individual does not in fact risk passing the disease to his children, *he cannot know that this is true.* And even thirty years of healthy life may well be seriously shadowed by anticipation and fear of the disease. Thus the fact that the disease develops late does not diminish its horror. If it could be shown that these factors could be adequately circumvented, my claim that there is a *class* of genetic disease of such severity that it would be wrong to risk passing them on would not be undermined.

   It might also be thought that Huntington's chorea is insufficiently common to merit such attention. But, depending on reproductive patterns, the disease could become a good deal more widespread. Consider the fact that in 1916 nine hundred and sixty-two cases could be traced from six seventeenth-century arrivals in America. (Gordon Rattray Taylor, *The Biological Time Bomb,* [New York, 1968], p. 176.) But more importantly, even if the disease did not spread, it would still be seriously wrong, I think, to inflict it unnecessarily on *any* members of new generations. Finally, it should be kept in mind that I am using Huntington's chorea as an example of the sort of disease we should try to eradicate. Thus the arguments presented here would be relevant to a wide range of genetic diseases.

4. *The Merck Manual,* (Rahway, N.J.: Merck, 1972), p. 1346.
5. Hymie Gordon, "Genetic Counseling," *JAMA,* Vol. 217 No. 9 (August 30, 1971), 1217.
6. Charles Smith, Susan Holloway, and Alan E. H. Emery, "Individuals at Risk in Families — Genetic Disease," *J. of Medical Genetics,* 8 (1971), 453. See also Townes in *Genetic Counseling* ed. Daniel Bergsma, *Birth Defects Original Article Series,* Vol. VI, No. 1 (May 1970).
7. J. H. Pearn, "Patients' Subjective Interpretation of Risks offered in Genetic Counseling," *Journal of Medical Genetics,* 10 (1973) 131.
8. Pearn, p. 132.
9. There are many important and interesting points that might be raised with respect to future generations and present society. There is no space to deal with them here, although I strongly suspect that conclusions regarding them would support my judgment that it is wrong for those who risk transmitting certain diseases to reproduce — for some discussion of future generations, see Gerald Leach, *The Biocrats,* (Middlesex, England: Penguin Books, 1972), p. 150; M. P. Golding, "Obligations to Future Generations," *Monist* 56 (Jan. 1972) 84-99; Gordon Rattray Taylor, *The Biological Time Bomb* (New York, 1968), esp. p. 176. For some discussions of society, see Daniel Callahan, "The Meaning and Significance of Genetic Disease: Philosophical Perspectives," *Ethical Issues in Human Genetics,* ed. Bruce Hilton et al., (New York, 1973), p. 87ff.; John Fletcher, "The Brink: The Parent-Child Bond in the Genetic Revolution," *Theological Studies* 33 (Sept. '72) 457-485; Glass (supra 2[a]); Marc Lappé, "Human Genetics," Annals of the *New York Academy of Sciences,* Vol. 26 (May 18, 1973) 152-59; Marc Lappé, "Moral Obligations and the Fallacies of "Genetic Control," *Theological Studies* Vol. 33, No. 3 (Sept. '72) 411-427; Martin P. Golding, "Ethical Issues in Biological Engineering," *UCLA Law Review* Vol. 15: 267 (1968) 443-479; L. C. Dunn, *Heredity and Evolution in Human Populations,* (Cambridge, Mass., 1959), p. 145; Robert S. Morison in *Ethical Issues in Human Genetics,* ed. Bruce Hilton et. al., (New York, 1973), p. 208.
10. *The New York Times,* September 30, 1975, p. 1. col. 6. The Joseph family disease is similar to Huntington's chorea except that symptoms start appearing in the twenties. Rick Donohue is in his early twenties.
11. There may be a price for the individuals who refrain from having children. We will be looking at the situation from their point of view shortly.
12. This is in fact the basis for certain parental duties. An example is the maternal duty to obtain proper nutrition before and during pregnancy, for this is necessary if the child is to have normal health when it is born.
13. One might argue that as many persons as possible should exist so that they may enjoy life.
14. Some thinkers have qualms about the use of some or all of these methods. They have so far failed to show why they are immoral, although, naturally, much careful study will be required before they could be unqualifiedly recommended. See, for example, Richard Hull, "Genetic Engineering: Comment on Headings," *The Humanist,* Vol. 32 (Sept./Oct. 1972), 13.

15. *Essays in Pragmatism,* ed. A. Castell (New York, 1948), p. 73.
16. For example, see Leach, p. 138. One of the ways the dilemma described by Leach could be lessened would be if society emphasized those aspects of family life not dependent on "blood" relationships and downplayed those that are.

FURTHER READINGS

Adams, J.
"Confidentiality and Huntington's Chorea," *Journal of Medical Ethics* 16:4 (1990) 196-99.
Annas, George
"Righting the Wrong of 'Wrongful Life,'" *Hastings Center Report* 11: 1 (Feb. 1981).
Bayles, Michael D.
"Harm to the Unconceived," *Philosophy and Public Affairs* 5:3 (1976).
Benkendorf, J. and K. Fitzgerald
"Genetic Counselling for Addicted Obstetric Patients," *Journal of Clinical Ethics* 1:2 (1990) 156-57.
Fletcher, J., et al.
"The Price of Silence," *Hastings Center Report* 20:3 (1990) 31-35.
Goodman, M.J and L.E. Goodman
"The Overselling of Genetic Anxiety," *Hastings Center Report* 12:5(1982)20-27.
Hicks, E.K. and J.M. Berg, eds.
The Genetics of Mental Retardation: Biomedical, Psychosocial and Ethical Issues. (Boston: Kluwer, 1988).

CHAPTER 20 GENETIC ENGINEERING

INTRODUCTION

In the eyes of many people, the ultimate aim of developing genetics is not merely to be able to tell whether we carry deleterious genes, but to "fix" these genes. This fixing is usually called genetic engineering. It involves excising the relevant sections from the genes of a particular person and replacing them with appropriate others. The technology already exists; the question is, should we do it?

Not surprisingly, there are several reactions. One is entirely negative: we should leave well enough alone, because we cannot foresee the ultimate consequences, or because we would be "playing God," etc.

Another approach is cautious acceptance, but only for defects that are coded on a single gene and that can be corrected by a simple substitution — and above all, only if this substitution occurs in somatic cells: cells that are not involved in human reproduction. In that way, the defect would be corrected in the individual who is affected, but the corrected trait would not be passed on.

Still another view is that not only this sort of limited somatic-cell manipulation should be permitted, but also research on reproductive, or germ line, cells. The reason is that genetic manipulation is a mode of therapy, and therefore should be developed like all others: cautiously, but developed nevertheless. Not to do this would be to deprive those who will be seriously affected by defective genes of something that could have prevented their suffering.

The selection from the Medical Research Council of Canada reflects current Canadian thinking in this area, from the standpoint of a regulatory body. It is narrowly focused on somatic-cell gene therapy.

The second selection presents the position of the Canadian Medical Association. It sets the two techniques next to each other and suggests cautious advance in both areas.

Guidelines for Research on Somatic Cell Gene Therapy in Humans

Medical Research Council of Canada

2. ETHICAL ISSUES

A physician should only undertake therapy outside standard medical practice when the outlook for the patient otherwise is dismal, and when the scientific team and the physician are able to master all the aspects of the proposed therapy. Research on somatic cell gene therapy demands a team of highly specialized scientists, preferably including the patient's physician. Since many of the questions and concerns in this complex new area demand research, the Working Group believes that the use of gene transfer techniques in humans should be viewed as research at this time, and that any proposal to use gene transfer techniques in a human subject be considered for ethical acceptability as a research proposal before being implemented.

Change to the genome of treated individuals has implications that need to be carefully weighed and there is a clear need for the information obtained to be scientifically valid. It is therefore the view of the Committee that all gene transfer techniques used in human subjects fall within the context of clinical research, and thus require approval of the Research Ethics Board (REB) as defined in the *MRC Guidelines on Research Involving Human Subjects* (1987).

The Committee also hopes that provincial Colleges of Physicians and Surgeons and other local levels of medical authority will take the same view if approached by physicians who wish to treat desperately ill patients under the rubric of innovative therapy.

2.2.1 Background

While it is true that some genetic diseases do not express themselves to the same degree and at the same age in each individual, the diseases which meet the criteria for suitable candidates for research on somatic cell gene therapy afflict patients in very similar ways. The damage caused is often progressive, cumulative, and fatal at an early age. This leads to a dilemma. On the one hand it seems appropriate to treat individuals as soon as they have been diagnosed to maximize the potential for therapeutic benefit if gene transfer is successful; the risks of performing gene transfer will not be reduced by waiting, and delay will almost certainly cause greater harm to the patients through irreversible accumulation of the effects of the disease. On the other hand, the younger the subjects, the less able they are to consent. A basic principle of the ethics of research is that competent subjects should be chosen if possible; however, patients with some candidate genetic diseases do not attain the age of consent, or even meaningful assent.

Medical Research Council of Canada, *Guidelines for Research on Somatic Cell Gene Therapy in Humans*, Chapter 2, "Ethical Issues." (Ottawa: Minister of Supply and Services, 1990) pp.24-33.

2.2.2 The Elements of Informed Consent

It is a fundamental principle that human beings can only be involved as research subjects if they have freely consented after fully understanding the research to be undertaken and their role in that research. This principle and the difficulties of implementing it when the patient is a child are fully described in the 1987 MRC Guidelines. Briefly, and at the very least, a potential research subject, or the person (proxy) who is to give consent on behalf of the subject, must understand:

(i) the reason(s) he or she has been selected to participate in the proposed study;

(ii) the nature and objective(s) of the research;

(iii) the harms and benefits associated with participating or refusing to participate in the research;

(iv) the available alternatives and the harms and benefits associated with these;

(v) the probability that any of the potential harms or benefits will manifest themselves;

(vi) the qualifications/experience of the researcher(s) involved; and

(vii) that the consent to participate can be withdrawn at any time with no adverse effects to ongoing medical care.

2.2.3 Consent with Special Populations

a) Research Involving Children

The elements of informed consent by the subject outlined above may not be completely met in the case of research on gene therapy, for several reasons. First, the most suitable candidate diseases are usually lethal, or cause mental retardation, at an early age; proxy consent is therefore essential. Since clinical trials on severe early onset disease necessarily involve very young children, there is an ethical dilemma; restricting research on gene therapy to those subjects able to consent will exclude the most severely affected patients in whom there is early onset of the disease and rapid deterioration. These have been identified above as probably the most suitable candidates. The greatest potential benefit of research on gene therapy is before deterioration is irrevocable. However, these are the subjects least able to consent for themselves. The Working Group is very conscious of the problem this dilemma poses. Within the context of research, it is clear that there is the potential of gaining the most knowledge in these diseases if trials are carried out on the earliest diagnosed patients even though these are just the individuals who are least able to give consent or even assent. The potential benefit to the individual child is also greatest before irreparable damage from the disease has occurred.

A unique aspect of research on human gene therapy concerns the option of withdrawing. The insertion of genetically modified cells cannot be undone; the gene transfer is irrevocable, so for some aspects a consent cannot be withdrawn. Further, long term monitoring is important to assess potential harm to the patient or to third parties. By withdrawing, the patient will not only lose the benefit from early recognition of harms to himself which might only manifest themselves later on, but will also deny any future subjects the benefits of the information to be derived from long term monitoring for harmful effects, and will make it difficult to assess the hazards to the community.

While the rights of the individual prohibit enforced compliance, it seems appropriate that, at the least, the prospective research subject, or the person giving a proxy consent, understand the potential long-term risks prior to consenting to increase compliance after the initial intervention. Proxies must understand that they may not have the right to withdraw a child from those portions of a protocol to which they have committed the child and which are therapeutically indicated. The situation could then be subject to the common law duties of a parent to provide medical necessities to the child. If remaining in the trial is in an incompetent subject's best interest, then this might be upheld in court. Since there are possible harms to others, it is appropriate to persuade the subjects to continue in long term follow-up. In the absence of settled law on this point, what would happen if a person nevertheless withdraws is open to question. In cases where there is possible harm to others, public policy might well overcome the individual's right to withdraw.

Full disclosure of risks is required for the subject to provide a valid informed consent to research. The risk of a harm should not only be quantified as accurately as possible but the harm itself described; the patient's or proxy's perceptions of potential harms may differ markedly from those of the physician, and a high risk of trivial harm may be acceptable, whereas a low risk of a very serious harm may not.

As children cannot provide a legally or ethically valid consent to research, consent must be sought from the parents or guardians. The decision by a parent or guardian to permit a child to participate in research on somatic cell gene therapy must be based on the same information which would be given to competent prospective research subjects. Because the proposed genetic intervention may be the child's last hope, parents and guardians may be willing to ignore the risks and to focus instead on the possible good; they may therefore be too eager to consent to their child's participation in the research. Their hope must be tempered by an adequate understanding of the risks involved. Feelings of guilt about transmitting a genetic disease may influence some parents to downgrade the risks of gene transfer. On the other hand some parents may inadvertently become over-protective and thus over-rate the risks. Provision should therefore be made in the protocol to ensure the availability of in depth counselling to ensure full understanding by the subject or legal guardian of what is proposed in the protocol.

Though parental consent is necessary for research on children, it is not binding. A child may express a desire not to participate and this expressed wish should be respected. The *MRC Guidelines on Research Involving Human Subjects* stipulate that "parental consent may be a necessary condition of engaging the child in research, but it is not necessarily a sufficient condition; the child's negative preferences in such cases should be respected" (p. 29). Given this, children should be encouraged to participate in the consent process to the extent to which they are capable. Unfortunately, this proviso may not be relevant to the children suffering from diseases suitable for research. For example, research with possible therapeutic benefit for ADA deficiency must be started with infants or young children; the severe mental retardation often present in those patients with recessive diseases who will be candidates for gene transfer may make it impossible for the child to register either assent or dissent. In addition, some provinces have particular rules with regard to the consent process regarding adolescents and minors.

b) Research Involving Human Fetuses

In the future, if somatic cell gene therapy is shown to be effective and safe, it may become an appropriate strategy for diseases which result in irreversible damage by the time of birth. In this situation, the proposed genetic intervention would have to take place early enough to benefit the patient, but late enough to ensure that the germ cells would not be affected (i.e. the gonads had already fully formed.)

In the view of this Working Group, research in somatic cell gene therapy for the conceptus *in utero* should not be done at this time; it would be irresponsible to incur the added risks to the mother involved in prenatal therapy without convincing evidence that somatic cell gene transfer can be effective in individuals after birth.

The 1987 *MRC Guidelines on Research Involving Human Subjects* clearly stipulate that the foreseen benefits must outweigh the foreseen risks in order for any research proposal to be approved. Accordingly, the probable safety and effectiveness of a proposed research project will have to be carefully evaluated with particular attention given to the potential risks for both the individual and society at large before approval is given. This is a difficult area in which to make judgments, as not only do risks and benefits to an individual and to society have to be weighed, but the balances of benefits to society and risks to individuals, and vice versa, need consideration.

2.3.1 Risks for the Individual

Gene transfer using somatic cells, in humans, though potentially beneficial, has important potential risks:

— Viral vectors used to deliver the gene of interest to the host cells may recombine with undetected viruses and regain their infectious properties or perhaps affect endogenous DNA sequences and produce malignancy. Thus, information addressing these risks is needed. The risk of malignancy as a result of treatment is not confined to this new approach; it also is a consideration in radiation therapy for cancer, immunosuppressive therapy used in transplantation, and the use of drugs with the risk of causing cancer, such as the antibiotic chloramphenicol.

— There is the possibility that a functioning host gene may be interrupted by the random integration of a foreign DNA sequence, and thus have negative consequences for the patient.

— The presence of bacterial contaminants in the DNA inserted into the patient's cells could cause unwanted side effects.

— The use of strategies designed to help the engineered cells establish themselves in the patient may have hazards which will need to be considered in the assessment of risks.

— There is a possibility that the inserted gene might inadvertently become transferred to their germ cells and might affect their offspring in an unanticipated way.

— If insufficient gene product is produced by the genetically modified cells, the genetic disorder may be only partially corrected so that the lethal genetic disease could be converted to one where the individual survives but suffers greatly.

2.3.2 Risks for Society

The risk of viral vectors again becoming infectious during somatic cell gene transfer must also be considered from a community perspective. These viruses might then be transmitted inadvertently to persons with whom the patient is in contact, for example, relatives, friends or health care personnel.

The possible impact on the composition of the human gene pool must also be considered. If individuals with rare lethal genetic disorders are successfully treated by means of somatic cell gene transfer, they may choose to reproduce. As discussed in the previous chapter, this would increase the number of abnormal genes in the gene pool since they may pass on the abnormal genes to their progeny. However, as noted, since human gene transfer is likely to focus on recessive disorders, the population impact would be extremely small. It could also be argued that any medical treatment of genetic disorders, including prenatal diagnosis, has some impact on the human gene pool. In fact, somatic cell transfer could be expected to have less of an impact on the gene pool than many other medical interventions.

The most serious risk for society concerns the possibility that the new genetic information will inadvertently be transferred from somatic to germ cells, and thus to the next generation. In the short term this could mean that an individual's offspring would be adversely affected by some unintended mutation. In the long term, the consequences are unknown. The impact is likely to be very small since only children of the small number of treated individuals could contribute to the gene pool. The human gene pool could be altered but the increase judged in the context of the total numbers of mutations that are constantly occurring would be infinitesimal. It is not appropriate to approve any protocol where the germ line is foreseen to be altered, even though this is not the primary intention of transfer.

2.3.3 Minimization of Risk — Maximization of Benefit

a) Safety and Efficacy

Before a proposed trial for somatic cell gene transfer involving humans is approved, the likelihood of benefit to the research subject must be well documented. This means that both the safety and the efficacy of the proposed genetic intervention must have been carefully assessed. The proposal should show that cells with the transferred gene have obtained and are capable of producing an active gene product. Data with regard to efficiency and appropriate expression in target cells *in vitro* and *in vivo* are needed. Whenever possible, a human gene should be used. However, in some circumstances it may be acceptable to propose a non-human DNA sequence for transfer. As noted under 3.3.2, if this is the case, then the reasons why a human gene is not appropriate should be clearly documented. In this case it is important to remember that the objective is therapy to return toward normal function.

Both technical and animal data must be provided showing that every possible precaution has been taken to assess and to minimize the risks. For example, to reduce the risk of infection and/or malignancy, all vectors used must have been shown to have been disabled so that they cannot replicate themselves. Information regarding the risk of unintended transfer of the vector to the germ line must be available.

b) Animal Models

Ideally, the safety of any proposed research protocol involving humans should be assessed on the basis of animal trials designed to study both the short term and long term impact. One important study will be to assess the risk of infection and malignancy by assessing whether the foreign DNA remains and functions in the host cells without harming them or other cells; another will be to observe treated laboratory animals throughout their life span to address the risk of cancer; it will also be important to study the offspring of these research animals to determine possible effects on subsequent generations and if there has been any transfer to germ cells. However, safety demonstrated in studies on animals does not guarantee lack of harm when used in humans. Ideally these trials should be conducted not only on mice and other small animals but also on primates, from which the findings may be more relevant when extrapolated to humans. There should be demonstration of correction of the disease if appropriate animal models exist.

There are no known animal models for the enzyme deficiency diseases which are likely to be early candidates for trials of somatic cell gene transfer in humans. For example, mice carrying the gene defect responsible for Lesch-Nyhan syndrome seem to function quite normally. Consequently, the potential for success may have to be assessed as far as possible on the basis of tissue cultures and research with animals. For other genetic disorders, however, it may be possible to assess efficacy on the basis of animal trials. As a minimum requirement prior to clinical studies, research with animals would have to show that:

1) new curative genes can be directed to specific cells and remain there long enough to be effective;
2) the inserted genes can express their product in the target cells at an appropriate level; and
3) no harm results to the treated cells, to the test animal or to its offspring.

Researchers should therefore provide the Research Ethics Board (REB) with detailed information about the precautions taken to minimize the various risks, and provide animal and cellular data relevant to whether the proposed research would benefit the patient.

c) Selection of Candidate Genetic Diseases

Obviously, research involving human subjects should only be undertaken if the anticipated benefits are expected to outweigh the possible harms. This means that initial trials for somatic cell gene transfer should only be considered for persons afflicted with serious genetic disorders (i.e. severely debilitating and/or rapidly lethal diseases) for whom there is no effective conventional treatment. Only if the burden imposed by the inherited disease on the afflicted individual is great and no satisfactory therapy is available, or the available therapy entails greater risks and less benefits, might clinical trials for somatic cell gene transfer be justified. There should be demonstration of accessible and appropriate target cells and of the possibility of amelioration if a functioning gene could be inserted into these cells. If the clinical trials for devastating diseases prove to be effective and safe, then research on somatic cell gene therapy might be considered in the future for less burdensome diseases such as haemophilia or PKU for which there are alternative treatments. It is clear that in the foreseeable future, research on somatic cell gene therapy should be limited to serious and untreatable genetic disorders for which there is no effective alternative treatment.

d) Selection of Research Subjects

The selection of research subjects must take into consideration the numbers of individuals to be treated in the first trials, and whether treatment should be restricted initially to one candidate disease. Experience has shown that it is very rarely possible to predict the success or failure of a new therapy on the basis of one or two cases. Beneficial approaches might not succeed in the first few subjects, or might even show harm; conversely an actually unacceptable method may be highly successful in its first few attempts. The arguments are essentially statistical; throwing heads three times in a row does not allow the prediction that the next 97 times will also be heads. For such reasons, a decision to start research on gene transfer in patients must recognize the intent in principle to treat a number of individuals, even though there can be no doubt that each patient must be studied very carefully to discover unexpected outcomes or to apply what can be learned from this experience to the next patient.

It has also been suggested that studies should be undertaken initially only on treatment for one genetic disease meeting the criteria outlined above. The Working Group rejects this view with one opinion to the contrary. Most committee members felt that, because these diseases are different, the genes added to human somatic cells to treat different diseases cannot be expected to behave in similar ways. However, experience with one means of therapy may provide useful information about risks associated, for example, with the method of inserting the new gene into the cells, and this information should be taken into consideration in later decisions.

One member believes it is contradictory to say that important information about risks of gene insertion can be learned from an experiment about one disease and applied to other diseases, while saying that each study protocol should be treated independently of protocols on other diseases. In that member's view, ethical requirements that the risks of research be minimized and scientific value and validity be maximized require that, in the initial stages of somatic cell genetic manipulation in humans, the early results of each approved protocol be reviewed and analyzed by an independent team before any further protocols are approved.

Since the genetic diseases for which research on somatic cell gene therapy may be suggested are rare (1/15,000-1/100,000) it is possible that research groups may be in competition to attract prospective subjects to their particular research centre. Alternatively, since centres trying the new methods are also likely to be few, it is possible that there will be more affected individuals than can properly be incorporated into trials of a new therapy. Hence, equitable criteria for selecting research subjects are important.

In summary, the selecting criteria should be clearly documented and submitted to the REB for approval.

e) Selection of Genetic Sequence

The Working Group is of the opinion that the DNA sequence to be transferred should preferably be of human origin. The ethical concern regarding a non-human sequence arises with respect to those sequences designed to be integrated as a functional portion of the subject's genome, the so-called 'target gene', or 'gene of interest', as opposed to those sequences, commonly derived from viruses, employed as a delivery system into the genome. The use of permanently functioning non-human genetic sequence in somatic cell manipulation differs from other therapeutic uses of non-human materials, (e.g. animal-derived insulin) in its irreversible alteration of the subject at the most fundamental genetic level. Most important, while the restriction of gene alteration to normal human sequences would confine such manipulation to therapeutic use, allowing the insertion of a non-human sequence would blur the crucial ethical distinction between therapy and enhancement. Therefore, the review body should apply an enhanced requirement of scientific justification to protocols intending the insertion of a non-human genetic sequence as the functional target gene. However, circumstances can be envisaged under which it may be appropriate to approve research protocols in which the gene to be transferred is from a non-human source. It might be desirable, for example, to use additional bacterial DNA sequences that would convey resistance to certain drugs and hence facilitate selection of cells in which gene transfer has occurred. Also expression of transferred genes might require, or be better controlled by, use of non-human regulatory sequences. If a non-human sequence is to be used, the reasons why this is proposed and why human sequence is not as likely to be of benefit must be fully documented, and the above concerns taken into consideration.

f) Long Term Monitoring

With this research, there is a potential for harm to third parties, to the subjects themselves after many years (e.g. late development of cancer), and to the offspring of the subject. The proposal should address the issue of long term monitoring of the research subjects and the outcome of their reproduction. Details on how long monitoring will be carried out, how adverse outcome will be evaluated and what strategies will be followed to handle it should be given.

Analysis

Canadian Medical Association

The Canadian Medical Association is convinced that the issue of genetic manipulation is one of the most important that face humanity at the present time. The Association is also persuaded that it transcends national boundaries because it touches the reproductive stability of the human species as a whole. It ought, therefore, to be approached with extreme caution because, in its effects, it concerns the survival of the species itself.

However, the Association also believes that the issue of genetic manipulation must be examined from another perspective. Does it really bespeak the acceptance of an instrumentalistic view of humanity and the objectification of the human person?

These considerations should engender caution, and the Association is concerned that their importance not be underestimated. However, the Association also believes that caution ought not to stifle an attempt at reasoned understanding and at a cool and, insofar as that is possible, an unprejudiced examination of the issues themselves. The Association, therefore, suggests that a start in that direction may be made by drawing a distinction that should be fundamental to the whole discussion: the distinction between somatic vs. germ line manipulation or therapy.

Somatic vs. Germ Line Therapy

Germ line therapy is the manipulation of human genetic material in such a way that the genetic changes will be passed on to the germ cells of a developing embryo.

Canadian Medical Association, "Analysis," from *The New Reproductive Technologies: A Preliminary Perspective of the Canadian Medical Association.* (Ottawa: Canadian Medical Association, 1991) pp. 127-135.

Therefore, the effect of such therapy would touch future generations.[207]

Somatic cell genetic manipulation, on the other hand, has far more restricted implications. This sort of manipulation only affects the genetic structure of a population of somatic cells that can be isolated and treated, and its effects would be confined to the individual who is treated. Gene therapy aimed at sickle-cell anemia would be an example. Bone marrow cells would be removed from the marrow of the affected person, the genetic structure of these cells would be altered and the treated cells would be returned to the original person. These cells would then continue to reproduce and would produce healthy red blood cells.[208] Because these cells are not involved in reproduction, changes that are made in them would not be passed on to future generations. The use of somatic cell gene therapy has been characterized by the President's Commission as follows:[209]

> Gene therapy carried out on somatic cells, such as bone marrow cells, would resemble standard medical therapies in that they all involve changes limited to the cells of the person being treated. They differ, however, in that gene therapy involves an inherent and probably permanent change in the body rather than requiring repeated applications of an outside force or substance. An analogy is organ transplantation, which also involves the incorporation into an individual of cells containing DNA of "foreign" origin.

It will be clear that considerations relevant to an evaluation of germ cell therapy and manipulation do not automatically apply to somatic cell manipulation and vice versa. In each case, relevance has to be established on separate and independent grounds.

Conceptual Considerations

Furthermore, although the Association is persuaded of the seriousness of many of the considerations that have been raised in regard to the use of genetic manipulation, intellectual honesty compels it to suggest that not all of these considerations carry equal weight.

For example, the Association cannot accept the thesis that in and by itself, the use of genetic engineering for germ line therapy means that people are treated as objects, or that it necessarily bespeaks an instrumentalistic view of humanity. This position would be valid only if being a person were the same as being a human being, and vice versa.

As the Association has averred on several occasions, and as it has pointed out in its brief on Bill C-43, the two are not the same. The human body is not identical with the person. For example, a human embryo is undoubtedly a human being from the moment of conception; however, that does not mean that it is a person from that very point. Instead, a human embryo becomes a person at some later stage in its development.

Furthermore, in somatic gene therapy, it is the human body that is the target of alteration, not the person. In germ line therapy, it is the body of the future offspring not the person that does not yet exist.

These are not idle considerations that touch only conceptual clarity. They go to the very heart of the issue of genetic manipulation. The destruction of human embryos in the course of developing gene therapy is implicated. The considerations that the Association has just adduced entail that, although the development and application of such therapy would indeed involve the destruction of human embryos, and although it would be true that to some extent it will involve treating them like pieces of organic matter, this does not mean that it would involve treating human persons as pieces of organic matter. The two are not the same.

The distinction between human being and human person, therefore, allows the Association to suggest that *if* the development of gene therapy can be defended on other grounds, then there must be a developmental limit beyond which human embryos may not be involved in the relevant protocols: a limit that finds its basis in the concept of a person. That is far different from the conclusion that is otherwise suggested.

Furthermore, the Association is concerned that the import of ethical principles and values not be misconstrued. In particular, the Association would like to focus on the value of respect for human life. As the Association has already observed, this value mandates a respectful approach to human beings. It requires that any undertaking that involves human beings be justifiable in terms of fundamental ethical principles, and that even if the destruction of human life is allowable, it occur only for the most weighty of reasons and in an appropriate way.

As to the *Principle of Respect for Persons,* the principle entails that human persons should be treated as ends in themselves, never as means. Therefore, the Principle prohibits an instrumentalistic approach to people. However, neither somatic nor germ line therapy need involve a violation of that principle. When somatic therapy is approached appropriately, the changes that are contemplated in the bodily functions of the relevant people are contemplated precisely because the individuals are considered as people whose suffering should be alleviated and whose needs should be met. As to germ line therapy, the reason for engaging in it is not some instrumentalistic perception of human bodies, but respect for the future offspring as people. The perception is that their suffering should be prevented or alleviated if at all possible.

The Association agrees that it would be ethically objectionable if the techniques of genetic manipulation were to be used for another purpose. They would then not be used as therapy, but as means to satisfy curiosity or to fulfill some other objective. Although such an approach might be acceptable in other contexts, the Canadian Medical Association would have to condemn it in the human setting in the strongest possible terms.

Furthermore, the Association would allow that techniques of genetic manipulation may lend themselves to such abuses. To that extent, it is persuaded by the slippery slope argument and by the considerations that it contains. However, the Association also believes that to condemn the development of these techniques for this reason may well be short-sighted. The Association submits that the cause of such misuse should not be sought in the techniques themselves, but in the people who would misuse them. Any medical or scientific development may be misused by unscrupulous people. To place the blame on the technique is to close one's eyes to the true causality of the matter.

As to the consideration that the application of gene therapy would impugn the dignity of those who are the subjects of such therapy, the Association can do no better than to quote the words of the President's Commission on the Study of Ethical Problems in Medicine and Biomedical and Behavioral Research:[210]

> An analogy is organ transplantation, which also involves the incorporation into an individual of cells containing DNA of "foreign" origin.

In this context, the Association is reminded that a similar objection of indignity was originally advanced against the development and use of techniques of transplantation. In the meantime, it has become apparent that such a critique was unjustified in that context. The Association submits that the same critique may also be unjustified in the genetic setting.

Gene therapy would be undignified if the dignity of the individual lay in the fact of suffering. However, to argue that would be to misrepresent the situation. The Association is fully persuaded that there may be dignity in the way in which some people respond to the suffering that they experience. However, the dignity of that response notwithstanding, the Association believes that there is no dignity in the suffering itself. Suffering is a curse. That is why society strives to alleviate it, and why physicians do their best to alleviate or ameliorate its cause. Nor does the Association believe that the people who are relieved of their suffering have any less dignity as people because they no longer need to suffer. If that were true, medical intervention in any context would lessen the dignity of humanity.

The Association also accepts the point that if the use of gene therapy were not to be properly controlled and approached in the appropriate manner, a stigma might come to be attached to those who have been "improved." There is no way of knowing. Stranger things have happened. However, the Association also believes that a stigma may come to be attached to all sorts of things. Therefore, in the estimation of the Association the problem — if problem there is — need not lie in these things themselves. It may also lie in the attitude toward them and in the social context that allows the problem to arise in the first place.

The Association, therefore, suggests that, as a matter of principle, the solution to such an issue should not necessarily be sought in prohibiting the relevant action and thereby leaving those who might be stigmatized in a disadvantaged position. That might well be to deprive these people of the possibility of relief from what otherwise would be a burdensome lot.

Instead, the Association proposes that, at least on occasion, a solution may more properly be found by dealing with the root of the problem that requires correction. In the case at issue, this means addressing the social process of stigmatization itself. Stigmatization is a form of discrimination. The Association submits that this is what requires correction, not the technology at issue.

As to the suggestion that the introduction of these techniques will soon turn something that is a matter of choice into a matter of obligation, the Association accepts that this may be possible. Certainly, in the eyes of the Association, it is something that should be guarded against. However, before it accepts the thrust of this consideration in the present context, the Association would like an answer to the following questions. Is there any reason to suppose that use of these techniques would in fact become a matter of obligation? Are there any data to support the position that is here expressed?

The Association can imagine a situation in which the projected scenario might indeed come to pass. For example, if gene therapy became cheaper and more effective than any other health care method available, and if at the same time its use would not offend the dignity of the person, society would require the use of it where appropriate and as a matter of course. However, the Association submits that if that were the case, then such techniques would be reduced to the status of other effective health care measures which society condones as a matter of obligation at the present time: measures such as vaccination and the like. Under such circumstances, the fact of obligation would be no more onerous, or objectionable, than the fact of obligation in other connections.

In sum, the Association submits that there can be no question but that techniques of genetic manipulation are liable to abuse. However, the Association also submits that is not something unique to genetic engineering. The same thing can be said about all sorts of scientific developments. Medical, pharmacological, and biological techniques can all be misused. Furthermore, they can all be misused in ways that have horrendous consequences: consequences whose magnitude would be as great as those that are painted for genetic engineering. When these other areas are considered in retrospect, it is possible to construct all sorts of slippery slope arguments against their introduction and use. Something as harmless as antibiotics would even fall into that category. For example, it could have been argued that they might be used only selectively, i.e., their use might have been confined to those who were deemed politically acceptable. It could have been argued that their use would initiate a lowering of our sensibilities toward suffering because we could deal with it so easily. It could even have been argued that their use would lead to a stigmatization of those who required them because they obviously lacked the inherent genetic mechanisms of resistance to infection. These arguments may be considered fanciful. However, they bear a close resemblance to some of the arguments that have been raised against genetic engineering.

To reiterate, the Canadian Medical Association does not intend to dismiss the slippery slope argument out of hand. It has a valid point to make. However, so far as the Association is concerned, its point is not logical but heuristic. The argument sounds a warning. Techniques of genetic engineering should be controlled and used with care because they carry the potential for disaster.

At the same time, the Association believes that this holds true of many biological, medical, pharmacological and engineering techniques. In fact, to a greater or lesser degree, it holds true of just about everything that humanity has developed. The invention of something as simple as the wheel is a case in point. The fact that something may be misused does not mean it should not be developed and used under appropriate circumstances. If it did mean that, humanity would still be in the caves. Hence, the Association urges this Commission to approach such considerations from a perspective of balance, rather than from a preconceived position of prohibition.

The avowed purpose and function of techniques of genetic manipulation are to assist in the delivery of health care. They should therefore be viewed from the same perspective and according to the same rules that are used in all other cases. In other words, they should be evaluated without preconceived bias as merely another set of weapons in the armamentarium of modern medicine. It may be that in the end they are too dangerous to use because we cannot evaluate them sufficiently. That would be a valid objection. It also may be that their development would require too many resources. That, too would be a valid objection, based on pragmatic concerns. It may even be that their development and use would contravene fundamental ethical principles. That would be the most important reason of all. However, the Association submits that none of these considerations can be assumed. The issue is too important for that. They have to be shown.

The Association has no wish to ignore the suggestion that the relevance of a specific genetic component may be misidentified, and that the therapy recommended on the basis of that information might be mistaken. Such errors have occurred, as in the XYY problem, and may occur again. The Association also has to admit that something may be developed in the arena of gene manipulation that will have serious negative consequences that cannot be controlled.

However, the Canadian Medical Association does not believe that these considerations entail the conclusion proposed. In particular, they do not entail that society should refrain from developing the relevant techniques or that it should refuse to use them. Instead, the Association believes that the conclusion is one of caution. If society does not attempt to develop and employ these techniques appropriately, the arsenal of health care will be impoverished, and the health of humanity will suffer needlessly.

The Association believes that society should allow the development and use of the relevant genetic manipulation techniques, but only under stringent controls. These controls should find their basis in statutory requirements and should be spelled out in nationally generated and enforced regulatory mechanisms. The Association is aware that because of the nature of the Canadian nation, the implementation and enforcement of such statutes and controls may present constitutional problems. However, the Association also believes that, unless consistent and nationally enforced regulatory mechanisms are in place, neither development nor application should be allowed to proceed. The Association believes further that the nature of these controls and the nature of these mechanisms should be accompanied by appropriate sanctions.

Finally, the Association believes that deliberate cloning of human cells for the purpose of research should be allowed if the protocols for such research meet otherwise applicable ethical standards. However, the Association also believes that deliberate cloning of human cells for the purpose of reproduction should be prohibited.

There remains the complex of questions that centre around decision-making. What conditions should be targeted for treatment? Under what circumstances? With what safeguards? Who should decide? The Association has no ready answers to these questions. All it can do is suggest that the problem is not unique to bio-engineering. It is something that faces the development and application of all new health care technologies. Society has begun to develop some ways of dealing with it. It has begun to institutionalize the notion of ethics review boards for all experimental procedures involving human subjects; it has begun to establish a national mechanism for developing ethical guidelines for experimental and innovative procedures; and so on. All levels of government concerned with the delivery of health care have struck committees, commissions have been set up, and the various professions have started to keep a watchful eye on these developments from their own perspective.

These developments suggest that in the end, it is probably society itself that will make the relevant decisions. The Canadian Medical Association would support such a development. As the Association has indicated on several occasions, the issues that are here at stake are issues that centre around ethical principles and social values. Therefore, the best that the Association can do in this connection is offer the perspective of the medical profession, with no preconception that this perspective should carry the day.

However, the Association would aver that to make decisions properly, society needs information. The Association would, therefore, suggest that as a start, it is here that there should be a concentration of effort on making relevant information available to the public, and in a way that the public can understand. The Association believes that this will provide at least some assurance that the decisions made in this arena will be made in an informed fashion by those who are intimately and ultimately affected.

The Association would also suggest that this Commission incorporate some of the Association's previous recommendations into its own deliberations. In particular, the recommendation that the development and use of techniques of gene manipulation should be closely controlled and subject to national guidelines based on statutory requirements grounded in law and backed by appropriate sanctions. Finally, the Association suggests that this Commission recommend the complete prohibition of experiments involving the combination of human and non-human genetic material except in contexts that are merely diagnostic in nature.

NOTES

207. USA, President's Commission (1982, note 187) pp. 45-48; German Bundestag (note 192) Section C:6, Section D.
208. Roblin R: Human genetic therapy: outlook and apprehensions. In Chacko GK (ed), *Health Handbook,* Elsevier-North Holland, New York, 1979: 108-112. For a failed early experiment along these lines, see Anderson WF: Genetic therapy. In Hamilton MP (ed), *The New Genetics and the Future of Man,* William B. Eerdmans, Grand Rapids, Michigan, 1972: 109 and 118.
209. *Supra,* note 187, p. 45. For a similar position, but one which was ultimately rejected, see German Bundestag (note 192) at 188a.
210. USA, President's Commission (1982, *supra,* note 187).

FURTHER READINGS

American Fertility Society
"Ethical Considerations of the New Reproductive Technologies," *Fertility and Sterility.* 46: 3 (Sept., 1986) Supplement, H.B.

Anderson, W.F.
"Genetic Therapy" in *The New Genetics and the Future of Man,* Ed. Hamilton, MP, Grand Rapids, Mich.: William B. Erdmans Pub., 1972: 109-118.

European Medical Research Council
Draft Guidelines for the Application of Gene Therapy to Human Beings. (Strasbourg: undated)

Fletcher, Joseph
The Ethics of Genetic Control. (New York: Doubleday, 1974).

Fowler, Gregory, Eric T. Juengst and Burke K. Zimmerman
"Germ-Line Gene Therapy and the Clinical Ethos of Medical Genetics," *Theoretical Medicine* 10: 2 (June 1989) 151-165.

Holmes, B., B. Hoskins and M. Gross, eds.
The Custom-Made Child? Women-Centered Perspsectives. (Clifton, N.J: Humana Press, 1981).

Knoppers, B.M.
Human Dignity and Genetic Heritage. Study Paper for the Law Reform Commission of Canada. (Ottawa: Law Reform Commission of Canada, 1991).
Lappé, M.
"Ethical Issues in Manipulating the Human Germ Line," *Journal of Medicine and Philosophy* 16 (1991) 621-639.
Law Reform Commission of Ontario
Report on Artificial Human Reproduction and Related Matter. (Toronto: Ministry of the Attorney General, 1985).
Milunsky, A. and G.J. Annas, eds.
Genetics and the Law. (New York: Plenum Press, 1976).
Perry, Clifton
"Wrongful Life and Comparison of Harms," *Westminster Institute Review* 1: 4 (1982), 7-9.
Ramsey, Paul
Fabricated Man: The Ethics of Genetic Control. (New Haven and London: Yale University Press, 1970).
Sacred Congregation for the Doctrine of the Faith
Instruction on Respect for Human Life in its Origin and Dignity of Procreation. (Rome: Vatican, 1987), 14H.
Society of Obstetricians and Gynecologists of Canada
Submission to the Royal Commission on New /Reproductive Technologies, "Genetic Manipulation." (SOGC: Toronto, 1990).
Suzuki, D. and P. Knudtson
Genethics: The Clash Between the New Genetics and Human Values. (Cambridge, Mass.: Harvard University Press, 1989).
Walters, L.
"The Ethics of Gene Therapy," *Nature* 320 (1986) 225-227.
Wertz, D.C. and J.C. Fletcher
"Moral Reasoning Among Medical Geneticists in Eighteen Nations," *Theoretical Medicine* 10: 2 (June 1989), 123-138.
World Council of Churches, Working Group Sub-Unit on Church and Society
"Manipulating Life," *Church and Society*, 1982 (Sept./Oct.).
Zimmerman, B.
"Human Germ-line Therapy: The Case for its Development and Use," *Journal of Medicine and Philosophy* 16 (1991) 593-612.

PART 6 CODES OF ETHICS

CHAPTER 21 CODES OF ETHICS FOR CANADIAN HEALTH CARE PROFESSIONALS

INTRODUCTION

The standards we expect of professionals in their actions are higher than what we expect from ordinary people. This is true whether we consider their actions as professionals or as moral agents. For example, if a parent gives acetylsalicylic acid (aspirin) to an asthmatic child who is running a temperature and the child has an adverse reaction, we will not condemn the parent for not knowing that aspirin is contraindicated for asthmatics. But if a physician were to give aspirin to that same child, we would hold the physician responsible. We expect physicians to know these things. That is part of their training. Similarly, we would not condemn a patient for failing to report a physician whose breath smelled of alcohol during office hours, whereas we would condemn the physician's colleague for not taking appropriate steps.

There are several reasons why we expect such higher standards from medicine. The first reason is simply the fact that medicine is a profession. This means that, like all professions, it is self-regulating: it has the right to set the standards that someone must meet in his or her role as physician.

However, with that right goes the duty to make sure that these standards are met in actual practice. That is why in each province there is a regulatory body whose function it is to oversee the licensure of new physicians, to check the credentials of physicians who move into the province and want to set up a practice, and to enforce the requirements that the professions itself has set. In most provinces, it is the College of Physicians and Surgeons. In Québec, it is the Corporation Professionelle des Médecins du Québec; in Newfoundland, the Newfoundland Medical Association; in the Yukon, the Yukon Medical Council;

and in the Northwest Territories, the Licensing Department of the Department of Justice and Public Service.

The second reason is that medicine is a legally entrenched service monopoly. This means that by law, only someone who meets the requirements set by the profession itself may practise medicine. This puts the profession into a uniquely privileged position, because, in effect, it allows the profession to control health care at the delivery level. Such control imposes a tremendous obligation on the profession in a material as well as in an ethical sense. It must ensure that health care is provided appropriately, adequately, equitably and universally.

A third reason why we expect more from medicine is that it is a fiduciary profession. This means that the physician-patient relationship is characterized by an ineluctable element of trust. In order for a physicians to be able to exercise his/her profession, s/he must know the patient's medical history and current medical condition. This involves knowing details of the patient's personal life which the patient normally would not reveal to anyone — or at least not to someone with whom the patient did not have a close and intimate personal relationship. That imposes certain ethical constraints on the physician. Confidentiality is clearly central here. Unless there are overwhelming ethical reasons that derive from a higher obligation that the physician owes to other patients or to other members of society, the physician may not divulge what is told to him/her in confidence.

A fourth reason for expecting higher standards from physicians is that usually a patient comes to the physician when the patient is ill. However, the fact that the patient is in a position of need, that s/he must divulge extremely personal details to the physician, that s/he is dependent on the physician — even the simple fact of illness itself — all exert a powerful compromising effect on the abilities of the average person to make decisions. Sometimes even their ability to understand is interfered with. Therefore, when the patient comes to see his/her physician, the physician is in a position of psychological power. Physicians have a special duty not to take advantage of this.

Finally, physicians are incomparably more knowledgeable about health, illness and appropriate treatments than the ordinary person. Such knowledge is the physician's stock-in-trade. Knowledge, however, is power — certainly when it comes to decision-making. What decision is made frequently depends on what information is given and how it is divulged. The physician must be very careful not to abuse that power.

All of these considerations find reflection in the Code of Ethics of the Canadian Medical Association, reprinted below. For instance, the obligation to be properly prepared finds its expression in the clauses that enjoin physicians to "teach and be taught," and the injunction to consult with their colleagues in matters that fall outside of their own area of expertise. The obligations that derive from the fact of monopoly find expression in the obligation not to refuse service in emergency circumstances, not to engage in unethical discrimination, to be responsible in setting fee schedules, and so on. The obligations that are entailed by the fiduciary nature of the physician-patient relationship are expressed in the various clauses governing confidentiality and related matters, and the duties that derive from the unique power position in which physicians find themselves by virtue of the compromised position of the patient are reflected in the clauses that deal with informed consent.

However, the codes and the clauses that it contains are not mere expressions of how the profession would like its members to behave. Although the various clauses that the Code contains are not laws — they have not been passed by any parliamentary legislative body — they do have the force of law. The reason is that in Canada, the practice of medicine is regulated by provincial legislation specific to medicine. Included in this legislation is usually some reference to the standards of the profession as accepted either by the relevant provincial College of Physicians and Surgeons or the appropriate provincial Medical Association. These bodies have the legal power to enforce their rulings on members who have been found guilty of an infraction against them, by striking them from the roles of individuals allowed to practise, or by levying a fine or exacting some other form of punishment. The Code of Ethics of the Canadian Medical Association should therefore be considered carefully from this perspective. Is what it enjoins really ethically appropriate?

The reason for including the Code of Ethics the Canadian Nurses' Association is that physicians do not practise in isolation. Physicians depend on nurses in their everyday practice. It is therefore important to have some idea of how nurses see their ethical position. Comparing and contrasting the two Codes may help to bring out areas of strength and weakness that might not be apparent when we look at the Code of the CMA in isolation.

One of the things that should become clear is that the two professions approach the relationship with patients from somewhat different perspectives. While nursing tends to approach the relationship with the patient more in the sense of co-adventuring in order to maximize the health potential of the patient, medicine tends to be much more concerned with the physician as professional and with the actions of the physician as independent agent. The mutuality of action that is characteristic of nursing seems to recede into the background. This of course has important implications for the way in which the ethical relationship between nurses and patients, as opposed to physicians and patients, is ethically perceived.

The Code of Ethics of the Pharmaceutical Manufacturers' Association of Canada (PMAC) is included because the delivery of health care involves more than professionals in the primary health care fields. Functionally speaking, it requires an integrated interaction with those manufacturing sectors of our society that provide the products and services that make the delivery of health care possible in a material sense. The pharmaceutical industry in particular is implicated. The pharmaceutical industry has become conscious of the responsibility it thus bears towards society, and has begun to regulate the actions of its members. Its Code of Ethics represents its most current efforts in that direction. It may be interesting to compare the code of the PMAC with those of Canadian health care professionals. Here it should be borne in mind that, unlike health care professionals, pharmaceutical manufacturers do not stand in a fiduciary relationship with patients, nor is their primary concern the latter's welfare. Yet it could be argued that they do owe an obligation to Canadian health care consumers, as well as to the health care professionals who provide the professional interface with patients. What are the lines of obligation here? How are they defined?

When reading the codes that follow, it might be useful to keep the following questions in mind:

What is the difference between the ethos of a health care profession and its ethics?

Why should different health care professions have different codes of ethics?

Is there a good ethical reason why the health care professions of different countries should have their own distinctive codes of ethics?

What happens when the personal ethical convictions of a health care professional conflict with what is in the code of ethics of the profession?

What is the ethical perspective of the codes below? Are they utilitarian, deontologically, agapistic or religiously oriented? Would they be different if they were written from a different perspective?

The Canadian Medical Association Code of Ethics

Principles of Ethical Behaviour for all physicians, including those who may not be engaged directly in clinical practice.

I

Consider first the well-being of the patient.

II

Honour your profession and its traditions.

III

Recognize your limitations and the special skills of others in the prevention and treatment of disease.

IV

Protect the patient's secrets.

V

Teach and be taught.

VI

Remember that integrity and professional ability should be your best advertisement.

VII

Be responsible in setting a value on your services.

GUIDE TO THE ETHICAL BEHAVIOUR OF PHYSICIANS

A physician should be aware of the standards established by tradition and act within the general principles which have governed professional conduct.

The Oath of Hippocrates represented the desire of the members of that day to establish for themselves standards of conduct in living and in the practice of their art. Since then the principles established have been retained as our basic guidelines for ethical living with the profession of medicine.

The International Code of Ethics and the Declaration of Geneva (1948), developed and approved by the World Medical Association, have modernized the ancient codes. They have been endorsed by each member organization, including The Canadian Medical Association, as a general guide having worldwide application.

The Canadian Medical Association accepts the responsibility of delineating the standard of ethical behaviour expected of Canadian physicians.

An interpretation of these principles is developed in the following pages, as a guide for individual physicians and provincial authorities.

RESPONSIBILITIES TO THE PATIENT

An Ethical Physician

Standard of care

1. will practise the art and science of medicine to the best of his/her ability;
2. will continue self education to improve his/her standards of medical care;

Respect for Patient

3. will practise in a fashion that is above reproach and will take neither physical, emotional nor financial advantage of the patient;

The Canadian Medical Association, *Code of Ethics*. (Ottawa, 1987).

Patient's Rights

4. will recognize his/her professional limitations and, when indicated, recommend to the patient that additional opinions and services be obtained;
5. will recognize that a patient has the right to accept or reject any physician and any medical care recommended. The patient having chosen a physician has the right to request of that physician opinions from other physicians of the patient's choice;
6. will keep in confidence information derived from a patient or from a colleague regarding a patient, and divulge it only with the permission of the patient except when otherwise required by law;
7. when acting on behalf of a third party will ensure that the patient understands the physician's legal responsibility to the third party before proceeding with the examination;
8. will recommend only diagnostic procedures that are believed necessary to assist in the care of the patient, and therapy that is believed necessary for the well-being of the patient. The physician will recognize a responsibility in advising the patient of the findings and recommendations and will exchange such information with the patient as is necessary for the patient to reach a decision;
9. will, upon a patient's request, supply the information that is required to enable the patient to receive any benefits to which the patient may be entitled;
10. will be considerate of the anxiety of the patient's next-of-kin and cooperate with them in the patient's interest;

Choice of Patient

11. will recognize the responsibility of a physician to render medical service to any person regardless of colour, religion or political belief;
12. shall, except in an emergency, have the right to refuse to accept a patient;
13. will render all possible assistance to any patient, where an urgent need for medical care exists;
14. will, when the patient is unable to give consent and an agent of the patient is unavailable to give consent, render such therapy as the physician believes to be in the patient's interest;

Continuity of Care

15. will, if absent, ensure the availability of medical care to his/her patients if possible; will, once having accepted professional responsibility for an acutely ill patient, continue to provide services until they are no longer required, or until arrangements have been made for the services of another suitable physician; may, in any other situation, withdraw from the responsibility for the care of any patient provided that the patient is given adequate notice of that intention;

Personal Morality

16. will inform the patient when personal morality or religious conscience prevent the recommendation of some form of therapy;

Clinical Research

17. will ensure that, before initiating clinical research involving humans, such research is appraised scientifically and

ethically and approved by a responsible committee and is sufficiently planned and supervised that the individuals are unlikely to suffer any harm. The physician will ascertain that previous research and the purpose of the experiment justify this additional method of investigation. Before proceeding, the physician will obtain the consent of all involved persons or their agents, and will proceed only after explaining the purpose of the clinical investigation and any possible health hazard that can be reasonably foreseen;

The Dying Patient

18. will allow death to occur with dignity and comfort when death of the body appears to be inevitable;
19. may support the body when clinical death of the brain has occurred, but need not prolong life by unusual or heroic means;

Transplantation

20. may, when death of the brain has occurred, support cellular life in the body when some parts of the body might be used to prolong the life or improve the health of others;
21. will recognize a responsibility to a donor of organs to be transplanted and will give to the donor or the donor's relatives full disclosure of the intent and purpose of the procedure; in the case of a living donor, the physician will also explain the risks of the procedure;
22. will refrain from determining the time of death of the donor patient if there is a possibility of being involved as a participant in the transplant procedure, or when his/her association with the proposed recipient might improperly influence professional judgement;
23. may treat the transplant recipient subsequent to the transplant procedure in spite of having determined the time of death of the donor;

Fees to Patients

24. will consider, in determining professional fees, both the nature of the service provided and the ability of the patient to pay, and will be prepared to discuss the fee with the patient.

RESPONSIBILITIES TO THE PROFESSION

An Ethical Physician:

Personal Conduct

25. will recognize that the profession demands integrity from each physician and dedication to its search for truth and to its service to mankind;
26. will recognize that self discipline of the profession is a privilege and that each physician has a continuing responsibility to merit the retention of this privilege;
27. will behave in a way beyond reproach and will report to the appropriate professional body any conduct by a colleague which might be generally considered as being unbecoming to the profession;
28. will behave in such a manner as to merit the respect of the public for members of the medical profession;
29. will avoid impugning the reputation of any colleague;

Contracts

30. will, when aligned in practice with other physicians, insist that the standards enunciated in this Code of Ethics and the Guide to the Ethical Behaviour of Physicians be maintained;
31. will only enter into a contract regarding professional services which allows fees derived from physicians' services to be controlled by the physician rendering the services;
32. will enter into a contract with an organization only if it will allow maintenance of professional integrity;
33. will only offer to a colleague a contract which has terms and conditions equitable to both parties;

Reporting Medical Research

34. will first communicate to colleagues, through recognized scientific channels, the results of any medical research, in order that those colleagues may establish an opinion of its merits before they are presented to the public;

Addressing the Public

35. will recognize a responsibility to give the generally held opinions of the profession when interpreting scientific knowledge to the public; when presenting an opinion which is contrary to the generally held opinion of the profession, the physician will so indicate and will avoid any attempt to enhance his/her own personal professional reputation;

Advertising

36. will build a professional reputation based on ability and integrity, and will only advertise professional services or make professional announcements as regulated by legislation or as permitted by the provincial medical licensing authority;
37. will avoid advocacy of any product when identified as a member of the medical profession;
38. will avoid the use of secret remedies;

Consultation

39. will request the opinion of an appropriate colleague acceptable to the patient when diagnosis or treatment is difficult or obscure, or when the patient requests it. Having requested the opinion of a colleague, the physician will make available all relevant information and indicate clearly whether the consultant is to assume the continuing care of the patient during this illness;
40. will, when consulted by a colleague, report in detail all pertinent findings and recommendations to the attending physician and may outline an opinion to the patient. The consultant will continue with the care of the patient only at the specific request of the attending physician and with the consent of the patient;

Patient Care

41. will cooperate with those individuals who, in the opinion of the physician, may assist in the care of the patient;
42. will make available to another physician, upon the request of the patient, a report of pertinent findings and treatment of the patient;
43. will provide medical services to a colleague and dependent family without fee, unless specifically requested to render an account;

44. will limit self-treatment or treatment of family members to minor or emergency services only; such treatments should be without fee;

Financial Arrangements

45. will avoid any personal profit motive in ordering drugs, appliances or diagnostic procedures from any facility in which the physician has a financial interest;
46. will refuse to accept any commission or payment, direct or indirect, for any service rendered to a patient by other persons excepting direct employees and professional colleagues with whom there is a formal partnership or similar agreement.

RESPONSIBILITIES TO SOCIETY

Physicians who act under the principles of this Guide to the Ethical Behaviour for Physicians will find that they have fulfilled many of their responsibilities to society.

An Ethical Physician

47. will strive to improve the standards of medical services in the community; will accept a share of the profession's responsibility to society in matters relating to the health and safety of the public, health education, and legislation affecting the health or well-being of the community;
48. will recognize the responsibility as a witness to assist the court in arriving at a just decision;
49. will, in the interest of providing good and adequate medical care, support the opportunity of other physicians to obtain hospital privileges according to individual personal and professional qualifications.

"The complete physician is not a man apart and cannot content himself with the practice of medicine alone, but should make his contribution, as does any other good citizen, towards the well-being and betterment of the community in which he lives."

Code of Ethics

Canadian Nurses Association

CLIENTS

I

A nurse is obliged to treat clients with respect for their individual needs and values.

Standards

1. Factors such as the client's race, religion, ethnic origin, social status, sex, age or health status may not be permitted to compromise the nurse's commitment to that client's care.

The Canadian Nurses Association, *Code of Ethics*. (Ottawa, 1987).

2. The expectations and normal life patterns of clients are acknowledged. Individualized programs of nursing care are designed to accommodate the psychological, social, cultural and spiritual needs of clients, as well as their biological needs.
3. The nurse does more than respond to the requests of clients, by accepting an affirmative obligation to aid clients in their expression of needs and values within the context of health care.
4. Recognizing the client's membership in a family and a community, the nurse, with the client's consent, attempts to facilitate the participation of significant others in the care of the client.

II

Based upon respect for clients and regard for their right to control their own care, nursing care should reflect respect for the right of choice held by clients.

Standards

1. The competent client's consent is an essential precondition to the provision of health care. Nurses bear the primary responsibility to inform clients about the nursing care that is available to them.
2. Consent may be signified in many different ways. Verbal permission or knowledgeable cooperation are the usual forms in which clients consent to nursing care. In each case, however, a valid consent represents the free choice of the competent client to undergo that care which is to be provided.
3. Consent properly understood is the process by which a client becomes an active participant in care. All clients should be aided in becoming active participants in their care to the maximum extent that circumstances permit. Professional ethics may require of the nurse actions that exceed the legal requirements of consent. For example, although a child may be legally incompetent to consent, nurses should nevertheless attempt to inform and involve the child in treatment.
4. Force, coercion and manipulative tactics must not be employed in the obtaining of consent.
5. Illness or other factors may compromise the client's capacity for self-direction. Nurses have a continuing obligation to value autonomy in such clients, for example, by creatively providing them with opportunities for choices, within their capabilities, thereby aiding them to maintain or regain some degree of autonomy.
6. Whenever information is provided to a client, this must be done in a truthful, understandable and sensitive way. It must proceed with an awareness of the individual client's needs, interests and values.
7. Nurses should respond freely to their client's requests for information and explanation when in possession of the knowledge required to respond accurately. When the questions of the client require information beyond that of the nurse, the client should be informed of that fact and referred to a more appropriate health care practitioner for a response.

III

The nurse is obliged to hold confidential all information regarding a client learned in the health care setting.

Standards

1. The rights of persons to control the amount of personal information that will be revealed applies with special

force in the health care setting. It is, broadly speaking, up to clients to determine who shall be told of their condition, and in what detail.

2. In describing professional confidentiality to a client, its boundaries should be revealed:
   a) Competent care requires that other members of a team of health personnel have access to or be provided with the relevant details of a client's condition.
   b) In addition, discussions of the client's care may be required for the purpose of teaching, research or quality assurance. In this case, special care must be taken to protect the client's anonymity.

   Whenever possible, the client should be informed of these necessities at the onset of care.
3. An affirmative duty exists to institute and maintain practices that protect client confidentiality, for cxamplc, by limiting access to records.

Limitations

The nurse is not morally obligated to maintain confidentiality when the failure to disclose information will place the client or third parties in danger. Generally, legal requirements to disclose are morally justified by these same criteria. In facing such a situation, the first concern of the nurse must be the safety of the client or the third party.

Even when the nurse is confronted with the necessity to disclose, confidentiality should be preserved to the maximum possible extent. Both the amount of information disclosed and the number of people to whom disclosure is made should be restricted to the minimum necessary to prevent the feared harm.

IV

The nurse has an obligation to be guided by consideration for the dignity of clients.

Standards

1. Nursing care should be carried out with consideration for the personal modesty of clients.
2. A nurse's conduct at all times should acknowledge the client as a person. For example, discussion of care in the presence of the client should actively involve or include that client.
3. As ways of dealing with death and the dying process change, nursing is challenged to find new ways to preserve human values, autonomy and dignity. In assisting the dying client, measures must be taken to afford as much comfort, dignity and freedom from anxiety and pain as possible. Special consideration is given to the need of the client's family to cope with their loss.

V

The nurse is obligated to provide competent care to clients.

Standards

1. Nurses should engage in continuing education and in the upgrading of skills relevant to the practice setting.
2. In seeking or accepting employment, nurses should accurately state their areas of competence as well as limitations.
3. Nurses who are assigned to work outside of an area of present competence should seek to do that which, under the circumstances, is in the best interests of their clients. Supervisors or others should be informed of the situation at the earliest possible moment so that protective measures can be instituted.

As a temporary measure, the safety and welfare of clients may be better served by the best efforts of the nurse under the circumstances than by no nursing care at all.

4. When called upon outside of an employment setting to provide emergency care, nurses fulfill their obligations by providing the best care that circumstances, experience and education permit.

Limitations

A nurse is not ethically obliged to provide requested care when compliance would involve a violation of her or his moral beliefs. When that request falls within recognized forms of health care, however, the client should be referred to a more appropriate health care practitioner. Nurses who have or are likely to encounter such situations are morally obligated to seek to arrange conditions of employment so that the care of clients is not jeopardized.

VI
The nurse is obliged to represent the ethics of nursing before colleagues and others.

Standards

1. Nurses serving on committees concerned with health care or research should see their role as including the vigorous representation of nursing's professional ethics.
2. Many public issues include health as a major component. Involvement in civic activities may afford the nurse the opportunity to further the objectives of nursing as well as to fulfill the duties of a citizen.

VII
The nurse is obligated to advocate the client's interest.

Standards

1. Advocating the interests of the client includes assistance in achieving access to quality health care. For example, by providing information to clients privately or publicly, the nurse enables them to satisfy their rights to health care.
2. When speaking to public issues or in court as a nurse, the public is owed the same duties of accurate and relevant information as are clients within the employment setting.

VIII
In all professional settings, including education, research and administration, the nurse retains a commitment to the welfare of clients. The nurse bears an obligation to act in such a fashion as will maintain trust in nurses and nursing.

Standards

1. Nurses accepting professional employment must ascertain that conditions will permit provision of care consistent with the values and standards of the Code. Prospective employers should be informed of the provisions of the Code so that realistic and ethical expectations may be established at the beginning of the nurse-employer relationship.
2. Accurate performance appraisal is required by a concern for present and future clients and is essential to the growth of nurses. Nurse administrators and educators are morally obligated to provide timely and accurate feedback to nurses, and their supervisors, student nurses and their teachers.

3. Administrators bear special ethical responsibilities that flow from a concern for present and future clients. The nurse administrator seeks to ensure that the competencies of personnel are used efficiently. Working within available resources, the administrator seeks to ensure the welfare of clients. When competent care is threatened due to inadequate resources or for some other reason, the administrator acts to minimize the present danger and to prevent future harm.
4. An essential element of nursing education is the student-client encounter. This encounter must be conducted in accordance with ethical nursing practices, with special attention to the dignity of the client. The nurse educator is obligated to ensure that nursing students are acquainted with and comply with the provisions of the Code.
5. Research is necessary to the development of the profession of nursing. Nurses should be acquainted with advances in research, so that established results may be incorporated into practice. The individual nurse's competencies and circumstances may also be used to engage in, or to assist and encourage research designed to enhance the health and welfare of clients.

The conduct of research must conform to ethical nursing practice. The self-direction of clients takes on added importance in this context. Further direction is provided in the Canadian Nurses Association publication entitled, *Ethical Guidelines for Nursing Research Involving Human Subjects.*

HEALTH TEAM

IX

Client care should represent a cooperative effort, drawing upon the expertise of nursing and other health professions. Acknowledging personal or professional limitations, the nurse recognizes the perspective and expertise of colleagues from other disciplines.

Standards

1. The nurse participates in the assessment, planning, implementation and evaluation of comprehensive programs of care for clients. The scope of a nurse's responsibility should be based upon education and experience, as well as legal considerations of licensure or registration.
2. The nurse accepts a responsibility to work with others through professional nurses' associations to secure quality care for clients.

X

The nurse, as a member of the health care team, is obliged to take steps to ensure that the client receives competent and ethical care.

Standards

1. The first consideration of the nurse who suspects incompetence or unethical conduct should be the welfare of present clients or potential harm to future clients. Subject to that principle, the following should be considered:
    a. The nurse is obliged to ascertain the facts of the situation in deciding upon the appropriate course of action.
    b. Institutional mechanisms for reporting incidents or risks of

incompetent or unethical care should be followed.

c. It is unethical for a nurse to participate in efforts to deceive or mislead clients regarding the cause of their injury.

d. Relationships in the health care team should not be disrupted unnecessarily. If a situation can be resolved without peril to present or future clients by direct discussion with the colleague suspected of providing incompetent or unethical care, that should be done.

2. The nurse who attempts to protect clients threatened by incompetent or unethical conduct may be placed in a difficult position. Colleagues and professional associations are morally obliged to support nurses who fulfill their ethical obligations under the Code.

3. Guidance concerning those activities that may be delegated by nurses to assistants and other health care workers is found in legislation and policy statements. When functions are delegated, the nurse should be satisfied regarding the competence of those who will be fulfilling these functions. The nurse has a duty to provide continuing supervision in such a case.

THE SOCIAL CONTEXT OF NURSING

XI

Conditions of employment should contribute to client care and to the professional satisfaction of nurses. Nurses are obliged to work towards securing and maintaining conditions of employment that satisfy these connected goals.

Standards

1. In the final analysis, the improvement of conditions of nursing employment is often to the advantage of clients. Over the short term however, there is a danger that action directed toward this goal will work to the detriment of clients. Nurses bear an ethical responsibility to present as well as future clients and so the following principles should be noted:

   a. The safety of clients should be the first concern in planning and implementing any job action.

   b. Individuals and groups of nurses participating in job actions share this ethical commitment to the safety of clients. However, their responsibilities may lead them to express this commitment in different, but equally appropriate ways.

   c. Clients whose safety requires ongoing or emergency nursing care are entitled to have those needs satisfied throughout the duration of any job action. Members of the public are entitled to know of the steps that have been taken to ensure the safety of clients.

   d. Individuals and groups of nurses participating in job actions have a duty of coordination and communication to take steps reasonably designed to ensure the safety of clients.

RESPONSIBILITIES OF THE PROFESSION

XII

Professional nurses' organization recognize a responsibility to clarify, secure and sustain ethical nursing conduct. The fulfillment of these tasks requires that professional organizations remain responsive to the rights, needs and legitimate interests of clients and nurses.

Standards

1. Sustained communication and cooperation between the Canadian Nurses Association, provincial associations and other organizations of nurses, is an essential step towards securing ethical nursing conduct.
2. Professional nurses' associations must at all times accept responsibility for assuring quality care for clients.
3. Professional nurses' associations have a role in representing nursing interests and perspectives before non-nursing bodies, including legislatures, employers, the professional organizations of other health disciplines and the public media of communication.
4. Professional nurses' associations should provide and encourage organizational structures that facilitate ethical nursing conduct.
   a. Changing circumstances may call for reconsideration and adaptation of this Code. Supplementation of the code may be necessary in order to address special situations. Professional associations should consider the ethics of nursing on a regular and continuing basis and be prepared to provide assistance to those concerned with its implementation.
   b. Education in the ethical aspects of nursing should be available to nurses throughout their careers. Nurses' associations should actively support or develop structures designed towards this end.

Code of Marketing Practices

Pharmaceutical Manufacturers Association of Canada

1. GENERAL PRINCIPLES

The Canadian innovative pharmaceutical industry is conscious of its unique position as a partner in the provision of prescription medicines and services to the public. The Industry promotes the concept of good health, and a positive, health-oriented approach to daily living.

Recognizing that its medicines have been, and will continue to be an important factor in modern therapy, the Industry undertakes:

- to provide medicines that conform to the highest standards of safety and quality;

Pharmaceutical Manufacturers Association of Canada, *Code of Marketing Practices*. (Ottawa, 1988).

- to ensure that its medicines are supported by comprehensive technical and informational services in accordance with currently accepted medical and scientific knowledge and experience;
- to use candour in dealing with the healthcare professions, public health officials, and the general public.

The Industry is committed to the rational use of medicines by informed consumers, and urges that its products be used only in accordance with the directions and advice of healthcare professionals.

Observance of the PMAC Code of Marketing Practices is to be in spirit, as well as in letter.

All companies that are engaged in pharmaceutical marketing but are not members of the PMAC, are also urged to adhere to this CODE to ensure the good health and best interests of the Canadian public.

The member companies of the PMAC pledge themselves to the following principles and/or practices of ethical pharmaceutical marketing, and recognize that adherence to these principles and/or practices is a condition of membership in the Association.

2. ADVERTISING & INFORMATION DISSEMINATION

2.1 The prescription medicines researched, developed, manufactured and/or marketed by Canada's innovative pharmaceutical industry are available primarily through pharmacies and hospitals. Advertising of these products is directed to healthcare professionals only.

2.2 Advertising

2.2.1 All PMAC member companies agree to abide by the Code of Advertising Acceptance of the Pharmaceutical Advertising Advisory Board (PAAB).

The PAAB comprises equal representation from those organizations representing the healthcare professions and institutions, consumers, pharmaceutical manufacturers (both international and Canadian owned), the Association of Medical Media, the Canadian Advertising Foundation and non-voting observers from the Pharmaceutical Marketing Clubs of Quebec and Ontario.

The PAAB establishes policy for the administration of its Code of Advertising Acceptance, selects its own Chairman, and retains a permanent Commissioner of Pharmaceutical Advertising. The Commissioner is responsible to the Board for clearance of pharmaceutical advertising based on compliance with the requirements of the PAAB Code.

The Health Protection Branch (HPB) of Health and Welfare Canada acts as an advisor and resource body to the Board. The HPB can request suspension of any PAAB-accepted advertising material which the Branch deems to constitute a potential hazard to health under terms of the Food and Drug Act and Regulations. Procedures following this action are indicated in the PAAB Code.

Copies of the PAAB Code can be obtained from PMAC, or from the PAAB, 345 Kingston Road, Pickering, Ontario, L1V 1A1.

2.3 New Product Information

2.3.1 As the primary source of information on their products, PMAC members are cognizant of the fact that, in today's media-oriented society, news of the availability of new prescription medicines could sometimes reach the general public before it has been communicated by the industry to the healthcare professions.

PMAC members shall therefore follow the procedure outlined below in order to obviate such situations:
2.3.2 Essential professional product information (eg. the official product monograph or appropriate portions thereof) shall be mailed a minimum of two weeks prior to market launch.
2.3.3 The information shall be mailed to all known Drug Information Centres, Poison Control Centres, and faculties of medicine and pharmacy throughout Canada.

3. CLINICAL EVALUATION PACKAGES ("SAMPLES")

3.1. General Principle

3.1.1 The PMAC holds the view that the judicious distribution of clinical evaluation packages (samples) to healthcare practitioners, in accordance with the requirements of the Food and Drug Act, is beneficial to the patient and the healthcare professional.
3.1.2 Clinical evaluation packages shall be used by the healthcare practitioner to initiate immediate therapy, if necessary. When appropriate, these packages can be used to determine clinical response to drug therapy before a full course of therapy is prescribed.

3.2 Definition

3.2.1 For the purpose of this CODE, a clinical evaluation package is defined as a package containing a limited quantity of a pharmaceutical product sufficient to evaluate clinical response, distributed to authorized healthcare professionals free of charge, for patient treatment.
3.2.2 In addition to the Food and Drug Act and Regulations respecting the manufacture, packaging, storage, and distribution of clinical evaluation packages, the following regulations will apply:

3.2.3 Distribution

(i) Clinical evaluation packages shall be provided only at the request of an authorized healthcare professional upon completion of an appropriate clinical evaluation package request form. Such request forms shall be properly completed before being presented for the signature of an authorized person.

(ii) Complete prescribing information for communication by the healthcare professional to his/her patient shall be provided as an essential part of the clinical evaluation package service.

(iii) All free goods (clinical evaluation packages or stock packages) supplied to a healthcare practitioner as part of an order must be included on the invoice or documented on a separate NO CHARGE invoice.

(iv) The quantity of clinical evaluation packages supplied shall not be considered excessive where the said quantity is deemed to be appropriate by the healthcare professional for the proper evaluation of clinical response.

(v) The provision of clinical evaluation packages in hospitals shall conform with individual hospital regulations. Clinical evaluation packages shall only be distributed if authorized by the Chief Pharmacist.

(vi) The provision of clinical evaluation packages at conventions is considered inappropriate.

(vii) It is unethical, and cause for dismissal, for a representative to sell, trade or otherwise dispose of clinical evaluation packages or stock packages for any purpose other than authorized by company policy.

3.2.4 Storage

(i) Effective controls and procedures to guard against theft and diversion of clinical evaluation packages shall be maintained at all times.

(ii) All clinical evaluation packages shall be stored in cabinets, storage areas, or rooms which are appropriately secured and accessible only to company representatives or other authorized persons.

(iii) Companies shall direct their employees to store clinical evaluation packages under conditions that will maintain their stability, integrity and effectiveness.

3.2.5 Disposal

(i) PMAC member companies shall ensure the return of excess and/or expired clinical evaluation packages of their own manufacture.

3.2.6 Inventory

(i) Companies shall require that a complete and accurate inventory of all clinical evaluation packages in the possession of a company representative be conducted at least annually by an agent of the company other than the representative in possession of the clinical evaluation packages.

4. CONTINUING HEALTH EDUCATION

4.1 General Principle

Symposia, congresses and other activities for continuing health education are indispensable for the dissemination of knowledge and experience to the healthcare professions. The principal objective in organizing such meetings shall be the enhancement of healthcare for all Canadians.

4.1.1 The organization, content and choice of speakers must be determined by the healthcare professional organizers.

4.1.2 Disposal of funds must be the responsibility of the individual designated as the principal organizer.

4.1.3 Wherever required, member companies must ensure that the principal organizer is aware that it is necessary to inform the local scientific or professional body regarding the meeting. This will avoid conflicts and duplication and will allow proper study credits to be issued to participants.

4.1.4 The value of limited social functions at Continuing Health Education meetings is recognized. However, they shall neither compete with nor take precedence over the central events, and shall be the responsibility of the healthcare professional organizers. Sponsorship of company specific social functions is strongly discouraged.

4.1.5 While grants or honoraria may be provided to participating healthcare professionals, they shall not, however, be extended to include a spouse or family member.

4.1.6 Representatives of member companies attending any Continuing Health Education meeting shall abide by the standards specified in the Sections of this CODE entitled "General Principles", "Pharmaceutical Representatives" and "Clinical Evaluation Packages".

5. CONVENTION/CLINIC DISPLAYS

5.1 General Principle

Convention/Clinic displays provide a means whereby valuable interaction between healthcare professionals and the pharmaceutical industry can be enhanced. The principal objective of the display shall be to disseminate accurate information concerning the properties of the products being displayed.

5.1.1 A convention/clinic display shall be attended at all times by at least one suitably qualified representative of the displaying company.

5.1.2 Where no exhibit space is available, no contribution towards a convention display shall be made.

5.1.3 Promotional and educational materials available at the display shall not present information or claims that are at variance with those contained in the appropriate Product Monograph(s).

5.1.4 Reprints of scientific and medical papers may be distributed at the display, provided they are reprinted verbatim, and are not presented in a manner which could reasonably be construed as implying claims that are at variance with those contained in the appropriate Product Monograph(s).

5.1.5 The distribution of clinical evaluation packages at convention/clinic displays is considered inappropriate.

5.1.6 Representatives attending a display shall abide by the standards specified in this CODE for pharmaceutical representatives.

5.1.7 Fees paid for exhibit space shall not include additional donations to the association holding the convention. Additional donations shall be reported as such.

5.1.8 If a member company sponsors a public relations event associated with a convention, the sponsorship shall not exceed the cost of a single exhibit. Sponsorship of company specific social functions is strongly discouraged.

5.1.9 No payment or donation shall be made for regular exhibits at clinic/hospital displays.

6. DONATIONS

6.1 General Principle

As responsible corporate citizens, PMAC members have an obligation to financially support worthwhile community and professional activities. It is imperative that such financial support be able to successfully withstand public and professional scrutiny.

6.1.1 Under no circumstances shall accessibility to a healthcare professional be contingent on a donation/fee.

7. PHARMACEUTICAL MANUFACTURERS REPRESENTATIVES

7.1 General Principle

7.1.1 Pharmaceutical manufacturers' representatives personify their company and the pharmaceutical industry as a whole in the eyes of healthcare professionals. They are the primary interface between the industry and other partners in Canada's healthcare system.

7.1.2 Accordingly, the industry shall establish and maintain high standards of recruiting and selection within the principles of employment equity to ensure the acquisition of well-qualified personnel. Representatives shall ideally be graduates of universities or community colleges or hold a designation in the healthcare field.

7.2 Standards for Employment and Training

7.2.1 An appropriate period of supervised initial training shall be provided to every representative immediately following employment. New representatives shall acquire adequate technical and scientific information to qualify them to competently present the technical aspects of their companies' products. They shall be familiarized with the principles of ethics and standards of conduct established in the Code of Marketing Practices.
7.2.2 Member companies shall implement periodic refresher courses for all representatives and encourage them to undertake courses of study and self-improvement.
7.2.3 Representatives shall qualify under the programme of the Council for the Accreditation of Pharmaceutical Manufacturers Representatives of *Canada or an equivalent* as a means of elevating their professional competency.
7.2.4 Representatives shall display the highest professional and ethical standards at all times, as reflected by their conduct and appearance. Representatives shall acquaint themselves with, and abide by the established standards of conduct and courtesy in physicians' offices, clinics, hospitals, retail pharmacies and wherever they may appear in a professional capacity.
7.2.5 Representatives shall provide full and factual information on products, without misrepresentation or exaggeration. Representatives' statements must be accurate and complete and must not be misleading, either directly or by implication. Their assertions must be scientific and consistent with the existing product monograph and current Canadian medical thinking.
7.2.6 Under no circumstances shall representatives be required to pay a fee in order to gain access to a healthcare professional.

8. POSTMARKETING STUDIES

8.1 Definition

8.1.1 Postmarketing studies are defined as any study that is conducted after the issuance of a Notice of Compliance in respect of the medicine being studied

8.2 General Principle

8.2.1 The principal objective of a postmarketing study shall be to obtain and evaluate safety and efficacy data on the controlled use of the medication.
8.2.2 Postmarketing studies must provide a scientific framework for the investigation of the medicine in broader or special populations.
8.2.3 All postmarketing studies shall have a clearly defined medical objective which is amenable to scientific review and testing.
8.2.4 The company shall ensure that control of postmarketing studies is administered by qualified personnel, in a manner analogous to the control exercized over other scientific studies.
8.2.5 Postmarketing studies shall be conducted in accordance with applicable legislation and guidelines of the Health Protection Branch and the Medical Research Council of Canada, including approval by the local Ethics Review Committee.
8.2.6 Postmarketing studies shall be conducted in accordance with a written protocol acceptable to both the company and the investigator.
8.2.7 Data shall be collected by the investigator in accordance with the protocol and retained on file with the company for at least two years.
8.2.8 The company shall provide the investigator with a scientific evaluation of the data after completion of the study.

8.2.9 The investigator shall be reimbursed by the company in proportion to the scientific services provided. Reimbursement may be in the form of a monetary grant, travel to attend scientific and medical meetings not sponsored by the company, or equipment, provided the latter is essential and appropriate for the study.
8.2.10 Reimbursement for the study shall not be conditional on continuing administration of the study medicine to patients after they have completed the study protocol.

9. PRICE-RELATED MATTERS

9.1 All member companies must abide by Federal and Provincial laws and regulations relating to market pricing. PMAC supports the principle of Actual Acquisition Cost (AAC) and all member companies shall cooperate with provincial governments to enforce this principle.
9.2 Simply put, Actual Acquisition Cost is considered to be the true transaction costs reflecting direct and/or indirect benefits to the purchaser.

10. SERVICE-ORIENTED ITEMS

10.1 Member companies shall refrain from distributing service-oriented items and from conducting "special promotions" which cannot be justified if subjected to professional and public scrutiny.
10.2 Member companies shall comply with those Sections of the PAAB Code dealing with "Other Media Promotions" and "Other Media Advertising."
10.3 Guidelines on acceptable criteria relative to service-oriented items are available from the PMAC.

11. AUDIT OF CORPORATE COMPLIANCE

11.1 In order to address company-specific issues, individual PMAC members are urged to conduct an internal audit of corporate compliance with this CODE, to review and evaluate their marketing practices on a periodic basis.

12. ENFORCEMENT

12.1 Complaints regarding any infraction of the provisions of the PMAC Code of Marketing Practices are to be communicated to the PMAC Marketing Practices Review Committee (c/o PMAC Director of Publications) for adjudication. The Committee will render a decision and will communicate same, in writing, to the parties involved.
12.2 Should the decision prove unsatisfactory to either party, or should the Committee be unable to render a decision, either party involved in the complaint will have recourse to an appeal body.
12.3 The appeal body shall be constituted as follows:

- A representative of each of the two parties involved in the complaint.
- A Chairman, selected and agreed upon by both parties involved.

12.4 The decision of the appeal body shall be final, and adherence to the decision is a condition of continued membership in the PMAC.
12.5 Any costs incurred by the respective representatives will be for the account of each of the two parties involved in the appeal. Costs resulting from the appointment and participation of the Chairman, will be for the account of the party who lost the appeal.

FURTHER READINGS

Bandman, E.L. and B. Bandman
"Moral Implications in Codes of Nursing," in Bandman and Bandman, *Nursing Ethics Through the Life Span*. (Norwalk, Conn: Appleton and Lange, 1990) 23-39.

Beauchamp, T.L. and L.B. McCullough
Medical Ethics: The Moral Responsibility of Physicians. (Englewood Cliffs, NJ: Prentice Hall, 1984).

Bonds, Curley
"The Hippocratic Oath: a Basis for Modern Ethical Standards," *Journal of the American Medical Association* 264:17 (Nov.7, 1990) 2311.

Engelhardt, Jr., H.T.
The Foundations of Bioethics. (New York: Oxford University Press, 1986).

Feinberg, Jocl
Social Philosophy. (Englewood Cliffs, NJ: Prentice Hall, 1973).

Flaherty, J. and L. Curtin
Nursing Ethics. (Bowen Maryland: Bradey, 1982).

Glick, S.
"Comparison of the Oaths of Hippocrates and Asaph," *Koroth: A Bulletin Devoted to the History of Medicine and Science* 9:3-4 (Spring, 1986) 297-302.

Jacob J.M.
Doctors and Rules: A Sociology of Professional Values. (New York: Routledge, 1988).

Jameton, A.
Nursing Practice. (Englewood Cliffs, NJ: Prentice Hall, 1984).

Jecker, N.S.
"Integrating Medical Ethics with Normative Theory: Patient Advocacy and Social Responsibility," *Theoretical Medicine* 11:2 (1990)125-139.

Khan, M.I.
"The Oath of Hippocrates updated by Muslim Physicians," *Plastic and Reconstructive Surgery* 83:3 (1989) 579.

Muyskens, J.
Moral Problems in Nursing: A Philosophical Investigation. (Towanda: Rowman & Littlefield, 1982).

Sawyer, L.
"Nursing Codes of Ethics: an International Comparison," *International Nursing Review* 36:5 (1989) 145-148.

May, R.
"Code and Covenant or Philanthropy and Contract?" in S.J. Reiser, A.J. Dyck and W.J. Curran, eds., *Ethics in Medicine: Historical Perspectives and Contemporary Concerns*. (MIT Press: Cambridge, Mass., 1977) 65-76.

Pence, Terry and K. J. Cantrall, eds.
Ethics in Nursing: An Anthology. (New York: National League for Nursing, 1990).

Thompson, J.E. and H..O. Thompson,, eds.
Professional Ethics in Nursing. (Malabar, Fla.: Krieger, 1990).

World Medical Association
"An International Code of Medical Ethics," *World Medical Association Bulletin* 1: 3 (1949).

ACKNOWLEDGEMENTS

PART I: HEALTH CARE AND BIOETHICAL PRINCIPLES

CHAPTER 1

1. Reproduced by permission of WHO from: *Basic Documents. Thirty-Ninth Edition.* Geneva: World Health Organization, 1992, pp. 1-2.

2. Daniel Callahan, "The WHO Definition of Health", *The Hastings Center Studies* 1:3(1973).3. C. Whitbeck, "A Theory of Health," in A.L. Caplan, H.T. Engelhardt, Jr. and J.J. McCartney, eds., *Concepts of Health and Disease: Interdisciplinary Perspectives* (Reading, Mass.: Addison-Wesley Publishing Co., 1981) pp. 611-626.

4. Lennard Nordenfeldt, "A Welfare Theory of Health," from Lennard Nordenfeldt, *On the Nature of Health: An Action-Theoretic Approach* (Dordrecht: D. Reidel Publishing Co., 1987)pp. 76-80.

CHAPTER 2

2. Benjamin Freedman and Françoise Baylis, "Purpose and Function In Government-funded Health Coverage." *Journal of Health Policy, Politics and Law* 1987 (Spring) 12:1; 97-112.

3. E-H.W. Kluge, "The Canada/US Free Trade Agreement," *Business and Professional Ethics Journal* 10:3 (Fall, 1991)29-52.

CHAPTER 3

1. Benjamin Freedman,and the McGill/Boston Research Group, "Nonvalidated Therapies and HIV Disease," *The Hastings Center Report* 19:3(June 1989)14-20.

2. Alvin H. Moss and Mark Siegler, "Should Alcoholics Compete Equally for Liver Transplantation? *JAMA* 265:(March 13, 1991) 1295-1298.

PART II: THE PATIENT AND THE PROFESSIONAL

CHAPTER 4

1.Robert M. Veatch, "Models for Ethical Medicine in a Revolutionary Age," from *The Hastings Center Report*, vol 2(June 1972).

2. Ronald J. Christie and C. Barry Hoffmaster, "The Physician-Patient Relationship," from Ronald J. Christie and C. Barry Hoffmaster, *Ethical Issues in Family Medicine.* 1986. (New York and Oxford: Oxford University Press, 1986), chapter 2., pp.19-31.

3.Martin Lakin, "Whose Agent is the Therapist?" from Martin Lakin, *Ethical Issues in Psychotherapy*. (New York: Oxford University Press, 1988), pp. 8-13 and 21-25.

CHAPTER 5

1. *Reibl v. Hughes*, 16 O.R. (2d)306, 78 D.L.R. (3d)35, reversed 21 O.R.(2d) 14,6 C.C.L.T.,227, 89 D.L.R.(3d)112; reverse [1980] 2 S.C.R. 880, 14 C.C.C.T.I., 114 D.L.R.(3d)1, 33 N.R., 17.

2. "Informed Consent: Ethical Considerations for Physicians and Surgeons," *Annals of the Royal College of Physicians and Surgeons of Canada*, 21:1(January 1988).

3. Benjamin Freedman, "A Moral Theory of Informed Consent," *The Hastings Center Report* 5:4 (August 1975); 32-39.

CHAPTER 6

1. Medical Research Council of Canada, *Guidelines on Research Involving Human Subjects 1987*. (Ottawa: Minister of Supply and Services, 1987).

2.Barry Hoffmaster, "The Medical Research Council's New Guidelines on Research Involving Human Subjects: Too Much Law, Too Little Ethics," *Health Law In Canada* 10:1(1989) 146-155.

CHAPTER 7

1. *McInerney v. MacDonald*[1990] N.B.J. No. 106 Action No. 74/89/CA

2. H.Brody, "The Lie that Heals: The Ethics of Giving Placebos," *Annals of Internal Medicine* 97:1(1982).

3. Stephen A. Kline, "Release of Information: Mental Competency Considerations," *Health Law in Canada* 10:1(1989)144-145.

CHAPTER 8

1. *Re S.D.* (1983)3 W.W.R. 618 (B.C.S.C.).Reproduced with the permission of Thomson Canada Ltd.

2. *Re Eve* (1987), 3 D.L.R.(4th) 1 (S.C.C.).,[1987] 2 S.C.R. 388 (S.C.C.).
3. Eike-Henner W. Kluge, "After 'Eve': Whither Proxy Decision-Making?" *Canadian Medical Association Journal* (1988) 5 pp.

CHAPTER 9

1. Law Reform Commission of Canada, Working Paper 61 *Biomedical Experimentation Involving Human Subjects*. (Ottawa: Minister of Supply and Services, 1989).

2. Barry F. Brown, "Proxy Consent for Research on Incompetent Elderly," from James E. Thornton and Earl R. Winkler, eds., *Ethics and Aging: The Right to Live, The Right to Die*. (Vancouver: The University of British Columbia Press, 1988) 183-193.

PART III: DELIBERATE DEATH

CHAPTER 10

1. Revised from *Editorial, Newsletter of the Association of Medical Women of Canada*: "Say No to Fetal Personhood." 1990. Reprinted with the permission of the author, Dr. Frances Rosenberg.

2. Canadian Medical Association, "The Status of the Human Foetus," from *Proceedings of the 123rd General Council, 1991,* pp.4-14.

3. *R.* v. *Green.* Vernon Registry No. 18024 [1988] B.C.J. No. 1807.

4. *R.* v.*Kitching and Adams* (1976) 6 W.W.R. 697 (Manitoba Court of Appeal). Reproduced with the permission of Thomson Canada Ltd.

5. Roland Pucetti, "Does Anyone Survive Neocortical Death?" in Richard M. Zaner, ed. *Death: Beyond Whole-Brain Criteria.* (Dordrecht: Kluwer Academic Publishers, 1988) pp. 75-90. Reprinted by permission of Kluwer Academic Publishers.

CHAPTER 11

1. Law Reform Commission of Canada, "The Need for Reform," from Law Reform Commission of Canada, Report 20, *Euthanasia, Aiding Suicide and Cessation of Treatment.* (Ottawa: Minster of Supply and Services, 1983) pp. 7-13, 17-20, 22-28.

2. James Rachels, "Active and Passive Euthanasia," *New England Journal of Medicine*, 292:2(Jan 9,1975) 78-80.

3. Richard Doerflinger, "Assisted Suicide: Pro-Choice or Anti-Life?" *The Hastings Center Report* 19:1(Jan/Feb. 1989) suppl. 16-19.

4. S.H. Wanzer, D.D. Federman, S.J. Adelstein ,*et al.*,"Letter," *New England Journal of Medicine* (1989) 320:844-849.

CHAPTER 12

1. *Malette* v. *Shulman*, (1990) 72 O.R. (2d) 417 (C.A.).pp. 17-42.

2. R.H. Fisher and E.M. Meslin, "Should Living Wills be Legalized?" *Canadian Medical Association Journal* 1990; 142:23-26.

3. Canadian Medical Association, Policy: "Advance Directives for the Resuscitation of Patients and Life-Saving or Sustaining Measures"

CHAPTER 13

1. *R.* v.*Morgentaler*, [1988] 1 S.C.R. 30, 63 O.R.(2d.)281, 26 O.A.C. 1, 44 D.L.R.(4th) 385, 82 N.R. 1, 3 C.C.C.(3d)449, 62 C.R.(3d)1, 31 C.R.R.

2.L.W. Sumner, "Toward a Credible View of Abortion," *Canadian Journal of Philosophy* 4 (September 1974) 163-181.

3. Robert C.Cefalo and H.T.Engelhardt,Jr.,"The Use of Fetal and Anencephalic Tissue for Transplantation," *The Journal of Medicine and Philosophy* 14:1(1989) 25-43. Reprinted by permission of Kluwer Academic Publishers.

PART IV: HUMAN REPRODUCTION

CHAPTER 14

1. Ontario Law Reform Commission, "Is There a Right to Procreate?" from Ontario Law Reform Commission, *Report on Human Artificial Reproduction and Related Matters*, 2 vols. (Toronto: Ministry of the Attorney General, 1985) 41-45.

2. Kathryn Paulyn Morgan, "Of Woman Born? How Old-Fashioned! — New Reproductive Technologies and Women's Oppression," from Christine Overall, ed., *The Future of Human Reproduction*. (Toronto: The Women's Press, 1989) pp. 62-79.

3. The Canadian Medical Association, "The Right to Have Children," from *The New Reproductive Technologies: A Preliminary Perspective of the Canadian Medical Association* (Ottawa: Canadian Medical Association, 1991) 42-49.

CHAPTER 15

1. *Re Eve* (1987), 31 D.L.R.(4th) 1 (S.C.C.).,[1987] 2 S.C.R. 388 (S.C.C.).

2. E.-H.W. Kluge, "Sterilization of the Mentally Severely Handicapped: A Violation of the Right to Have Children?" *Ethical Problems in Reproductive Medicine* 1989; 1:1, 12-15.3. Raanan Gillon, "On Sterilizing the Mentally Handicapped," *Journal of Medical Ethics* No. 13 (2) 1987; 59-61.

CHAPTER 16

1. Christine Overall,"Introduction," from Christine Overall, *Ethics and Human Reproduction*, pp. 1-2 and 5-16. Reprinted with permission of the publishers, Routledge, Chapman and Hall, Inc.

2. Canadian Medical Association, "Background Considerations," from *The New Reproductive Technologies: Preliminary Considerations of the Canadian Medical Assocation* (Ottawa: Canadian Medical Association, 1991)1-9.

CHAPTER 17

1. Law Reform Commission of Ontario, "The Surrogate Mother," *Report on Artificial Human Reproduction*. (Ministry of the Attorney General, 1985) pp. 239-260.

2. The Canadian Medical Association, "Surrogate Motherhood," from *The New Reproductive Technologies: A Preliminary Perspective of the Canadian Medical Association*. (Ottawa: Canadian Medical Association, 1991).

3. Conseil du Statu de la Femme, "Preconception Contracts," from Gouvernement du Québec, Conseil du Statu de la Femme, *General Opinion of the Conseil du Statu de la Femme in Regard to New Reproductive Technologies*. (Québec, 1989) pp.19-21.

CHAPTER 18

1. Bartha Knoppers, "Towards Genetic Justice," from *Human Dignity and Genetic Heritage*, Study Paper prepared for the Law Reform Commission of Canada, Protection of Life Series. (Ottawa: Law Reform Commission of Canada, 1991), pp. 1-4.

2. Marc Lappé, "The Limits of Genetic Inquiry," *The Hastings Center Report* 17:4 (1987) 5-10.

CHAPTER 19

1. Richard West, "Ethical Aspects of Genetic Disease and Genetic Counselling," *Journal of Medical Ethics* 14:4 (1988) 194-197.

2. Raanan Gillon, "Genetic Counselling, Confidentiality, and the Medical interests of Relatives," *Journal of Medical Ethics* 14:4 (1988) 171-172.

3. L.M. Purdy, "Genetic Diseases: Can Having Children Be Immoral?" in *Genetics Now: Ethical Issues in Genetic Research* ed. by J.J. Buckley, Jr. (Washington, DC: University Press of America, 1978) 6 pp.

CHAPTER 20

1. Medical Research Council of Canada, *Guidelines for Research on Somatic Cell Gene Therapy in Humans*, Chapter 2, "Ethical Issues." (Ottawa: Minister of Supply and Services, 1990) pp.24-33.

2. Canadian Medical Association, "Analysis," from *The New Reproductive Technologies: A Preliminary Perspective of the Canadian Medical Association*. (Ottawa: Canadian Medical Association, 1991) pp. 127-135.

PART VI: CODES OF ETHICS FOR CANADIAN HEALTH CARE PROFESSIONALS

CHAPTER 21

1. The Canadian Medical Association, *Code of Ethics*. (Ottawa, 1987).

2. The Canadian Nurses' Association, *Code of Ethics*. (Ottawa, 1987).

3. Pharmaceutical Manufacturers Association of Canada, *Code of Marketing Practices*. (Ottawa, 1988).